Margaret and Charley

For Jill

H BM Best

Margaret and Charley

The Personal Story of Dr. Charles Best, the Co-Discoverer of Insulin

Henry B.M. Best

THE DUNDURN GROUP
TORONTO · OXFORD

Proofreader: Jennifer Bergeron
Design: Jennifer Scott
Printer: Transcontinental

National Library of Canada Cataloguing in Publication Data

Best, Henry B. M. (Henry Bruce Macleod)
    Margaret and Charley : the personal story of Dr. Charles Best, the co-discoverer of insulin /
    Henry B.M. Best.

Includes bibliographical references and index.
ISBN 1-55002-399-3

1. Best, Charles Herbert, 1899-1978.   2. Medical scientists — Canada--Biography. 3. Diabetes--Research — Canada — History. I. Title.

R464.B397B48 2003   616.4'62027'092   C2003-902295-9

1   2   3   4   5   07   06   05   04   03

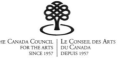

THE CANADA COUNCIL | LE CONSEIL DES ARTS
FOR THE ARTS | DU CANADA
SINCE 1957 | DEPUIS 1957

Canada

ONTARIO ARTS COUNCIL
CONSEIL DES ARTS DE L'ONTARIO

We acknowledge the support of the **Canada Council for the Arts** and the **Ontario Arts Council** for our publishing program. We also acknowledge the financial support of the **Government of Canada** through the **Book Publishing Industry Development Program** and **The Association for the Export of Canadian Books,** and the **Government of Ontario** through the **Ontario Book Publishers Tax Credit** program, and the **Ontario Media Development Corporation's Ontario Book Initiative.**

Care has been taken to trace the ownership of copyright material used in this book. The author and the publisher welcome any information enabling them to rectify any references or credit in subsequent editions.

J. Kirk Howard, President

Printed and bound in Canada.⊕
Printed on recycled paper.
www.dundurn.com

Dundurn Press   Dundurn Press   Dundurn Press
8 Market Street   73 Lime Walk   2250 Military Road
Suite 200   Headington, Oxford,   Tonawanda NY
Toronto, Ontario, Canada   England   U.S.A. 14150
M5E 1M6   OX3 7AD

To Margaret and Charles Best
for inspiring me to write their story,
and for teaching me to respect the past.

To Janna Ramsay Best
whose devotion, clear judgment, and wise advice
have given me the support I needed to undertake
and complete the writing of this volume.

Table of Contents

Introduction

This is the story of two people, Charles Herbert Best and Margaret Mahon Best, the story of their lives together, their family, their friends and colleagues, their travels, the events with which they were connected. It is even more the occasion to tell the tale of two vital people and their very full lives.

Some readers will turn immediately to the chapters that tell about the discovery of insulin and the saga of the Nobel Prize. This is perhaps unfortunate, but it is also inevitable. The documentation for this period is considerable, particularly regarding differing views on the role of the major participants.

The amount of documentary material for any one period obviously varies greatly. After their marriage in 1924, Margaret and Charles Best were seldom apart, so the exchange of letters was rare except during the Second World War, when he was away frequently. Their 1925–6 and 1928 stays in Britain and on the Continent are especially well documented because of numerous letters to and from their parents in West Pembroke and Toronto. Throughout their marriage and even before, Margaret Best told of their lives in her diaries as she saw it — and often, it appears, as she wanted it to be seen. From the eighty-four volumes, spanning six decades, a reasonably clear picture of their history emerges.

The organization of the Best family papers before any research or writing could be done took many months to accomplish. Then the writing was spread over several years, interrupted by bouts of serious illness. Perhaps the most difficult part was the editing of the manuscript to one-third its original length; here the contribution of a professional editor in the person of John Parry of Toronto was important. My research assistant, Claire Lecoupe, my wife, Janna Ramsay Best, my daughter, Dr. Mairi Best, and my son, Bruce Best, helped me edit the final work.

The major lecture and research trips that the Bests made to South Africa, South America, and Australia really deserve a volume to themselves, not only because of Best's scientific activities and gruelling lecture schedules, but because of Margaret's observations of people, places, plants, and art. Her 200-page account of the six-week scientific and cultural safari in South Africa in 1949, the 300 pages covering their two months in South America in 1951, as well as 600 pages recounting the almost four months in Australia in 1952, deserve much more attention than I have been able to give them.

Why write a joint biography? For fifty-three years, Margaret and Charles Best were inseparable, but more than that, they were an especially good team. Margaret was proud of the fact that she and Charley fell in love and were engaged in 1920, before he became celebrated. They discussed not only all decisions concerning their life and family, but also everything else, from his work, through people and the arts, to public affairs.

Margaret graduated from the University of Toronto in botany in 1923. She remained a keen and active botanist all her life, but she denied any scientific pretensions. She did not belong to any women's organizations other than her sorority — the Thetas — and politely refused invitations to join a bridge club or anything of that sort. She always said that she was too busy with her husband, and later on, with their two sons.

The principals were addressed in various ways. I did not call my parents by their first names, nor did many of their colleagues. First names were less widely used during most of their lives than is now the case. A close scientific and personal friend, Dr. Jessie Ridout, called Margaret by her first name, but called Charley "Dr. Best" to his face or "The Professor" in his absence. Some people in the Department of Physiology or the Banting and Best Department of Medical Research referred to him as "The Chief." The Best family often used initials when referring, especially in writing, to each other. "CHB" and "MMB" are obviously the most frequent, but the glossary on page 492 gives a list of all initials and abbreviations I have used.

Charles and Margaret Best wanted to write their own story. They started their memoirs in the late 1950s, but did not get beyond the mid-1930s. As well as my mother's eighty-four diaries, there are: fifty-one large scrapbooks, chock full of letters, newspapers clippings, magazine articles, greeting cards, souvenirs and memorabilia from their travels; well over 100 binders of correspondence, postcards, theatre programs, and various clippings; and at least fifty photograph albums. As she said with pride in the last years of her life, "Quite a record of a family." Beyond what has already been mentioned, in the course of this project, all that was collected and that make up the Best Family Papers has been further organized into thirty-three feet of cabinet drawers holding files for individual people, subjects, and institutions. A list of names counting over 5,500 entries was compiled to help identify the people in the archives.

For the present volume, I use as much as possible what my parents wrote, adding, verifying, and commenting on their words. In so doing I have had to balance my professional role as a historian with my relationship to the subjects. Unattributed quotes are, as indicated, from Margaret Best's diaries. Early on, it became clear to me that I was in a unique position, especially with respect to my mother's diaries. Even if many of the early volumes cover a period before my birth, I am still probably the individual best able to know what she is writing about. I grew up hearing constant references to many of the events and people.

Yet another published volume is possible — an edited version of Margaret Best's diaries. I remember the flurry in June 1951, when Little, Brown & Company and Houghton Mifflin Company, both of Boston, competed to obtain the rights to publish the diaries. My mother responded that she intended to keep them for the book that she and my father would write someday.

The original diaries and most, if not all, of the other papers — including much original and/or handwritten correspondence — will go to the University of Toronto, for use by future researchers, while some items will be on semi-permanent loan to the university's Department of Physiology and the Banting and Best Department of Medical Research, and to the office of the dean of medicine, for display. The Ontario Archives and the Public Archives of Canada were anxious to obtain the collection, and Sir Alan Hodgkin, president of the Royal Society, London, from 1970 to 1975, expressed the opinion that the Society's archives would be the ideal repository.[1]

In considering the extensive material that comes from the pen of either Margaret or Charley, the reader may often wonder whether they were conscious of the impression that their accounts would make. I think that certainly this was the case. They set out to preserve and to inform. They were usually careful not to insult or to shock. At times, Margaret, in her diaries, does allow herself to make negative judgments about people, but not too often. Charley gave vent to critical assessments in some of his letters and in interviews recorded in the 1950s and 1960s, but generally they were both quite careful people, not apt to make rash judgments, especially in public.

It has been interesting for me to read biographies of individuals written by members of their own family, especially sons or daughters. The circumstances vary greatly. Some are obviously hagiographies; others try to prove how independent the author is by emphasizing the "warts." I do not intend this volume to be either but to give an account of the full and fascinating lives and times of two people. That it is a labour of love requires no excuses. Someone else will write a very different kind of life of Margaret and Charley Best — and so it should be.

Thus, I realize that I am not the only person able or keen to write a biography of Charles H. Best. Someone with thorough scientific training is better able to judge the professional aspects of my father's career. The role of the historian in making scientific judgments, or judgments about scientists, is a fascinating one. Historians assess politicians, soldiers, churchmen, and many others, so why not scientists? One reply is that we should not judge those whose lives have been of note in such fields without relevant preparation in their particular profession. If this view were followed, many historians would be out of business. I believe, however, that there are particular dangers in non-scientific evaluations of scientific accomplishments. Certainly, in my own case, although I spent my early university years in science, I felt obligated to canvass various professional opinions before arriving at any conclusions here.

No biography of Charles Herbert Best has appeared to date. After Best's heart attacks in the mid-1950s, Dr. William R. Feasby, an MD and a medical historian, began writing a biography. Before his health prevented him from carrying on, he had prepared eighteen chapters, leading up to 1928. He was given free access to many papers, to the draft chapters of their reminiscences prepared by Margaret and Charley, and to many of the diaries, at least those that had been typed, up to 1935. Feasby tried to be as objective as possible. He read a great deal of the background material and interviewed many people. The result is of considerable interest, sometimes for his conclusions and often for the accounts of interviews with people who are no longer available. However, I am aware that he took great pains not to offend either of the Bests.

Understandably, insulin played a major role in the lives of Margaret and Charles Best. The excitement and drama surrounding the discovery of insulin, the fact that insulin has saved so many lives since 1922, and the highly emotional occasions when my parents met with diabetics and their families, singly or in groups that sometimes numbered in the hundreds and even thousands, inevitably loom very large. Diabetics, unlike those whose lives have been saved by blood transfusions, penicillin, heparin, or other drugs, are reminded every day of the miracle of insulin.

There are, however, at least three other major scientific developments in the career of Charles Best that would have put him in the front line of achievement in medical research even without insulin. These are the discovery of the enzyme histaminase in 1929; discovery of the role of the lipotropic factor choline, one of the B vitamins in 1932; and the purification of the anticoagulant heparin in 1935. The number of cases where heparin has been used since it first became available for human use in the late 1930s and early 1040s is difficult to calculate, but there is no question that thousands of heart operations that have taken place in recent years would have been and still would be impossible without it. The importance of the choline work is less easy to illustrate to the public, but the scientific value is considerable. Histaminase is an enzyme that breaks down histamine, and again, its value is not so much clinical as scientific.

Other achievements of importance include the launching and development of the dried blood serum project in 1939, the Red Cross blood donor clinics, and the work done by the Royal Canadian Navy's Medical Research Division headed by Best on night vision, seasickness remedies, clothing, and rations for servicemen dealing with the frigid conditions of the North Atlantic. Charles Best's research interests covered a very broad area. He is usually identified as a physiologist, but he could be called a biochemist. He was involved in basic science but was always interested in the clinical applications of this work. He once remarked, "Physiology is a conveniently broad label, but I am not one who would defend it or any other similar appellation very vigorously."[2]

Many people will not realize just how young Margaret and Charley Best were when the most dramatic events of their lives occurred. At the time of the momentous events of the early twenties, they were twenty-three and twenty-four years old, respectively. For the first half of this volume, they were both under forty years of age. It was hard for many to believe that at twenty-two he could be the co-discoverer of insulin.

Chapter One
Salt in Their Veins, 1899–1920

The Bests and the Fishers

Charles Herbert Best was proud of his roots in the Maritime provinces of Canada. Six generations before Charley, the first Best in Nova Scotia was William, a master stone mason, whose name appears in the records of Fort Louisbourg in 1747. When Louisbourg was returned to France, William Best and his close friend Sergeant John Burbidge, both originally from Hampshire, England, moved with the rest of the garrison to take part in the founding of Halifax in 1749. Both men were merchants and builders, and both were elected wardens of St. Paul's Church of England, the first non-Catholic church in Acadia. William Best, master mason in charge of building the foundations, billed Governor Cornwallis, "To your order for the masons to drink on your laying the foundation stone of the church — 3 pounds," and added a reward for a rescue from the outhouse: "To cash ordered to Daniel Dunn for [fetching] your Honrs watch out of the Little house — 5 shillings."[3] Later first Burbidge, then Best moved to Cornwallis on the Minas Basin in the Annapolis Valley, but they both represented Halifax in the first elected assembly in British North America, which met in Halifax in 1758–9. John, a son of William, married a niece of John Burbidge.

Their great-grandson John Burbidge Best II was the grandfather of Charles Herbert Best. At Grafton, further up the Annapolis Valley from Cornwallis, he had an orchard and engaged in mixed farming. His wife, Isabella Adalia Woodworth, came from a New England "Planter" family, one of those that emigrated from the Thirteen Colonies to take up lands from which the Acadians had been expelled.

Their son, Herbert Huestis Best, was born in 1871, the eighth of eleven children and the seventh boy. He taught school in Grafton and Woodville and then attended Dalhousie University in Halifax in 1893–4, intending to transfer to McGill University in Montréal to study medicine, but a bout of typhoid fever forced him to drop out. He then went to New York City, where his sister Anna was a nurse, and she was able to help him with his expenses. He enrolled at the University of the City of New York, receiving a diploma in operative surgery in 1895, and became an MD in 1896.[4]

While in New York, Herbert Best met a second cousin who had been born on a farm near Waterville, just a few miles from his own home at Grafton. She was Luella May (Lulu) Fisher. Her father, James E. Fisher, died of sunstroke when she was only one year old; her mother, Eunice Louise Woodworth, was a first cousin of Herbert Best's mother. Both women suffered from depression. Lulu Fisher was raised by Harmon Newcomb and his wife, Isabella Fisher, sister of Lulu's late father. Newcomb was a ship's carpenter, and the family lived in a small house that he had built on the mud banks of the Cornwallis River at Port Williams.

When she was a young adult, Lulu Newcomb, as she became known, crossed the Minas Basin, possibly from Apple Tree Landing (now Canning) or from Kingsport, to Advocate Harbour in Cumberland County, where she taught school for two years.

Herbert Best and Lulu Newcomb married in New York on 4 May 1896, the day before the fifty-fifth annual commencement of the University of the City of New York Medical Department, held in Carnegie Music Hall. Almost immediately, the young couple set off for the State of Maine where Dr. Herbert Best began his long career as a country doctor. For a short time he was in partnership with his older brother, Dr. O. Fletcher Best, in Patten, but for most of his life he was in sole practice further north in the state at West Pembroke. West Pembroke is situated on Cobscook Bay, off Passamaquoddy Bay, twenty-eight miles south by road from the international border at Calais, Maine and St. Stephen, New Brunswick. By the time Herbert and Lulu arrived, the ship building, lumbering, and iron works were gone. It was not a rich area with the inhabitants involved in a combination of farming, wood-cutting, and fishing. Sardine packing was an important source of employment between 1885 and 1960.

At first, Herbert and Lulu Best lived in the rented "McLaughlin House" in West Pembroke. There, Charley's sister, Isabella Hilda Best, was born on 23 February 1898. "Lulu confined. Baby born at 6:30 am. Dr. Byron up. Both well. Greatest storm of the season. Hail, sleet, and wind." In May, there is another entry, "Baby Hilda is ten weeks old today. Well and strong. Lulu really well."[5]

15

On 6 November 1898, the Bests moved across the road to the "Murray House,"[6] a typical rambling New England house, painted white with green shutters. It was there that Charles Herbert Best was born on 27 February 1899: "At 10:40, Dr. A.T. Lincoln brought our boy along. I helped and Lulu was more comfortable. Gave chlorol and chloroform. Boy is a good-sized bouncing baby and rests well. Lulu rests well."[7]

Dr. Arthur Lincoln of nearby Dennysville, a medical graduate of Harvard University, was Dr. Herbert Best's closest friend. He was a descendant of General Benjamin Lincoln, who had received Lord Cornwallis's sword in 1781 at Yorktown, Virginia, in the Revolutionary War. He rarely practised his profession, though he had attended Charley's birth. He became a gifted artist and a great expert on the flora and fauna of the area. John James Audubon named the Lincoln sparrow in honour of his father. Arthur Lincoln's wife, Anna Maxwell, had auditioned for Sir W.S. Gilbert, Sir Arthur Sullivan, and Richard D'Oyly Carte, and became a principal in the first of their touring companies on the European continent, where she met Dr. Lincoln in Vienna.

Lulu Best was very musical and loved to sing in a clear soprano voice, accompanying herself on the piano or the pump organ. She could play anything by ear and was much in demand at weddings and funerals. Herbert Best especially loved his college songs, spirituals, and hymns, and the two would often sing together. All his life, Charles Best loved the "old songs" — hymns such as "The Old Rugged Cross," "Unto the Hills Around," and "Abide with Me;" love songs such as "Silver Threads among the Gold" and "I Cannot Sing the Old Songs;" southern songs such as "Carry Me Back to Old Virginny," "My Old Kentucky Home," and, his favourite, "Old Black Joe."

Dr. Herbert Best once drove his team of trotting horses as far as eighty miles in twenty-four hours to deliver babies in widely separated areas of the large region covered by his practice. He delivered over 1,500 children into the world, and took his seriously ill patients to the Chipman Hospital in St. Stephen, New Brunswick, where there were better facilities. His pocket diaries that have survived give some idea of what he charged — $5 for a confinement and the delivery, which was often paid in kind: a cord of wood, a chicken for the pot, fish or produce.

Robert P. Tristram Coffin, professor of English at Bowdoin College,[8] wrote the poem "Country Doctor" with Dr. Herbert Best in mind. Later, Professor Coffin prepared a hand-written copy of the poem, illustrated it, and sent it to the delighted son of the subject, "For Charles H. Best, whose father was a country doctor."

> Through rain, through sleet, through ice, through snow,
> He went where only God could go,
> He drove his old mare out of breath,
> Between a baby and a death.
>
> He left an old man in the dark
> And blew up a tiny spark
> In a young man two feet long
> To carry on the dead man's song.
>
> ...
>
> Our farms so lonely and spaced far
> Could never have grown this nation we are
> But for this man, come sun, come snow,
> Who went where God alone could go.[9]

> — Robert P. Tristram Coffin

Next to the doctor's office was the main body of the house, then the wood shed, the barn, the carriage house, and finally, in later years, the garage. From the age of seven, Charles Best, with the aid of a step ladder, was able to unharness the team, rub down the horses, feed and water them, and have a new team ready for the next trip, while his father went into the house to have something to eat.

Many of Charley's earliest recollections were about horses. When he was just four, he and his father brought a racing mare, "Topsy," to West Pembroke from the Annapolis Valley. Charley remembered "driving with him from Kentville to Digby, Nova Scotia. The mare was then put on the ferry from Digby to Saint John, New Brunswick, and we drove her in two days the one hundred miles to West Pembroke via St. Stephen and Calais."[10]

"My grandparents and their ancestors for many generations had lived in the Annapolis Valley and fast trotting horses were a part of their lives. I remember the birth of a colt when I was four years old. He was named 'MacDougal' but we called him 'Maxie.' When he was only a few days old, his mother was led from her stall and the lower half of the Dutch door was

17

closed. Maxie was excited and ran around the large box and then to our amazement, he half jumped and slid over the door and triumphantly joined his mother."[11]

"My Father and I raced our horses not only in the summer on the tracks or straightaways, but during the winter months when I was home for the Christmas vacations. On the four-mile course, the horses trotted almost all out with the exception of good breathing spaces while going up several long hills. The most exciting racing was on the ice of Pennamaquan Lake … Horses properly shod can travel faster on smooth ice than they can on a perfect racetrack. One must set a course and hold to it or the sleigh or sulky will slew, and that can be dangerous. The recollection of the fascinating racing rhythm created by the 'never-slip' shoes of the horses, chipping the crisp ice, exhilarates me."[12]

Herbert Best was a restless man and became dissatisfied with his practice in the small community. On two occasions, he moved his practice elsewhere but soon returned to West Pembroke. In 1904, they moved to Eastport, where, for at least part of the time the nurse was Dr. Best's older sister, Annie Best Jenkins (Aunt Anna). After two years, the Bests went back to West Pembroke. Apparently, the hospital was not a great financial success. Also, Lulu said that young Charley was getting into trouble "in the city," having been one of the young boys suspected of setting fire alarms so that they could see the fine team of horses dash out of the fire hall pulling the pumper.

A few months later, Herbert Best decided to accept an invitation to set up practice in Easton, Aroostook County, Maine, 150 miles north, near Presqu'Ile, the Saint John River and Perth-Andover in New Brunswick. "We went in two carriages. My mother and father drove in one and led the colt, Maxie. My sister and I and Cousin Iomene Newcomb from Port Williams, Nova Scotia, were in the second. We had two horses — one in the shafts and a second which was tied to the harness of the other. As I remember it, at age seven, I did most of the driving in our carriage although my cousin was a competent horsewoman." They arrived at their new residence, "a house about a mile south of Easton. The house was painted yellow and had windows, the top half of which were coloured red. It was a comfortable dwelling but not very attractive. The stable was attached, also the wood shed and carriage house in the New England manner."[13]

Herbert Best soon had a busy practice in prosperous Aroostook County. "Traffic on the roads was chiefly two-horse teams which carried

potatoes from the half-buried storage places at the farms to the high potato barns at the railway stations. In winter, the drivers urged the horses to
a fast trot to shorten the time of exposure of their precious and well-cov-
ered cargoes. Boys of my age and older would catch rides on the fast-mov-
ing sleds and would go for a mile or two in one direction and then find an
empty sled for the return journey."

Charley Best recalled a near disaster: "I went to a school which was
about one mile away straight across the fields, much farther by the roads.
I used snowshoes in the winter and had no difficulties except on one occasion when I was overcome by the cold and wind. I fell in the snow and was
unable to get up. Fortunately, my father saw me and came to the rescue.
My face and fingers were frozen."[14]

Dr. Herbert Best did much better financially in Easton, but the family missed the sea, and after two years they returned to Pembroke for good.
With them went Charley's first dog, a collie named Carlo. "When Carlo
arrived at the sea he rushed in and began to drink the water. He quickly
learned to distinguish between sweet and salty water. He was a fine animal
and soon learned to draw me on a sled." A wealthy farmer in Easton had
been very impressed with Maxie, who "had made a reputation for himself
on the roads and at the race track in nearby Presqu'Ile." He wrote to Dr.
Best offering $400 for the horse; the two men met halfway and exchanged
horses, and the doctor came home with a good profit. He said that Maxie
really belonged to Charley and thus the nine year old was able to open his
first bank account.

When Charley was twelve, his father bought one of the first cars in the
village: an open, red Buick roadster. Dr. Best was away on a call, so the dealer taught Charley how to drive the vehicle. His father was wary of the
machine, but a call about an accident at the sawmill in Whiting, nine miles
away, prompted him to ask Charley to drive him there. The only comments
he made were, "Can't you go faster? I could have made better time with my
horses." Years later, Charley added, "That was not entirely accurate, as we
proved a few days later. We raced car against horse for the twelve miles to
Eastport. He passed me again and again by running his mare up the hills
while I was in low gear. I passed him on the downgrades and eventually
coasted down the hill to the main street of Eastport ahead of him."[15]

Charles Best never forgot Captain William Eldon Leighton, who had
commanded the local contingent that went to the Civil War. He owned
and operated the Leighton Organ Company from 1880 to 1885, making

600 cases for pump organs that graced many a church, hall, and home. The Best family still has a Leighton organ and also a violin made by the captain from a tabletop.

Herbert Best often used Captain Leighton's former cottage on Leighton's Point, four miles from the village. In 1921, he acquired the lease on the property for $500. The cottage overlooked the narrow channel where the tide sped through to fill the passage all the way to Whiting, six miles away. Seals played among the rocks. Lulu Best loved "The Point," and in winter she would go there on snowshoes, sometimes staying overnight with Albert and Keziah Leighton at their farm nearby. When Captain Leighton became very ill, she looked after him. Charley recalled his mother sitting in the kitchen making over for him a suit that the captain had given her, saying that he would never need it again. Eleanor Mahar Hurst, who went to school with Hilda and Charley in West Pembroke, recalled, "The Bests had no money at all, you know. They were always hard-up. Charley Best always wore the same knickerbocker suit. He got new underwear and socks but he always had the same brown knickerbocker suit."[16]

Nevertheless, CHB recalled that "the whole family went to New York for several weeks in 1912. We travelled by ship, the *Calvin Austin*, from Eastport to Boston and on to New York City on the Fall River Line of Steamships. We had a wonderful time and saw some of the art galleries, several plays, the Natural History Museum, and a circus in Madison Square Gardens. One of the sights which impressed me most was the horse-drawn fire engines going at full speed down Fifth Avenue."[17]

Both Herbert and Lulu had been raised as Anglicans, but there was no Episcopal congregation in the area, so they joined the People's Methodist Church. Lulu held various posts in the Order of the Eastern Star and the Rebekah Lodge. Both she and Herbert were buried from the Union Church.[18]

Charley Best went through both public and high school in Pembroke. At the Head of the Tide school, Mrs. Earl Bridges was the teacher. Then came grammar school, where Mr. Carrol Fisher was the principal, followed by high school with Principal Everett Peacock, "a stern disciplinarian," who encouraged Charley to work at Latin until he really loved it.[19] Classmate Eleanor Mahar recalled young Charley jumping from ice floe to ice floe at the mouth of the Pennamaquan River: "That Charley Best was a card. He was some number. He'd jump ice cakes in the river when the ice broke up. If you fall between the cakes, you're gone.

His parents didn't know. If they'd known he'd have been in trouble — their only son, jumping ice cakes!"[20]

Charley Best and Harold Blackwood were lifelong friends. One day they set out to row down the Pennamaquan River and over Cobscook Bay to Eastport, twelve miles away. On the way they stopped at Red Island; they wrestled there all day and then rowed home. Another time they took the train to the fair at St. Stephen, New Brunswick, where they had such a good time that they missed the last train and had to walk the twenty-one miles home by the back road. Blackwood became a judge and principal of the high school.

Styles Bridges, oldest child of Charley's first teacher, had to take on family responsibilities early when his father died. During the winter holidays, he and Charley cut wood on the Bridges' wood-lot, "four miles across the snowy country on Big Hill,"[21] which Charley always thought could have been the inspiration for Robert Frost's well-known poem, "Stopping by Woods on a Snowy Evening." On one occasion the two young woodsmen decided to improve on the usual method of felling trees. They cut those at the bottom of the hill part way through, hoping for a domino effect when they felled those at the top. It was quite a job, however, to disentangle the result, and in the end, they saved no time or effort.

Styles Bridges went on to serve as governor of New Hampshire and dean of the American Senate. His brother, Ronald, became executive director of the Federation of Protestant Churches of America. The three friends received honorary degrees from the University of Maine.

Charles Best was fascinated by the Indian place names in Maine and New Brunswick. On all possible occasions he quoted the poem "The Maiden of Quoddy," by James De Mille, professor of English at Dalhousie University in Halifax.

> Sweet maiden of Passamaquoddy
> Shall we seek for communion of souls
> Where the deep Mississippi meanders
> Or the distant Saskatchewan rolls?
> Ah, no! in New Brunswick we'll find it —
> A sweetly sequestrated nook —
> Where the swift gliding Skoodoowabskooksis
> Unites with the Skoodoowabskook.[22]

Eventually, in 1915, it was time to leave his enchanted east coast to further his education in Toronto. "My first trip to Toronto was in the autumn of 1915," wrote Charles Best in "My Early Years." "I travelled by way of Boston and came in to Toronto from the West. I have been turned around ever since. East seems West to me."[23]

He had decided to attend a Canadian university at least partly because his father's younger sister, Lillian, lived in Toronto. In 1904, she married the Rev. William T. Hallam, professor of Greek and Hebrew at Wycliffe College, a low-church Anglican theological college federated with the University of Toronto. Charley's Aunt Lillie and Uncle Will had met while classmates at Dalhousie University in Halifax, graduating in 1901. In Toronto Charley lived with the Hallams first at 89 Wilcox Street and then at lodgings in the college.

In later years, Charley loved repeating Uncle Will's story of how he met Aunt Lillie. "Did I ever tell you how I married your Aunt Lillie? She and I were classmates at Dalhousie. In the first year, she stood first and I stood second, and this happened again in the second and third years. However, in the fourth year, I worked very hard and I stood first and she stood second." At this point, the elderly gentleman would shake with laughter and say, "But, she beat me after all, she married me!"

For a year, Charles Best went to Harbord Collegiate in order to make up subjects such as Canadian history and French that were not part of the high school curriculum in Pembroke. He had happy memories of several of his teachers: Miss Lawler in English, Mr. Glassey in Latin, and Mr. Irwin in French. "It was a profitable year and I particularly enjoyed the Latin and English and only wish that I had devoted myself a little more diligently to French!"[24] Mr. Hagarty, the principal, was recruiting for a Young Soldiers Battalion, but Charley was not old enough.

Charley spent the summer of 1916 in Maine, working with Captain George Hershey on a small two-masted boat with a seven-horsepower motor, carrying general cargo around Cobscook and Passamaquoddy bays. In the autumn, he entered the general arts course at the University of Toronto. "I gained some valuable experience in conducting meetings of various kinds as I had been elected president of the year." Lorne Hutchison, later in 1923 to work closely with Charley, was one of the counsellors. Best recalled that it was a "very disturbed time. Our thoughts were constantly on the fighting in France."[25]

All first-year students at the University of Toronto had to write an essay about themselves for their English class. Charley sent home a copy of "Who I Am and Why I Came to College." "Dear Mama, Thinking that you and Dad would like to know why your son came to college, I am sending you this essay. I may not write anything else but a card or two. This one also was the best of the boys. Lovingly, C."[26]

In the essay, he wrote, "During the last two years of my high school my father, who is a medical man, spent a large proportion of his leisure moments perusing the catalogues of the various medical colleges of the United States and of Canada, and in talking with my mother about the life work of their only son. When I was asked what calling I should choose for myself I answered that I wished to become a physician. Both my natural inclination and that paternal hero-worship which is present in the heart of every lad prompted me to make that choice." He then had to decide on a university: "Harvard, Johns Hopkins, Yale ... were discussed; but, as my parents are both Canadians, they resolved to have me enter one of the universities of Canada. McGill, Dalhousie, and Toronto were all proposed. My father suggested Dalhousie but I objected very strenuously. My visits in Halifax, though very pleasant, did not make me desire to live there for a large portion of four or five years. The decision was therefore to be between McGill and Toronto. McGill University was very highly esteemed by both my parents, but realizing that the City of Toronto excelled Montréal in many ways, and being persuaded by several relatives who are connected with the University of Toronto, they finally decided I should enter the latter as soon as I was prepared."

Family illness helped direct Charley's research interests. On 24 May 1917, his Aunt Anna (Annie Best Jenkins) died of diabetes. She had trained at the Massachusetts General Hospital when the diabetes specialist, Dr. Elliott Joslin, was a houseman there, and after she was diagnosed with the condition in 1913, she became patient no. 875 under his care at the Deaconess Hospital, also in Boston. The family has correspondence about her care with various relatives and four pages of charts giving details of her treatment. In a letter to Dr. Joslin in February 1917, Dr. O. Fletcher Best, an eye specialist, asked about his sister's condition and "what her chances are for recovery."[27] In later years, Charles Best often recounted how his aunt had helped his father through medical school and had worked with him when he had the hospital in Eastport, Maine. Her illness and death had a profound influence on Charley.

23

He spent the summer of 1917 on the ranch of his uncle Clarence Best at Huron, South Dakota, stopping on the way at Faribault, Minnesota, to see his uncle Homer Best. In Huron, Charley soon settled into the ranch life, ploughing with six horses abreast, and cultivating mile-long fields of corn. Uncle Clarence was away most of the time in Pierre, the state's capital, where he was a state senator. Charley made friends with his cousin, Eva, later Mrs. Milo E. Smith of Fort Lauderdale, Florida, and together they rode bareback over the prairie. His male cousins seemed to resent him, particularly as he was a university student. At the end of the summer, he took the train to Boston and the boat to Eastport and had a week at home in West Pembroke before returning to Toronto. Two months into his second year, Charley transferred into first-year physiology and biochemistry. He sent home a photograph of the YMCA executive of the University College branch, 1917–8, where he was listed as "conference promoter."

In December 1917, the *Pennamaquan Guide*, the student paper of Pembroke High School, published an article by Charles H. Best, class of 1915, entitled "The Effect of a Great War upon a Canadian College." He wrote of the end of invitations, dances, dinners, and theatre parties and of the much larger proportion of girls in the classes, of absent faculty members, and of uniforms on campus. Pembroke was only thirty miles from Canada, and many residents had relatives across the border. In writing to his sister Lillie on 30 March 1918, Herbert Best said, "We hope for better news from France. Fearful fighting. Poor boys. Will Germany ever give up? When she can get a good excuse or is compelled to do so?"[28]

In late 1917 and early 1918, Charley had difficulty being accepted for the army because of a systolic murmur caused either by scarlet fever or measles. For some time he wore an "AR" button, meaning "Applied, Rejected." Finally, he found a recruiting officer on duty at the Toronto armouries, Dr. Pat Hardy, a homeopath, who simply looked at him and pronounced him perfectly fit. He later noted that Hardy was the doctor who looked after the Hallams "and gave them little white pills with nothing in them."[29]

Charley joined the 70th Battery of the Horse Artillery and in the spring of 1918 was sent to Camp Petawawa on the Ottawa River. "My riding experience stood me in good stead and I won the horseback wrestling championship of the Camp and competed in the mounted swimming races. I have always felt that it was due to my achievements in those fields that I was made a Sergeant!"[30] His cards home talked mainly of his fellow soldiers and of the food, and he extended thanks for the packages of "eats." He asks for a suit of BVDs.

Riding appeared in each letter home. On 12 June 1918, he wrote, "There are about 2,300 artillery horses in camp and sometimes they are all out at the same time." On 19 June, he added, "I can vault into the seat with one spring now when the horse is trotting or cantering. We were also bending down and touching the ground with horses at the walk." On 26 June, "We have been out on the guns today." There was a possible promotion for him to lance corporal: "I will go where I get the stripe first," but he added on 4 July, "I don't care much about the stripe really." And on 9 July, "I have been camp mounted orderly all day. I did not do much in the morning, but this afternoon I was riding pell mell all over the camp, delivering over twenty-five telegrams and taking all kinds of rush orders. My horse was fast and I had some difficulty in keeping within the speed limits."

Postcards showed the tents for the men and tethering posts in lines for the horses, with a few spruce boughs for shade. On 10 July, a photo of the whole battalion was taken. Two such photos have survived, currently in metre-wide frames. Charley wrote on 31 July about a possible transfer to the university's Canadian Officers' Training Corps (COTC). On 5 August, "I drove a lead team today for the first time and especially during the fast manoeuvres I enjoyed it immensely. We gave a little show to some big boys today. The whole brigade was at a close interval (four feet between the teams) and the orders came for the trot, gallop, then run. Believe me, it was some sight and some fun to see the whole bunch on the dead run. My nags were stretched out to the limit."[31]

On a few days of leave, Charley went home, taking his university friend Clark Noble to see the ocean for the first time. The *Eastport Sentinel* of 28 August 1918 reported: "Private Charles Best, Camp Petawawa, Ontario, arrived Friday to spend a brief furlough with his parents ... accompanied by his friend Clark Noble ... Miss Hilda Best gave a party in the evening at Leighton's Cottage ... where a large circle of young people gathered. Moonlight dance on the veranda was much enjoyed."[32]

Henry Marsh, another good friend from university, was mentioned frequently in cards from Petawawa. Marsh graduated from Wycliffe and was later bishop of the Yukon. On 4 September, "A sudden order came in the p.m. for twenty-five volunteers for an immediate draft overseas. I did not volunteer because Henry was not here." On 5 September, "A draft for France was picked yesterday and cancelled today. The fellows are leaving for Siberia soon." Other cards discussed the merits of the tank corps, the horse artillery, and the infantry. A card dated 18 September to his sister Hilda implied an impending move. Henry Marsh had received a transfer to the COTC. Charley had not, and he was disappointed.[33] Before leaving for overseas, he had a short leave in Toronto. His uncle, Professor Hallam, remarked in a letter to Herbert and Lulu that "in spite of a cold, he had clear eyes and skin and his muscles were like iron."[34]

Charles Best went to England in early October 1918 as part of a draft for the 2nd Canadian Tank Battalion. He wrote to his mother on 3 October, "On the way now. Enjoying trip great. Lots of eats." The next day there were three cards, one saying that some of the fellows have "grippe" but no "Spanish flu." He was not sure whether they were bound for Quebec or for Halifax. From Quebec on the fourth, Charley wrote, "We are on the boat now. I have good quarters and the Sergs are OK. Several Varsity boys are in the bunch. I was not sick a bit on the train and will be Jake on the boat. One warship is here already, HMS *Donegal*. We are on the *Victoria*, a 5,000-ton transport. Everything looks ready for a pleasant trip." Then, "We are leaving tomorrow for overseas direct, I hope. I have been in Canada over four months and desire a change. I am Orderly Sergeant on the trip over and that means a lot of work, but I like to be busy and don't mind having authority so will be Jake."[35]

Out of the one hundred men in his unit on the seventeen-day voyage, nine were lost to influenza and buried at sea. The vessel had no doctors or nurses and few medical supplies. Charley believed that he survived because he was on mast duty for several hours each day and slept on the top deck.[36] The destination was Kinmel Park Camp at Rhyl in north Wales, painted in 1918 by Canadian war artist David Milne ("Pte. Brown Writes a Christmas Letter," and "The Camp at Night.")[37] Infantry drill kept the men occupied. They went on long marches to the foothills of Mount Snowdon. The authorities wanted to keep the men busy and out of trouble. Charley had his introduction to Canadian football, playing flying wing. He particularly mentioned Sergeant Worsick who was a "tough bird," but Charley liked him; the older man had joined him to sleep on deck on the trip over. Later in Wales he was ill, and Charley was made an acting sergeant major in his place.

With Armistice on 11 November 1918, discipline evaporated. Sergeant Best and another sergeant hired a car for a week to tour southern England. In London, with overcoats to cover their uniforms, they "borrowed" two officers' caps with braid and enjoyed being saluted. When they returned from the unauthorized leave, Sergeant Mel Wilson, later a lawyer in Toronto, fixed the records. They also toured some of the Welsh surroundings. In Rhyl a Welsh choir gave a concert, "the best voices, I think, I have ever heard." Charley's thoughts must have been like those of many a young soldier: "I shall always be sorry that I did not get as far as France but am glad to be so near."[38]

He witnessed the Rhyl riots, when veterans objected to recent arrivals who had not seen action in the grim trenches of France but were being sent home first. "Tempers ran very high. The Arsenals were raided and for a week or more the Camp was in an uproar and we found ourselves in the midst of vicious skirmishes."[39]

Charley's unit arrived home in December 1918 on the *Aquitania* from Southampton to Halifax. In Halifax, he thought that he would go and see his Aunt Minnie Megeny, his mother's sister, on Barrington Street, and he missed the troop train. A kind conductor gave him a berth on a regular train, and he rejoined his unit at Quebec. Leave soon followed, so he returned to his studies. He started his courses in mid-December, before going home for Christmas. It was a joyful homecoming. Dr. Herbert Best drove up to meet the Canadian Pacific Railway (CPR) train at St. Stephen. Either Lulu or his sister Hilda played the piano or the pump organ for carol singing at church and at home. Charley and his father raced the horses on Pennamaquan Lake.

When Charley was discharged from the army in February 1919, he had enough money to keep him going for a short while. He took classes most of the summer and completed his second academic year, but it was not easy to catch up. Professor F.C.A. Jeanneret, later chancellor of the university, recalled, "I remember him well in a second-year reading course in scientific French, and would like to think that his imagination was then stirred by Louis Pasteur."[40] The first of the many of his class notebooks still extant starts on 11 December 1918, for second-year chemistry. The last entry is for 23 April 1919. The next two sets of notes are for third-year biochemistry and physiology. On 15 January 1919, Charley wrote home, "The work is very hard for me and I will probably have to remain for several weeks or months after convocation to complete the work." Two days later, "I am studying hard now for the Christmas (delayed) exams. I am not expecting to make much in them but one is a final so will have to plug at that."[41] He bought a copy of *The Practitioner's Medical Dictionary*, "containing all the words and phrases generally used in medicine and the allied sciences, with their proper pronunciation, derivation, and definition."[42]

Adaptation to university life after military service spent outdoors was not easy. Clark Noble and Charley thought of applying for posts as fire rangers in northern Ontario. "I would be through by June 15th, and home in the middle of August. The work is fine and the pay fairly good. I am getting to dislike indoors more all the time." Further letters were about exams: "It is hard to work because there are so many things going on." On 23 January 1920, "We have our final on the bones one week from next Wednesday. Final of dissection of rabbit is next Wednesday. We started the dissection of the human yesterday. There promises to be a lot of interesting work. I will have to study some next summer."[43] So he did, but he also went back to Pembroke.

For his third year of the physiology and biochemistry course (1919–20), most of his notes in both subjects survive. In physiology, the instructor was Dr. A.C. Redfield, an assistant professor who had been trained at Harvard and Woods Hole, Massachusetts. Best recalled that "Redfield told Noble and myself that if we came back in the summer and got well ahead of the medical students, that we could get posts as demonstrators and junior research workers in the following year on a part-time basis." There were not sufficient funds yet, "but the plan was definitely made that we should come back early that autumn, about a month ahead of the beginning of the academic year, and prepare to demonstrate to the medical students."[44]

For Charley Best, however, life was not all work and no play. "The most fortunate event of my life occurred on February 28th, 1919, when I attended a sorority party and met Margaret Mahon, a lovely 18-year-old girl."[45] Margaret and Charley found that they had been born ten miles apart, as the gull flies, she at St-Andrews-by-the-Sea, New Brunswick, and he at West Pembroke, Maine. When he went home later that summer, Charley went to see Margaret, who was visiting friends in St. Andrews. The Grey Dort that Dr. Best gave Charley was very helpful for such excursions. He drove the car to Boston in one day, "something of a record over the gravel roads."[46]

The next summer after exams were over in the spring of 1920, Clark Noble and Charley Best started work building a golf course at Georgetown, thirty miles northwest of Toronto, owned by a well-known real estate dealer, J.A. Willoughby. The young men worked and played hard. Charley was the catcher on the Georgetown baseball team, while Clark played third base. They won the championship of their league:

Acton, Brampton, Georgetown, and Milton. After the final game, the fans carried Percy Blackburn, the pitcher, and Charley Best from the ball park down the main street of Georgetown. Premier E.C. Drury came to town to have his picture taken with the winning team.[47] Margaret Mahon was often at these games. Meanwhile, the Mahon house on Brunswick Avenue in Toronto became a second home to Charley.

The Mahons and the Macleods

Margaret Mahon was equally proud of her Maritime background. Her paternal ancestors arrived in Nova Scotia from Ulster in 1761. They owned farms in Nova Scotia on the shores of Cobequid Bay in the contiguous townships of Truro, Onslow, and Londonderry in Colchester County. Many members were shipbuilders and captains of sailing ships. More than one gravestone reads "Lost at Sea." A house in Great Village bought by Captain James Albert Mahon sat on Mahon land but for many years was occupied by the Rev. Alexander Wylie, for whom Margaret's father was named.

When Alexander Wylie Mahon was young, his father, named James after his seafaring ancestor, bought Fort Belcher Farm at Onslow, up the bay from Great Village. Both James Mahon and his wife, Charlotte McCullough, died when Alex was still young. The boy then lived with his brother David and his wife, Margaret. From the latter he learned his love of gardening. Across the bay at Noel lived the O'Briens, one of whom became the great-grandmother of Charles Herbert Best. Margaret later wrote of the "very pleasant link between the English, Established Church and Tory Best family and the Irish, Presbyterian and Whig Mahon family."[48]

Alex Mahon studied Latin and rhetoric at Dalhousie in 1874–5. He went next to normal school in Truro and then taught at the Protestant St. Ninian Street School in predominantly Catholic Antigonish. Back at Dalhousie, Alex Mahon received prizes in metaphysics, French, constitutional history in 1878–9, and in psychology and French in 1879–80. Mahon's name appeared frequently in the *Dalhousie Gazette* during 1879–80. On 15 November 1879, he was elected president of the student body. From this date until April 1880, he was an editor of the paper. He published several articles and took part in meetings of the Sodales, or debating society. From 1880 to 1884, Alex Mahon was a student at Pine

Hill Theological Seminary, which had recently moved to new quarters overlooking the North West Arm in Halifax.

John Scott Macleod, paternal grandfather of Margaret Mahon's mother, arrived in Prince Edward Island in 1820 at the age of seven, with his mother, Matilda Graeme Macleod, probably from Dumfries in Scotland. He became a farmer and a Liberal, a supporter of Robert Poore Haythorne, champion of the tenants' league against the mainly absentee landlords. Henry Morpeth Macleod, a son of John Scott and his wife, Mary MacDonald, taught in Charlottetown. Henry wed Sarah Ann Stewart, daughter of John Stewart and Flora Cameron Stuart, whose father was reportedly an officer who had served with Wolfe at Quebec. They were married at Five Mile House on St. Peter's Road by the recently ordained George Munro Grant, later principal of Queen's University in Kingston, Ontario. They and their first four children moved in 1868 to a farm at Dunstaffnage in Lot 35 in Queen's County. A small courthouse was built on the farm where he held the post of clerk for many years. Henry Macleod was proud to have a rail line through his property with a halt where the presiding judge could alight. There are many stories of picnics and parties with music and dancing on the lawn at the Macleod house.

Of their ten children, several died young, and most of the others left to pursue further education. Mary Agnes, a teacher, died of tuberculosis in 1891 at twenty-five. Herbert Stewart went to Prince of Wales College in Charlottetown and then to McGill to study medicine; he died of TB at twenty-three in September 1892. Ambrose "Amby" Watts also went to Prince of Wales and was a graduate of Dalhousie and Pine Hill Theological College; he was about to receive his PhD from Harvard when he died of TB in June 1893 at the age of twenty-nine. Henry Stainforth "Stainey," the eighth child, also studied at Prince of Wales College, and he went on to McGill where he received his BA in philosophy in 1898. After their father died in January 1899, Stainey replaced him as clerk of the court until he too died of TB in January 1902, at twenty-six. The family was decimated by tuberculosis and only three Macleod children survived beyond their twenties: Flora Cameron, Margaret Mahon's mother; Bruce Morpeth; and Sarah Melinda.[49]

The family belonged to St. Columba's Presbyterian Church in Marshfield, a short distance along St. Peter's Road towards Charlottetown. It was to this parish that twenty-nine-year-old Rev. Alexander Wylie Mahon ("A.W." to his family) was inducted and ordained on 4 October

1883. His sister, Eliza Ann, known as "Lydie," had taught in Heart's Content, on Trinity Bay, Newfoundland, during 1881–2, and then returned to keep house for her brother. She painted in oils and gave classes to young ladies, including sixteen-year-old Flora Cameron Macleod. She died of tuberculosis in 1890, aged thirty-four. In 1893, Mahon went to the theological seminary in Princeton, New Jersey, where he received his bachelor of divinity degree. He was listed as a graduate student, "Pursuing Special Studies in Addition to the Regular Course: Special Course in Higher Criticism of the Hexatench (the first six books of the Old Testament), and Special Course in Early Aramaic Inscriptions," given by John D. Davis, editor of the *Westminster Dictionary of the Bible.*

On 26 June 1895, Rev. Alexander Wylie Mahon wed Flora Cameron Macleod in the parlour of her parents' home in Dunstaffnage. He had been inducted a month earlier into Greenock Presbyterian Church, St-Andrews-by-the-Sea, New Brunswick.

Greenock Kirk, completed in 1824, is a fine, two-storey Georgian church built of wood, and no nails were used in the construction. Captain Christopher Scott from Greenock, Scotland, was very involved in the building of the kirk, and he had a large green oak carved on the front of its tower. Margaret recalled the serious debate between those who wanted to introduce an organ into the church and those who regarded it as "an instrument of the devil."

Margaret Hooper Mahon was born on St. Andrew's Day (30 November) 1900, in a cottage opposite the Georgian court house, where her older brother, Henry MacLeod, was born three years earlier. In 1901, Margaret's godmother, Mrs. George Hooper of Montréal and St. Andrews, had the manse designed and built by Edward Maxwell, the well-known Montréal architect, who also had a summer home in the popular seaside town.[50] Here, Emma Linda was born in 1905.

Margaret's memories of life in the manse were very happy. She claimed that she could remember events from a very early age. One grisly incident made a lasting impression on her: a moose tried to jump the graveyard fence, was impaled on the spikes, and died.

The parlour of the manse held the piano — a wedding gift from Flora's parents that took them two years to pay off. Other furniture included Henry Morpeth Macleod's armchair, made probably in Charlottetown, Sarah Macleod's spinning wheel, a rocking chair with a bird's-eye maple balloon back, and a large barometer inscribed "Daniel Brennan,

Charlottetown." Pictures on the wall were from Flora's brush or from that of Eliza Mahon, A.W.'s late sister.

On the ground floor was the study, where the family would go after supper. It was a comfortable sitting room, lined with bookshelves, and usually had a fire burning in the open grate. There, Margaret's father would read to his children, instilling in them a lifelong love of literature. A.W. started a Canadian literature club in St. Andrews in 1905 and contributed articles to the original *Acadiensis* and other journals. In 1908, he published a small book entitled *Canadian Hymns and Hymn-Writers*, printed by the *Globe* in Saint John. In his foreword, he wrote: "It has been said that we might as well look for a needle in a haystack or for snakes in Ireland, as for good writers in Canada … Persons who talk in this way speak unadvisedly with their lips."

A.W. wrote an undated article headed "Howe and Tupper." "There were giants in Nova Scotia in those days. The first time I ever saw Sir Charles Tupper, and the only time I ever saw Hon. Joseph Howe was when as a boy I attended one of the greatest political meetings ever held in Nova Scotia." At thirteen, young Alexander was taken by his father on 4 June 1867 to the big Drillshed in Truro to hear the two men debate Confederation. "They spoke alternately, from two p.m. until dark, to an immense audience."[51]

As a minister, A.W. Mahon created an ecumenical atmosphere that influenced his family as well as his parish. At one stage he decided to invite another local clergyman to preach on a Sunday evening at Greenock Kirk once each month, but both the Anglican and the Catholic bishops forbade their priests from participating. At the infrequent communion services, he invited "all members of the Church catholic to join with us in Holy Communion."

A.W. Mahon had a green thumb, and his favourite form of exercise was gardening. From the manse garden came a bountiful supply of fresh vegetables, "very early green peas and little new potatoes," and beautiful flowers — an abundance of sweet peas, dahlias, and sweet-scented stocks.

A newspaper clipping from 1910, headed "The Leaders in Schools: Names of Pupils Who Occupy Honour Rolls" shows Henry Mahon at the top of the list for grade eight and Margaret first in grade five. Margaret was less successful in music. Once a new student at their school turned to her while the class was singing and said, "Less noise and more music please." Margaret observed, "I was quite hurt at the time but for many years I have realized that she spoke the truth."

Skating and snowshoeing, skiing and sledding were popular winter sports for the Mahons. Margaret often accompanied Miriam Mowat and her fiancé, Dr. Herbert Everett of St. Stephen, on outings. In the summer, the couple would take Margaret to the Mowat family farm on the St. Croix River to see Grace Helen (Nellie) Mowat, who started the Charlotte County Cottage Craft, where women spun wool and wove fabric in their own homes. They gave the vegetable dyes of the material names evocative of the area, such as Briar Rose, Quoddy Blue, Spruce Green, and Yellow Birch. On one of their many walks Margaret confided to Miriam, "When I grow up, Miriam, I am going to write a book." Her friend replied, "Then I shall read it to the bitter end." Judge Melville Cockburn and his family of St. Stephen were also obviously close friends as they appear often in the diaries and photographs of the period.

The young girl was neither athletic nor a tomboy, but she was independent and enjoyed climbing trees. On at least one occasion, passing women went to the door of the manse to report that Margaret was seated reading in a fork of a tree. Her mother thanked the callers but did not chastise her daughter. Margaret inherited her mother's independent spirit and willingness to be different.

Two special people in the family's life were A.W.'s brother, Joseph Crowe Mahon, and Flora's only surviving brother, Bruce Morpeth Macleod. Uncle Joe Mahon owned Bible Hill Farm, near Truro, where he raised trotting horses, which he sent to Ireland and possibly Austria. He owned the Sussex Bottling Works and would send his nephew and nieces barrels of bottled soft drinks — orangeade or ginger ale — packed in excelsior. One time, he asked Margaret if she would like a fur coat. Her mother sent off the measurements, and a few weeks later a "beautiful, gray squirrel coat, lined with blue satin, arrived."

Uncle Bruce Macleod also loved horses but could not afford to breed race horses; however, he owned one or two, which he raced when he was acting manager of the Bank of Nova Scotia in Woodstock, New Brunswick, in 1904. He would sometimes take Margaret for a ride in his sulky, but once when he did not take her, she said the most cutting thing that she could think of: "The Bank of Nova Scotia is no good." Uncle Bruce taught Henry to play golf and gave the children a fox terrier called "Colonel Bogey," who would run after the doctor's carriage and chase chickens. Colonel Bogey was accordingly dispatched to live on the Island of Grand Manan, but he returned home on the boat a few days later.

The household included a young woman named Lizzie Henderson, daughter of a black father and a white mother. Lizzie helped do everything from preparing meals and making taffy for church sales to looking after the children. Flora Mahon recalled that on several occasions visiting women asked whether it was suitable to have a mulatto girl looking after the minister's children. She spiritedly rejected their concern.

St-Andrews-by-the-Sea became a favourite summer home for many people of means, both Canadian and American. The Mahons knew most of these summer visitors, many of whom attended Greenock Kirk. Some stayed at the Algonquin Hotel, built in 1889 and bought by the Canadian Pacific Railway Company in 1902. Sir William Van Horne, president of the CPR, lived at "Coven Hoven" on Minister's Island, accessible by road only at low tide. He built a grand house, had gardens and orchards planted, and raised Dutch belted cattle. He was also an artist, and once, when Margaret was visiting with her parents, he took them upstairs to see the charming frieze that he had just painted in his grandson's nursery. He also showed Margaret the handsome door-knockers, one on each side of the fireplace. "I had those placed there," he said, "so that I can hold on and toast my toes." Margaret remembered Lady Van Horne as a "slim and lovely old lady."

Probably the summer home that the Mahons visited most frequently was "Clibrig," the residence of Senator and Mrs. Robert Mackay of Montréal. Margaret's favourite person there was their daughter, Cairine, fifteen years her senior. In 1909, she married Norman F. Wilson, an Ottawa lumberman and farmer, who was MP for Russell County from 1904 to 1908. Cairine later often recalled her fiancé's asking little Margaret if he had her permission to marry "her" Cairine, which she solemnly bestowed.[52]

In the autumn of 1912, when Margaret was almost twelve, A.W. and Flora Mahon moved their family from St. Andrews to Toronto. A.W. had a poor heart, and was advised to see specialists there. The choice of schools available for the children in Toronto was also a factor, as were the several good friends who lived there.

For Henry, Margaret, and Emma Linda, the train trip west was exciting. The first winter, the family stayed in a rented house at 13 Barton Avenue, near St. Alban's Cathedral, belonging to William Houston, an editor for the *Globe*, legislative librarian, and constitutional expert. The house was full of books. Margaret remembered one evening when Houston was having dinner with them. "As we were enjoying our soup a great crash came from the kitchen and a pile of Houston dinner plates was gone. My mother remained calm and said in her charming way that it was an open pattern."[53] Henry attended the University of Toronto School, and Margaret and Emma went to Huron Street Public School. Margaret found that the students knew less history than pupils in St. Andrews but that they were more expert at mental arithmetic.

After another summer in St. Andrews, without any improvement in his health, A.W. retired from that charge. Uncle Joe Mahon paid $7,000 for a house in Toronto at 370 Brunswick Avenue at the corner of Lowther for his younger brother and his family. In his will, he left the house to A.W., along with any money beyond what went to his wife.

In the autumn of 1913, Margaret attended Harbord Collegiate. The next summer, she started her first diary. She regretted that they were not back in New Brunswick, on the ocean. There was a list of the books that she read that year — volumes available at home or at the public library on College Street. Her father's interest in Canadian literature was reflected in Stephen Leacock's *Sunshine Sketches of a Little Town*, W.S. Wallace's *The United Empire Loyalists*, several other volumes from the *Chronicles of Canada* series, and Marjorie Pickthall's *Little Hearts*. Classics included George Eliot's *Silas Marner* and Charles Dickens's *Oliver Twist*. Other authors recorded were Jane Austen, Rupert Brooke, Ralph Connor, Arthur Conan Doyle, W.T. Grenfell, Robert Service, and Henry Van Dyke.

The summer of 1914 was busy. The Tennis Club at Walmer Road Baptist Church was close by, and Margaret passed many happy hours there with Tracy and Ordway Lloyd and George Gilmour, later president of McMaster University. There were picnics in High Park and on Toronto Island. On 3 August 1914, Margaret wrote, "The world is greatly excited — Germany is given 'till midnight tonight to decide whether she will march through Belgium or not. If she does, England has to go into the war." And on 14 August, "We have no very definite news of what is going on. The Belgians are doing wonderfully but the Germans seem to be gaining." Flora Mahon was stocking up on food items. "Mother got a barrel of sugar, a lot of tea, cocoa and Postum."

In February 1916, Henry Mahon registered at University College, University of Toronto, but transferred to the Royal Military College in Kingston, which gave him a special commission on 22 August 1917.[54] He went to England and was attached to the Fifth Battalion of the Middlesex Regiment as a lieutenant and then joined the Royal Flying Corps.[55] He sent an undated card accompanied by a silk scarf for Margaret in the

Middlesex colours. A photo showed him standing beside his plane, which had gone off the runway and ended up with its nose in the mud and its fuselage straight up in the air. On 7 November 1917, Lieutenant Mahon wrote that he was being moved to a base near Newcastle for training in flying heavy bombing aircraft. Apparently, the young pilot reported to a rail depot to take the train north and was sent with a guide to find his train, which was about to leave. Moving between two stationary trains that then suddenly started to move, Henry was crushed and badly injured. There are letters from his base at South Carlton, Lincolnshire, and from Mount Vernon Hospital in Hampstead, London. Other photos showed him recuperating at an unidentified country home in Ireland.

Margaret fell ill with scarlet fever in November 1917. David Glassey, the classics teacher at Harbord who had also taught Latin to Charley, telephoned her home almost every evening and gave a report on her progress to the class the next morning. Margaret kept a letter that she received dated 20 November written in Greek by Glassey and his pupils, including Robert Finch, academic, poet, and artist.[56] Margaret was obviously popular, certainly spoiled, and she enjoyed both. From a young age, she kept track of compliments. Back in school for the winter of 1917, Margaret enjoyed her year. For English, she had Mr. Carlyle, grand-nephew of Thomas Carlyle, the great literary critic and historian; for history, Miss Robinson; and for French, Mr. Irwin — "a very fine group of teachers." Among Margaret's fellow students were Arthur Kelly, later a well-known doctor, and Dalton Wells, who became a prominent jurist. A few students had gone into the armed forces. David Pratt, wearing the ribbon of the Croix de Guerre, caused a stir when, "resplendent in his Air Force uniform," he came home from the war and visited the school.[57] Margaret's junior matriculation diploma gave little information, except that she did not write papers in physics and chemistry nor in German authors and composition.

Margaret entered University College (UC) at the University of Toronto in October 1918. She started a new diary on 9 October. Shortly after the term began, all classes were cancelled for a month because of the influenza epidemic. Theatres were closed, and churches had only one service on Sundays. Flora Mahon had a light case of the flu, and Margaret served as housekeeper. Capable in the kitchen but never really very interested in cooking, Margaret learned at least to make simple meals for her family.

Back at university again, Margaret was the only woman in the Greek class given by Professor Carruthers. The others were theological students from Wycliffe and Knox colleges. Margaret considered her instructors "characters": W.J. Alexander for English; Alfred Baker, "who always donned a glove when he used chalk," for geometry; and Alfred De Lury for algebra. At meetings of UC's Women's Literary Society, Principal Maurice Hutton gave a talk on the Irish playwrights Synge and Shaw.[58]

Margaret wrote on 13 November 1918: "Great things have happened since I wrote on Sunday. The Armistice was signed and all fighting stopped at 11 o'clock Paris time on Monday (Nov. 11) and 6 a.m. our time. At about 5 o'clock, I was wakened by the whistles and bells and felt sure that the news must be correct this time. Boys were going up and down with big feather dusters and cans of powder. They sprinkled the dusters well and then powdered people's faces. It must have been a hard day on those whose boys won't come back." On the following Sunday, John Philip Susa's Band of American Sailors performed in Queen's Park, and the crowd sang, "There's a Long, Long Trail a-Winding" and "Over There."

Margaret's life was very full. University activities included an autumn tea, a Modern Discussion Group, and the Modern Languages Club. "Monsieur De Champ gave a talk on Alsace Lorraine, or I think that was the subject. He spoke entirely in French. He is the wildest looking creature, I am sure I would be overcome if he said anything to me, especially as he always talks in French." There were sorority events, as well as invitations to the movies and to dances. Should she accept one young man's invitation to go to the theatre, or another's to a dinner dance at the Westminster Hotel? Church functions included a supper at the university for the "First-Year Presbyterians" from out of town.

More and more the Mahons, who had at first attended nearby Bloor Street Presbyterian Church, were transferring their affiliation to St. Andrew's Presbyterian Church at King and Simcoe streets in downtown Toronto. This connection was to become more formal as A.W. became pastor-in-charge while Dr. Thomas Eakin, the minister, went overseas with the "Khaki University." Mahon served there for the next eleven years — an onerous undertaking for one whose health was none too good. Margaret remembered, "When my father visited the new Canadians on Peter and John Streets, many of them from Scotland, the children ran along the street calling, 'The minister is coming!' They all loved him. He was far from strong yet he was constantly coming and going on foot and by streetcar to comfort and help his very scattered congregation. My mother watched over him tenderly and the whole family became very involved in the affairs of St. Andrew's Church."[59]

At St. Andrew's Institute, Margaret taught children from the downtown area. "The youngsters belong to poor families and are as nice as they can be. I am teaching them about Moses. They were telling me all they knew about Moses and one little fellow said that, 'Pharaoh's daughter went down for a swim and found Moses in the rushes.'" As late as 1930, the year her father died, she submitted to the church the report of the Social Service Committee, which assisted the deaconess with her work among women and girls.[60]

Christmas dinner 1918 centred around a goose sent from Prince Edward Island; New Year's featured a duck. Also from the Maritimes came a large box of Ganong's chocolates. A parcel arrived "express" for Margaret from Miss Olive Hosmer of Montréal and St. Andrews. Inside a blue Birks box was a "darling little gold watch. I have simply been in ecstasies over it ever since. It is octagonal in shape with a gold face and on a black band with gold clasps. The very latest thing in a watch." The Mahons did not have much money, but many people, particularly parishioners in St. Andrews and in Toronto, were generous.

Over the Christmas holidays, her new sorority held a picnic. On 12 December, Margaret had accepted the invitation to join the Kappa Alpha Thetas. "They say that that is the high-brow — the very learned bunch — they believe in hard study — to begin with they invite, as a rule, the professors' daughters ... [They] must think that I am learned because I take Greek." Fellow initiates included Adelaide Macdonald and Lorena Wellwood, along with Frieda Fraser, Elizabeth Maclennan, and Catherine MacLeod — names that were to reappear in Margaret's diaries.[61] For the picnic, "We went to Stop 81[62] on Yonge Street and then about two miles into the woods by the Don River. It was frozen over and we crossed the river and made a fire. We fried bacon and eggs."

Margaret had turned eighteen on 30 November 1918, and "for the first time, that year I was allowed a good deal of freedom to go to dances and theatres." There were dances at the university's Women's Union, and Margaret met all sorts of people, including many young men, still in uniform. She surprised many of her friends one evening by dancing with a Jewish man — "awfully nice." UC, the only college without a religious affiliation, was where most Jewish students registered. On Saturday, 22 February 1919, UC held its First-Year Reception — the first dance that she attended where "programmes" were used. Margaret was pressed to speak but firmly refused.

On 24 February, Margaret wrote: "On Friday of this week our sorority is giving a dance at Margaret Walton's, 10 South Drive, Rosedale. I had no evening dress to wear. Mother was over on Madison for tea with Mrs. Watt, and Mrs. Watt said she had just the thing. She got it in the misses' department at Eaton's and only wore it once this winter. So she sent it down for me. It is pink and the prettiest thing imaginable. It is silk with a wide girdle of pink with a band of silver ribbon. The neck is square in front and pointed in the back. The sleeves (what there is of them) are white net with pink and silver. I am going to get a pink tulle scarf."

She went on to describe the evening: "Then I had the tenth, the supper dance, with Charlie Best and strange to relate, we discovered that Charlie used to live in Maine, right across from St. Andrews. He was down there for a while last summer and was even in St. Andrews for a day, the very same time I was there. Then, the year I was in IIIA at Harbord, he was in the Fourth Form, but I don't remember him. His best friend is Clark Noble and Clark was down with him for a couple of months last summer. We had supper on the third floor in the billiard room, along with about a dozen other people. As soon as we ate, Ross Webster played the piano up there, and we danced around the billiard table. Charlie asked if he could take me home and, as I had the last dance with Bob Robertson, I didn't know what to do, but as I thought Bob might have taken a girl to the party, I accepted … [Margaret, of course, knew exactly what she was doing.] The eighteenth I had with Bob Robertson and he asked me where we could meet when I got my hat and coat on, so I had to tell him I was going home with Mr. Best." Best and the two Noble brothers, Clark and Warwick, got a taxi. "First, we took Barbara Finlayson and Eleanor Harbord home, so I had four gentlemen, counting the chauffeur, to get me home safely." Charley brought her home "at 3 o'clock, a fascinating hour to be out and about." Little wonder the last sentence of that entry reads, "On Sunday, Mother took my Sunday School Class."

Charley Best's name appeared frequently in Margaret's diary, but he was not her only beau. He took Margaret to the Princess Theatre to see *Tiger Rose*. "His father is a doctor. Clark Noble was along with Miriam Morden, the Rev. Morden's daughter. The play was great and we went to Bingham's afterwards and managed to arrive home at three minutes before Sunday morning. Clark and Charley are in second-year Arts and Medicine."[63] A week later, "Clark Noble took me down to see *Seventeen* at the Royal Alexandra. Charley Best was there with another minister's daughter, Helen Skey. The play was very funny. They changed the story a good deal from the way it is in the book. As far as I can make out from Charley's remarks, Clark is just eighteen." A few days later, Clark called to say that, since Charley was going home to Pembroke on 28 May, the friends had agreed to change nights, so Charley took Margaret to the theatre and gave her a box of Laura Secord candies. Next day Clark came to play tennis and then back in the evening to go to the Marie Allen Theatre on Bloor Street to take Margaret to see Dorothy Gish (Lillian's sister) in *Peppy Polly*. Craig Hamilton, an engineering student and an organist, was also very much in the picture. One evening they went to the Bloor Street Allen to see Tom Moore in *One of the Finest*. "The picture was very good and we had a fine time." A few days later, "I went over to the Island with Craig Hamilton and we went to Hanlan's Point to hear the Station Band from Atlantic City."

A sorority party was held for five days at Lake Simcoe. The girls went out on the Yonge Street radial to Stop 96[64] and walked a short distance to the rented farmhouse right on the water. They all took turns cooking for the seventeen present. Margaret had taken along a book to read — *Greatheart* by Ethel Dell. "It turned out to be very slushy — they all wanted to censor it by reading it themselves. Some parts of it were wild. I read them short extracts such as 'she palpitated in his arms.'"[65] One sorority girl had brought her nine-month-old baby — "a rather modern idea."

Margaret got second-class honours that year; only two students, both boys, got first class. She then had a busy summer in St. Andrews, her old home. Many friends, old and young, entertained her. Robert Cowley, chief inspector of schools for Toronto, and his family met Margaret at the station. Her "honorary aunts" Sue and Annie Campbell, welcomed her to "Elm Corner," their genteel guest house. Every Sunday she went to Greenock Kirk. Edwin Ganong of the St. Stephen chocolate family took her to movies, to the casino to dance, and for a ride in his Cadillac — "He talks as though he were twenty, at least." Margaret played tennis at the Algonquin Hotel, visited old friends such as the Maxwells from Montréal on the Bar Road and the Cockburns, the Everetts, and the Mowats.

Charley Best, who was visiting his family in Pembroke, Maine, could not resist a trip to see her. "Charley came over here with his family a week ago Sunday but I had not yet arrived. Mr. Rollins informed me that a young divinity student from Maine was trying to find me. I couldn't think for a minute who he meant. I had a letter from [Charley] yesterday and he wants to come over the end of this week some day." Warren Skey, Helen Skey's brother, had been visiting Pembroke, and he had given Hilda Best a diamond ring. The trip "was about fifty miles around, I think, perhaps a little more. Hilda is a dear. Charley looked just the same as ever and it was fine to see him. We went out to Joe's Point. We put our food in a cool place and walked around to the Biological Station. Charley discovered a chap from the University of Toronto whom he used to work with. The chap showed us all the collections and we signed the Visitors' Book. Dr. Huntsman was in his office, so I spoke to him and reminded him of the birthday cake he once brought me from Elm Corner to Toronto."[66]

Good news arrived about Henry Mahon. A.W. forwarded two letters to Margaret, saying that her brother had his discharge and was awaiting passage. "It's the best news I've heard for a long time. He expects to get the money from the university to put him through, but it must be in a foreign country so he chose Harvard."

An excursion organized by the Cowleys took Margaret to Grand Manan, an enchanted island off the coast of New Brunswick inhabited by fishermen, birds, seals, whales, and summer visitors — many of them American. They stayed at "Rose Cottage," described by an islander: "There ain't very many roses about and it's certainly not a cottage." Margaret remarked that the people staying there "weren't very congenial, mostly Yankee school teachers. The beds remind me of so many to be found in small guest houses and hotels, 'hills and valleys.'"

A telegram from her father on 10 August changed Margaret's plans. Henry had arrived home from England, and she wanted to go back to Toronto right away.

"Henry (in his uniform) was at the station to meet me. We have been having an uproarious time since then." Henry practised walking and then running at Varsity Stadium at the University of Toronto. With his veteran's credits, he was to go to Harvard University, where he won his letter in track. There were many happy parties and evenings at the movies, interspersed with a boat trip to Niagara, a ball game at the Island, and best of all, the visit of the Prince of Wales. Margaret saw him several times, when he passed Avenue Road and Bloor Street, at the Exhibition Grounds, and in Convocation Hall at the University of Toronto when he received an honorary degree. "He replied so very nicely. Then Henry and I saw him at about seven o'clock at Lowther and Avenue Road. He was holding his hat in his hand and sat on the back of the car. They were going very slowly and when the car came right to us the Prince looked down right at us. I said 'Hello' and kissed my hand at him. He held his hat high above his head and leaned out of the back of the car and smiled at me, turning back as the car went along. Henry and I were both so excited that we yelled and the people about us laughed."

Because of her good first-year marks, Margaret was able in the autumn of 1919 to transfer into second-year political economy. "Henry was very anxious for me to change. There are so many people taking general course work and this is an age of specialization anyway. The work is pretty difficult. We have a great many essays. This afternoon I wrote one for Professor Alexander, whom I have for English, on 'The Advantages and Disadvantages of My Course.' I have Professor W.P.M. Kennedy for group work in English constitutional history and I have to write an essay for him next week on 'William the Conqueror and the Church.' Then a big economics essay on 'My Home City' of two thousand words that has to be in by November 12th." For the essay on Toronto, a trip to the Harbour Commission's office and to the Canada Steamship Company elicited a lot of help. Margaret found actuarial science difficult. There were very few young women in her course; among the men were Dalton Wells and Warren Skey, Hilda Best's fiancé.

Charley Best and Clark Noble were back in Toronto, so there were invitations to the movies. Charley took Margaret to a Women's Art Association dance being run by his aunt Lillie Hallam. Margaret wore her new rose taffeta dress made by a dressmaker who came to the house. She had "a great time and Mrs. Hallam's awfully nice." Margaret had become convener of the social committee for the Young Women's Christian Association (Y.W.C.A.) on campus, and this meant much time spent on organizing a party for the "freshies" and other events. At a college "circus," Adelaide Macdonald dressed as "Galli-Screechi," a take-off on the great opera singer, while Margaret was a "snake charmer and had a peach of a costume. Everyone said it was stunning."

Charley took Margaret to Canon Cody's church, St. Paul's Anglican, to hear Canon Frederick George Scott of Quebec, CMG, DSO. Margaret was impressed: "I liked him immensely." Another Sunday, they went to Holy Trinity to hear the Rev. Ralph Sherman. One evening, they went to the university's newly opened Hart House, where the Players Club was presenting *The Queen's Enemies* by Lord Dunsany, the Irish soldier-playwright. On 30 November, Henry Mahon sent his sister a Harvard pin for her nineteenth birthday, and a sweater with a large "H" on it that she proudly wore. Charley Best gave her a box of chocolates.

One evening, Craig took Margaret and Emma to the Mock Parliament at Convocation Hall. "The third-year skit was a Students Administration Council Meeting and Clark and Charley were both in it. Charley was the W.C.T.U. [Women's Christian Temperance Union] representative and was dressed as a lady in a green silk petticoat and a green hat with white spots, a cape and fur, white gloves with a diamond ring on the left hand over the glove and a little bag. He made a great hit — according to *The Varsity*, he was the hit of the evening. After the third-year skit he went about the audience and sat beside different boys ... and got them all considerably fussed 'by making love to them.'"

Margaret reported triumphantly that she came fourth in the whole class in the constitutional history exam before Christmas, and first among the girls. "Of course, there are only four or five girls, but there must be sixty or seventy boys. Everyone seems to be dumbfounded that I got so much as they think I never study."

During the early weeks of 1920, Margaret went to the Harbord Collegiate Graduates Dance with Alec McAlpine, from St. Andrew's Church, and to the engineering school's dance at Hart House with Craig Hamilton. Then she attended the Arts dance, also at Hart House, with Charley: "It was just about the best dance I have ever been at, except the Theta dance last year," where she had first met CHB.

McAlpine took Margaret on 7 February 1920 to Hart House Theatre to see Ben Johnson's *The Alchemist* with Charley Best playing Dame Pliant, a production that Margaret did not seem too enthusiastic about. Although she came down with the flu, she was soon well enough to go with Charley to see Euripedes' *The Trojan Women* at Hart House. Edith Gould and Clark Noble were in the party.

On 29 February, Margaret wrote in her diary, "Friday was Charley's birthday and the two of us had a little birthday party. He was twenty-one years old, which is getting on. I bought him a pretty pink rosebud and a spike of pussy willow for his buttonhole and he liked it very much. We went to Shea's and then to Bingham's and had a fine time."

For a month or more, Margaret had jaundice, was very ill, and remained very weak afterwards. Her father applied for aegrotat standing for her in her university courses. She later commented, "I probably did a little too much partying and so became ill." When she was better, there were plans for her to go to Boston or to Winnipeg for a trip. Meanwhile friends took her for rides to York Mills and other places. Charley came for a visit one afternoon and for dinner one evening. Both her parents and Charley persuaded her that her academic program was too heavy for the good of her health, so she registered in the general course, taking courses in botany and also in history. She kept her text, Carlton Clark's *Nature and Development of Plants* (1922), and probably used *How Plants Grow* (1872) by Asa Gray, the best-known American botanist of the nineteenth century, a copy of which was in her father's library.

Years later, Margaret Best recalled: "There were a good many very nice boys coming and going at our house and I am shocked when I find in my diary the number of dances and theatres we attended." She added, "But, it is evident as I look back that Charley Best was becoming more and more special for me." Charley proposed to her on 12 July 1920 at the Noble family farm at Norval, just east of Georgetown. Thus, their "betrothal day" — The Glorious 12th — had a double meaning for them; the Mahons were Presbyterians from Ulster, though not Orangemen. Margaret was nineteen, and Charley, twenty-one. He bought the diamond engagement ring with money earned playing baseball at Georgetown. There were many discussions about their future. Charley was undecided as to his field of specialization — physiology or surgery. They even considered going to South America, where there might be opportunities for a young doctor. But within a year, unexpected events were dramatically to change the course of their lives for ever.

Chapter Two

The Discovery of Insulin, 1921–1925

The discovery of insulin was certainly the most important event in the life of Charles Herbert Best. One can talk of fate or chance, or of being in the right place at the right time, but the fact is that he accepted an opportunity to work on fundamental research of a very important medical problem, with a young doctor of apparently limited potential who had a burning desire to succeed where many others had failed. The result could well have been just another footnote in the long battle to defeat the scourge of diabetes, perhaps adding a few details to the accumulated knowledge on the subject. Instead, within a matter of a few months in the middle of 1921, Fred Banting and Charles Best discovered the hormone insulin.

The succeeding months and years brought many improvements in the purity of the substance, methods of mass production and distribution, and later refinement of different kinds of insulin with longer periods of release. Many people contributed to the development and improvement of insulin and deserve great credit for their accomplishments. Given the magnitude of such a discovery and the heady atmosphere that resulted, there were many conflicting claims.

The story has three stages: discovery/announcement (summer/autumn 1921); development, purification, and manufacture (1922); and recognition for the people involved (1923). The emphasis here is on Charles Best, his scientific contribution, his association with Frederick Banting and other professionals in the unfolding drama, and his relationship with his fiancée, Margaret Mahon. This chapter continues with their personal lives, through Charley's MA in 1922, Margaret's BA in 1923, their wedding in 1924, and Charley's MB in 1925.

The many accounts of the discovery of insulin include: the very readable and thorough study by Professor Michael Bliss;[67] a very balanced account by Dr. Barbara Hazlett;[68] the factual and non-confrontational *The Story of Insulin* by Wrenshall, Hetenyi and Feasby;[69] the short but widely distributed *Insulin* by Leibel and Wrenshall,[70] prepared as part of the University of Toronto's celebration of the fiftieth anniversary of the discovery of insulin; and numerous commentaries attempting to assess the role of the various participants.

Only a few of these are referred to here: instead, contemporary letters and documents are cited extensively. Charles Best's own account is obviously central to this telling of the drama, along with his views on the roles of others.

The written history of diabetes begins in the second millennium BC. Then in 1869, a twenty-two-year-old medical student, Paul Langerhans of Berlin, described the group of cells in the pancreas that were later found to produce insulin. In 1889, Joseph von Mering and Oskar Minkowski in Strasbourg made a considerable advance in knowledge by removing the pancreas of a dog and thus producing diabetes. Eugene Opie in Baltimore, Claude Bernard in France, Georg Zuelzer in Germany, and others added to the growing body of knowledge of the condition. Dr. Frederick Allen, in New York, the best-known advocate of virtual starvation as a way of treating the illness, had discovered by extensive research that not only carbohydrates, but also fats and proteins, were harmful to diabetics.

Several researchers attempted to make a pancreatic extract that would cure or control the condition. Many came close. One of the sadder chapters in the search was that of E.L. Scott of Chicago in 1911. If he had not been discouraged from continuing his work, he might well have become the discoverer of insulin. His story, as told by his wife, is pathetic because of the absence of support and resources for his research.[71]

A campaign has been underway recently to recognize Nicolas Paulesco, professor of physiology at Bucharest, as the discoverer of insulin. Unfortunately, he did not continue his early experiments, and his reports of promising results with "pancreine" in 1921 failed to arouse the attention of other researchers.

At this point, two unlikely candidates for scientific glory enter the stage. Frederick Grant Banting was an Ontario farm boy and graduate in medicine from the University of Toronto who went overseas during the First World War as a medical officer, was wounded, and received the Military Cross for bravery. After his return to Toronto, Banting served a surgical residency at the Hospital for Sick Children and then attempted to set up a general practice in London, Ontario. His practice did not thrive, and he was pleased to accept a part-time job paying $2 an hour as a demonstrator in surgery and anatomy at the University of Western Ontario.

46

On 30 October 1920, while preparing a seminar on carbohydrate metabolism, the process by which the body converts food to energy, Banting read an article that was to change his life and the lives of millions of others. Assistant Professor of Pathology Moses Barron at the University of Minnesota reported on the results of blockage of the pancreatic ducts by gallstones.[72] Blockage of these ducts, which drain the pancreatic digestive juice into the intestine, does not cause diabetes. It damages cells in the pancreas that make the digestive juice, but not the other cells in this organ, the Islets of Langerhans. It was well known that removal of all of the pancreas from dogs would produce severe diabetes. During the night, Banting woke up and jotted down in a notebook: "Oct 31/20. Diabetus. Ligate pancreatic ducts of dog. Keep dogs alive till acini degenerate leaving Islets. — Try to isolate the internal secretion of these to relieve glycosuria."[73]

Colleagues in London, including Professor F.R. Miller, head of the university's Department of Physiology, advised Banting to go to see Professor J.J.R. Macleod. This scientist from Aberdeen, Scotland, a world expert on carbohydrate metabolism, headed the Department of Physiology at the University of Toronto. Macleod, understandably, was not very encouraging, but he eventually agreed to give Banting laboratory space and minimal equipment: "It was worth trying," and, "Even negative results would be of great physiological value."[74]

Macleod knew the long history of other researchers' failure to find an internal secretion of the pancreas. Did he really have a sense that Banting's idea might lead to something, or did he just give in to the persistence of the young surgeon? In retrospect, if he had seen any possibility of positive results, he might have been more helpful.

In April 1921, Macleod arranged for Banting to have an assistant, Charles Best, who had just completed an honours degree in physiology and biochemistry. Macleod had suggested that Best and Clark Noble might collaborate with Banting, even though the professor had apologized to his two new graduates, telling them that he considered that "it would likely all go up in smoke but would be a good operative training, and we must leave no sod unturned."[75] Noble had other immediate priorities, but Best agreed to work with Banting from mid-May to the end of June, when he was due to attend militia camp. The oft-repeated story of a coin being tossed to decide which man should first join the project was, according to CHB, the product of a journalist's imagination, but it became part of the folklore.

During their fourth year of studies (1920–1), Best and Noble had demonstrated to third-year medical students in physiology. They also undertook a research problem involving the production of diabetes in turtles. A pin-prick at a certain point in the brain of an unconscious turtle produced signs of diabetes — a phenomenon first described by Claude Bernard. In 1921, Best and Noble sought to determine the pathway of the nerve impulses produced by the pin-prick to see what caused the illness. In the course of this work, they learned about the Myers and Bailey modification of the Benedict procedure[76] for estimating the amount of sugar in small quantities of blood — the principal chemical procedure used in the research leading to the discovery of insulin.

Best's knowledge of carbohydrate metabolism and diabetes was certainly fresh in his mind, because Macleod had given a two-hour talk each week to the fourth-year students on "The History and Present Knowledge of the Use of Sugars in the Body." Best could have had no better preparation for the work that awaited him. His physiology notes for Macleod's course — one of thirty-four sets of his university notebooks to survive — contain the following entries:[77] "Utilization of Sugar in the Tissues on Assimilation Test ... New Method: Inject intravenously known amount of dextrose at a known velocity ... Woodyatt at Chicago used above on many patients ... Woodyatt injection method should be accompanied by blood sugar estimations." Mention followed of the work of H.C. Hagedorn of Copenhagen and of Francis Benedict of Boston, both leading researchers in carbohydrate metabolism.

The entry for 31 January 1921 described more of Macleod's tests and refers to "Allen — starvation theory." There were many references to the importance of the blood sugar and discussions on the "mechanism by which blood sugar is maintained constant ... Nervous or Hormone — maybe this, maybe that — these are speculations." On 21 February 1921, there were notes on how to determine the "degree of diabetes," blood sugar levels, and sugar in urine, with constant mention of other researchers such as Epstein,[78] August Krogh, Jacques Lépine, E. Pflüger, and R.T. Woodyatt. Macleod mentioned the work of Lépine on several occasions and disagreed with his observations, as he did with those of several other researchers.[79]

Supporting the theory of "nerve control," there was a discussion of family characteristics of people with diabetes, especially nervousness. The incidence of diabetes fell in Berlin during the last two years of the war, but this might have been explained not by "nervous strain, but low food.

In the States, diabetes has risen — no nervous strain and large quantities of sugar. More dietetic than nervous." This led to a look at "Control thru Hormones," and a list followed of all possible glands that might be studied. The first mentioned is the pancreas, with a detailed description of how its removal from an animal produced diabetes. "This discovery is extremely important. We can produce experimentally a condition like that in a clinic."

On 28 March 1921, the notes covered reflexes, carbohydrate metabolism, and the pancreas again. Perhaps the "pancreas may produce an internal secretion." Bernard, Pavlov, Pflüger, and W.G. MacCallum were cited. Then, "Macleod does not believe the point proven between internal secretion and detoxification. A great many people have tried to get a prep. Macleod has shot holes in many of them." Finally, "Pancreatic extract is only way, says Macleod." There were certainly contradictions between some of the statements.

Several pages further on Best noted: "Relation of the Isles of Langerhans — Pathological and Histological evidence — Disease of pancreas likely to be found in patients who died of diabetes. But might be effect rather than the cause." There follows a reference to H.H. Dale of London, and a note: "Macleod thinks that the isles have a close connection with carbohydrate metabolism. Can not change symptoms of diabetes by any extracts of pancreas."

Charles Best's copy of the 1918 edition of Professor Macleod's textbook has the following paragraph marked:

> The removal of some hormone necessary for proper sugar metabolism is, however, by no means the only way by which the results can be explained, for we can assume that the pancreas owes its influence over sugar metabolism to some change occurring in the composition of the blood as this circulates through the gland — a change which is dependent on the integrity of the gland and not on any one enzyme or hormone which it produces.[80]

Macleod left Canada for Scotland in mid-June 1921, a month after the two young researchers had begun work. He had suggested what route to follow, but he did not take any direct part in the research during the next three months.

1921: Summer

The twenty-two-year-old Best wrote his last exam on 16 May 1921 and started work on the diabetes project the next day. The first task for Banting and Best, after a thorough cleansing of the filthy laboratory, was to consult the literature on the method by which to make dogs diabetic. Best had some knowledge of French (although he always regretted his weakness in the language) and neither man knew any German, so they depended on abstracts and translations. Banting brought his surgical expertise to the enterprise; Best, his knowledge of carbohydrate metabolism and relevant chemical methods. As time went on, each learned from the other.

At the beginning of June, Best wrote a jubilant letter to his father, who had just been wired Charley's examination results by his uncle Will Hallam. "I am quite pleased. I worked hard and was lucky to beat the fellows I did." Only one person was ahead of him — Henry Borsook, later a professor at Caltech.[81] "Margaret called me up before seven this morning to tell me. The paper came to their house long before ours arrived. You can give her a lot of the credit for my rank. She has been simply great all the year." The love and support of Margaret and her family meant a great deal to Charley. "I am having a lot of trouble refusing to have meals at the Mahons. Mrs. Mahon would like to have me come up there all the time. They are well-known people in the Presbyterian Church. Mr. Mahon writes a lot." Best did not think that he would be working very long with Banting: "I don't know yet what I will do during July and August. Work is rather scarce. I will find something."[82] In order to save money, Best, Noble, and Marsh had their graduation photograph taken together.

Money was short that summer of 1921, as neither Banting nor Best received a stipend. Fred loaned Charley money to cover expenses. Charley moved to the Nu Sigma Nu fraternity house on St. George Street. Dr. Nelles Silverthorne, later a senior pediatrician in Toronto, was living at Nu Sigma Nu that summer and described CHB as "quiet, never made wild statements." Charley had "the highest IQ and most rational mind" that he had ever known.[83] In July, he stayed with Margaret's brother and sister, Henry and Emma Mahon, at 370 Brunswick Avenue, when the rest of the family was on holiday.

Margaret was away a good deal that summer, regaining her strength after her winter illness. First, she stayed with her friend Elizabeth Maclennan at Lake Joseph, in the Muskoka region north of Toronto, where her parents later joined her. She spent August with Jack and Ethel Robertson, cousins of Margaret's mother, and their children in Coniston near Sudbury, but she and Charley kept in close touch by mail.

According to Banting, "At the end of three weeks [early June] it was decided that Best should continue to assist because it was both inconvenient for Noble to return to the city and inconvenient for Best to go out of the city. (Each one of them subsequently married the girl.)"[84] Charley fulfilled a commitment at the end of June to go for two weeks to a militia camp at Niagara-on-the-Lake, where he hoped to earn a little money training with the Governor General's Horse Guards. He was the medical sergeant, but he had very few duties. He spent most of his time riding horses that others found difficult to handle.[85]

Banting on his own in the laboratory obtained conflicting and erratic results. He blamed Best for leaving "filthy glassware" and for inaccurate solutions and soundly berated him on his return in early July. According to Banting, Best spent the whole of that night cleaning the lab and the glassware. The next morning, Banting found everything "spick and span. We understood each other much better after this encounter."[86]

The summer heat in the small room in the Medical Building was a real problem, and the two found it difficult to keep diabetic animals alive long enough to permit tests with the extracts that they made. Time was very precious, and infection in the first series of animals operated on increased the pressure. In his report to Colonel Albert Gooderham[87] in September 1922, Banting described the working conditions: "The place where we were operating was not fit to be called an operating room. Aseptic work had not been done in it for some years. The floor could not be scrubbed properly, or the water would go through on the laboratories below. The walls could not be washed for they were papered and then yellow washed. There were dirty windows above the unsterilizable wooden operating table. The operating linen consisted of towels with holes in them. It was made more difficult to get things because I had been given six weeks [mid-May to the end of June] to get results, and overtime was not in any person's line, and, worst of all, no one took me seriously, since the professor has said that 'it would likely go up in smoke.'"[88]

Charley wrote to Margaret from the Mahons' house, "I hope you are a lot cooler than we are here. I stayed up here last night. Henry and I slept on the balcony. I don't know how much longer I will be staying in the city — a week more at least and perhaps the rest of the month as we had thought." The results of the experiments were discouraging. "I found two of my dogs dead this morning and expect more to depart. I will be all caught up on my work tomorrow and for the first time for five weeks won't have to work on Sunday."[89] A couple of days later the weather had improved. "We have had a very refreshing rain this afternoon. I worked in the lab this morning and finished up for the weekend."[90]

On 10 July, "I am going to work in the Lab again this week. The weather will not be as bad as this past week ... I have not heard from Clark or any of the connection since he left town."[91] Charley reported that for his militia service he had received $10.25, but $7.75 had been deducted. He did not explain why.

CHB spent all his spare moments away from the lab in the company of Margaret's brother Henry and their fifteen-year-old sister Emma. "We are continuing to thrive on Emma's meals. She is a great girl in every way."[92] Sometimes, Henry and Charley played tennis, or went swimming, or all three would go to Toronto Island to escape the heat. In every letter Charley reiterated how much he missed Margaret and how much he wished she were in Toronto.

Things went slowly at first. On 17 July Charley said, "I really do not work very hard in the Lab these days. For quite a while now I have been taking several afternoons a week off. I will begin working harder again tomorrow. It is difficult to say when I will be through."[93]

But the work certainly did intensify. Encouraging results emerged on 30 July. A pancreatic extract ("isletin") prepared with the greatest care and kept frozen until just before it was used, produced a lower blood sugar count in one diabetic animal, dog no. 410. This result was not the sort that would persuade the scientific world, but it was very encouraging to Banting and Best.

On 3 August, at the suggestion of Best, Banting abandoned the time-consuming, two-stage pancreatectomy — the Hédon method — and did a total pancreatectomy on dog no. 408 which was a success. Dog no. 408 was given the pancreatic extract which caused the blood sugar to fall, whereas extracts of liver and spleen had no effect on the blood sugar. After surviving for four days on the "isletin," the dog died on 7 August of widespread abdominal infection. The same day, Sunday, 7 August Charley wrote to Margaret, "This is the first spare moment I have had. I worked Sat. until about five-thirty and went up to 370 for tea — I went back to the Lab at eleven p.m. and we worked all through the night and to-day until two. We got fine results. The prize dog [no. 408] died to-day at about twelve."[94] This was the dog in Henry Mahon's oft-reproduced photograph of Banting and Best on the roof of the Medical Building in early August 1921.

On 9 August, Banting and Best each sent a handwritten letter, with Banting countersigning Best's report, to Professor Macleod in Paisley, Scotland, giving their results to date. Banting was excited, "I have so much to tell you and ask you about that I scarcely know where to begin."[95] But Best was more cautious: "We have delayed writing you because until recently we have not been able to secure any significant results."[96] After explaining that their extract "invariably causes a decrease in the percentage of blood sugar and in the excretion of sugar in diabetic dogs,"[97] both men emphasized their problems. They wrote, "Infection has been our great trouble. We have found it next to impossible to keep a wound clean during the very hot weather. Conditions in the animal room also are not very good, as you know … We have had very heavy casualties among the 'duct tied' dogs during the hot weather."[98]

Banting outlined fifteen items for Macleod's consideration. "Especially during the hot weather, we have been so greatly hampered by infections despite our utmost care, and since we have lost so many dogs, I strongly desire more help to keep the place clean and gloves and gowns and a thorough fitting up of our operating room. I told Dr. [C.L.] Starr of my difficulties and he has secured the use of the surgical research operating room (for operations only) and I will take the dogs down and bring them back when the operation is over. Mr. Best has expressed the desire to work with me and I should be more than pleased to have him. His work has been excellent and he is absolutely honest, careful and impartial, and has taken a great interest in the work. He has assisted me in all the operations and taught me the chemistry so that we work together all the time and check up each other's readings."[99]

In a letter to Margaret dated 10 August, Charley wrote, "We are doing identical operations on the dogs. We are going to give one the extract and the other none and study the conditions of each — how long each one lives, etc. It will be quite a crucial test for our 'Isletin.' I am glad you asked to hear about the dogs, dear. I know you are not interested in them apart from my work. It will be a great help, Margaret mine, when we are married to have you interested in the things I am doing. You could read any articles I might write about cases I may have and help me make them understandable for people."[100] Margaret did contribute in this way many times.

Momentum was mounting. The next day Charley wrote, "We are spending tonight in the Physiology Department; have done five operations to-day and are due to work day and night for several days."[101] By 15 August, the pace was beginning to take its toll. Charley wrote, "I have not had a minute these last few days to write you, but I know you will have understood. It is about midnight of the fifth consecutive night up and I am getting the disease called insomnia. I can not sleep even when I have the chance … Everything is going fine in the lab. The dog which had no extract [no. 409] is dead and the other one [no. 92] is as lively as can be."[102] They obtained these results by using the whole gland extract of a dog's pancreas. Six months later, Charley informed his father: "Our notes show that we worked 14 nights and 31 days in August. And at one time five days and nights without more than one hour's sleep a night."[103]

Meanwhile, Margaret had a very active summer in Coniston with the warm and hospitable Robertsons, going down into the Worthington mine, playing tennis, trying to learn to drive, going with groups of friends for picnics by Lake Ramsey and to movies in Sudbury. But she missed Charley and thought about him often. "Mother said that you are working so hard — night and day. I think about you so many times every day, Charley, wondering how you are getting along, but most of all at night before I go to sleep. I wonder if we will be like Ethel and Jack [Robertson], loving each other all the time and so happy."[104]

In his letter dated 23 August, Macleod, if not "very excited" by their results as CHB said later, was guardedly optimistic. "You know that if you can prove to the satisfaction of everyone that such extracts really have the power to reduce blood sugar in pancreatic diabetes, you will have achieved a very great deal." He sensibly suggested that they would have to establish a solid body of proof to respond to potential criticisms of their results. The problems were not insurmountable; the criticisms "can be satisfactorily met and your results are definitely positive, but it is not absolutely certain." Macleod was glad that Banting had decided to stay on in Toronto and reassured him: "I will do all in my power to help you. In Best's letter it is proposed to run two depancreatized dogs side by side, one receiving injections of extract. That is admirable, go ahead with it." In fact, they had already done this. "Tell Best that I am very pleased with the way he appears to be doing his work and give him this letter to read so that he may meet my criticisms by using data on other dogs."[105]

On 6 September, Charley let Margaret know: "We have had a letter from Dr. Macleod. He is very excited about our results. He said that my work and plans 'were admirable.' We are going to start a day and night drive about Thursday morning I expect."[106] By the time they received the professor's letter, they had already completed many of procedures that he suggested.

Autumn 1921

When Macleod arrived back in Toronto in September, he found that Banting and Best had already completed the tests that he had required and had carried on without him. Instead of being pleased, Macleod appeared to resent their success in an area in which *he* was the expert. Despite his promise of support of 23 August, he did nothing to help. He appeared dissatisfied and had some reservations about the work. To assert his authority, Macleod refused to provide either a salary to Banting or any of the necessary improvements to working conditions. Banting was furious and threatened to leave the university and go to the United States. Then Macleod changed his mind after the intervention of Professor Velyien Henderson, head of the Department of Pharmacology, and Dr. Clarence Starr, chief surgeon at the Hospital for Sick Children, who had both taken an interest in Banting and Best's work during the summer. Appearing more conciliatory, Macleod offered Banting a small room to work in, a "lab boy," and some improvements to the operating room, but no position in his department.

Henderson offered a position to the penniless Banting starting 1 October. Neither man had consulted Macleod, who was put out that such an arrangement had been made without his knowledge. Macleod, however, had never offered any post to Banting, nor had he given him any financial support; by his not supporting Banting and by the latter's acceptance of Henderson's offer, the professor inevitably lost some control.

Henderson's offer was indeed very important to Banting. Later he said, "It was because of Henderson that I stayed ... It was he and he alone who kept me in Toronto and in Canada. Were it not for Henderson I believe insulin would have been a product of the United States. Henderson had a thousand times more to do with the discovery of insulin than had Macleod. In the first place he knew more about it. In the second place he was consulted before every series of experiments and he advised, criticized or commended. In the third place he remained and still remains the trusted friend with whom there are no secrets, who guides and advises from behind the scenes."[107]

Charley dictated to Margaret several pages of the manuscript of the first presentation on insulin. She was always proud that these historic pages were in her hand. The paper was given at a meeting of the Physiology Journal Club in the department's library on 14 November 1921. Banting was to present the paper, and Best to show the charts. They had asked Macleod to introduce them, but he presented the salient points of the research, thereby undercutting their presentation and giving the impression that it was really his work. "Professor Macleod in his remarks gave everything that I was going to say and used the pronoun 'we' throughout. The following day students were talking about the remarkable work of Professor Macleod," Banting later complained to Colonel Gooderham.[108]

It was after this presentation that Macleod asserted his authority over the investigations. Writing to E.P. Joslin a week after Banting and Best's presentation Macleod guardedly stated, "It is true that we have been doing work on the influence of pancreatic extracts which has yielded most encouraging results, but I would rather hesitate to attempt the application of these results in the treatment of human diabetes until we are absolutely certain of them. Dr. Banting and Mr. Best, who have been doing this work, are to report their findings at the meeting of Physiological Society at New Haven, by which time we expect to be in a position to come to a definite conclusion. I may say privately that I believe we have something that may be of real value in the treatment of Diabetes and that we are hurrying along the experiments as quickly as possible."[109] Macleod's attitude to the exciting discovery was ambivalent, using the pronoun "we" (which so annoyed Banting) yet, at the same time, crediting "Dr. Banting and Mr. Best."

Macleod immediately began assigning problems arising from the work to others in his department, including Dr. John Hepburn, Dr. J.K. Latchford, and Clark Noble, but he did not consult the two primary researchers, Banting and Best. Later Best, however, did emphasize that these other scientists made valuable contributions to the development of insulin for human diabetics.

Best prepared the first paper on the internal secretion of the pancreas for publication based on the presentation of 14 November. He noted at the top of the manuscript, "The hand-written paper was then typed and sent as the first report on Insulin to the *Journal of Laboratory and Clinical*

Medicine.[110] The article, submitted in December 1921, appeared on 3 February 1922, as "The Internal Secretion of the Pancreas" by F.G. Banting, MB, and C.H. Best, BA.[111] "In the course of our experiments we have administered over seventy-five doses of extract from degenerated pancreatic tissue to ten different diabetic animals. Since the extract has always produced a reduction of the pancreatic sugar of the blood and of the sugar excreted in the urine, we feel justified in stating that this extract contains the internal secretion of the pancreas."[112] There has been a suggestion that not all seventy-five injections showed good results as claimed, and this may well be the case, but the conclusion is clear that the data were positive and "this was the essence of the discovery of insulin."[113]

Margaret celebrated her twenty-first birthday on 30 November 1921. A note accompanied Charley's present to her, expressing his continued devotion. "I often think that you and I should never be unhappy — we are so sure of each other. You have been wonderful to me ... It has meant more than I can tell you to have one person just 'out for me' in the lovely way that you are."[114]

Banting and Best continued their research. They obtained potent extracts from the pancreas of unborn calves. Further tests were obviously needed. At the suggestion of Dr. Norman Taylor, they undertook a longevity experiment. They depancreatized the most famous of all the dogs used, Marjorie, dog no. 33, on 18 November. On 6 December, they began treating her with extract from fetal calf pancreas. Within an hour, her urine was sugar-free. Each researcher took a subcutaneous injection of the extract himself without any negative reaction.

> The main feature of the work at this time was a depancreatized dog that had been kept alive for 70 days on extract. All depancreatized dogs that had not received extract in our experience had died within a week. Macleod thought that this dog's condition and survival were due to the fact that the pancreas had not been totally removed. Seventy days was ten times longer than our longest control. This dog had become a great favourite. It was becoming very thin and weak. It had received some bad extract at times and had developed abscesses at the site of injection. Furthermore it required a great deal of extract and it was felt that we could learn more by utilizing this precious and

scarce substance in more acute experiments. Consequently it was decided to take a picture of the dog for record and [on 27 January 1922] after chloroform, that an autopsy be done immediately by an independent and impartial pathologist. Dr. William Robinson was consulted and he consented to make an exhaustive search for pancreatic tissue by serial section. Best and I were present and it was a very great relief when the dog was opened to find not the slightest trace of anything that even resembled pancreas. We all wanted to be doubly sure, so serial sections were done/cut. This revealed a microscopic group of cells so small that it was agreed that they could not be responsible for the survival of the dog.[115]

They found that adult beef pancreas, available in adequate quantities and thus a cheap potential source of the extract, yielded insulin when it was extracted with acid alcohol. Banting and Best started an experiment on 12 December "the whole pancreas of a cow was chopped in 0.3% hydrochloric acid in 95% alcohol, mascerated, filtered evaporated, emulsified in saline, and given intravenously to dog no. 35. Blood sugar fell from 0.28 to 0.11 in four hours. This was the first whole gland extract of beef pancreas."[116] For the next forty years, whole-gland extract of beef pancreas was to be the source of most insulin. On injecting this extract in dog no. 35, they obtained positive results.[117]

Starting in November 1921, Professor J.B. Collip, a well-trained and brilliant biochemist on leave of absence from the University of Alberta and employed on a Rockefeller grant in the University of Toronto's Department of Pathological Chemistry, repeatedly asked Banting if he could be involved studying pancreatic extracts. H.M. Tory, president of the University of Alberta, suspected him of always looking for a better position elsewhere. Apparently, Tory had months earlier questioned Collip's motives for spending his year's leave at Toronto. He told him bluntly, "… in spite of the many good qualities of mind you possess, you can never overcome that disposition of seeing matters only in the light of your own desires, a disposition which is recognized by all your old friends."[118]

Banting was very keen to involve Collip in their work. Best did not think that they needed another person; he wanted to have the chance to do the biochemical studies himself, without what he saw as the interference of the more experienced Collip. Initially, Macleod opposed the addition of Collip, perhaps because he was not in his department, but eventually he acquiesced.

About this time, in mid-December 1921, Banting invited Collip to help estimate glycogen content in the liver. Banting recalled, "He told Professor Macleod the results. This occurred about one week before the Christmas holidays. Collip began working on the biochemistry of the extract about this time."[119] It is difficult to be exact about dates because Collip's notebooks are missing.

The Collip Papers at the University of Toronto include a handwritten note headed, "To Prepare Insulin, Collip Process, Dec 22/21." A card attached has a hand-printed message: "The procedure for extracting insulin was written by Dr. Collip, and left in the possession of his wife in case something should happen to him. Mrs. Collip kept this sheet in an envelope, on which she wrote, 'Original Collip process for preparing insulin. Dec 22/21.'"[120] First, in December 1921, the term "insulin" had not yet been adopted for the pancreatic extract. It was called "Isletin" by Banting and Best in August 1921, and "Insulin" was not used until April 1922. Collip's procedure of December 1921 must have been the improved formula for small quantities, not for greater clinical use. Particularly, given the date, Collip may have written down the procedure after he duplicated Banting and Best's method of obtaining extract from whole beef pancreas using alcohol. Banting later described this occasion:

> One afternoon when Collip came in I showed him the effect of adding 99% alcohol to 70% extract. When about four or five volumes of the former were added to the latter the solution became bluish and hazy due to an extremely fine precipitate. Collip could stand it no longer. The following evening at five he came in again. He said, "There is something wrong with this whole piece of work." Best replied, "What makes you think that?" Collip answered, "Well, I made some extract and did not get the results which you got." We enquired how he made it. After many questions we found that he had sent his lab boy to the abattoir to ask for sweetbreads. As a consequence he had obtained thymus or thyroid glands because up to that time the pancreas was not even removed but was discarded and

made into fertilizer. We told him to get pancreas gland and that he would then get the same results. Thus Collip started a little show of his own.[121]

Others were becoming interested in the extract. On 15 December, a group of physicians at the Toronto General Hospital (TGH), including Drs. Walter Campbell, Duncan Graham, and Almon Fletcher, took part in a discussion with the researchers. Shortly afterwards, Banting gave insulin orally to his classmate Dr. Joseph Gilchrist, a severe diabetic, but to no effect. In January 1922 Gilchrist was the second person to receive an injection of insulin with positive results.

Certainly by December 1921 Banting and Best believed they had discovered insulin. Just before Christmas Margaret's sixteen-year-old sister, Emma Linda, wrote to their uncle Bruce Macleod with the exciting news about her future brother-in-law:

> Charley is not going home this Christmas but he and a Dr. Banting, with whom he was doing research work all summer, are going to speak before the American Medical Society by invitation. I tell you what, old dear, they are stirring up a lot of excitement in this city. They have completed a cure for diebeaties (????) Just now they are trying to get the "stuff" so that it can be drunken. They have it so they can put it under the skin but that is sort of painful so they are trying to see how it can be taken by mouth. Imagine those two. One twenty-two and the other twenty-nine. Dr. Banting was the one who set my leg for me.[122]

A week later Margaret, obviously proud of Charley's achievements, also wrote to their uncle Bruce. She said Charley had spent part of the Christmas holidays with the Mahons:

> … but he had to leave on Monday evening for New York and New Haven. He is to speak tomorrow before an American Medical Convention at Yale. Since early last spring Charley and Dr. Banting have been working as partners on a diabetes cure. He is getting his M.A. this year and does nothing but research work. They have had wonderful

success. The thing isn't perfected yet but it seems that they have got much farther ahead than any other investigators. They spoke before a meeting of the surgeons here a few weeks ago and now they are speaking at Yale. If you would care to see it I will send you a copy of their first paper when it appears in the Medical Journal. Charley wrote the paper ably assisted by your niece. He dictated parts to me and I have developed a real interest in diabetes.[123]

The first international presentation of the Toronto research took place at a meeting of the American Physiological Society at Yale University in New Haven, Connecticut, on 30 December 1921. Macleod chaired the meeting. His name had not appeared on the oral presentation on 14 November in Toronto, and it was not to appear on either of Banting and Best's first two articles, "The Internal Secretion of the Pancreas" and "Pancreatic Extracts," published in February and May 1922, respectively, in the *Journal of Laboratory and Clinical Medicine*. His name was, however, added to the Yale paper, and months later Macleod said that, "at Banting's request, I agreed that my name should appear. Banting said he wished this because it would call attention to the paper since I was known as an authority on experimental diabetes."[124] This paper was essentially a "preliminary communication" or "summary"[125] sent to the *American Journal of Physiology* in advance of the Yale presentation, but it appeared in print about a week before Banting and Best's first article, which they submitted months earlier to the *Journal of Laboratory and Clinical Medicine*. According to Best, the Yale paper "should, perhaps, not be considered to constitute priority although it has performed this function in several strategic places."

Banting, nervous and unused to speaking in public, gave the paper, outlining the work that meant so much to him. He became incensed when Macleod fielded all questions following the presentation, "using the term 'we' throughout the discussion. I was the only one who gave a paper to the Physiological Section who was not asked to respond to his paper."[126] For the second time, Banting felt that Macleod had taken the credit for the work that Banting considered was really his and Best's. Once again there were bitter recriminations; Banting resented the senior man's apparent attempts to steal his thunder. In all of this, Best was involved, but he remained relatively silent. He was torn between loyalty to his colleague and respect for his professor.

Reaction to the paper was cautiously positive, but there were many questions from the experts, such as clinician Dr. Frederick Allen from New York and Professor Anton Carlson, a well-known physiologist from Chicago. Many people wanted to find out more about the new extract. One of those interested in the work was G.H.A. Clowes, director of research for Eli Lilly and Company of Indianapolis; another was Elliott P. Joslin of Boston, a physician who specialized in the treatment of diabetics. Years later Joslin recalled the New Haven meeting: "Dr. Banting spoke haltingly, but we could gather that really something had happened and that the sugar in the blood of a dog had dropped. It was a little difficult to catch the whole story, but later this was emphasized and beautifully told by Dr. Macleod, with little praise or congratulation, and a moderate amount of friendly but serious criticism of the work. The physiologists present deeply resented the interest and enthusiasm of us clinicians who were there, and evidently hinted that never again would we be invited to come to their meeting."[127]

In succeeding years, there have been harsh criticisms of the weaknesses in the early papers. Flaws there were, certainly, but the result was of world-shaking importance, and that is what mattered. The lack of experience of Banting and Best, the initially poor working conditions and lack of financial and other support make their achievement all the more impressive.

1922: Purification, Development, and Manufacture

On 11 January 1922, the first insulin was given by injection to a severely ill patient, Leonard Thompson, by Dr. Edward Jeffrey, a resident physician on Dr. W.R. Campbell's service at the Toronto General Hospital. Banting, especially, was insistent that the first clinical trial be made with extract prepared by himself and Best. Best made a batch from beef pancreas and tried it on "Marjorie," and they gave each other injections. Hospital protocol forbade them even to be in the room when Leonard Thompson received the first insulin given to a human patient, and they were refused a urine specimen. The extract, in a relatively small dose, had a positive effect on lowering the blood sugar level, but, as had occurred with the dogs, there was a problem with abscesses at the site of injection because of impurities that it contained.

Banting described the results: "A 33% fall in the blood sugar followed the administration of the first dose of the extract to a human being.

Unfortunately, this extract contained too high a percentage of protein and other solids, and an aseptic abscess followed its administration."[128] Best said, "We obtained 25% lower in the blood sugar, but the material produced severe local reactions."[129] Despite the discouraging appearance of an abscess, this was a landmark occasion. It was the first application of insulin to a human diabetic patient that lowered the blood sugar level. It can be argued that the administration of extract to Thompson was premature. Obviously, further refinement was necessary. In their second paper, "Pancreatic Extracts," Banting and Best stated that their "method of preparation is being materially improved by various important modifications which are being worked out by Dr. J.B. Collip."[130]

Macleod had put Collip in charge of purifying insulin from the raw extract prepared by Best. Collip reported to Macleod regularly. His work was progressing well. Using a similar method, but with major improvements to that of Banting and Best, he prepared larger amounts of purer and more potent extract. According to Macleod, "As a result of Collip's researches a non-irritating, highly potent preparation of insulin was supplied to the medical clinic."[131] It was this extract that was used in the first series of treatments of diabetic patients at the TGH, lasting just over one month.

The Connaught Antitoxin Laboratories, founded in 1914 by Professor J.G. FitzGerald to produce diphtheria antitoxin and similar products, had made a grant to Banting, Best, and Collip to work on production of insulin in larger quantities to respond to the ever-increasing demand. Best received an appointment as director of insulin production at Connaught effective 1 January 1922, but Macleod assigned him to work with Dr. John Hepburn on the topic for his master's thesis, "The role of pancreatic extracts in the utilization of carbohydrates by diabetic animals," due 1 May 1922. However, according to his report of September 1922 to Colonel Gooderham, Best instead spent most of his time "superintending the collection and initial concentration of material which was then handed over to Dr. Collip for completion."[132]

On 25 January 1922, Collip wrote to Dr. Tory in Edmonton, accepting his offer of the chair of biochemistry and confiding his latest success in research:

> Last Thursday Jan. 19th I finally unearthed a method of
> isolating the internal secretion of the pancreas in a fairly
> pure and seemingly stable form suitable for human

administration. It was tried out on one case in the clinic with such encouraging results that today $5000 has been placed at our disposal to secure apparatus, four assistants, etc. to rush the work for the next four months in the hope that we may establish a block of clinical evidence which will prove either the value or the worthlessness of this substance in treating diabetes in the human. There are three of us associated with Prof. Macleod in this work. Dr. Banting a surgeon and Mr. Best a recent graduate first demonstrated the feasibility of use of pancreatic extracts. I was invited to share in the future developments and definitely took over the chemical side as well as part of the physiological side of the problem.[133]

Collip credited the discovery of insulin to Banting and Best, while welcoming the chance to take part in its development.

About this time, an astonishing incident apparently took place. It involved a threat by Collip to abscond with his latest, positive results (referred to in his letter to Tory), followed by a fierce altercation with Banting. According to Banting, this incident constituted "a breach of a gentlemen's agreement amongst Dr. Collip, Mr. Best and myself, as we had agreed amongst ourselves to tell all our results to each other. Dr. Collip discussed this new preparation with Professor Macleod and secured the consent of Professor Macleod to keep the process a secret. I believe that Dr. Collip at this time endeavoured to patent this process, and was only prevented from doing so by Professors Macleod, [Andrew] Hunter and Henderson."[134]

Banting later elaborated on the "breach": "Collip had become less and less communicative and finally after about a week's absence he came into our little room about five-thirty one evening. He stepped inside the door and said, 'Well, fellows, I've got it.' I turned and said, 'Fine, congratulations. How did you do it?' Collip replied, 'I have decided not to tell you.' His face was white as a sheet. He made as if to go. I grabbed him with one hand by the overcoat where it met in front and almost lifting him I sat him down hard on the chair. I do not remember all that was said but I remember telling him that it was a good job he was so much smaller — otherwise I would 'knock hell out of him.' He told us that he talked it over with Macleod and that Macleod agreed with him that he should not tell us by what means he had purified the extract."[135]

Best's version is only slightly more dramatic. He claimed that after hearing Collip's announcement, he put a chair against the door and sat on it to prevent Collip from leaving. When Banting arrived, Collip repeated his boast, and Banting jumped him and tried to throttle him. Best pulled them apart, prompting him to say later, "I may have helped to save millions of diabetic lives, but I know of one life I saved for certain — Bert Collip's."

In writing to Tory a few days later, Collip made no reference to the incident, but he did say, "On the advice of Prof. Macleod and others I am keeping the process an absolute secret. We have decided not to patent it but to offer it to the University."[136] Why did Macleod not want Collip to share his secret with Banting and Best? Why did Collip risk a confrontation by going to them to boast that he had "got it"? If he was looking for a reaction, he certainly got one. Macleod showed that he was aware of the "angry and confusing confrontation"[137] when he mentioned that he had noticed in January "a strain between Banting and Best on the one hand and Collip on the other."[138]

Dr. FitzGerald arbitrated the quarrel. On 25 January 1922, the same day that Collip had written to Dr. Tory in Alberta, an agreement was drawn up between Banting, Best, Collip, Macleod, and the Connaught Laboratories. The four researchers agreed that none of them separately and independently would patent insulin. Instead, they all agreed to co-operate with the Connaught Laboratories. It was for this purpose that Connaught assigned the funds for staff and equipment. The storm seemed to have abated, and everyone worked very hard for the next few weeks to produce insulin to send to the wards for the clinical trials.

Charley Best wrote to his father on 12 February, "We have our new Lab. fairly well completed. We began work yesterday p.m., but one of the stills blew up at the first trial so we are held up again temporarily … Allen of New York and Dr. L.F. Barker of Johns Hopkins are both working on pancreatic extracts. We will have to hurry to keep ahead of them. I hope we get our stills working well soon."[139] Referring to the sleepless nights of the previous summer, he added, "We don't work thru the night now, but the days are from 9 a.m. to 11 p.m. quite often."[140] The previous Sunday, however, he had gone to church with Margaret in the morning and had had dinner with Dr. Henderson.

Competition with scientists elsewhere finally convinced the researchers in Toronto that some kind of patent was necessary. Banting had opposed this step, which seemed to him to go against medical ethics. Macleod had been reluctant. In a letter that July from St. Andrews, New Brunswick, where he had gone to work at the Marine Biological Station on the use of fish pancreas for insulin, he wrote to Dr. J.J. Mackenzie: "I was at first opposed to the idea of taking out any patents whatsoever but was compelled to change my point of view when I saw that in no other way could we effectively control the proper manufacture and sale of insulin."[141] It was proposed that a patent be taken out in the names of Banting, Best, and Collip, on behalf of the University of Toronto. The patent, issued in 1923, was to ensure that, "when the details of the method of preparation are published anyone would be free to prepare the extract, but no one could secure a profitable monopoly."[142] The university then could "license manufacturers under a small royalty (5 percent of the sales). The money thus collected by the University will be used to establish a research fund ... No person directly or indirectly participating in the work on insulin will receive any part of these royalties."[143] In the spring of 1922, Eli Lilly and Company of Indianapolis received the first exclusive one-year licence to manufacture insulin.

Charley Best prepared his MA thesis amid the confusion and frenzied activity of the winter and spring of 1922. He was so busy with the preparation of scientific papers and the production of insulin that he had little time to spend on the thesis. He stated at one point that he had written the text the night before it was due. A bound copy, "The Role of Pancreatic Extracts in the Utilization of Carbohydrates by Diabetic Animals," was filed in the department, and another with the university.[144]

Collip's role, after signing the agreement with Connaught, was described in his three colleagues' reports to Colonel Gooderham in September. Macleod stated, "In February the Connaught Laboratories undertook to prepare insulin in larger quantities and it was arranged that Dr. Collip should devote all of his spare time to this work."[145] Why Macleod says "spare time" is not explained. Best said, "In my opinion the principal work which Dr. Collip performed was to determine the highest concentration of alcohol in which the active principle was soluble."[146] According to Banting, "Dr. Collip refined the extract, which was made by Mr. Best, sending the refined extract to the wards for clinical tests."[147]

Then a very strange mishap occurred. In mid-February, Collip "lost" his improved method. He had apparently not written it down, not wanting anyone else to know it. In his letter of 25 January to Tory, he had given 19 January as the day when he had found a successful method for purifying insulin. So, how did he lose his method?

Macleod glossed over this event when writing to Gooderham: "After an initial success, the yield became unsatisfactory and finally failed entirely."[148] Banting recorded, "On February 19th, Dr. Collip found that he was unable to refine the extract by his method and was unable to keep up his supply to the wards. During the following six weeks, or longer, no extract was available for clinical tests. I believe the reason for this to be that Collip, wishing to keep his process a secret, had not kept careful records."[149] Best simply told Gooderham: "For a long period, Dr. Collip was unable to obtain any active material."[150]

Collip never gave any explanation. In three different documents, he outlined his contributions to the development of insulin; each account differed.[151] In early June 1922, Collip returned to Edmonton to take up the chair in biochemistry. The University of Toronto's accounts for 1921–2 contained a notation saying that he resigned.[152] Best and Scott stated that Collip's "method of purification worked out satisfactorily for a short time, on a small scale. Large scale experiments were not successful and subsequently it was found impossible to duplicate consistently the earlier results. For a period of two months scarcely any insulin was available."[153]

A doctoral thesis on Collip written by Alison Li, under the direction of Professor Michael Bliss at the University of Toronto, adds considerably to our knowledge and understanding of Collip the man, and his career. However, despite her thesis director's later emphasis on the importance of Collip's contribution, this thesis of 289 pages has only ten and a half pages on the discovery of insulin. Li's account skims over what happened in Toronto in late 1921 and early 1922: "For a period of several months that spring [1922], Collip was faced with the bleak fact that he had lost the ability to make potent extract. The cause of this problem is difficult to ascertain, but variations in vacuum pressure, temperature, and distilling time can wreak havoc on the preparation of biological products. Also Collip's haphazard way of notetaking did nothing to help."[154]

In fact, the exact method that he developed for large-scale production is not known. Some of his recommendations for small-scale purification were used by Best and his colleagues as they evolved a method for large-scale production during an intensive six-week period starting in mid-May 1922. After much trial and error, Best and his colleagues at Connaught Laboratories succeeded in finding a method of providing purified insulin in sufficient quantity to meet the clinical and experimental needs in Toronto for the next three months.[155]

In his volume *Carbohydrate Metabolism and Insulin,* Macleod gave great prominence to Collip's method, which was successful in producing small batches of insulin as described above. He mentioned only in one sentence the subsequent development of large-scale production under Best at the Connaught Laboratories in Toronto, and at Eli Lilly and Company in Indianapolis.[156]

In his copy of Macleod's book, Best made many corrections and comments in the margins, as in the following example. Macleod dedicated several pages to the research on producing insulin from fish islets carried out by N.A. McCormick, E.C. Noble, and himself and concluded that, under certain conditions, "fish should prove a profitable source of manufacture." CHB jotted in the margin, "— far more cost than beef pancreas."[157]

If Collip were so crucial to the large-scale production of insulin, surely President Sir Robert Falconer and Dr. FitzGerald would have insisted that he stay on at the University of Toronto. Dr. Tory could have made alternative arrangements for Collip's courses for the following year. Tory and Falconer had excellent relations, as is clear in their letters. Tory had written to Falconer about the offer of the chair in biochemistry to Collip, asking about any arrangement that the University of Toronto might have made with Collip. Sir Robert replied, "Though we are glad to keep Dr. Collip, I hope you will understand that he has always approached us rather than we him. We had no desire to interfere with your arrangements, though as I say if he chooses to stay here at a salary that we can give him, we shall be glad to have him. I believe that lately he has been interested along with others in a piece of research which he thinks may prove valuable and may have to be developed."[158] This research was presumably Collip's purification of the extract on 19 January. Tory responded, "I never had any doubt about your relation to Collip. I always believed that he was doing the manoeuvring himself, not anyone else. He has a fatal gift of interpreting a hint as an offer for the simple reason that he cannot see things outside their relation to himself."[159]

Recalling this period, Banting wrote of the isolation he felt:

> It was an extremely trying time for me. Best was still intimate with MacLeod and the others about the laboratory. I was out of the picture entirely. MacLeod had taken over the whole physiological investigation. Collip had taken over the biochemistry. Professor Graham and Dr. Campbell had

taken over the whole clinical aspect of the investigation. None of them wanted anything to do with me … During the latter part of February and the whole of March, I almost ceased to work. The whole affair was too much for my nervous system. The only means by which I could get to sleep was by taking alcohol. I did not always have enough money to buy it. On two occasions I actually stole a half a litre of pure 95% alcohol from the laboratory, diluted it with water and drank it in order to sleep. I do not think that there was one night during the month of March 1922 when I went to bed sober. About 10.30 on the night of March 31st Best came to my room at 34 Grenville. It was blue with smoke. I was partially finished with my preparation for sleep. Best sized up the situation and proceeded to give me a setting out. He told me that MacLeod was vexed because he was not getting extract with which to work. Collip was unable to make an extract as he had not written down his procedure so was unable to repeat it. Campbell was held up entirely and Professor Fitzgerald had offered to advance $5,000 for the provision of a laboratory in the basement of the medical building if we would commence work again. I told Best I was not interested, that they could have the whole show and that I would finish the teaching term with Henderson and then look for a place where there were decent people to live with. Then Best said possibly the only thing that would have changed my attitude, "What will happen to me?" "Your friend MacLeod will look after you," I said. Best replied, "If you get out I get out." There was silence for some moments. I thought of all the joy of the early experiments which we had known together. Here was loyalty. I emptied my glass. "That is the last drink which I will ever take until insulin circulates in diabetic veins. Shake on it Charlie. We start in tomorrow morning at nine o'clock where we left off." Best was pleased. We sat down and as we had done hundreds of times, planned experiments. For the succeeding months it was back to the old hard grind. Best and I worked in the sub-basement of the old medical building day and night. Time, meals, sleep

— all were of secondary consideration. We had to get insulin into a form that was refined enough for continued clinical use. The atmosphere was different. We were happy. To Best must be given the greatest amount of credit for this phase of the development. It was he more than anyone else who bridged the gap between the test tube and the beaker and later the large-scale production.[160]

On 10 May 1922, Charley Best wrote to his father in West Pembroke: "I will have a lot to tell you when I see you about our work. There has been a lot of trouble, quarrels, etc., but we are getting on. Collip has not played fair. He was in charge of making the extract. Banting and I were going along with the clinical and physiological, respectively. He [Collip] was kicked out yesterday and I am in charge of making the dope. It means a lot of work, long hours, etc., but I hope to get it standardized before July."[161]

Best and his team at the Connaught Laboratories started right away working on the problem. He had the full support of FitzGerald and Defries and the assistance of Jessie Ridout and David Scott as well as Donald Fraser, Peter Moloney, and Arthur Wall[162] as technician. Meanwhile, Banting had been appointed to the Christie Street Military Hospital in charge of the diabetic clinic. It was there that he carried out clinical trials from 16 May to 21 September 1922.[163]

Several Americans showed early interest in the production of insulin, including Dr. W.D. Sansum of Santa Barbara, California, and Dr. Rollin T. Woodyatt of Chicago. G.H.A. Clowes, the English-born research director of Eli Lilly, who had heard the presentations at Yale on 30 December 1921, also expressed interest. Eli Lilly's solid reputation, coupled with the Toronto group's respect for Clowes and for his colleague George Walden, led to the choice of that firm as the first U.S. producer — an unusual co-operation between a commercial firm and a university that was to be very productive for both partners. The personal friendship that developed between people at Eli Lilly and Banting and Best was crucial to this whole arrangement. Lilly insulin helped fill the gap in supply when there were production problems in Toronto.

Best made nine trips to Indianapolis in the summer of 1922 to consult with Clowes and his colleagues. Writing to Margaret from the Claypool Hotel, Charley remarked on the luxury of his accommodation, "with a private bath and all conveniences," and on his impressions of Eli

Lilly, which had "a very large and well-equipped plant here."[164] By the end of June, with Lilly's practical help and advice, many production problems were being solved in Toronto.

Charley was anxious to go home to Maine, as he had not been there since Christmas 1920. This long absence had originally been planned so that he could finish his undergraduate degree and work during the summer of 1921. "I will be rather sorry to leave," Charley had written on 31 December 1920, from West Pembroke, "because I am not planning to go back again before a year from next summer."[165] His mother had not been at all well. In one letter, he had suggested to his father that she should come to Toronto to see a specialist.

By early July 1922, the insulin work was sufficiently established that he could leave Toronto. He had kept his father informed of all events. Dr. Herbert Best had come to Toronto to take the first clinical course in diabetes, given at the TGH. Dr. Roscoe Graham "took my dad under his wing and was really wonderful to him."[166]

Charley and Clark Noble collected a new, open, four-door Studebaker car in Detroit that had been bought by Dr. Herbert Best, and the two young men set off for the east coast with Margaret and her mother, who were going to St. Andrews. Charley was to be away from Toronto about a month. It was Margaret's first visit to West Pembroke. She said that it took them five days to get there, as they stopped off "for all sorts of reasons … such as swimming in Lake Champlain. Clark played the mouth organ and the journey was quite jolly."[167]

Arthur Wall kept Best up to date by letter with news from the lab. In Best's absence, Dr. David Scott was in charge of production, and while Dr. Defries was on holiday at Port Carling, Dr. Donald Fraser was acting head of the laboratory. Up to 10 July, Wall stated, "We have sent 236 cc. of Xtract, exclusive of Physiology, all of which has been washed and centrifuged. This last process takes extra time, of course, but seems to remove the cause of reactions, as we have had no complaints so far." The manager of the Harris abattoir, which supplied the beef pancreas, appeared to be trying to hold them to ransom for the formerly worthless glands, saying that he wanted "definite arrangements made about the Pancreas — said that someone else was after it." Further in the letter, Wall added, "Dr. Fraser was telling me that Harris's will be shutting down on us in the near future. They claim there's a market for Pancreas now. Which by the way, this Lab created."[168]

On the same day, Banting also wrote to Best in Maine, "You are a lucky one to be out of the heat that prevails here at present, and even worse than the heat as a disturbance is that diabetics swarm around from all over and think that we can conjure the extract from the ground. Everything is going as well as can be expected. We miss you a great deal, especially Arthur I think … I was in to see Prof Graham and got another brow-beating this morning because I have two patients in the Pavilion and now the Hosp. think that if those patients can be cared for there that there is no need for any alterations. Poor 'Dunc' [Duncan Graham] is always in trouble over this work of ours."[169]

A couple of days later, Wall reported that Harris's was going to send all its animal glands to England, packed in ice. "We are starting to collect at the Civic Abattoir today."[170] In his previous letter he had reported, "They showed great willingness to give us the glands, but conditions there are not the best for collecting (entrails fall on the floor)."[171] On Monday 17 July, Wall wrote, "Work here had been going along well until Thursday afternoon when we had two weak lots in succession. This put us out a little, but Saturday's extract was OK so have quit worrying." Still concerned about the supply of pancreas, the technician said, "Harris's shut down on us this morning. They have a couple of girls collecting the glands and packing them in ice … With the idea of getting more pancreas, I sent Lowe down with Coull to the Civic Abattoir today instead of working nights. He caught on to the way of getting the glands so he is to be at the Civic tomorrow while Jim is at Davies … I am seeing about collecting at Gunn's tomorrow. We are getting so little pancreas that it is a mighty difficult job to keep the regular patients going. But trust me to get it somewhere. What do you think about paying for the glands?"[172] Wall suspected that if they had paid Harris, they would not have lost this reliable source of supply.

Supply of the raw material was but one problem that Wall mentioned. In his letters, he described many details of different aspects of the production process and the problems that they were encountering. He had earlier written, "We were a little short last Sat. Banting and Christie St. had been using quite a lot. B. wanted some badly in the afternoon before the sterility tests were up. Fraser, being new, & also nervous, made B. sign a declaration of responsibility before letting it out."[173]

A letter had arrived from Eli Lilly concerning its experiments and tests and discussing the sample of "Iletin" that it had sent to the Connaught Laboratories for tests. On Monday, 17 July, Wall wrote that Dr. Clowes of

Eli Lilly had been in the office on Saturday, "but he refused to tell anything of their process, beyond that they placed acetone a second time on the minced glands. Also, they were pig's glands. Were they not supposed to co-operate with this Lab. in making the Xtract?"[174]

After his visit to Toronto, Clowes wrote to Best that he had talked about reactions and impurities with Banting and Fraser, making some suggestions as to the cause. He continued, "I understand that you intend to return to Toronto August 1st and am glad to hear that you will be in charge of the production of Insulin for the Connaught laboratory." Clowes suggested that Best meet him in Boston on his way back to Toronto, "so that we may have a chance to talk over the latest developments in Indianapolis and Toronto and make some plans for the future."[175]

Banting wrote again to Best on 21 July 1922. "Dr. Defries was down yesterday and we had a meeting and decided that Scott and I should go to Indianapolis. We had a letter from Dr. Clowes in which he said that we should almost 'scrap' our plant and install a vacuum system. I am having a copy forwarded to you. We thought it better to go to Indianapolis because I have a hunch that Clowes, since he would not tell us how that batch was made, is holding back a little, and furthermore since the extract we are making here is pretty rough I think they might supply us with more of theirs, for the patients are needing extract very badly. Dr. Defries is taking up the pancreas problem and getting legal option on it. Dr. Moloney is working on the chemistry and refining. Scott is doing his best with the production."[176]

On his return from Indianapolis, Banting reported to Best that he and Scott had been well received and that Lilly had given them all the information that it had. Scott had received details of a high-vacuum pump; Banting got permission from the university's board of governors to order one for the Connaught laboratory, and hoped that Best would be back in time to install the new equipment. In spite of Wall's worries about problems with reactions and impurities in the extract, Banting was quite positive: "The lab have not turned out one cc. of really objectionable stuff since you left."[177]

Banting decided to go to New York to raise money for the new vacuum pump. "Banting is getting 500 cc. a week from Eli Lilly and is all tickled to death," Wall told Best. "He is away to N.Y. at present after money. Says he won't come back unless he gets $15,000 or $20,000."[178]

In July 1922, J.J.R. Macleod went to the Marine Biological Station in St. Andrews, New Brunswick. He found the facility "a perfectly ideal place both for work and for recreation."[179] Macleod hoped that the ductless glands of fish would provide a good source of insulin. For recreation, he played golf. He apparently did not see Margaret Mahon and her mother, who were on holiday there. The next year he sent Clark Noble and N.A. McCormick to continue the research into fish pancreas, which proved to be very rich in insulin, but there were problems in collecting it.

Best was enjoying his visit home. Charley's friends decided to have a party in his honour. Prohibition was in effect but it was very difficult to police the many coves and inlets of Passamaquoddy Bay. At the gathering in a local hall those who were revenue officers agreed to be locked in the hall from midnight to 1 am to allow their companions, who were rum-runners and had provided the drink for the party, time to disappear in their cars or boats. Everyone had a good time and no arrests were made.

Best returned to Toronto at the beginning of August. Both Connaught and Lilly began producing fairly reliable supplies of insulin. Two of the earliest American clinicians to receive supplies were Elliott Joslin in Boston and Frederick Allen in New York. On 4 August an elated J.K. Lilly wrote to Clowes: "I am almost overwhelmed with this tremendous situation, and experience some difficulty in keeping my feet on the ground and my brain in normal operation."[180]

Problems could arise quickly. In several ways September 1922 was not an easy month. Best was preoccupied by the problems of insulin production. On the fifth of the month, Charley wrote to Margaret at the St. Andrew's Church Holiday House at Lefroy on Lake Simcoe, Ontario, saying that things were going well at the lab. But a few days later he reported, "It was blue Monday for sure. The rain had flooded us out. Christie Street and Banting both had returned lots of extract as unusable. Macleod was raving for more dope and better, etc. Scott was on edge."[181] For a couple of weeks, Best was in the lab every night and all day Sunday. But by late on the nineteenth, the problems had been overcome, and a tired Charley was able to report that they had had a very fine day with the "dope."[182] Shortly afterwards, he wrote that Banting and he had been awarded "some prize for the best piece of research work ($50) and also a patient of Banting insisted upon presenting me with $25 so I'm $50 up."[183]

Best's life in 1922 was exceedingly busy. Officially, from 1 January 1922, he had also been director of Insulin Production at the Connaught Laboratories — a position that earned him $2,000 per year. For the first few months of 1922, he had prepared the crude extract, which Collip refined. After 10 May and Collip's subsequent return to Alberta, Best was in charge of all aspects of development, purification, and production of insulin. His work took him out of town a good deal that summer, especially the nine times to Eli Lilly in Indianapolis.

This hectic schedule continued in September when he started his medical studies. Best used the medical text by Osler and McCrae,[184] and Llewellys Barker's *Clinical Medicine, Tuesday Clinics at Johns Hopkins Hospital* (1922). Classmates took notes for him, particularly fellow members of the Nu Sigma Nu fraternity, where he had moved from the Hallams' house at Wycliffe in 1921. He tried to attend as many clinics as possible. He recalled as being particularly helpful Harold Couch, later a general surgeon in Toronto, with whom he was paired in clinics. Best had been Couch's demonstrator in physiology. Other classmates were Grégoire Amyot, Walter Carscadden, Frieda Fraser, Harris Gray, F. Carlyle Hamilton, and Art Kelly. At Nu Sig, Charley Best shared a room with Don MacLean, later a colleague at the Connaught Labs. In 1923 Best was elected a member of the Alpha Omega Alpha Honor Medical Society. In spite of his busy schedule at the insulin lab and a great deal of travel, especially to the United States, he managed to keep his marks up and achieved As and Bs throughout his medical studies.

In Canada, there was great public interest in insulin. Quite a number of press reports described it as a "cure" for diabetes, and many gave the major credit to Macleod, as he was the most senior of the group. Banting's already raw relations with Macleod worsened. As a result of confusion about credit for the discovery, not only in the newspapers but among some people who should have known better, Fred Banting gave a statement in September 1922 to the *Toronto Star*:

> It would appear from articles that have appeared in some papers that Mr. Best was not associated with me in my research work until after some progress had been made. I would like to correct that impression. Mr. Best was with me from the first. The idea came to me in November 1920, while I was on the staff of the Western University, London, Ontario. In May, 1921, Mr. Best and I made the first experiment and we have been working together ever since.
>
> While the idea, it is true, is mine, Mr. Best must have equal credit for the success we have attained. I never would have been able to do anything had it not been for him. We

have worked together side by side, sharing ideas and developing them together, and but for his unflagging devotion and his enthusiasm and his patient and meticulous work we would never have made the progress we have.

From the very beginning it has been a case of Banting and Best and if our hopes are realized I desire to see Mr. Best given all the honour that will be his due.[185]

In an attempt to calm the waters, Colonel Albert Gooderham, who chaired the Insulin Committee of the University of Toronto's board of governors, attempted to mediate. He asked Banting, Best, and Macleod each to give a "typewritten statement of your understanding of the discovery of 'Insulin' right from the very start and its production to day ... I would then compare these statements and see wherein they differ, and ask you three gentlemen to meet at an early date with a view to harmonizing these statements with me."[186]

Banting listed the six points that indicated "a lack of trust and co-operation on the part of Professor Macleod."[187] Macleod, he showed, had repeatedly tried to appropriate credit, thus depriving Banting, and to some extent Best, of their due.

Macleod submitted his report entitled, "History of the Researches Leading to the Discovery of Insulin," and a five-page letter, expressing concern for the university's reputation. Although he gave Banting "full credit for suggesting the experiment of using extracts of duct-ligated pancreas and for successfully carrying it out with Mr. Best's collaboration," he did not want to imply that he "gave these gentlemen complete credit for the Discovery of Insulin as now used in the treatment of diabetes."[188] Macleod wanted to be sure that Collip got recognition: Collip had secured a "purer extract, which he succeeded in doing by the method now in use."[189] "Now in use" is inaccurate. As we saw above, very many crucial changes in the method had occurred between May and September 1922 without any input from Collip, and in any case, no one was certain what Collip's method had been.

Best's factual report was by far the shortest, which was not surprising, considering the long hours that he was working in the lab. Young and optimistic, he noted at the end that he had given less detail than he had intended, as a result of "conversation with Dr. Banting and Dr. Macleod. I am sure there will be very few contravening points."[190] In this he misjudged the situation or, rather, wished to minimize the disagreements. Dr. Barbara McKinnon Hazlett wrote recently, "Best wrote a fair account, giving credit to Macleod for suggesting alcohol extraction and immediate chilling, and to Collip for determining the highest concentration of alcohol in which the active principle was soluble."[191] She added, "The relationships between the four men are the most interesting — jealousy, greed, paranoia, and innocence, intermingled with hard work in dreadful conditions and brilliance"[192] — a good description of the situation.

Meanwhile, Macleod wrote to Collip that he had prepared a "statement of all the steps which have led up to the completed discovery,"[193] and would ask Gooderham's approval to send a copy to him. Gooderham did not attempt to reconcile the three statements. In the light of later disagreements, it was perhaps a pity that he did not make some effort to do so. He may have seen little likelihood of clearing up "all your misunderstandings."[194] In fact, his action might have emphasized the differences, with Banting and Best on one side and Macleod and Collip on the other.

Interest in the events in Toronto was becoming intense all over the world. In the autumn of 1922, the Medical Research Council in Great Britain asked Drs Henry Dale and Harold Dudley, from the National Institute for Medical Research, to go to Toronto, "to report to them on the progress of this remarkable discovery and on the initial results of its practical application … We arrived in Toronto towards the end of September and the evidence put before us carried immediate conviction that a genuine discovery of great potential importance had been made. … Professor J.J.R. Macleod had organized a team of workers to reinforce the activities of the original discoverers, in work directed to the improvements of methods for estimating the amount of insulin present in extracts, and to the production of purer preparations in a higher yield. The practical production was, indeed, still in its infancy."[195] This is a clear account of the situation in Toronto at that time, with a definite distinction between the discovery of insulin and its development.

Macleod's research team — aside from Banting and Best — included initially Bert Collip, John Hepburn, J.K. Latchford, N.A. McCormick, and Clark Noble. The insulin production team, however, was led by Best at the Connaught Laboratories, and Banting was involved in the treatment of patients and instructing physicians in the clinical application of insulin.

By the beginning of October 1922, Best was back in Indianapolis, where he had a busy time at Eli Lilly and Company. In a hasty note to Margaret, written at 5:30 a.m. from the Hotel Lincoln (450 rooms, 450 baths!), he said that he was about to go to the station to meet the English scientists Henry H. Dale and Harold W. Dudley, who had been in Toronto a few days earlier.[196]

Another important visitor to Toronto that autumn was Professor August Krogh from Copenhagen. He had recently won "the Nobel prize for his work on Capillary Circulation" and lectured "on Friday, November 23rd from 5 to 6 p.m. in Room 22, Mining Building (College Street). He will show a cinematograph film of some of his experiments."[197] Krogh and his diabetic wife stayed with Professor and Mrs. Macleod for the three days they were in Toronto.

Many articles on insulin appeared in the press. This publicity made difficulties for the University of Toronto workers who were deluged with requests for insulin and treatment.[198] For those diabetics who were lucky enough to be treated with insulin there were no bounds to their gratitude. Both Banting and Best received touching letters. On 14 December 1922, eight-year-old Frederick Gerrier wrote from the Deaconess Hospital, Boston, to the University of Toronto: "Dear Doctors, I want to thank you for making serum. It has helped me along well. I am getting lots more to eat and am feeling better."[199] The next day, Patrick W. Coffey, a patient of Dr. Joslin, wrote to Best from Northampton Massachusetts: "Thank you and Dr. Banting for the discovery of the wonderful 'I'latin'[sic] and for the personal benefit each of us has received from its use. Perhaps to me, a father, with a wife and two little boys, it is more fitting to say that my relief has been fourfold."[200]

On the same day Richard Whitner wrote from Rock Hill, South Carolina: "Dear Mr. Best, I have just returned to my home from Boston where I have been under the care of Dr. Joslin, he has been giving the extract that you and Dr. Baning [sic] have given to the world and I am so thankful to you for what you have done for me that I wanted to write and tell you so. I have been almost starved to death and now to be able to have enough food to satisfy makes me so thankful and gratiful [sic] to you. You and Dr. Baning [sic] have done so much for the world and all diabetics are thinking of you with love and gratitude. With every good wish for you I am your young friend, Richard Whitner."[201] For the rest of their lives Banting and Best constantly received such heartfelt letters of thanks for the gift of insulin. No two people would have been more delighted than these partners if they, or someone else, had found a cure for diabetes, but insulin was a wonderful improvement on the previous situation. Neither saw the advent of humulin — synthesized insulin — but Best often said that he dreamed of a way to accomplish this.[202]

Charley went home to Maine for Christmas. His mother was still not well and was nervous about further treatment in Baltimore. On the way down east, accompanied by Dr. Arthur Van Wort of Fredericton, Best spent one day in Montréal, where he visited the Montreal General and Royal Victoria hospitals. "Insulin is a magic word. The man in charge of the diabetics, Dr. Rabinowitch (he needs no other description) nearly turned himself inside out to entertain us. We toured the hospital, lunched there and eventually rode in a prepaid cab to the Royal Vic. Mason[203] is the man in charge there. He had received several impotent lots of 'Isletin' and was a bit sceptical at first, but thawed and gave us a very busy and interesting afternoon."[204]

1923: Recognition

Best was back in Toronto by the end of December 1922, when he and Clark Noble "demonstrated the effect on rabbits of insulin" at the meetings of the Federation of American Societies for Experimental Biology.[205] Also attending the gathering was Professor Robert Bárány from Uppsala, Sweden, who had won the Nobel Prize in 1914. Bárány wrote to Macleod on 3 January thanking him for his hospitality and saying that he wanted to talk with him concerning insulin: "I thought that this discovery is of such importance that it should be awarded the Nobel prize."[206] A few days later in Buffalo where he was to make his train connection for Indianapolis, Charley wrote a quick note to Margaret. "Some of the scientists returning from Toronto are on this train so I have not had an opportunity to write you. They have been talking continuously."[207]

Later in January, Macleod and Banting gave the Beaumont Foundation Lectures of the Wayne County Medical Society in Detroit. In two lectures on the scientific aspects of carbohydrate metabolism and insulin, Professor Macleod spoke of his special interest in fish insulin, and took care to mention Best, Collip, and Noble. Banting spoke more of the clinical side. He mentioned Best several times as well as Macleod, Collip, Gilchrist, and several other clinicians.[208]

By February 1923, 250 physicians, 60 clinics, and 1,000 patients in Canada and the United States were receiving insulin. By mid-September,

25,000 U.S. diabetics were on insulin. Arrangements for production followed in other countries.

The Ottawa Branch of the University of Toronto Alumni Association held its Annual Dinner at the Château Laurier Hotel on 13 February 1923. "Dr. Fred G. Banting and Charles Best were the guests of honour ... whose insulin treatment for diabetes is bringing hope and life and health to hundreds of thousands of people throughout the world."[209] Sir Robert Falconer was present. The next day, the visitors had lunch with the governor general and Lady Byng of Vimy.

Perhaps as a result of the attention given to Banting and Best during this visit to Ottawa, Thomas L. Church, Conservative MP for Broadview in Toronto since 1921, raised the matter of an annuity for Banting and Best. On Best's twenty-fourth birthday, 27 February 1923, Church said in the House of Commons, "I think something like a $7,500 annuity should be provided in the Supplementary Estimates or some substantial financial aid be given to men like Dr. Banting and Mr. Best."[210]

Best's aunt Lillian Hallam in Saskatoon wrote to Banting on 6 March 1923, requesting clarification of the role of her nephew. She had been reading "strange accounts of the way in which 'Insulin' was discovered ... Then comes a Canadian despatch, headed up 'Pay for Banting?' But speaks of Dr. C.H. Best as one of the discoverers, but in every report there sounds a note of discrimination, as if you really did all the work that brought about the present preparation."[211] Banting noted on his calendar for 10 March, "Got a rotten letter from Charlie's aunt, Mrs. Hallam." Her letter upset Banting, who replied that he had always tried to give Best due credit. He particularly praised Best for his work in re-establishing the manufacture of insulin after Collip had lost the secret.[212]

Meanwhile, Macleod wrote to J.B. Collip in Edmonton. "You may rest assured, however, that I am doing all in my power, quietly, to place things in their proper relationship and to see to it that your part of the work in the preparation of insulin is given full recognition."[213]

Shortly after these exchanges, on 23 March 1923, the Toronto Academy of Medicine enthusiastically acclaimed the work of both Banting and Best, recording its "deep appreciation of the signal contribution of Dr. F.G. Banting and Dr. C.H. Best to Science by the discovery of Insulin, and to humanity at large, by virtue of its successful application to the treatment of Diabetes Mellitus; and further, commends the admirable manner in which they have acted in giving it freely to the medical and scientific world, thereby maintaining the traditional ideals of our profession with respect to observations or discoveries tending to the prevention, cure or control of disease, or the amelioration of human suffering."[214]

The awarding of another honour illustrates very well the role of politics in the whole insulin story. On 27 March 1923, Sir William Mulock, the seventy-nine-year-old chief justice of Ontario, sent a handwritten letter to Prime Minister William Lyon Mackenzie King concerning "the question of a dominion grant for Dr. Banting the discoverer of insulin treatment for diabetes."[215] (Mulock, as Canada's first minister of labour in 1900, had appointed King as his deputy minister, the latter's first position in the Canadian public service.) Mulock continued, "The good to the world resulting from Dr. Banting's discovery is simply incalculable. It is recognized throughout the world as the product of a Canadian brain, and it seems to me fitting that Canada as a whole should identify itself with it by making a substantial gift towards one of the greatest benefactors in all ages."[216] It may have been to counter the Toronto prejudice against Best because he was born in the United States that his father, Dr. Herbert Best, certified that he himself had been born in Nova Scotia: "I am now and always have been a Canadian — a British subject, not having been naturalized as an American citizen."[217] Mulock sent a second letter on 27 March 1923 attaching an unidentified and undated statement by Banting[218] given to him by an equally unidentified, "eminent and worthy citizen of Toronto" — possibly Dr. G.W. (Billy) Ross. Banting's statement does nothing to encourage King to include Macleod in any annuity scheme. Banting, however, is positive about Best, but Mulock does not mention his name. Billy Ross was a son of Sir George W. Ross, premier of Ontario from 1899 to 1905. He was on staff in the department of therapeutics at the University of Toronto. For many years, he lived at 79 Old Forest Hill Road in Toronto, across the street from the Bests. Ross told many people that he was writing a biography of Fred Banting.

King replied on 6 April, returning Banting's statement, "My colleagues appear to be in hearty sympathy with the proposal which I have made of recommending to Parliament recognition in the form of an annuity of between $5,000 and $10,000." He had secured the support of Arthur Meighen, leader of the opposition, and had also consulted with John D. Rockefeller, Jr., in New York City to obtain further appreciation of Banting's work from the Rockefeller Institute of Medical Research.[219] In March 1923, Dr. Ross also wrote to the prime minister in support of an annuity for Banting, attaching letters of recommendation from Drs Frederick Allen, Elliott Joslin, Russell Wilder, and Rollin Woodyatt.[220]

Tommy Church was among the MPs who, on 27 June, approved the resolution to honour Banting, but he observed: "I notice that the resolution does not include the name of Mr. C.H. Best, Dr. Banting's co-worker and associate."[221]

On the same day, J.G. FitzGerald, in his capacity as secretary of the university's Insulin Committee, wired the prime minister that he had just read in the Toronto *Globe* that the supplementary estimates were to recognize Banting's work. He continued, "Banting and Best worked together from the beginning of the research problem, which led to the discovery of insulin. Best was not an assistant but a collaborator who supplied the necessary chemical knowledge. The Toronto Academy of Medicine has officially recognized Banting and Best as the discoverers of insulin. Banting has energetically supported Best's share in the discovery. In his absence in England and in the interests of accuracy and fairness, I venture to bring these facts to your attention."[222]

King replied, "In considering the recognition accorded Dr. Banting, the Government had occasion to consider also representations on behalf of Mr. Best, and Dr. Collip of the University of Alberta. It was apparent that if anything in the way of national recognition was attempted, it would have to be limited to one person, and that, in associating Dr. Banting's name with the Discovery of Insulin, the Government would be only following the general consensus of professional and scientific opinion."[223]

On the day that Banting received notice of his award, ($7,500 per year for life), he wrote from London. "Dear Charlie, I have just had a marconigram telling about the Dominion Government. I wish they would give you an equal amount. Surely blessings are falling on us fast enough now. We must keep our heads. Fred."[224] Charley wrote to Fred on 28 June 1923, congratulating him on the annuity. He said that he had talked to FitzGerald, who had wired the prime minister. He continued, "It was rather disconcerting to me, after the way my side of the story has been supported, especially by you, to have the government acknowledge you as the discoverer, with no reference whatever to my help. However, this is an old story now." CHB said that he could plainly see Ross's hand in the matter and added, "You say that Dr. Ross is a friend of mine. I can not see it. If it had not been for you, he would never have connected me up in the Academy thing. Perhaps, however, the idea was to keep well outside of the range in which

Collip figures." He finished on a happy note, looking forward to visiting Margaret at Lake Simcoe. "I am enjoying your car. Had it all fixed up."[225]

On 15 July, Banting replied from London. He had talked the matter over with Velyien Henderson, adding, "Only this I can assure you that you will be looked after in some way." He thought "the Connaught Labs should take some of that on themselves. You will be given due place in the Exhibition thing which I wish was in hades." (Banting and Best were both fêted at Toronto's Canadian National Exhibition that summer, but Banting was the only one to speak.) Banting concluded, "All I want in the world at present is to get down to work quietly and uninterruptedly in a lab. Any person can have any damned thing they like if I can only be left alone. I have some new remote ideas in a new field and am going to give up practice and everything pertaining to insulin, as I am sick of it all."[226]

Earlier, while all the correspondence was going on about the annuity, Banting showed his support of Best in a letter dated 4 April 1923 to Ontario Premier E.C. Drury, where he discussed formation of the Banting and Best Department of Medical Research and other provincial support. "I feel that it would be an injustice, not only to me but also to Mr. Best, if our names were not coupled in this matter, since we worked together, as I explained, from the very beginning. Furthermore, Mr. Best differs from all other associates, in that he worked with me before the discovery was made. I urge this matter particularly because of the friendship that exists between us, and our desire that we may continue working together."[227] The third reading of an act setting up an annual grant to the University of Toronto to promote Medical Research took place on 4 May 1923. "This Act may be cited as the *Banting and Best Medical Research Act, 1923.*"[228]

Margaret's brother, Henry Mahon, graduated from Harvard in the spring of 1922 and immediately went west to take up a position as superintendent of schools in the Yukon. In Boston, he had become engaged to Lydia Arnoldson, whose parents had emigrated from Sweden to the United States. In June 1923, Lydia visited Henry's family in Toronto. She then travelled west by train to Vancouver where Henry joined her and they were married on 26 June 1923, the twenty-eighth anniversary of Henry's parents' wedding. Henry and Lydia left immediately for Dawson City, Yukon, where they thoroughly enjoyed the next twelve months.

Best spent much of August 1923 in the United States, and, as usual when they were apart, he and Margaret wrote to each other almost every day. He and Lorne Hutchison, the newly appointed executive secretary of the Insulin Committee, went to visit firms that were interested in procuring a licence to manufacture insulin — the task that Best had told Banting he was not looking forward to.[229] In Detroit they saw the representatives of Stearns Co., Digestive Ferments Co., and Parke-Davis.[230] In Chicago, they inspected Wilson's "immense plant." Hutchison, who was the same age as Best, was scandalized when Best, following the example of their host, removed his coat and walked around the plant in his shirt sleeves. "Lorne himself was quite proper in coat, hard collar and <u>vest</u>." At the end of his letter Charley told Margaret how much he missed her and that when they were married the following year she would always travel with him.[231] Charley then went to Boston and from there visited his parents in Pembroke, Maine. By the end of the month he was in New York, where he and Hutchison were to meet a Japanese representative, Mr. Takamini, who wanted to secure the rights to make insulin in Japan. Lorne was worried because Charley again was in shirt sleeves.[232]

In October 1923, CHB was invited to Boston to speak at Harvard University. Margaret wished that she could be a medical student at Harvard so that she could hear his talk to the students.[233] After the visit to Boston, Charley wrote to her from Indianapolis, where he was staying with Dr. Clowes. He described the Harvard visit to Margaret:

> I arrived in Boston about noon Friday and went directly to Dr. Joslin's house on Bay State Road. Uncle Fletcher whose picture you have seen at Aunt Lillie's was there. There were a number of other doctors. We had lunch and had a talk afterwards. It seems that the Boston papers speaking rhetorically and otherwise had heralded the coming of "The Most Famous Medical Student in the World." It has to be the most something.
>
> I went to the Peter Bent Brigam [Brigham] Hospital at 2.30 and stayed there until nearly four. Went then to the Harvard Medical School where the students had congregated. The largest Hall available was filled to overflowing. President Elliot or Eliott or otherwise [Charles William Eliot] who is over ninety introduced me. He said that Dr. Banting, a surgeon, had come to Toronto to investigate a problem but that I had supplied the necessary knowledge to enable the problem to be investigated

therefore I was the real discoverer of insulin. Hurrah! cried the students. They really gave me a great reception both before and after my little talk.

At the end of my talk Dr. Joslin read a telegram he had just received from Banting saying, "I assign to Best equal share discovery Insulin. Hurt that Nobel Trustees did not so acknowledge him. Will share with him. Please read this telegram at any dinner or meeting. Banting."[234] Dr. Joslin read it again at the dinner at night.[235]

In the meantime, Margaret had already seen the announcement about the award of the Nobel Prize to Drs. Banting and Macleod. "I doubt if Dr. Macleod gets any joy from the use of that $20,000 because it doesn't belong to him. The honour, and the money, too, would have been wonderful, Charley, but it wouldn't have made me love you any more. So that's the main thing."[236]

A month later Margaret wrote to her uncle Bruce Macleod in Lethbridge, Alberta, with her comments on the awarding of the Nobel Prize:

Dr. Banting is a fine fellow and he and Charley discovered insulin. Dr. Macleod was head of the department they worked in but he was absent in Europe when Insulin was discovered. They sent hopeful reports to him in Scotland but he sent back word for them not to be over-confident. Dr. Macleod is an extremely clever man who had a big reputation. Ever since the experiments proved successful he has shoved himself to the front. He spent this summer in Europe and just returned to the university after the Nobel Prize was awarded. If the Nobel Prize was given for the Discovery of Insulin he should have received no part of it. Dr. Banting asked President Falconer or any other man to put their finger on one thing that Dr. Macleod had done towards the Discovery of Insulin.

As for Collip — Dr. Banting and Charley think he is beneath contempt. He came here, after Insulin was discovered, to assist in the purification. He was given all information about making Insulin — and when he thought he had discovered a means of greater purification he actually made

85

an attempt to leave for the States, to patent the whole thing. He was an awful ass and people here paid no attention to him until Dr. Macleod handsomely divided his share of the Nobel Prize. In the clipping you sent me, Dr. Macleod remarked that Collip was "entitled to an equal share of credit for his part in the work." The next day a little paragraph appeared: "The statement that Dr. Collip was entitled to an equal share of credit for his part in the work was not quite properly phrased," said Dr. Macleod. "It might be more accurate to say that he is entitled to a fair share of the credit. I would be glad to correct any misapprehension. If I used the word equal I should not have done so."

All this sounds as if I were fearfully bitter on the subject but I don't think about that side of it much. Charley has really had a great deal of credit and has made a great name for himself already. Ex- President Elliot of Harvard introduced him as "the greatest medical student in the world." Charley is working very hard, as always. He is in his fifth year in Medicine and has complete charge of the manufacture of Insulin.[237]

The Nobel Saga

The story of the Nobel Prize for physiology and medicine in 1923, given for the discovery of insulin, has been told and retold. The process of awarding the prize failed to operate properly in 1923 and is most responsible for the unfortunate result that has embarrassed the Nobel Committee ever since.

The first event in the process was the visit to Toronto of Professor August Krogh and his diabetic wife from 23 to 25 November 1922, when they were the guests of Professor and Mrs. Macleod. Krogh, professor of zoophysiology at the University of Copenhagen, had won the Nobel Prize in 1920 for his outstanding work on capillaries. Macleod had written to Krogh a month earlier inviting him to visit Toronto "to spend a day or two with us. I should like very much to go over our Insulin work with you and get the benefit of your advice and cooperation."[238] Macleod had ample occasion to emphasize his own role to his house guest at 45 Nanton Avenue. He could hardly avoid mentioning Banting, but he did not make

Best's role clear. Macleod was obviously elated by Krogh's visit, mentioning it as the reason he could not attend to other matters in letters to England and to the United States.[239]

Neither Banting nor Best at the time understood the real significance of Krogh's visit. They were not aware that he was one of very few people allowed to make nominations for the Nobel Prize of 1923. Banting was somewhat overawed by him. Best, the young medical student, knew only that he was an eminent visitor, a distinguished lecturer interested in insulin. A memo in Fred Banting's hand dated 24 November 1922, recorded, "Last evening had dinner at York Club. The guest of honour was Professor Krogh of Copenhagen." There followed an account of a medical discussion between the two men: "Prof. Krogh does not believe that hyperaemia causes hypersecretion of gland substance. He believes secretion to be the result of a hormone or nerve stimulation. On being questioned he could not give me any proof that this law which has been established for glands of external secretion maintains in glands of internal secretion. I still believe that hyperaemia of the glands of internal secretion causes an increased production of the secretion." Then Banting added, "To-day, November 24, I had the honour of showing a number of patients to Prof. Krogh, of giving a paper to a group of surgeons at the Hospital for Sick Children, of listening to Prof Krogh's lecture. Tomorrow at 9 a.m., the following group of doctors will meet for a clinical conference on use of insulin: Rollin T. Woodyatt of Chicago; Elliott P. Joslin of Boston; Frederick M. Allen of Morristown, New Jersey; Russell M. Wilder of the Mayo Clinic in Rochester, Minnesota; John R. Williams of Rochester, New York; G.H.A. Clowes, Arthur Walters, John A. MacDonald, and Irvine Page of Indianapolis; and Joseph A. Gilchrist, Charles H. Best, W.R. Campbell, Almon Fletcher, Duncan Graham, and Frederick G. Banting of Toronto. Luncheon Hart House and dinner York Club."[240]

Best was introduced to Krogh along with the others who attended the seminar, but he certainly had no opportunity to speak to him at length. There is no evidence that Krogh met J.G. FitzGerald, although he must have been interested in the purification and production of insulin — the main purpose of his visit to Toronto. Marie Krogh, a medical doctor, was a diabetic, and they were intending to set up insulin production facilities in Copenhagen. Krogh did not contact Henry Dale, who, on behalf of Britain's Medical Research Council, had visited Toronto at the end of September 1922. Krogh had been, however, in Washington and Cleveland prior to coming to Toronto, giving him the occasion to talk to Crile and Stewart, and perhaps to Benedict — the other three who nominated either Macleod or Banting. If the Nobel Committee had taken the time to consult more widely their decision might well have been different.

"The special regulations concerning the distribution of prizes from the Nobel Foundation by the Caroline Medico-Chirurgical Institute given June 29, 1920," set down several points regarding those who were to be asked for advice on the prize for physiology and medicine, including: "The qualification requisite for the right to nominate candidates for the Nobel prize competition shall be held to be possessed by: Members of the Medical Faculties at the Universities of Uppsala, Lund, Christiania, Copenhagen and Helsingfors" — thus two in Sweden and one each in Norway, Denmark, and Finland. Also eligible were "Members of at least six other medical faculties, to be selected by the Staff of the Caroline Institute in the way most appropriate for the just representation of the various countries and their respective seats of learning."[241]

The institute received four nominations in connection with insulin. First, Krogh nominated Banting and Macleod:

> I hereby recommend the Nobel Prize for Physiology goes to: Dr. F.G. Banting and Professor J.J.R. Macleod, Toronto, for their discovery of the pancreas hormone, Insulin, and the research of its physiological and clinical trials.
>
> As the reasons for my recommendation, I refer to my attached manuscript of a lecture to the Copenhagen Medical Society. It is my opinion, that the discovery, production and research of insulin, is an achievement which eminently meets the qualifications, which Alfred Nobel set for this Prize. It concerns a discovery of enormous theoretical breadth and of very great practical significance, as made clear in my aforementioned lecture. I have convinced myself of the accuracy of the basic research and produced insulin according to some of the formulae.
>
> Since the Papers published to date concerning insulin have developed as a result of the joint work of several authors, I must emphasize why I feel the Prize should be awarded to Professor Macleod and Dr. Banting, foregoing all other researchers.[242]

In paragraph five of Krogh's communication the particularly interesting sentence was, "However, he [Banting] would probably not have been able to carry through with the research on his own which from the beginning and through all stages, was led by Professor Macleod." It is true that Banting could not have discovered insulin alone; he needed the participation of a physiologist, and Charles Best filled that role. Macleod did not lead the research "through all stages." He was out of the country from mid-June until late September 1921 — the crucial months. Krogh did not recommend Collip for inclusion in the prize, but he was apparently unaware that Best, not Collip, produced the insulin that he saw used in Toronto in November 1922.

Second, Dr. George Washington Crile nominated Banting. Crile was a professor of surgery at Western Reserve University in Cleveland, Ohio, from 1893 to 1924. He was co-founder of the Cleveland Clinic, which was modelled on the Mayo Clinic in Rochester, Minnesota. Crile became a colonel in the U.S. Army Medical Corps in the First World War, serving in France. His letter of nomination reads in part: "The initial investigations of the value of this product appear to indicate that the expectations of Dr. Banting and his co-workers are justified."[243] Macleod was head of the Department of Physiology at Western Reserve from 1902 to 1918.

Third, Dr. George N. Stewart, JJRM's predecessor at Western Reserve, nominated Macleod. Stewart was born in London, Ontario, but grew up in Scotland. At the University of Edinburgh he received a DSc in 1887 and his MD in 1890. In 1894, he was called to the chair of physiology at Western Reserve. He spent four years as a professor of physiology at the University of Chicago and then returned to Western Reserve as professor of experimental medicine. He was the first at Western Reserve to initiate a full-time physiology laboratory dedicated to research.

Stewart stressed Macleod's "thorough and sustained investigations on metabolism, particularly carbohydrate metabolism, and the functions of the internal secretion of the pancreas"[244] — all of which was certainly true. Stewart mentioned no other name in his recommendation. Where did he and Crile get their information? Did they decide to each nominate the name in their own field? Unfortunately, there is no documentation in Cleveland to help us. Neither Stewart nor Crile had had any personal experience with insulin.

Fourth, Dr. Francis G. Benedict submitted the longest letter of recommendation, nominating Banting. A Harvard graduate, he obtained his

PhD from the University of Heidelberg, Germany, in 1895. He was director of the Boston-based Nutrition Laboratory of the Carnegie Institution of Washington, DC, from 1907 to 1937. Benedict asserted that none of Banting's colleagues "contributed anything near an equal share in these researches." He nominated Banting as:

> … the one man preeminent above all others who should be considered for his remarkable work on the isolation of a pancreatic extract that will reduce blood sugar and has made marvellous changes in the treatment of diabetes. My only question was, first, should any of Dr. <u>Banting</u>'s colleagues or confrères be mentioned as having contributed anything near an equal share in these researches? To this I find the answer is "No." Second, since there are a number of people in America working on the pancreatic extract, is there any one else whose claim for priority is liable to be seriously considered by scientists as a whole? To this I can also answer "No." Under the circumstances, therefore, I feel very confident in naming Dr. <u>Banting</u>, and trust that the committee will be able to secure all the information they desire with regard to his work.[245]

On 26 October 1923, news reached Toronto that Banting and Macleod had received the Nobel Prize for physiology or medicine for the discovery of insulin. Charles Best, as we saw above, was lecturing at Harvard. Banting's anger about Macleod's inclusion was understandably great. His loyalty to Charles Best was evident. He considered rejecting the prize. Two older and wiser heads, Professor Velyien Henderson and Colonel Albert Gooderham, persuaded him to think of the University of Toronto and of Canada, as the Nobel Committee would never be moved.

The reasons given for Best's exclusion from the prize were given over thirty years later by Professor Gøran Liljestrand, secretary of the Nobel Committee for many years, who pointed out that "Best's name was not nominated at all,"[246] and thus could not be included in the prize. In 1991, the author conducted an interview with Professor Rolf Luft, then secretary for the Nobel Committee. Then in a letter, Luft reiterated: "I can say that, with reservations, I think that it might have been fair to give the prize to Banting, Best, and Paulesco."[247]

At the time of his lecture at Harvard, Best's immediate reaction seemed to be astonishment and pleasure at the enthusiastic acclaim of the medical students who cheered him to the rafters. Margaret was the one who commented that Macleod did not deserve the prize. Both Margaret and Charley wrote to each other about the awarding of prize but then went on to other, ordinary things.[248]

In a "brief sketch of the work which led to the discovery of insulin," written in June 1924, Macleod summarized the work of all those involved in the discovery and development. He concluded "I may say that my share in the work was that of directing it and of devising the types of experiments and the methods of carrying them out and, of course, in connection with this it was usually necessary for me to take an active part in the various investigations in their early stages until the preliminary technical difficulties had been overcome and the sources of inaccuracy eliminated."[249] Macleod, of course, had not taken "an active part in the various investigations in their early stages" during the summer of 1921 when Banting and Best were working by themselves. By the time Banting and Best had received the professor's letter of 23 August 1921 they had already carried out the experiments that Best had proposed in his letter of 9 August to Macleod.

Professor Macleod delivered his Nobel Lecture in Stockholm on 26 May 1925. He stuck to an account of the history of diabetic research. His references to the research that was being honoured were very diplomatic and he did not make the claims in the account of June 1924 that he had sent to Professor Darmstaedter. He recounted: "F.G. Banting … with the aid of C.H. Best, and under my direction."[250] He mentioned J.B. Collip briefly and also McCormick, Noble, and others. It was a careful scholarly account.

"To Charlie — Fred." Thus Banting inscribed a copy of his Nobel Lecture entitled, "Diabetes and Insulin," delivered on 15 September 1925, in Stockholm. Banting gave a brief account of the history of diabetes research. He described how he got the idea for his approach and how his and Best's researches proceeded. He recounted the first tests on human diabetics in 1922 and the involvement of Macleod, Collip, and FitzGerald. "Dr. Collip took up the biochemical purification of the active principle and ran the scale of fractional precipitation 70% to 95% alcohol and succeeded in obtaining a more improved end product. But, unfortunately, his method was not applicable to large scale production. Dr. Best then took up the large scale production and contributed greatly to the

91

establishment of production and purification. This work was carried out in the Connaught Laboratories under Professor FitzGerald who is kind enough to be here today."[251]

Best was in London working with Dr. Henry Dale when Banting gave his lecture. Had he and Margaret considered going to Stockholm? Probably not. They were newly arrived in London and very busy adapting to their new life there. FitzGerald wrote them a card from Trondheim in Norway on 10 September: "We expect to arrive in London September 18th ... will be at Almond's Hotel, Clifford Street, W1."[252]

On 26 November 1923, at a special convocation, Banting and Macleod received honorary degrees from the University of Toronto. The banquet following seated four hundred at Hart House. An account published in the *Globe* the following day included a photograph of the head table: Sir William Mulock, the chief justice, sat between Banting and Best. Macleod was three seats away from Banting, between Sir Edmund Walker, the chancellor, and President Falconer. Canon Cody, chair of the board of governors, presided. W.F. Nickle, the provincial treasurer, Colonel Gooderham, Dean Primrose, J.G. FitzGerald, and Dr. L.F. Barker of Johns Hopkins, representing the University of Toronto's graduates in the United States, were among the other dignitaries.[253]

The *University of Toronto Monthly* stated: "Dr. Banting extended his thanks to Mr. C.H. Best, who had been associated with him from the beginning, and also to Professor V.E. Henderson, whom he describes as, 'The truest friend and the best guide of all.' Dr. Macleod said, 'I can only assume that I have been chosen to represent the many co-workers,' and he mentioned in particular the work of Dr. J.B. Collip of the University of Alberta."[254]

One of the most thoughtful publications about the insulin controversy is the last article written by the late Geza Hetenyi, emeritus professor of medicine at the University of Ottawa, and previously a colleague of Best and professor in the department of physiology at the University of Toronto from 1957 to 1970. Hetenyi was co-author with G. A. Wrenshall and W. R. Feasby of *The Story of Insulin* published at the time of the fortieth anniversary of the discovery of insulin.[255]

In the article entitled, "Why Can't We Get It Right? Notes on the Discovery of Insulin," Hetenyi judged that Banting, Best, Collip, and Macleod should all be recognized as members of a team. He complimented Professor Michael Bliss for the "balance" in *The Discovery of Insulin* (1982), but, Hetenyi added: "Disregarding his own judgment that to allocate individual credits among team members is gratuitous, Bliss not only tried to do this, but did so with bias in two subsequent papers. Again, it seems that the temptation to allocate individual credits to one or two favored team members at the expense of others became too strong to be resisted." Then, "a further revision followed in 1993. The focus shifts to Best and his efforts to promote Banting's and his role in the discovery at the expense of Macleod's and Collip's. The paper is written with animus, for example, it is insinuated that Best and not Banting should have been on the plane that crashed in Newfoundland. No mention is made about Best's accomplishments during the war, such as directing the work on dried blood serum for military use and his service in the Navy as of 1940 ... Even if occasionally Best went too far to promote his (and always Banting's) role in the discovery of insulin, this does not diminish his achievements."[256]

Thus ended an extraordinary two and a half years at the University of Toronto, beginning with the pioneering work of Banting and Best in the summer of 1921, followed by the nerve-wracking, but exciting period of development, purification, and manufacture of insulin in 1922, to the roller-coaster ride of recognition, controversy, and honours in 1923.

A charming and unusual honour was accorded Banting and Best in 1925 when the Ontario government named two townships after them in the Temiskaming District, west of Latchford in the mid-north of the province. Best never managed to visit "his" township as it was quite inaccessible, except by canoe and several portages, but he always considered it a special honour.

1924–5

Margaret Mahon had graduated from the University of Toronto in the spring of 1923. Professor George Duff of the Department of Botany offered her a junior post but she declined. Under her photo in *Torontonensis* was written: "She has a world of capability for joy ... Her charm and graciousness, her gay enthusiasms and broad interests and her happy faculty of taking and giving pleasure make Marg an eager student and most companionable friend."[257] She did not like being called "Marg" and firmly discouraged the few classmates who persisted in so doing. Charley was continuing his studies in medicine, in addition to his full-time work in charge of insulin production. They were both looking forward to their wedding in September 1924.

On 3 September 1924, after an engagement of four years, Margaret Hooper Mahon and Charles Herbert Best were married by the bride's father, the Rev. Alexander Wylie Mahon, who had also written the order of service specially for them,[258] in "stately St. Andrew's Church, King Street," as one Toronto newspaper described it.[259] A dressmaker had come to the Mahons' home at 370 Brunswick Avenue to make Margaret's brocade crêpe gown, "long waisted in those days, with a girdle of pearl embroidery. My 'something borrowed' was Ruth Green Price's beautiful train of georgette lined with pink."[260] The attendants were all close family and friends: the bride was escorted by her uncle Bruce Macleod, with her sister, Emma Linda, and Charley's sister, Hilda, as bridesmaids. Henry Mahon was Charley's best man, and the ushers were Clark Noble, Ralph Salter (Hilda's fiancé), Gordon Cameron (a fraternity brother), and Joseph Gilchrist.[261]

Saturday Night described the event as one of Toronto's "most interesting early autumn weddings." The article included a full-length portrait of the bride, "a charming and popular Varsity graduate ... graceful in a gown of ivory brocade crêpe ... and the bridal bouquet was of white and pink cosmos," grown by the Rev. Mr. Mahon in his garden and arranged by Tidy's Flowers on King Street.

Following the ceremony, friends and family, some from as far away as the Maritimes and New England, were received by the Mahons in their garden, which Margaret remembers as "literally blossoming like the rose. My father had seen to that."[262] George Coles Limited catered for two hundred guests in a large tent decorated with six bags of rose petals. Tina and Berta MacLaren, who summered in St. Andrews, New Brunswick, had made the twenty-pound wedding cake, iced in Toronto.[263]

Margaret wore a stylish going-away outfit when the newlyweds left for the East Coast in their new Dodge touring car. Dr. L. Karczag from Budapest, who was studying the work on insulin in Toronto, asked, "What kind of car?" to which the groom replied, "Honeymoon Special." "Ah," said Karczag, "an American make."[264] The honeymooners left Toronto and headed for Pembroke, Maine, via Ottawa, Montréal, Québec, and New Brunswick. At St. Stephen they crossed the St. Croix River to Calais, Maine, and drove down to Pembroke. There, ten days later, Charley's sister, Hilda, married Ralph Salter, a Toronto lawyer, in her parents' church.

Margaret and Charley then drove down U.S. Route 1 to Boston. They stayed in Cambridge, Massachusetts, with Henry and Lydia Mahon,[265] and later in Oxford, with Dr. Elliott Joslin and his wife. With the Mahons they played golf at Sandy Burr Club, near Boston. For several years Margaret played with Charley, but rarely after her first son was born. Like riding, she did it because her husband wanted her to, but she did not really enjoy it. For the rest of their lives, Charley and Henry golfed whenever they met — in Toronto, Maine, or Massachusetts.

That autumn, Margaret and Charley, blissfully happy, moved into a five-room flat on the third floor of the York Apartments, over the Owl Drug Store, at the northwest corner of Bloor and Spadina. The flat was within easy reach of Margaret's parents at 370 Brunswick Avenue and the Toronto General Hospital, where Charley spent much of his last year (1924–5) in medicine, often on night duty in obstetrics. It was also near the old Y.M.C.A. building on Spadina Avenue, which served from 1923 to 1927 as the insulin plant, where Charley supervised the production of insulin.

Charles Best enjoyed this final year of medicine and was class president. In June 1925, he graduated with a Bachelor of Medicine degree.[266] He won the Ellen Mickle Fellowship of the Faculty of Medicine for the highest rank in the medical course[267] and the J.J. Mackenzie Prize for the highest grade in pathology. These awards, along with a grant from the Connaught Research funds and an eighteen-month fellowship from the Rockefeller Foundation, demonstrated that Charles Best was thought worthy of support. This funding was an important investment in a young man who had shown ability, hard work, and leadership in Toronto. Now he was ready to begin the next stage of his development as a research scientist on the international stage. Thus, in July 1925, Margaret and Charley embarked on a wonderful new adventure.

Chapter Three

Overseas Idyll,
1925–1928

When Dr. H.H. Dale visited Toronto in September 1922 to report on the discovery of insulin, Best had been fully occupied with the production of insulin at the Connaught Laboratories and his newly started studies in medicine. Best and Dale met at that time, and Dale suggested that when he had completed his degree in medicine, Best should consider leaving the hot-house atmosphere of the insulin research at the University of Toronto and obtain fresh perspectives further afield where he could broaden his experience in other scientific research. Towards the end of his final year in medicine, Best took up the suggestion and arranged to go to London in 1925 to study with Dale at the National Institute for Medical Research (NIMR).

In December 1924, Dr. J.G. FitzGerald, director of the Connaught Laboratories, had informed the University of Toronto president Sir Robert Falconer about a planned fellowship from the Rockefeller Foundation to enable Charles Best to study abroad in London and Copenhagen. FitzGerald suggested to Falconer that $2,500 be made available from the Banting-Best Research Fund for the same purpose.[268] In January 1925, the office of the Rockefeller Foundation's International Health Board (of which FitzGerald was the only Canadian member[269]) wrote FitzGerald announcing a fellowship for Best, conditional on his receiving his MB (Bachelor of Medicine) in June 1925.[270] (At that time, a medical degree was awarded as a bachelor degree, in the British tradition. In 1932 the MB was converted to an MD, which was the North American practice.)

A few days later Best received notice of the award as a fellow of the Rockefeller Foundation — he was to receive £182 each month for a year, later extended to eighteen months, starting on 1 July 1925, with additional funds for tuition and "necessary travel." The letter noted the recipient's intention of studying with Drs H.H. Dale and A.V. Hill in London and with Drs August Krogh, Johannes Lindhard, and Einar Lundsgaard in

Copenhagen. The Foundation requested details about work to be undertaken with each man and the time envisaged, which Best was to forward to its Paris office. It also supplied additional information about useful people to contact in France and in Germany.[271]

In spite of protesting that he was "not in the least bit excited over going as yet," Charley, full of enthusiastic anticipation, wrote to his parents that "the trunks are filled to capacity and we have two club bags, a hat box, golf bags and a briefcase in addition." His one regret was that they would not see their parents while they were away, "but everything will be fine as long as we are all well."[272] Their address in London at first would be the Charing Cross Hotel. People in Toronto were being helpful. "Col. [Keiller] MacKay, a friend of ours, has just brought over his Ford coupe for us to use today and tomorrow. Scotty also offered us his car."

Not long before leaving, Charley had his "first experience in broadcasting over a radio … Sir William Mulock, chief justice of Ontario and chancellor of the university, talked first and then I did on the research foundation [Banting's]. Over $300,000 has been collected so far. Banting was supposed to speak but at the last moment got cold feet and asked me to take his place. The talk was on medical research."[273]

Margaret described their sendoff from the North Toronto CPR Station at 10:45 p.m. on 9 July 1925.[274] Her parents had said goodbye at home. A.W. Mahon probably feared that he would be too emotional at the station. He gave them *A Wanderer in London* by E.V. Lucas; Linda, *The Thirty-Nine Steps* by John Buchan; and the Best parents, a cheque. "There were 25 people down to see us off," wrote Charley to his mother. "We were greatly pleased."[275] Amongst them were the Bantings, the David Scotts, the Salters, the Prices, and Keiller MacKay. Flowers, chocolates, and books were among the gifts.

Setting off on this trip to Europe was a very exciting step for the young couple. This was Margaret's first trip overseas, and it was their first opportunity to have a real break from Toronto since the discovery of insulin. Charley wrote to Maine that they sailed north of Anticosti and just south of Belle Isle. "The St. Lawrence was like a mill pond, but the first day outside made us feel a bit sick. We recovered quickly and have been fine ever since." They quickly made friends, some of whom they saw for many years. Dr. Healey Willan, the Toronto organist and composer, was at the next table in the dining room. Margaret won second prize at deck tennis; Norman Macleod, eighteenth Earl of Caithness, presented the prize — two silver candlesticks with "Montrose" on them. Margaret noted ships that they passed and described other passengers on the voyage to Liverpool.

CHB enjoyed the shipping in Liverpool harbour and recorded seeing the *Royal Daffodil,* the ferry boat that carried troops to the attack on Zeebrugge, near Bruges, in the war. From Liverpool, the Bests shared a compartment on the train to London with several friends they had made on board ship, "among them Mr. and Mrs. Sweny who are going to study in London for the winter. He [George] is a McGill man. She [Dorothy] is very nice and Margaret and she are great friends."[276]

Their first few days in the metropolis were very busy. With the help of Edgar McInnis, an old friend studying at Christ Church, Oxford, they found a place to live in Hampstead, convenient to Charley's lab at the NIMR. Their flat, in a block of six at 4 Yale Court, Honeybourne Road, Hampstead, was comfortable, with shops and the no. 13 bus to central London nearby. They had to sign for "one aspidistra in perfect condition" and "two chairs, slightly soiled; carpet, slightly worn, etc." Three months' rent in advance strained their cash flow. They got used to the gas heaters and used a coal fire for hot water. Charley commented, "Things are about 100 years behind hand here. There is no central heating. The hot water is heated from a coal fire. All the groceries, etc. come up on a lift which the delivery man cranks up. He whistles up through a tube to let us know he is there."[277] However, they had Maud Ballard come in four times a week, do the lunch dishes, clean the flat, prepare dinner and clean up afterwards — all for ten shillings a week. This left Margaret Best free to spend a lot of time in the museums, galleries, libraries, and antique shops and to gain an excellent education of the sort that only London offered.

Charley went up to the NIMR to see Dr. Dale. Experiments on blood pressure were to start right away. "Dale is probably the greatest authority in this field so my opportunity is great. He has also made a clinical connection for me with Sir Thomas Lewis of University College Hospital, probably the greatest heart specialist in the world. If the thing turns out clinically I will work a bit with Lewis."[278] As usual, Charley knew how keen his father would be to know about research at the institute. "The work is going to be intensely interesting at the NIMR. There is so much going on — the work on the cancer virus is very interesting. I had tea with Barnard, one of the men here, today.[279] The work is interesting not only because of its importance in cancer, but because the germs of many other diseases may possibly be recognised by the techniques developed."[280]

Protocol visits followed. They met Peter Larkin, the tea merchant and Liberal Party financier who was Canadian high commissioner in London from 1922 to 1930. On a visit to the Royal College of Surgeons, bearing a letter of introduction to Sir Arthur Keith, conservator of its Hunterian Museum, Best ran into Dean Primrose of Toronto, who was receiving an honorary fellowship. Sir Arthur took the young visitor around to meet the impressive fellows — "All are 'Sirs' or most of them. It was interesting to see the famous English surgeons."[281] Years later Best spoke of the impact of this period on him: "You could almost look up a list of the seniors or people who were to be senior physiologists and biochemists in England and we became close, personal friends."[282]

Best had great respect for Dale and his research. "He was the first to show that pituitrin causes contractions of the uterus." He also admired William Ewart Gye and his work on cancer at the institute. Gye told Best "that all the younger chaps give Banting and Best the credit for insulin. The older people favour Macleod."[283] Interestingly, Best mentioned to his father that Dr. G.H.A. Clowes had written to him asking for information on the cancer research, so the Eli Lilly Company wanted to have Best as their observer in London.[284]

Young and eager for new experiences Margaret and Charley enthusiastically set off to discover London. They started sightseeing right away by going to Westminster Abbey for a service and noting the tombs of William Pitt (both the elder and the younger), Charles Darwin, and Joseph Lister. Several times, Charley encouraged his parents to use their new Nelson's *Encyclopedia* to follow their travels and regretted having left his copy at home. Cleopatra's Needle impressed them, and they enjoyed museums, particularly the Victoria and Albert. Charley was thrilled to see original works by Raeburn, Millais, Landseer, Turner, Constable, Michelangelo, Raphael cartoons, sculptures by Rodin. "Your encyclopedia would tell you a lot about these things. You would be delighted with them."[285] He drew his parents' attention to a painting called *The Doctor*, by Sir Luke Fildes, reproductions of which hang in so many hospital and doctors' waiting rooms. "The original (at the Tate Gallery) was very fine."[286] At Liberty's on Regent Street, Margaret bought a silk shawl. "There were as many shawls the other night at the Theatre Royal, Drury Lane, as cloaks." When Margaret's cousins, Jack and Ethel Robertson, visited London, Margaret and Charley had tea with them at the Ritz, danced at the Cecil, and dined at the Grosvenor.

Margaret made an important diary entry on 22 August 1925. "On Wednesday evening Dr. and Mrs. Hoet spent the evening with us. They are Belgians. Dr. Hoet works at the institute. We spent one evening with them. Next week they plan to go back to Belgium for a time, but they will return for the winter. Dr. Hoet says that when he returns, 'I will look down on you, I will be a father.' They speak very good English." This meeting launched a very close friendship between the two families that is now into its fourth generation. Joseph Hoet received a PhD in pharmacology from Cambridge working with Professor Walter Ernest Dixon. Hoet, like Best, was on a Rockefeller Fellowship.

On Sunday, 23 August, the Bests went to Bournemouth for a few days with George and Dorothy Sweny from Vancouver, whom they had met shipboard. There they visited the chines — the wooded ravines running up from the sea — and played golf at a pretty course with purple heather growing everywhere. Dorothy and Margaret went to an antique shop called the King and Hangmans on Old Christchurch Road and Margaret made her first art purchases, Baxter prints. From Bournemouth, the two couples went to Southampton, where Charley gave a paper in two parts to the British Association for the Advancement of Science entitled "Preparation and Purification of Insulin/Lactic Acid in Insulin Hypoglycemia." He told his father that he was very much interested in the blood pressure work at the NIMR and had "two good ways of standardizing the active material now. There were no methods when I left Toronto." He was unsure what Macleod's reaction would be. But he added, "Dr. W.J. Macdonald is working in the Department of Physiology, University of Toronto, so Macleod may not like anyone else to get ahead with the physiological work. I don't care about Macleod, but it is Macdonald's work primarily and his wishes must be considered first. When I left Toronto, he was extremely anxious for me to work on these problems and I think he still will be."[287]

Dr. Macdonald, from St. Catharines, Ontario, had produced a liver extract that he at first thought was a cure for cancer, and then believed to lower blood pressure.[288] Best, given his own experience, was very sensitive to the situation of a young researcher working under Macleod in Toronto.

J.J.R. Macleod, who gave a talk on carbohydrate metabolism, and Sir Robert Falconer, president of the University of Toronto, were also in Southampton. Charley reported to his father, "I gave my paper last Thursday and got along very nicely. ... I have had a long talk with Macleod and he says that the blood pressure work is outside his line and that it can be done much better here. I will be able to go at it full speed."[289]

On his return to London Charley noted that the liver extract that he had been working on did not deteriorate even in his absence. He could standardize the extract quite accurately. Competitive as ever Charley told his father, "I am anxious to get ahead so that a lot of others who are working in this field will not get ahead of me."[290]

Margaret and Charley had a wonderful trip to the Isle of Wight where Charley's Burbidge ancestors came from. He enthused to his father, "The Isle of Wight is one of the most beautiful places I have ever seen."[291] Margaret gave Charley a Dunhill pipe for their first anniversary on 3 September. "It makes him ill to smoke it; his first pipe." Charley's present to her was a Slazenger tennis racquet. That week they went to Wembley to the British Empire Exposition and Charley wrote his parents, "There are many wonderful things to see. Banting's picture and mine have been there for two years now, to mention some of the wonderful things." The fair, he thought, was no better than the Canadian National Exhibition in Toronto.[292]

Charley showed impatience at the slowness of getting experiments going at the institute. Materials from Toronto had still not arrived. British Drug Houses (BDH) had offered to help. Francis Carr, the scientific director and a friend of Dale's, wanted some information from Best because BDH was getting only about one-quarter as much insulin from pancreas as was being obtained in Toronto. Charley wrote to his father, "He has invited Margaret and me to their summer home at Petersfield in Hampshire, not far from Portsmouth, for a few days. He is very nice and I don't mind capitalizing on my insulin knowledge a bit." Charley added that the "hypertension thing is drawing quite a bit of interest as you can see from the journal. I think that you might like an English journal. *The Lancet* ($11) and the *British Medical Journal* ($17) are both fine. I think it is fine to get the point of view of the English physician as well as the American. For condensed information that is reliable, Nelson's [*Loose Leaf Living Medicine*][293] cannot be beaten."[294] Herbert Best certainly enjoyed receiving the scientific information from his son, which he could then share with pride with other medical people in the area.

Charley worried about his parents. He tackled his mother's tendency to self-accusation: "There is one thing I wish to tell you, never write me again about 'I am to blame etc.' or any of that foolish nonsense. I told you about that when I was home."[295] At that time, Charley, like most people

101

who have not experienced depression, thought that positive thinking was the best antidote. To his father he wrote, "I think about you a lot, Dad, and the big job you are doing, giving Mother the care and treatment she would get in no other surroundings in the world. You must always remember that I am with you in everything and we will look forward to the time when we can be closer together. Take good care of yourself because we are going to have forty years of good times together."[296] Apart from her depressive condition, it is not clear what else was wrong with Lulu Best. Many years later, Charley talked of his mother's having had an operation — "a butcher job" — probably a hysterectomy that had gone wrong.

Henry Dale had been in Geneva at the League of Nations Conference on Physiological Standards. On his return he was very interested in Best's results. Charley asked his father if he has seen the editorial in the *Journal of the American Medical Association* (JAMA) on hypertension and the work being conducted by Macdonald in Toronto, and in Dale's lab in London. "Fishbein got most of his information from me. I would rather he had not mentioned my name. There are a number of Toronto people helping Macdonald. ... I must write a long letter to Macdonald soon. He will be able to get ahead much faster with a good method of testing. He was greatly worried because the material is so much like histamine. We have done a great number of experiments here and the extract cannot be distinguished physiologically from histamine. Chemically, however, we have observed some definite differences."[297]

Charley kept his father up to date:

> I have had a good week's work on the blood pressure problem. Everything is working out well. Dale is very interested. I have just sent off a long letter to Macdonald telling him of all the new results. I am hard at work on a paper Scotty and I are going to publish from Toronto.[298] We will have lots of results for a good paper from here very soon. Sir Thomas Lewis, the heart man, was in the other morning. He is greatly interested in this work. We did a couple of experiments to compare the effect of histamine and the extract re their power to produce wheels on intracutaneous injection. We injected a series of doses of histamine and the extract into Lewis' arm and into mine. The histamine wheels came up larger than the

extract and persisted longer. We have found a lot of little differences between histamine and the active substance of the extract but no very striking ones.[299]

Dale presumed that Best would want to leave Britain with a graduate degree. Dale was not associated with a university at the time, so he had contacted a colleague at the University of London and arranged to be appointed as an adjunct professor, so that Best's work could be credited towards a degree. "Dr. Dale is going to see what can be done to secure a DSc degree for me. I am very anxious to get one from London."[300] Best registered to begin work towards his London DSc in October 1925, to add to his three degrees from Toronto: BA (1921), MA (1922), and MB (1925).

Margaret made notes in a small book that would fit into her purse. Among other things, she wrote about lectures that she went to at various galleries. In a large book, she entered information either from her own observations or from lectures that she attended. The first section was on "Raphael and Michelangelo" at the National Portrait Gallery. The second, dated 1 October 1925, was on "British Portraiture." The next day, there was a session on "British Landscapes." Other topics included the "Spanish School" and "Dutch Landscape and Dutch Genre." At the National Gallery in November, she made notes on French art. In December, she went to the Victoria and Albert where she recorded comments about Rodin and English silver plate, complete with drawings. In March 1926, Margaret was back at the National Gallery studying masterpieces by Paolo Uccello, a fifteenth-century Florentine painter. She moved to the Wallace Collection to study Rembrandt, and then to the Tate Gallery for a session on Turner. When the Bests returned to London in 1928, Margaret went to the British Museum to see "The Elgin Marbles" and "Greek Vases." A Mr. Wilson lectured on Chinese porcelain at the Victoria and Albert in April. At the end of May, the National Portrait Gallery held an exhibition on "Victorian Women Writers."

For Margaret's twenty-fifth birthday on 30 November 1925, Charley gave her a pair of opera glasses. That evening they went for dinner — "very formal, but quite amusing" — to the Grosvenor Street home of Colonel Sir Bruce Bruce-Porter, a distinguished medical and military figure.

Before Christmas, they went to Nottingham as guests of another drug company, Boots, and were shown all the sights. "They did everything to give us a good time." They saw the "wonderful university, a gift from Sir

Jesse Boot in a wonderful location, out of the city, on the side of a hill, with an artificial lake in front," and met John Campbell Boot, soon to succeed his father as the second Baron Trent of Nottingham.

Back in London, the Bests had dinner at the Portman Hotel on Christmas Eve 1925 with Mary and Percy Herring from Wroxham, in Norfolk, relatives of the Herberts', close friends of Margaret and Charley from Georgetown, Ontario. They had Christmas dinner at home, opening many parcels from Canada. On Boxing Day, they took the Herrings to the Lyric Theatre in Hammersmith to see Isaac Bickerstaffe's *Lionel and Clarissa*, with Nigel Playfair. It was an opera "after the fashion of *The Beggar's Opera*," the first revival since 1768, and Margaret was very enthusiastic.

On 27 December, Margaret and Charley left for ten days on the Continent, a much anticipated and interesting first visit for both, along with Cousin Mary Scott from Winnipeg. They followed the time-honoured route from Victoria Station to Dover, arriving at Ostend at three in the afternoon, and then taking the train to Antwerp via Brussels. Joseph Hoet met them at the station and took them to his parents' house, very spacious quarters above the family pharmacy. His father had died recently, but his mother was there. Marguerite Hoet was also there, with "baby Joseph," their first child, only a few weeks old. Charley and Margaret had a large bedroom on the top floor with a sitting room. Margaret wrote, "Our bed was so enormous, with a great puff, like a feather bed on top."

Hoet took his guests on a tour of Antwerp to see the Rubens paintings in the cathedral; the van Dyck, Giotto, Memling, and van Eyck canvases in the museum; the Rubens house; and the Hôtel de Ville, where paintings by Hendrik Leys were specially lighted so that they could see them. The Hoets had a dinner party for them. One of the guests, who held the chair of therapeutics at the Université catholique de Louvain, was Professor Manille Ide, who was to be part of the team to operate the next day on Désiré Joseph, Cardinal Mercier, a pioneer of Neothomism at Louvain's famous Faculty of Theology.

They went to the theatre and saw a sad piece called *La Lépreuse*[301] — The Leper — "tragédie légendaire en trois actes." Although Charley was able to carry on scientific conversations if he spoke English and the other person French or German, neither of them was a linguist. Margaret read André Gide and André Maurois in French but never mastered the spoken language.

From Antwerp, the Bests went to Louvain to visit Professor A.K.M. Noyons, a Dutchman, head of physiology at the university. The destruction remaining from the war distressed them. They saw the remains of the university's library and the new building rising from the ruins. Joseph Hoet gave them an engraving of the old library. They travelled next to Brussels for a brief visit. Margaret and Mary both bought Brussels lace, and they visited the Palais de Justice and the Royal Art Gallery.

Then the travellers took the train to Paris, where they stayed at the Hôtel de Malte — "very comfortable and most central" — at 63 Rue de Richelieu, opposite the Bibliothèque Nationale, where Hoet had reserved rooms for them. It was New Year's Eve, and the three visitors walked about Montmartre. "There were crowds of people on the streets and when midnight arrived some of them shook hands and some kissed." On New Year's Day, they walked down the Rue de la Paix, the Place Vendôme, and the Rue de Rivoli and strolled along the Seine. Margaret remarked on the famous shops, such as Le Printemps, Les Galeries Lafayette, and Aux Trois Quartiers, where she bought an evening dress. They went to see *Cyrano de Bergerac* at the Théâtre de la Porte-Saint-Martin, where it was originally produced. Margaret had read the play "en français" at university. They had dinner at Marguery on the Boulevard Bonne-Nouvelle and enjoyed its "Sole Marguery."

On 2 January, they went shopping, and then paid their first visit to the Louvre — "too big and too wonderful almost to believe." The next day brought a "Cook's tour" to Versailles and Malmaison, down the Champs Elysées, and through the Bois de Boulogne. At Notre-Dame, they saw the magnificent view from the top of the tower. They had lunch at Gerny's on the Rue de Port-Mahon and thought that a lot of the diners looked like actors and actresses. That night they saw *La Tosca*, with Mlle Sibille as Floria Tosca, and *Cavalleria Rusticana*,[302] with Mlle Saiman-Gritti as Santuzza, at the Théâtre National de l'Opéra-Comique. They went to the Café de Paris for dinner, but Charley "had a slight disagreement with the waiter and we left to go to Gerny's. A woman there sang beautifully as she sat at supper. A man across the room drank to my health a couple of times." Margaret and Charley were increasingly noticed wherever they went, even if people did not know who they were. They gained confidence, and graciously accepted the compliments that they received.

The next day brought another visit to the Louvre to see the *Venus de Milo*, the *Winged Victory*, Corot's *Dance of the Nymphs*, and Millet's *Gleaners*. Dinner was at the Boeuf à la Mode on Rue de Valois. On 6 January came visits to the Sainte-Chapelle in the Palais de Justice and to the Rodin

Museum, a favourite. That night, the trio went for dinner to Prunier on Rue Daphot, noted for its fish. They took the train the next day to Calais, had a rough crossing to Dover, and then returned to London, to stacks of mail. Margaret received a letter from her sister announcing that Edith Gould and Clark Noble were to be married on 16 June. Unfortunately, Margaret and Charley would not be able to attend.

Margaret was not well for a few days but went to see the Sargent pictures at the Royal Academy of Arts. It was too soon, however, for she came down with bronchitis for ten days. Then she was able to go to dinner at Nellie Dale's at Mount Vernon House where the guests included Lady Bayliss, widow of Sir William, who had been professor of general physiology at University College, London, and sister of E.H. Starling, a colleague of Sir William's, a diabetes researcher and Foulerton Professor of the Royal Society, and Margaret Hill, wife of A.V. Hill and a sister of the economist John Maynard Keynes.

"We have become acquainted with a very nice couple, the Sparlings, from Toronto. We met them at the Hotel Cecil. We find that they live across the road."[303] One afternoon, Margaret and Carabelle Sparling went to the Strangers Gallery of the House of Commons and heard Ramsay MacDonald and Stanley Baldwin.

On 26 February 1926, CHB attended a meeting of the London branch of the Glasgow University Club at the Trocadero Restaurant, chaired by the Rt Hon. Sir Henry Craik, MP, who at various different periods was rector of the universities of Aberdeen, Edinburgh, Glasgow, and St. Andrews. On 27 February, Charley's twenty-seventh birthday, the Bests went to Oxford. Edgar McInnis met them at the train and showed them around. They visited Joe McCulley, later headmaster of Pickering College in Ontario, and warden of Hart House at the University of Toronto, at his rooms at Christ Church College. They attended a rugger match between Brasenose College and Queens, had tea with Cousin Norman Robertson, of Balliol College, and walked with McInnis in Christ Church Meadow — "glorious." Margaret liked New and Magdalene colleges, particularly the "Tom Quad" and the "marvellous little cathedral" at Christ Church.

Back in London, there was special interest in going to see Edwin Justus Mayer's comedy *The Firebrand*[304] at Wyndham's Theatre, starring Ivor Novello, Ursula Jeans, and Constance Collier. Collier, who played the Duchess of Florence, was a diabetic on insulin. Charley was always pleased to know of diabetics who were leading normal lives. His love of theatre, however, went back to his first visit to his aunt in New York at the age of twelve, and was fuelled during his student days at U of T when he participated in a fair number of productions himself.

Charley took friends to hear Elena Gerhardt, the Leipzig-born concert singer, at Albert Hall; Margaret and Cousin Mary were "indisposed." Margaret admitted, "No wonder my tummy gave out. Out of the eight nights from last Friday 'till the Friday before I had six dinners out and most of them were parties." She then listed their hosts from 19 to 26 March, "not to mention luncheons and teas … It was a bit too much for my inner workings." St. Andrews and Toronto had never been like this.

Attending the Oxford-Cambridge boat race was one of the "things to do." Standing on hogsheads near Hammersmith Bridge, Margaret and Charley cheered for Cambridge, who won. The Bests enjoyed visiting both universities but obviously had a preference for Cambridge, possibly because both of the senior researchers Charley worked with, Dale and A.V. Hill, were graduates.

At home in Hampstead after spending a few days in St. Albans, they watched the children sailing their boats on the Round Pond and played a set of tennis on the courts at the institute, with Margaret using her new Slazenger racquet. She never became an avid player, although she was anxious to please Charley by trying, as with golf and riding. The same day they went to the National Gallery to see the Dutch paintings, to the Isola Bella in Soho for dinner, and then to *Mr. Pepys*, a ballad opera,[305] at the Royalty Theatre. "The last act was a treat. It was a puppet show at Bartholomew Fair. The puppets sang a song, 'There was Catherine of Aragon — Pretty Ann Boleyn.' One puppet was Henry VIII, another Catherine Parr, and the third an astrologer. The dancing master sang a good song, 'I Do What I Can.'"

Margaret and Charley went on Easter Sunday to Westminster Abbey, and later, walked up Whitehall to Downing Street to see no. 10, "an unpretentious house in a row of houses — no sign of Premier Baldwin hovering about." They walked by Buckingham Palace, through Green Park to Piccadilly, and had lunch at the Criterion. Later in the day they had tea with the Dales.

The General Strike started on 3 May 1926 and lasted for nine days. Unemployment had soared when exports plummeted after Britain put sterling back on the gold standard at a pre-war rate. Over one and a half million workers in transport, electricity, printing, steel, and other industries went out on strike. For five days, Margaret worked at Finchly in an office registering volunteers for essential services. Charley was a special constable on point duty at Golders Green. He kept his whistle, stamped No. 40508, Metropolitan Police, made by J. Hudson & Co., 244 Barr Street, Birmingham. He was also assigned a billy to protect a march of protesters and prevent a clash between opposing groups. Margaret kept copies of the *British Gazette* for 12 and 13 May. This was the newspaper hurriedly created by the Baldwin government and sold for one penny. It not only gave news of the situation at home but quoted the comments of papers in Toronto, Montréal, and elsewhere.

In late May, Charley spoke to the Royal Society on "The Action of Insulin." Sir Ernest Rutherford, the Nobel Prize-winning physicist, was president at that time, and Henry Dale, secretary. Sir Walter Fletcher, secretary of the Medical Research Council and chairman of the NIMR, was also present. Best had four articles, all on insulin, published in the *Proceedings of the Royal Society of London* in 1926 — one of his own, the others with Dale, Hoet, and H.P. Marks as collaborators.

Fred Banting wrote to Charley giving family news. "I have just come back to the lab. After dinner, Marion and I went over to see your mother and father at Hilda's. Your mother looks well and your dad is even younger than the last time I saw him. He was down to see the old Y.M.C.A. lab the day before yesterday, and is coming down to spend the morning with me tomorrow."[306] Banting also mentioned that damaged equipment had arrived from London. Banting complained of other administrative headaches as well; "Next week I have to go to Ottawa as I'm up for fellowship in the Canadian Royal Society. I hope you will be up for fellowship next year or soon. The 25th of this month, Marion, Miss Gairns and I leave for Alaska — where we expect to spend two or three weeks and then go to Victoria to the Canadian Medical Association. The new Public Health Building is almost ready for roofing. It looks great. Fitz is as pleased as 'Punch' and wears a smile not unlike the historic gentleman. I must get to work, Charlie, As ever, Fred." Banting drew a cartoon of a smiling Dr. FitzGerald.

Charley's father-in-law, A.W. Mahon, also wrote giving family news. He and Emma were alone, as Flora, suffering from a persistent cough, was in Winnipeg where her sister Linda was forcing her to rest. A.W. had been reading a biography of a man who had had two serious nervous breakdowns. "He became greatly depressed, couldn't do anything, didn't want to see anybody. This lasted for a year or two and then he suddenly recovered. He said it was like raising a window-shade and letting the light in. ... Hilda tells me that it is descriptive of your dear mother's case. It would have done you a world of good to have seen your mother when she was here, she was so bright and deeply interested in everything." A.W. went on to say that Emma would tell them all about Clark and Edith Nobel's wedding.[307]

Best had requested a six-month extension of his Rockefeller grant and permission to go to Glasgow and Edinburgh to see scientists in universities there. In January of 1926, the Rockefeller office in Paris granted permission for the trip north, but this had to be delayed because of the General Strike. Later Charley recalled, "I really wanted to drive a bus — I applied to drive a bus but they said, 'You're a big fellow, we'll make you a policeman.'" He added, "My life was in danger constantly because the Cambridge undergraduates were driving the trams."[308]

They planned to spend part of the summer at the University of Freiburg for research, attend the International Physiological Congress in Stockholm, and visit labs in Copenhagen. The precise nature of the work done in Freiburg is not known, but the decision to go there was likely motivated by the fact that both Dale and FitzGerald had done work there. The latter had been a research student in bacteriology with Professor Ludwig Aschoff for several months in 1911. Preparing for the Continent, they gave up the flat in Hampstead and put all the items they would not be needing in two large wooden boxes. The meticulous landlord, inspecting the flat when they vacated, was surprised that they had had very few breakages of china.

On 25 May, Margaret and Charley left Liverpool station in London for their second visit to the Continent, sailing on the *Archangel* from Harwich for the Hook of Holland, near Rotterdam. The train left for Freiburg at seven o'clock on the morning of 26 May. They saw lots of windmills and men working in the fields wearing wooden shoes. They went through Rotterdam, Garda, Utrecht, Ede, and Arnhem and reached the German border.

Margaret wrote, "I do not remember the name of the place where we crossed the border,[309] but I will never forget our difficulties and our fear that we were going to be sent back because our passports had no special visa." A fellow traveller, a Scot named Murray who spoke fluent German, intervened. He had recognized the name Best and explained to the official that this was a famous scientist who was doing great work for people and that it would be a serious matter to hold him up. A customs man spoke to Best in German and was answered in English. A senior official said, "When I am in England, I have to speak English. When you are in Germany, you must speak

German." The same Mr. Murray came to the rescue, and the Bests' luggage was not opened. At Freiburg, Dr. H.B. van Dyke, an American endocrinologist studying at the university, met them at the station. At the beginning, Margaret did not think that she was going to like Freiburg or their hotel, the Minerva. They were both sick for several days, and it rained all the time, but things improved. Their room was comfortable, with a nice little balcony and wisteria vines, and they could see the Schlossberg Mountain from their window. They ate their meals on a terrace under a big chestnut tree. The owners of the hotel were pleasant — the "Her Ober" speaks "fine English." The spire of the red sandstone Munster dominated the town, with the market in its shadow. A religious procession wound for hours through the streets with children of all ages and church dignitaries in their robes — "the highest mucky-muck under a canopy."

Duelling bothered Margaret: "You see good looking chaps on the street with ugly scars on their faces. We are told they are very proud of their scars and try to keep wounds open so as to have more pronounced scars. I think it is dreadful! The nicest pictures in the photographers' windows are of university boys in their uniforms, with scars on their faces!" The Bests spent a lot of time walking in the region of Freiburg, enjoying the views and stopping at the beer gardens to drink Munchener Dunkel (dark) beer.

At the large State Opera House in Freiburg, the Bests enjoyed Wagner's *Das Rhinegold*,[310] *Parsifal*,[311] and *Die Walküre*, and Saint-Saëns's *Samson und Dalila*.[312] Margaret asked Cousin Mary to send two books in English on opera from London, which helped them understand what they heard.

Members of the university faculty invited the visitors for dinner, including Professor Paul Trendelenburg, director of the pharmacological institute. Also studying in Frieburg were Dave and Eleanor Pratt. Dave had won the Ellen Mickle Prize the year after Charley. The seventeen-year-old son of another faculty member, Dr. Naether, left an uneasy impression, as he was "very military — clicking of heels and low bows."

Each day the Bests, especially Charley, took a German lesson with Fraulein Waldkucher. Margaret kept a book of forty-six pages of notes on her lessons: *Guten tag, Guten morgen, Guten abend, Das ist sehr weit von hier.* She rarely had a chance to use German afterwards. At the last lesson, Margaret took the teacher a bunch of sweetpeas with baby's breath. Waldkucher said to Margaret that she was a flower herself. Margaret did not understand, and to Charley's amusement, said "Ja! Ja!" Dr. Franz Knoop, professor of biochemistry, and his wife also entertained them, offering "home-cooked apricots and red currants and different sorts of cakes and much wine."

Dr. Naether accompanied them on a trip to Basle, an hour and a half by train, from Freiburg, with the Black Forest on the left and the Rhine on the right. The fields had wild flaming poppies and enormous cherry trees. The Holbein pictures in the museum in Basle very much impressed them. The men went to the university while Margaret looked in the shops.

As they prepared to leave Freiburg, the Bests made the rounds to thank their new friends. The staff of the Minerva lined up in the hall to say farewell. Herr Schaupperle asked when they would be back, and when Charley said perhaps in two years, he replied, "Perhaps you will bring with you something small."

Charley had had a good few weeks with Drs. Trendelenburg and Knoop. Though he did little research in Freiburg, the time spent was no doubt a valuable experience for Best, meeting new scientists, and seeing how work was done differently on the Continent.

From Freiburg, the Canadians went to Heidelburg and Mannheim, where Charley wanted to see Dr. Ernst J. Lesser, who had been working on the action of insulin. In Frankfurt, Charley saw Professor Gustav Embden, an expert in cellular metabolism.

At the International Physiological Congress in Stockholm in August, the Bests realized that they were beginning to know more scientists. They had met some in Canada, the United States, London, Germany, and Belgium. One new friend was Dr. Richard de Bodo, a Hungarian who had been working with Starling in London. De Bodo later moved to the United States and worked at New York University on the action of insulin in relation to other substances.

The great social event of the congress was the banquet in the Gold Room of the City Hall. "We wore our best garments and had a scrumptious time. I was in my mauve chiffon dress that I got in Paris last winter and my silver shoes." She and Charley were several tables apart, "but we both had a fine time." Her place card read "Madame Best," but her neighbour introduced her to others as *Mademoiselle* Best since she seemed too young to be the wife of Dr. Best who, he assumed, would be much older. He asked if her *father* was with her and she replied she was not with her father but with her husband. When she pointed out her husband, her neighbour couldn't believe that this young man of twenty-seven was the co-discoverer of insulin.

111

Dancing followed in the Blue Room, "not blue at all, but a dull red brick." Margaret danced with several delegates, including Drs. Ulf von Euler and Yngve Zotterman of Stockholm and Dr. Robin Lawrence of London, a severe diabetic as well as a diabetic specialist on Harley Street. Diagnosed as diabetic in 1921, he had decided to face illness and death alone in a distant place. Word of insulin reached him in Venice, and he headed back to England immediately. Robin and his wife Anna were to become lifelong friends of the Bests. "The banquet was an eminently successful affair. We were all quite thrilled by it."

The Skansen open-air museum and park in Stockholm offered entertainment and restaurants. About twenty delegates went by boat to Saltsjöbaden, a favourite resort, and had dinner there, including Dr. and Mrs. Sohan Sal Bhatia of Bombay. He had won the Military Cross in the First World War and received his MB from Cambridge. "Mrs. Bhatia was quite a sensation at the Congress — only twenty-one and good looking, and wearing her striking native costumes of silk, peach coloured and flame coloured, and many others. He is about thirty-five, a tall and handsome man."

The Bests learned Swedish drinking customs — when to say "Skol" and when a speech is expected. "We all wrote our names on postcards and 'skolled' at a great rate." Dr. Gunnar Ahlgren was very particular and told Margaret that she should not take a drink until everyone did. Margaret danced all evening. A young physiologist, Dr. Wilhelm Raab of Prague, introduced himself. He asked Margaret to dance but then said that he could not dance. "I am afraid this is not a fox trot," he said, "I can only fox trot." He then confided that he had bought a book and practised in the evening to gramophone music. As one delegate noted, it was a "dancing congress."

The final meeting was at the University of Uppsala, home of Linnaeus, the naturalist. It was decided that the next congress should be held in Boston in 1929. From Stockholm, the Bests and Joseph Hoet left for Oslo, stopping along the way at Kil, which they christened the Swedish Pembroke, due to its similarity to Pembroke, Maine, where Charley was born. Writing to her uncle Bruce Macleod, Margaret observed, "Sweden is most like Canada."

Copenhagen was the next major stop. Best spent time in several Danish labs, including one directed by August Krogh, the Nobel laureate, whom he had met briefly in Toronto in 1922. Best worked with Professor Johannes Lindhard, who worked closely with Krogh. Lindhard was the expert on the physiology of muscular exercise. He worked on oxygen consumption of people doing various activities, like swimming across the Oresund.

While they were travelling on the continent, Henry Dale wrote a glowing letter to J.J.R. Macleod about the young Canadian: "Best has now left me, and gone to Freiburg for the summer. It was a great joy to have him here. We have never had anybody in the Department who was more generally popular, or who worked more consistently, modestly, quietly and unselfishly. I wish we could have kept him for good. I am quite sure that he is going to be a big man, and one of splendid influence in Toronto. We have practically given up worrying about liver extract, as such. I am very glad, however, that Best brought that particular investigation with him, as it reawakened interest and enterprise here, with regard to the chemical nature of depressor substances of tissues in general."[313]

That autumn, Best gave a series of lectures at the University of London. Margaret put the poster in her scrapbook: "Advanced lectures in Physiology, a course of four lectures on 'Insulin' will be given at University College, London, by Dr. C.H. Best, at 5 p.m. on Wednesdays, November 3rd, 10th, 17th, and 24th, 1926. The lectures are addressed to students of the university and to others interested in the subject. Admission free, without ticket." Best was now completing his fourth term as a DSc (Doctor of Science) candidate.

On 10 December 1926, after a splendid eighteen months of wonderful new experiences and meeting many interesting people, the Bests sailed from Liverpool for Saint John, New Brunswick, on the Canadian Pacific Steamship *Montnairn*. In Toronto, there was great excitement as the family gathered for Christmas.

On 26 January 1927, Best wrote to Dr. Clifford W. Wells, the fellowship adviser of the Rockefeller Foundation, expressing his "great appreciation and gratitude to the Council of the International Health Board for my appointment and to the executive officers for their courtesy and helpfulness and in particular to Mr. Gunn of the Paris office with whom I was constantly in touch."

He reported on his activities in London, in Scotland, and on the Continent, giving details of work that he did with Henry Dale, Harold Dudley, A.V. Hill, Joseph Hoet, H.P. Marks, and others:

> Our first researches were on the nature of the depressor substances present in certain liver extracts. These extracts

113

had been used in the treatment of hypertension. More recent clinical investigation has shown that the therapeutic properties of the extract were greatly overestimated, but our physiological studies were rewarded by the identification of histamine and choline. Subsequent investigators demonstrated the presence of histamine in normal tissue in much greater amounts than had hitherto been supposed. The results of these investigations are in press and will appear in an early number of the *Journal of Physiology* …

Although he enjoyed visiting a number of labs, "time is certainly more profitably spent, however, when one is able to do some active research. For this reason, my time spent with Dr. Dale was the high point of the extremely interesting and instructive eighteen months as a fellow of the International Health Board."[314]

While he was overseas, Best had been in contact with Professor FitzGerald about arrangements for the new Department of Physiological Hygiene at the University of Toronto, which Best, at age twenty-eight, was to head. Sir William Mulock, now also Chancellor of the university (in addition to being Chief Justice of Ontario), had laid the cornerstone of the School of Hygiene on 20 January 1926. Sir George Newman, a distinguished public health scientist from London and chief medical officer of Britain's Ministry of Health, opened the building in June 1927.

Amongst his first tasks as head of the department, Best gave lectures to doctors working on graduate diplomas in public health on ventilation, muscular exercise, ultraviolet light, and the effect on health of increased and diminished atmospheric pressure. Initially, his department consisted of himself as an assistant professor, and three research assistants, Jessie Ridout, Ruth Partridge, and E.W. McHenry. Then Dr. David Scott, also an early associate, moved to the new building. Best had arranged to bring a technician from England, William Parkinson, a brother of A.V. Hill's head technician. It was at this time in 1927 that Emma Linda Mahon, Margaret's younger sister, who now insisted on being called Linda, started working for Charley. The production of insulin, which had started in the basement of the Medical Building in 1922, and in the old Y.M.C.A. building, was moved to the Connaught Laboratories in the new School of Hygiene building in 1927.

Margaret and Charley were looking for a home. By spring, they were installed at 226 Rosedale Heights Drive in Moore Park, near several friends, the Van Wycks, the Lows, and the Janes. On 24 May 1927, they had a housewarming. Margaret wrote, "A first house must always be exciting for a young couple." They had learned much about furniture during their stay in England and now bought an old Scottish dining room table and a sideboard made in Tunbridge Wells, England. An old Yorkshireman who worked in a building off Yonge Street made dining room chairs of mahogany in a Chippendale pattern. It was a comfortable home, with plenty of space. They paid $12,000, $9,000 of which was Charley's half of Fred Banting's share of the Nobel Prize money. A.V. Hill was the Bests' first house guest on Rosedale Heights. He donned "running costumes" each morning before breakfast and ran through the streets, followed by small boys on bicycles.[315]

In the summer of 1927, Margaret and Charley took the elder Mahons and Linda to Maine, driving along the St. Lawrence. Herbert Best had three horses available, and Charley was delighted to be able to ride again. Judge William Cockburn and several of his family came from St. Stephen. The Bests had a supper party at the cottage at Leighton's Point, and the photos taken are the only ones to show both the Best and Mahon parents together. Margaret remarked on "the more mature ladies in ankle-length skirts and cloche hats." From Pembroke, the travellers drove to Boston, stopping at North-East Harbour on Mt. Desert Island to have lunch with Dr. and Mrs. George R. Minot. Minot, a severe diabetic, collaborated with George H. Whipple and William P. Murphy in the discovery of the liver treatment for pernicious anaemia. Proud of Minot's achievement, Best nominated him and Whipple for the Nobel prize, which they shared with Murphy in 1934.[316]

Margaret's brother Henry Mahon and his wife Lydia were their hosts in Boston. On 5 October 1927, Dr. Philemon Truesdale wrote to Charles Best inviting him, on behalf of the Alumni Association of Harvard Medical School, to be its guest at the dedication of Vanderbilt Hall, the new students' dormitory. It was modelled on Hart House at the University of Toronto, about which Best had spoken in Boston in 1923. It was "a monumental work achieved mainly through the untiring efforts of Doctor Elliott P. Joslin."[317] About this time, Joslin wrote to Best to say that a common room in Vanderbilt Hall was to be named for him. He also said that he had had a lantern slide made of a photo of the Bests with a pony at the Joslins' farm at Oxford, which he showed to students at the University of Pennsylvania. They "enjoyed seeing the girl who was bright enough to make a diagnosis and fall in love with you before you discovered insulin."[318]

The dedication of the Charles Herbert Best Room in Vanderbilt Hall took place on 14 October 1927. Present were the chief donor, Harold S. Vanderbilt of the great railway family, and Dr. George Vincent, president of the Rockefeller Foundation. In November, the president and fellows of Harvard College sent a formal letter to Banting and Best, thanking them for the donation of a leaf from their original laboratory notebook to the Medical Library. It was page forty-seven, recording the progress of dog no. 408 from depancreatization to its death from infection.[319]

After the winter in Toronto, Best wanted to finish his DSc at the University of London and he had a number of other projects in mind. He and Margaret, therefore, left Toronto for Boston on 22 March 1928, en route to Britain.

The travellers settled into their cabin aboard the SS *Celtic*, bound for Liverpool. Lord and Lady Elphinstone[320] were very agreeable companions; she was "the sweetest thing" and they twice invited them to their home, "Carberry Tower," near Edinburgh. "She wore lovely soft, powder blue clothes or sand — very sweet and simple, and scarcely any jewellery." An elderly man named Bonser from Nottingham wrote later to Best that he recalled with pleasure "your cheerful refreshing countenance and the handsome personality of your dear spouse." He added, "In the name of our common humanity and in that of the survival of the fittest it is up to you both to see that the name of Best shall not die out."

Arriving in Liverpool on 2 April, Margaret and Charley went to London and settled in at the Kingsley Hotel at 36 Hart Street in Bloomsbury Square where they stayed for a week. By 9 April, they were installed at the Rosslyn Lodge Hotel in Hampstead. They had seen Henry and Nellie Dale, Charles and Laura Lovatt Evans, and Harold and Mary Dudley. Cousin Mary Scott, who had travelled with them to the Continent in 1925, was now working in London, and the Bests were to see a lot of her.

Best had been made a temporary member of the Athenaeum Club, put up by Dr. Ernest William Brown of Oxford, FRS, a famous astronomer, and seconded by Sir Richard Gregory, also a well-known astronomer and the editor of *Nature,* who had made that review "a great, international institution."[321] Best enjoyed its facilities. There were more invitations than they could accept.

The Harvey Tercentenary was being celebrated in London that year in scientific circles. William Harvey's *De motu cordis* (On the Motion of the Heart and the Blood in Animals), describing the circulation of the blood, had first appeared in 1628. It was "an enormous week." Dr. R.D. Rudolf, professor of therapeutics at the University of Toronto, was the official Canadian delegate, but Sir John Rose Bradford, the president of the Royal College of Physicians, invited the Bests to all the functions.

Margaret went with a group of women to Lord Ellesmere's home, Bridgewater House, beside St. James' Palace and overlooking Green Park, which had Britain's finest private collection of pictures, including Raphaels, Titians, and Rembrandts. Miss Barlow, sister of Sir Thomas Barlow, the eighty-two-year-old past president of the Royal College of Physicians, invited Margaret to the Albemarle Club on Dover Street for dinner that evening, along with twenty other women from various countries. Margaret especially liked Mrs. Olaf Thomsen, wife of a pharmacologist who was dean of medicine in Copenhagen; they had recently lost a small boy, and Margaret was very sympathetic. After dinner, the party went to Lady Rose Bradford's at 8 Manchester Square, across from the Wallace Collection. Nellie Dale, Laura Lovatt Evans, and Margaret Hill were there as well. The men came from their dinner at the Grocers' Hall. Sir John Rose Bradford "was tall and very nice." Dr. William Arthur Winter, from Dublin, president of the Royal College of Physicians of Ireland, was full of admiration for Charles Best and told Margaret that "he thought the girls must have scratched my eyes out when I got Charley. He didn't know which of us was the proudest of the other." That evening the Bests met Dr. Otto Loewi from Graz, Austria, a future Nobel laureate whom they got to know well later.

The delegates went one evening to the Merchant Tailors Hall on Threadneedle Street. The Bradfords received, and the Prince of Wales attended, "looking very strained at first, but very young yet." Dr. Naether of Freiburg was there. Dr. and Mrs. Jan Van der Hoeve of Leyden made a good impression, as did Dr. Gøran Liljestrand and his wife of Stockholm. He was secretary of the Nobel Prize committee for physiology and medicine for an amazing forty-two years, from 1918 to 1960. Dr. Geoffrey Keynes was there — a surgeon, literary executor of the poet Rupert Brooke, and brother of the economist as well as of Margaret Hill, A.V.'s wife. "We wandered all about and had very delicious refreshments."

A film was shown about the work of William Harvey, which was a great success. Raymond Crawford, registrar of the Royal College of Physicians, wrote later to Best that it was available for £46-12-6, and was bought by the University of Toronto. The film proved most popular in Canada, and Best loaned it to a number of Canadian and American institutions.

The next scientific gathering was of the Physiological Society at Cambridge. A group of scientists and spouses travelled by charabanc on 17 May from Golders Green in London. At Downing College for lunch, Margaret and Charley met Professor Edward Mellanby and his wife May, both well-known researchers. Professor Mellanby was at the time professor of pharmacology at Sheffield. They also saw Keith Cannan, then a lecturer in biochemistry at London, and Dr. Alan Drury, the Cambridge physiologist who was later director of the Lister Institute. The Bests found the service and the music of the five o'clock service at King's College Chapel very moving. The service was followed by dinner in Trinity College, where they shared a table with A.V. Hill, Charles and Laura Lovatt Evans, Albert Szent-Györgyi, the Hungarian-born American biochemist who had just discovered vitamin C, and his wife, Nellie, and Harold and Hilda Channon. Harold Channon was involved in cancer research at the University of Leeds.

Charley's sister, Hilda, and her husband, Ralph Salter, arrived on the new *Duchess of Bedford* on 22 June 1928 and stayed in London at the Hotel Victoria. The four had dinner at Au Petit Savoyard in Soho and went to the Olympia to the Horse Show. The brothers-in-law rented a Wolseley for £45 per month. Charley took Ralph to the Athenaeum for lunch, while Margaret took Hilda to Swan and Edgar's department store.

When Linda Mahon arrived in London a few days later, Margaret did not want her to miss anything. The first day, they saw Trafalgar Square, made a brief visit to the National Gallery, did a little shopping, and visited some of the Bests' London friends. Later, the five dressed for dinner, which they had at home, so that Margaret could show off her culinary skills. The party went to the Drury Lane Theatre to see *Show Boat,* with Edith Day as "Magnolia" and Paul Robeson as "Joe," singing "Ol' Man River." Afterwards, they went to the Cecil for dancing and coffee. It was quite an initiation to London for Linda.

Charles Best's interest in the physiological changes that took place with the exertions of competitors in international track meets, particularly sprinters, started with work he did with A.V. Hill at the University of London and then with Johannes Lindhard in Copenhagen. This led him to seek permission to do a number of tests at the 1928 Olympic Games in Amsterdam. Charley, Margaret, and Linda stayed in a house very near the stadium where he was to carry out a number of tests on runners. Free passes let them into the stadium for each day, with seats in the front row at the finish line. They saw the Englishman David Cecil (Lord Burghley) win the 400-metre hurdles, and Percy Williams of Vancouver take the 100-metre dash, then the 200-metre. They went to the Holland Hotel where the athletes were staying and talked to several of them. Another day, they saw Douglas Lowe of Cambridge win the finals of the 800-metre flat race. Margaret noted that he was "such a good-looking chap." In the women's 100-metre dash, Bobbie "Fanny" Rosenfeld of Toronto came second to Elizabeth Robinson of the United States.

They all spent a good deal of time at the Games, although the weather was "dreadful" and the track "pretty rotten." The 3,000-metre steeplechase saw the Finns excel with Toivo Loukola winning. One evening, a group of scientists went on a boat trip through the canals and out into the harbour. The Bests sat with Dr. and Mrs. S. van Creveld of Holland (he was the first Dutch diabetic to use insulin.) The lights on towers and bridges in honour of the Olympic visitors were particularly fine.

On Sunday, 5 August, Canada won the 400-metre relay race for women, with Fanny Rosenfeld and Myrtle Cook[322] posting the best times. Ethel Catherwood of Canada won the high jump. Margaret wrote, "The Catherwood girl is very pretty and very self-possessed. When she came to sit with the other Canadians, she made for Williams and threw her arms around his neck and kissed him." The girls' team finished first overall for the Games. This was Charles Best's big day when he did tests on the marathoners. He completed his tests not long before midnight. Best carried on the work after he returned to Toronto and summarized the results in a paper that he wrote with Ruth C. Partridge for the *Proceedings of the Royal Society* for 1929, reproduced in *Selected Papers of Charles H. Best.*[323] One photograph from 1929 shows Best doing the 100-yard dash on the indoor track at Hart House at the University of Toronto. Another is of Dr. FitzGerald, Dr. E.W. McHenry, Best, and Dr. Neil McKinnon in running togs.

The Mahon sisters made a young autograph hunter happy by signing a book that he held out and writing "Olympiad's 1928." Linda wrote, "We left the small boy becoming quite assured he'd picked on two first-class champions."[324]

At the Olympic pool, the visitors saw races and a water polo game between Hungary and France, and they particularly enjoyed the diving. A lovely Delft tile with the Olympic flame and garlands reading simply "IXe Olympiade Amsterdam 1928" is still in the family.[325]

On they went to Berlin where a Dutchman came to the hotel to consult with Charley about his diabetic son, who was in Saskatoon, Saskatchewan. More and more frequently, people who had a diabetic in their family or who just wanted to talk to someone whose advice they respected contacted Best. He enjoyed this confidence, in the case of diabetics referring people to a clinician he respected and always turning down offers to pay for his counsel. Many did not understand that he did not have a licence to practice medicine and therefore could not accept fees. This was a conscious decision. As a scientist he felt that accepting fees from diabetics would compromise his position.

Charley and Margaret came back from Britain earlier than expected. J.J.R. Macleod was returning to Aberdeen, and FitzGerald, as head of the Department of Hygiene and Preventive Medicine, had written to Charley that they wanted him to take some lectures in the Department of Physiology.[326]

Macleod's health had been deteriorating with the advance of arthritis. The atmosphere in Toronto was not a happy one for him; friends of Fred Banting's resented what they saw as his intrusion into "their man's" fame. There is no record of friction with Best, but then Charley was away in Europe. As early as March 1928, Henry Dale in London had been in touch with Andrew Hunter, head of biochemistry in Toronto, about the situation there. On 21 April, Dale wrote, "I heard from Macleod of his application to Aberdeen, but found, when Best arrived here, that the latter had not heard of it at Toronto, so that Macleod could not have spoken widely of his intention to move." He proceeded directly to the point:

> I realise that [Best] is young and relatively inexperienced; but I have been watching with interest his rapid ripening during the last year or two. I have the greatest confidence that ultimately he will take high rank in medical science, and his natural bent seems to be toward Physiology. Circumstances have, of course, made his training up to the present an intense rather than a wide one. Under present conditions of Physiology, however, you will almost be bound to take a man who is something of a specialist in some direction, if he is to be any good at all. It may quite

120

well be that such a promotion of a local man, perhaps over
the heads of some who have been his teachers, might cause
personal difficulties which the University would not like to
face; but, speaking as an outsider, independent except as
regards a really good opportunity of judging Best's quality
and potentialities in comparison with those of men of this
own standing in this country, that is what I should do.[327]

Ten days later Dale wrote to Macleod, still in Toronto, expressing his
pleasure that the Scot was returning to Britain. Apparently, both Macleod
and university president Sir Robert Falconer had asked Dale's opinion on
how to find a replacement. He replied carefully, "I quite realise that my
particular suggestion may be inappropriate, from the local point of view,
in one way or another," but proceeded with a strong argument in favour
of his Canadian student, reiterating his points to Andrew Hunter:

[Best's] very real modesty made him inclined at the out-
set to put himself almost too much in the position of a
learner; but it has been both interesting and delightful to
see him get more certain of himself, and claim independence of thought and judgment, without losing a shade of
his modesty and self-criticism. Seeing him now again,
after an interval, one cannot miss the stride which he has
made since he left Europe more than a year ago. I find
him now prepared to stand up to A.V. Hill and to myself,
to each on the ground of one of our particular interests,
and to hold his own with quiet confidence in his own
facts and judgment, but without a trace of undue self-
assurance. He made the best kind of impression in
Germany, in the different centres which he visited; and I
feel more certain of his future than of that of almost any
other young man in Physiology at the present time.[328]

On 5 May, Oskar Klotz, professor of pathology and bacteriology at
the University of Toronto, wrote from London, "Best has in his favor a
well-trained mind, an attractive personality, an enthusiasm for work,
and initiative. Moreover he also has youth in his favor, with good
health. Best is in the midst of his productive period, and I fear he would

suffer the burden of administrative responsibilities if he was to assume a professorship."[329]

In June, Professor FitzGerald wrote to Best that a "committee, consisting of the President, Dean Primrose, Professors Macleod, Hunter, Henderson, Graham, Klotz, FitzGerald, and Dr. George S. Young[330] was constituted by the President to consider the question of a successor to Professor Macleod." The committee suggested that, instead of recommending a successor to Professor Macleod, during the academic year of 1928–29 the duties in the Department of Physiology be carried out by the members of that department with the assistance of Best, if he agreed to co-operate. FitzGerald said:

> I took the liberty of agreeing on your behalf (though, of course, this does not bind you in any way) to the proposal that, in your present capacity, you would assist in the work of the Department of Physiology during next year. Dr. Macleod is to go over the programme of work for next year with Professors Irving and Taylor and later with you, if assuming, of course, that you will be willing to co-operate. … The President requested and I agreed to arrange the work in such a way in the School of Hygiene and Connaught Laboratories that you would be free to give from one third to one half your time, if necessary, to the voluntary duties which you would assume in the Department of Physiology.[331]

This meant that Best would have to return to Toronto earlier than expected in September since he would need to spend a week or ten days before the opening of the session on 25 September 1928 to discuss departmental matters with Irving and Taylor. "The suggestion which I have roughly outlined was made in the meeting this morning with only the President, Professor Macleod, Prof. D. Graham and myself present, the others originally present having left."[332]

Best replied to FitzGerald agreeing to his proposal saying that he was willing to help in any way he could with the teaching of physiology during the next academic year.

> If the suggestion had been made to me by any member
> of the committee, other than yourself, I would not have

felt inclined to take from one third to one half of my time from the development of Physiological Hygiene and the continuation of productive research to apply it to teaching in a department with which I have no connection. I realize, however, that there are circumstances which make it seem advisable to you that I should do this.[333]

In a letter to President Falconer, Macleod said that he had discussed the running of his department after his departure with Irving and Taylor, and would do the same with Best when he saw him in Scotland. The proposal was for Best to give eight lectures on respiration to third-year medical students, and seven lectures on physiology in the nineteenth century in the history of physiology option; he would give the introductory lectures to the second-year students; one lecture in applied physiology to the sixth-year students; and, some laboratory work on respiratory chemistry to fourth-year B&M [Biological and Medical Sciences] students.[334]

Best wrote FitzGerald, "I am almost certain to see Professor Macleod somewhere in Scotland … If I see Prof. Macleod and find out in detail what teaching I will be expected to do I can make the necessary arrangements with Irving and Taylor by letter."[335]

Best also told FitzGerald that a notice of his DSc from the University of London had appeared in the papers. "I am very pleased to have finished with it. Leathes, Dale and Hill were the examiners. They are a critical trio so I have the satisfaction of knowing that the degree was well earned."[336] Examiner John Beresford Leathes was in his early sixties. A graduate of Oxford in classics, he had studied medicine at Guy's Hospital in London. In 1909, he had been appointed to the new chair of pathological chemistry at Toronto, staying there until in 1914 he became professor of physiology at Sheffield where he served two terms as dean of medicine. His inclusion in the committee was possibly because of the Toronto connection. In 1925 and 1926, Best served four terms (three in the academic year 1925–6 and one in 1926–7) towards this degree; he received credit for a fifth term when he was back in Toronto in 1927, and then completed his sixth in London in 1928.

On 1 July, the Bests, the Salters, and Linda Mahon left for a three-week motor trip covering a lot of ground: the fen country, the Yorkshire dales, Durham, the Scottish border country, Edinburgh, Perth and Braemar, Aberdeen, and then back to London. On the way south, Charley

123

took his relatives to Kimmel Park in North Wales where ten years earlier, he had been stationed as a sergeant in the Canadian army.

Best wrote to FitzGerald from the Ullswater Hotel in Patterdale, in the Lake District, thanking him for the financial help from Connaught.

> I met Prof. Macleod in Aberdeen. It was rather amusing that I should be the first to greet him on his arrival. He came a day before he was expected and I found out from Prof. Clark [Professor of Materia Medica Alfred Clark] in Edinburgh that he was going to motor to Aberdeen. Prof. Macleod left word with Clark that he would be glad to see me at any time in Aberdeen. We had dinner together last Friday and spent the entire evening discussing the teaching program for physiology in Toronto. Prof. Macleod told me that the committee had decided to look around for another year for a suitable man. Irving, Taylor and I are to elect one of ourselves as chairman of the committee of three.
>
> I had a very nice letter from Irving. He offered to make any arrangements for me with regard to the teaching. I am going to write him soon. I am planning, of course, to give the lectures we planned in Physiological Hygiene to the medicals the first week of October.[337]

Best knew that support for his being appointed professor of physiology to succeed MacLeod was not strong because he was very young. FitzGerald, although he had agreed to the proposal for Best to assist in the department of physiology for the year 1928–29, really hoped that his protégé would succeed him as director of the School of Hygiene and the Connaught Laboratories.

In early September, Margaret took ill and was not able to get out until they left for Canada on the *Duchess of Bedford* on 21 September. Nellie Dale, with daughters Alison and Eleanor, came to the train to see them off to the boat. Margaret had to be very quiet. Don and Mary Fraser were on the *Bedford* with their children, Donnie and Nancy. Mr. and Mrs. Charles Michie of St. Andrew's Church in Toronto were also on board as well as Geoffrey Keynes and Sir Thomas Peel Dunhill, both consulting surgeons at St. Bartholomew's Hospital, London.

For Margaret and Charley, the time in London and on the Continent introduced them to a whole new world. Margaret attended lectures on art and made detailed notes in her diaries about her careful observations in many galleries in Britain and on the Continent. For all her study, Margaret could have earned a degree in art history. Her years in London and on the Continent formed a very solid base that served her well wherever she and Charley travelled. Her artistic judgment was very good and she and Charley eventually built up a good small collection of Canadian, American, and Australian works.

Though the time spent in Europe was generally a very positive time for both, it was not all rosy. Apparently at some point during their stay in London, Margaret had a miscarriage. A cat that had got into their flat jumped out at her, and the resultant fright was blamed. This may account for her lifelong dislike of the species. The Bests always had a dog.

Charley's reputation for his work on insulin had gained him supervision by two giants of physiology, A.V. Hill and Henry Dale. With them Best added to his reputation through his work on histamine. In particular, Dale and his wife put them in touch with many of the most fascinating minds in Europe. The Bests' trip to the International Physiological Congress in Stockholm in 1926 showed them, to their considerable surprise, how well known *they* had become. The total of twenty-four months that they spent in Europe in the years 1925–8 launched them on their lifelong roles as unofficial ambassadors for insulin, for medical research, and for Canada.

Chapter Four

The Best Years of Their Lives, 1928–1941

Arriving back in Toronto in late September 1928, after six months away, the Bests settled into the house they had bought the year before, 226 Rosedale Heights Drive, which Joe and Mary Gilchrist kept an eye on during their absence. Their two-stage stay in Britain and on the Continent had been very important for Charles Best: it took him away from the scene of the discovery of insulin and allowed him to research different problems and meet and work with many of the world's greatest medical scientists.

While Best was studying with Sir Henry Dale at the National Institute for Medical Research, his first researches were on the nature of the depressor substances present in certain liver extracts. These extracts had been used in the treatment of hypertension. More recent clinical investigation had shown that the therapeutic properties of the extracts were greatly overestimated, but the physiological studies were rewarded by the identification of histamine and choline. Histamine isolated from lung seemed to play a crucial part as a depressor agent to lower blood pressure. Best found that histamine in lung tissue rapidly disappeared. Continuing his research on histamine in Toronto in 1929 he thought that this disappearance was caused by the presence in the tissue of an enzyme "histaminase." Later it was understood that "the disappearance of histamine from lung tissue was not the result of the action of a single enzyme" but Best's "observations were the starting point of many important investigations by others."[338]

Within months of his return to Toronto, Best began the chemical research on the anticoagulant heparin that would help save millions of lives. He continued studying histamine and later, with colleagues at the University of Toronto, identified choline as the active constituent of the lecithin molecule, an essential nutrient in the body associated with blood pressure and fatty liver. His work on heparin and choline would lead to his nomination for a Nobel Prize.

His DSc from the University of London completed the unusual double qualifications of a medical and a research degree; he later encouraged those who came to work with him at the University of Toronto to do the same. He was always interested in the clinical application of all research work. He became professor of physiological hygiene (public health) and head of that department at the university in 1928; the next year he succeeded J.J.R. Macleod as professor and head of the department of physiology. He was thirty years old. Assistant director of the Connaught Laboratories since 1925, he became associate director in 1931.

Margaret began volume five of her diaries with their departure on 15 June 1929, by Canadian Pacific Railway (CPR), for their first visit to Vancouver, where Charley was to lecture at the Summer School of the Canadian Medical Association (CMA). Charley had attended many scientific meetings before, but now, in 1929, he was attending these meetings as *the professor.* This trip to the Canadian West was almost as much of a revelation and education to Margaret and Charley as their experiences in Britain and Europe had been. With their good looks, energy, and intelligence, Margaret and Charley were a charismatic and dynamic young couple. Always interested in people and new experiences, on entering a room they instantly became the focus of attention.[339] Wherever they went they were showered with invitations from friends and relations, professional colleagues, and acquaintances old and new.

The working holiday to Vancouver set a pattern for much of their travel during CHB's career, and Margaret kept a lively account in her diary. A magnificent sunset along the north shore of Lake Superior delighted them. They stopped at Winnipeg where Aunt Linda and Uncle Walter Scott greeted them along with their daughter, Kirk Scott Wright (younger sister of Cousin Mary Scott whom they had seen so much of in London), who was the same age as Margaret, and her husband, Tom Wright, a lawyer.

Twenty-four hours later, they boarded the train again. Margaret wrote, "At first, I was desperately disappointed with the Prairies. There were low trees, poplars, and it wasn't as flat as I expected," although the golf courses were "pathetically flat." "Calgary looked like a very nice place to live."[340] The winding Bow River came into view, and the snow-capped mountains in the distance. On the trip to Banff, Dr. William E. Gallie, the new professor of surgery at the University of Toronto, and his wife, Janet, and Mrs. Angela Bruce were fellow passengers. Mrs. Bruce was the wife of Herbert

A. Bruce, a surgeon and founder of the Wellesley Hospital in Toronto and, later, lieutenant governor of Ontario from 1932 to 1937.

"Banff was marvellous. The hotel is very fine, with a beautiful lounge and great plate glass windows that frame the view like gorgeous paintings." A glorious rainbow appeared across the Bow River. At Lake Louise little yellow and orange poppies were growing in "great masses." On the Yoho Valley Road, the driver and the bus were both on their maiden trip, and the very large vehicle seemed too big for the road. "It was rather exciting to back to the edge of the canyon and realize that an inch or two might be fatal." Mountain flowers included Indian paintbrush, Indian tea, wild roses, and yellow columbine.

The Bests rejoined their train at Golden for Vancouver, where Dr. Wilfred Graham, a fraternity brother of Charley's, met them. After leaving their bags at the Hotel Georgia, they went to the Grahams' home. George and Dorothy Sweny, friends from London (whom they had met on the SS *Montrose* in 1925), were early visitors. The Bests, the Grahams, and Lyall and Lottie Hodgins spent the weekend on Vancouver Island — Lyall was head of the Vancouver branch of the Connaught Labs. Butchart Gardens, near Duncan, appealed especially to Margaret — "Roses, peonies, iris and poppies and all were a glorious sight. The Canterbury bells, foxgloves and columbine were wonderful too!" The Empress Hotel in Victoria "reminded us of an English Hydro — with red-faced military men sitting about."

They took the midnight ferry to Vancouver, and Charley gave a series of four lectures to the CMA's Summer School. Margaret was impressed by the way Dot Sweny looked after her two-year-old daughter Anne; she had a picture from Venice in Anne's room: "Pictures in children's rooms are so often silly and insipid." Dorothy drove Margaret around the grounds of the University of British Columbia — "a beautiful site beside the water, they have very few buildings, but I daresay it will grow." Stanley Park had its totem poles and dug-out Indian canoes. All in all, Vancouver was "ideally situated and a very beautiful city."

From Vancouver, they took the Canadian National Railway (CNR) train to Jasper, enjoying the views of the mountains from the open observation car. For three days at the Jasper Park Lodge, they stayed in a cabin, went canoeing, and danced every evening. One afternoon, Margaret donned Charley's white golf trousers, and they went riding. "Charley made my horse race along beside his and it was great fun. Charley had a frisky little horse, a darling, and the guide didn't like Charley racing around on it. He wanted us all to get in a line and follow him."

The Gallies were also staying at Jasper on the trip back to Toronto. The Bests went to a rodeo and took along young Allan Gallie and his friend Pierre Wilson of Toronto. The boys had taken dancing lessons, and Margaret danced with both of them. She asked Allan if his father did not like dancing. He answered, "Of course, he would like it better if it were not for his corns." When Mrs. Gallie talked of riding, Allan said, "poor horse," and made an up-and-down motion with his hands. Margaret added, "His mother is marvellous. She pays no attention to a remark like that."

After another short stop in Winnipeg to see the Scott relatives, Margaret and Charley went on to Fort William where they took the CPR steamship *Keewatin* across Lake Superior through the locks at Sault Ste. Marie to Port McNicoll on Georgian Bay. Margaret said they were very much disappointed in the boat trip. "The weather was rotten, rain and fog, with the foghorn going all night. There were uninteresting people on board and I am afraid I expected something more like ocean travel. The food was not good either. Altogether, we wished we had come by train."

They had been away just over three weeks, combining scientific business with pleasure. They would repeat this formula in varying degrees many times. Margaret almost always went on these trips, and Charley was more apt to accept invitations when her expenses were included.

In early August, exams for the fellowship in Britain's Royal College of Surgeons (FRCS) took place in Toronto. Best and James Playfair McMurrich, professor of anatomy and dean of graduate studies, were the two local examiners. From London, England, came two physiologists, Professors Charles Lovatt Evans and John Mellanby of University College and St. Thomas's Hospital Medical School, and two anatomists, Dr. W.E. Le Gros Clark, also of St. Thomas's, and Dr. William Wright, professor and dean of graduate studies in the London Hospital Medical College.

The visitors all stayed at the newly opened Royal York Hotel. The Bests took them and their wives to York Downs on Bathurst Street to play golf and to have dinner. Margaret invited some of the English visitors to dinner; as she usually did, she recorded the menu: "Sherry cocktails in the living room, fruit cocktails of honeydew melon and cantaloupe made into round balls with lemon and a thick syrup, lamb with mint sauce, potatoes and green peas, then apple tart and a melon mould of Cole's ice cream (vanilla centre and green water ice) and cheese straws. The fruit course was big black cherries and coffee was served in the living room."

In mid-August, Margaret and Charley and Linda Mahon travelled with Charles Lovatt Evans to Boston for the XIIIth International Physiological Congress. Lovatt Evans stayed in Vanderbilt Hall, as were many European delegates, the Bests and Linda, with Henry and Lydia Mahon. The first evening, Charley went looking for his Belgian friend Joseph Hoet and brought him back to the Mahons. They saw Drs. H.B. van Dyke, Gustav Embden, and Franz Knoop, whom they had met in Freiburg. Other delegates included Dr. Wilhelm Raab of Prague, who had danced with Margaret in Stockholm in 1926. Professor G. Mansfeld of Budapest, an "old, bold chap who kissed very hard, told Charley that he remembered me as the most beautiful woman at the Stockholm Congress." Margaret went to hear Charley's paper on histamine and complained that the ten minutes that he was allotted was not long enough — a chronic problem for all congresses.

While in Boston, Henry, Lydia, Linda, and Margaret went to Margaret's first "talkie" — *The Last of Mrs. Cheyney*, starring Montréal-born Oscar winner Norma Shearer. Margaret, who thought the film was good, had seen the play in London with Gladys Cooper and Sir Gerald du Maurier.

A telegram from their old friend Dr. Joe Gilchrist in Toronto informed them that A.W. Mahon had had a heart attack, but he was recovering. Nonetheless, they left Boston that afternoon and drove 181 miles to Albany, New York; the next morning, they departed at nine o'clock and drove the 400 miles to Toronto, arriving at midnight. They found A.W. to be doing very well. "Joe handed the case over to Charley at once." Earlier in the summer, Charley's mother, Lulu Best, had been in Toronto for the arrival of her daughter Hilda's first baby, Charles Ralph Best Salter, born 19 July 1929. Charley spent the day with his sister who, he said, "was very brilliant under the anaesthetic" — whatever that meant.

Some of the physiologists and their spouses who'd been in Boston followed the Bests to Toronto as planned. Charley went to Niagara to meet them, and they all came across Lake Ontario by boat. Margaret, who was not well, missed a garden party for the visitors at Connaught Farms, a big dinner at Hart House, and a luncheon at the Canadian National Exhibition. On 3 September 1929, the guests went on to Montréal by boat. It was Margaret and Charley's fifth wedding anniversary and he "gave me a gorgeous present, a combination radio and Victrola, electric!"

Best was busy both at the School of Hygiene and with the department of physiology. As an undergraduate in 1920 he first became interested in anticoagulants when doing research on turtles where he and Clark Noble had problems with blood clotting in their experiments. In Sir Henry Dale's lab at the NIMR in 1928 Best's assays on histamine and choline were complicated by blood clots. This problem rekindled his interest in anticoagulants. In 1929 Best launched research into the purification of the anticoagulant heparin, which had been discovered by Jay McLean in 1916 at Johns Hopkins University.

Also after his return to Toronto in September 1928, Best continued the work on histamine with Dr. E.W. McHenry. They were eager to use an effective anticoagulant with their "histaminase" work. No preparation was safe for clinical work and none was being used. Laurie Chute recalled a dramatic incident in 1929 when Best was demonstrating the effects of histamine. The labels had been accidentally switched and he got a dose of histamine some ten times larger than anticipated. "He naturally showed all the signs of sudden, acute, hypotension and shock which ... disturbed the class very greatly and myself in particular as I had been the one to administer the intravenous injection." Chute was impressed at the extent of Best's scientific interest by refusing to have any adrenalin or other counteracting material administered since he said nobody else would ever probably take a similar dose again and he wanted to be able to record the reactions.[341]

In the autumn of 1929, Margaret started to pickle and preserve — something she did regularly for more than thirty years. She bottled plums, crabapples, chili sauce, uncooked pickles, and so on, and family members still use her recipes. The uncooked pickles were the most unusual of all the recipes, given to her by Elizabeth Simpson. Margaret prepared a mustard sauce in a crock and added each vegetable as it ripened — beans, cucumber, cauliflower, onions. In addition to making pickles, she made several attempts to learn how to drive, but did not continue. Driving tired her greatly, and she obviously did not enjoy it.

Margaret and Charley went to the college football games in the autumn of 1929. Friends such as Joe and Mary Gilchrist and Edgar McInnis joined them. They also saw old friends at dances including the Rev. Henry Marsh, Charley's friend from University College, and from the time he spent during the war in Petawawa. Catherine Macleod, a lifelong friend of Margaret's, was dancing with Charley on one occasion and he told her not to keep her recently returned veteran suitor, Captain George Scroggie, waiting, she should marry him. So she did![342]

Ramsay MacDonald, Britain's Labour prime minister, was in Washington in October on a "Peace Mission" to President Hoover and came to Toronto to receive an honorary degree. Margaret and her father went to Convocation Hall, which was packed for the occasion. "When he received the degree, I believe that every professor in the university except Charley was on the platform. Charley and Don Fraser were out playing golf." Best had met MacDonald while in England, though he did not know him well. Not attending was not a slight; Best was never really interested in the "pomp and circumstances" of convocation, and would generally avoid such ceremonies. When he could not avoid them, however, because he was presenting or receiving a degree or an award, he did enjoy the occasions.

MacDonald's daughter, Ishbel, "seems to have won all hearts by her naturalness and sincerity." She gave a talk to the Women's Canadian Club on her work with poor children in London. When not at 10 Downing Street, the MacDonalds lived in Hampstead, right across from the NIMR, and Charley used to see the Prime Minister every morning when he went for an ultraviolet bath, which was supposed to be good for his health.

Toronto's artistic scene was busy, and in the autumn of 1929, the New York Theatre Guild played *Wings Over Europe* — "the story of a young scientist who tells the British Cabinet of his wonderful discovery about the power of the atom. He has discovered how to release the energy of the atom." The Hart House String Quartet, consisting of Géza de Kresz and Harry Adaskin, violins, Milton Blackstone, viola, and Boris Hambourg, cello, was very popular. Margaret had recently read everything written by Katherine Mansfield, the New Zealand-born writer known particularly for her short stories — for example, *Garden Party and Other Stories* (1922) — and attended a meeting of the Heliconian, a ladies' club in Toronto for those involved in or interested in the arts, to hear Katherine Hale, herself a well-known Canadian author, speak about Mansfield.[343]

Margaret went with Charley in late November 1929 for her first visit to Indianapolis, the headquarters of the Eli Lilly pharmaceutical company. Dr. G.H.A. Clowes, senior scientist with Eli Lilly, took them to see the land outside the city where he proposed to build a house. Margaret liked the site, the brook flowing through it, the tulip trees, the beeches, and the white thorns. She met the two Clowes boys, George and Allen. At a dinner party at the Clowes', Margaret met Mr. and Mrs. J.K. Lilly, Mr. and Mrs. Eli Lilly, and Mr. and Mrs. Nicholas Noyes. Margaret described J.K. as a "charming old gentleman." She noted that people whom they met in Indianapolis talked a great deal about the literary figures who lived there, such as James Whitcomb Riley, the poet, and Booth Tarkington, the novelist, who had twice won the Pulitzer Prize.

Back in Toronto, A.W. Mahon and Flora, neither of whom was well, were moving to an apartment. A.W. was selling many of his books and he gave Margaret a number of volumes, including James Bryce's *South America*. A.W. had met the author years before at Lord Shaughnessy's in St. Andrews.

Christmas 1929 saw nine guests around the Bests' table at 226 Rosedale Heights Drive: Margaret's parents, Linda, Ralph and Hilda, Uncle Bruce Macleod, Ruth and Vincent Price, and Vincent's brother, Colonel Price. Ruth Green was an old friend of Margaret's, from McAdam, New Brunswick. She married Major Vincent Price, who became the Bests' lawyer. For years, he did their legal work, never charging them anything for his time. The Prices were trusted advisers as well as very close friends. Wee Charley Ralph Salter was upstairs with his nursemaid. After the traditional meal came dancing and charades. Charley gave Margaret a bow-front mahogany chest. She and Charley gave A.W. the new *(Sir James) Barrie: The Story of a Genius,* by Sir John Alexander Hammerton, and Flora a cheque for $100 towards a fur coat.

The death of A.W. Mahon, aged seventy-five, on 3 August 1930, hit Margaret hard. She was very fond of her father; she believed that she was most like him in temperament and interests, and there seems to be no question that she was his favourite. She certainly believed that she was. He had borne his long years of heart trouble stoically, and from all accounts he was "a man of God." His years in Toronto had been happy. His parishioners respected and dearly loved him. His children had grown up healthy and happy.

By the mid twenties the University of Toronto needed more space for the Faculty of Medicine and it had been decided to build additional accommodation to be named in honour of Banting. On 16 September, 1930, the new Banting Institute building was officially opened at 100 College Street, between University Avenue and Elizabeth Street. Canon Cody, chairman of the board of governors of the university, presided at the opening. The new building would house the Banting and Best Department of Medical Research on one floor where Banting, as director of the department, would have his office. The remaining four floors were taken up by several departments of the faculty of medicine. Dean Primrose presented the representatives of Canadian and other universities, thirty in all. Lord Moynihan of Leeds, emeritus professor of surgery in the University of Leeds, a major-general in the Royal Army Medical Corps and president of the Royal College of Surgeons of England, spoke on "The Science of Medicine." In the afternoon, the Chancellor, Sir William Mulock, presented honorary degrees to Lord Moynihan, Professor T.S. Cullen of Johns Hopkins University, Charles S. Blackwell, chairman of the board of trustees of the Toronto General Hospital, and in absentia, to Dr. Davidson Black of the Geological Survey of China. Mulock said, "This is Doctor Banting's day." Banting, however, did not give a speech but was guest of honour at the reception. Lord Moynihan was the only person to mention Best, whose name "is forever linked" with Banting's.[344]

Banting's official portrait was painted by Curtis Williamson and presented by Banting's classmates from medical school. Fred gave Charley a black and white photograph of the portrait, signed "Alpha and Omega — Charlie, Yours, Fred." A great deal was said in those few words.

Margaret started a different sort of diary from 7 July 1931, the day on which she gave birth to Charles Alexander, "Sandy," weighing eight pounds, ten ounces. It was a hot day in Toronto, and there was no air conditioning in the Wellesley Hospital. It had been hot for some days, and Margaret had spent most of the time sitting in the basement at home. Dr. H.B. van Wyck was the obstetrician assisted by Dr. Don Low, both close friends of Charley's. Dr. Harry Shields was the anaesthetist. The number of medical people involved reflected Charley's concern for Margaret and his anxiety to spare her pain and discomfort. Margaret did not see Sandy until the next morning. He "had lots of dark hair and dark blue eyes and lovely skin, not a bit red and wrinkled." Margaret thought that he looked like her father.

She gave details of nursing the baby and was pleased that by the time he was five days old she was providing some of his nourishment. "For the first five days after Sandy was born, I was not allowed to have even a glass of milk, only ginger ale and water, ice and orange juice. Five days later, I was allowed a glass of milk and some fruit."

Almost two weeks later Margaret sat up for the first time "for ten minutes and felt terribly tired." Given the regimen she was on, no wonder she was tired. On the twenty-third, mother and baby went home. Proud grandmother Flora Mahon was there to welcome them to the flower-filled house. Miss Bastien, a registered nurse, stayed until Sandy was a month old when a nursemaid, Miss Maymie Harford, replaced her. Dr. Roy Simpson was Sandy's paediatrician. "He insisted that the baby have supplementary feedings of 'St. Charles' Unsweetened Evaporated Milk, Boiled Water and Dextra Maltose #1."

After seven years of marriage, Charley was ecstatic that Margaret had come through childbirth without a hitch and that they had a healthy son. The Best grandparents came from West Pembroke and Flora's cousin Dr. Bill Macleod from New York to see the baby. Several presents arrived, including a silver porringer from Sandy's godmother, Cairine Mackay Wilson, recently appointed as the first woman member of the Canadian Senate.

Margaret was able to go to Ottawa with Charley in November 1931 to the inaugural meeting of the College of Physicians and Surgeons of Canada. They enjoyed the reception at Government House, hosted by the Earl of Bessborough, the new governor general, and his wife. They stayed at Lac Lucerne in Québec and went on to Montréal before returning for Sandy's first Christmas. Flora Mahon made him a red suit with white angora, and she and Linda gave him a playpen. On Christmas morning, Charley and Margaret went riding at the Connaught Farms, took a pudding to the Scott Mission, visited Don and Mary Fraser, and had lunch with Flora and Linda at their apartment.

The matter of fellowship in the Royal Society of London (FRS) was, and is, of great importance to people of science. J.J.R. Macleod wrote to A.V. Hill agreeing to propose Banting as a fellow of the Royal Society "on the understanding that I am not expected to promote his candidature in preference to Collip's when the time comes." Macleod added that he hoped he might have the "privilege of proposing Best's name. I think, however, that this last step might not be taken for another year or so."[345]

In the new year's honours list Dr. Henry Dale received a knighthood. He wrote to Best saying "it *would* need a bit of an effort to get used to it." He referred to baby Charles Alexander "who looks an attractive person. My only quarrel with his parents is that they didn't give him 'Henry,' at least as a third name! However, I shall hope for better treatment on another occasion. I wish you were coming over again soon. You young people must make the most of your chances before professorial & family responsibilities begin to weigh heavily."[346]

In March 1932, Flora, unwell for some years, became very ill, with bronchitis and asthma battling for her small frame. Flora died on 20 March, aged sixty-four, and she was buried with her beloved A.W. in nearby Mount Pleasant Cemetery. Linda, who had been living with her mother, then joined Margaret and Charley at 226 Rosedale Heights Drive. She had been Charley's secretary since 1927; from 1932 onwards she became also an integral part of the Best household.

Charles Alexander Best was christened in St. Andrew's Church on 6 June 1932 by Dr. Stuart Parker. "He was very naughty, talking and laughing with a big voice." Three days later, Sandy was rushed to the Hospital for Sick Children with a strangulated hernia which was successfully treated. Because of this operation, and the fear of infection, later in June when the Bests left on the first of many family trips to Maine, Sandy was taken out of the car only at night.

By noon of the third day they arrived in West Pembroke. Small changes took place when Charley went "home." It was very important for him to be the "doctor's son." His father was *the Dr.* Best, while he was known as "Dr. Charley." Somehow, it put things in perspective. He slipped back into a Maine accent and swore more, both of which bothered Margaret. Charley always did pronounce words like "leisure" and "pleasure" with long vowels not known in Ontario.

That year Dr. Herbert Best gave his children Charley and Hilda jointly Schooner Cove Farm and the cottage at Leighton Point four miles from West Pembroke. The property was about eighty acres, part of it straddling the peninsula of Leighton's Neck with the sea on both sides. Schooner Cove, on the west, had two small islands, which the family later named Sandy's Island and Henry's Island. The tide rose and fell forty feet in the spring and autumn, a little less between. The bottom was mud, with many rocks — a good source of clams at low water. One part of the cove provided a good anchorage even when the tide was out. There was a weir (pronounced ware) — a large fishing trap for herring. The catch was taken to one of the sardine factories in Pembroke, Lubec, or Eastport, where women would do the canning.

The wooden buildings at Schooner Cove Farm had walls and roofs covered with cedar shingles. There was birch bark under the shingles instead of tar paper. The buildings consisted of a house, a coach house, and a barn with a tool shed attached. The house had a parlour, dining room, kitchen, pantry, wood shed, and small bedroom built off the parlour for a grandmother, so that she did not have to climb the steep stairs. Upstairs were three bedrooms, and over the kitchen was a boat loft, where one of the Leightons had built rowboats. The loft had large windows at one end, where a boat could be slid down poles to the ground, and from there down the hill to Schooner Cove. When Margaret and Charley acquired the property, there was a ladder from the kitchen to the loft, but later they cut a passage through from the bedrooms. Under part of the main house was an ice cellar filled with sawdust, where in late winter blocks of ice were stored, cut from one of the lakes inland from Pembroke. Margaret and Charley added a small, screened porch off the living room and later closed it in so that they had a dressing room as well as a bedroom on the ground floor.

The coach house was attached at one corner to the house. It contained Charley's study, in which he sat beside a window he had cut so that he could see the cove. Here every summer Charley spent mornings working on scientific papers and drafts of the physiology texts that he co-authored with Dr. Norman B. Taylor. An upper floor was built in the coach house so that visitors could sleep there. External doors led to another bedroom and a shower room, the water being pumped in above-ground pipes from a well in the pasture. The barn had four or five stalls for horses, a chicken coop, a hay loft, and space for a buggy and a sleigh. Drinking water came by pail from a spring over the fence in Mr. Mariner Leighton's pasture or from Dr. Best's well in West Pembroke. There were two wells near the house, one with a well-sweep — a cantilevered pole — to one end of which a pail was attached and lowered to get the water. In later years, these were both filled in for fear of a grandchild falling in.

The land was fairly rough pasture, but there was one decent hay field. On one side, a slope ran down to a rail fence that allowed the horses to cross through to a trough fed by pipe from Mr. Mariner's spring. Beyond lay Schooner Cove. The other side looked out over Cobscook Bay to Moose Island and Eastport.

At the Point was a small cottage. Its main feature was a large, screened porch, and off the main room was a kitchen with a lead sink. The Point was always an exciting place, with the tide racing by, seals playing, and the roar of Cobscook Falls just up the way. This was a reversible falls, unknown to most people, of great power and beauty. All the water that went up and down the eleven miles to Dennysville and to Whiting went through this narrow passage. At high and low tides, it was like a millpond, but at other times it was fierce, noisy, and dangerous. As a boy, Charley Best swam his father's horses to Cobscook Falls Island to be pastured. All ages of the Best family picked up driftwood to be used for steaming clams they had dug and for boiling corn. One never knew what surprises each new tide would bring.

Margaret Best had seen Schooner Cove Farm but had never been in the house before 1932. Some work had been done on the inside, but that summer Margaret, Charley, and Linda set to work painting, putting up curtains, and making dressing tables from orange crates. Schooner Cove was to become their favourite place in all the world.

Wherever they went, the Bests went to auctions and antique stores, looking for furniture or glass for Schooner Cove or for their home in Toronto. Margaret began to build a good collection of pressed glass — some American and some Canadian. The Bests did a lot of scraping to get layers of paint or varnish off the furniture. For some pieces, they knew the provenance; for others, the source was a mystery. A lovely birch dining table was discovered to have an inscription at one end only long after it had been added to the dining room: "M=A=C. I=C. April, 1852." Years later, an unused drawer in another table provided a 1920s-era Waltham car clock, mounted on hardwood. Charley knew that it came from one of his father's first cars, but was unsure which one. Charley was fascinated by "Yankee gadgetry." He had learned early how difficult it was to improvise new equipment for the lab. Over the years he bought clocks, three coffee grinders, ox-yokes, several gas light fixtures, two apple corers, and a variety of carpenters tools. He admired the ingenuity and resourcefulness of the smart people who had designed these objects. Margaret was often puzzled that he would buy a second or third example of the same thing, and he would say, "But this one's slightly different."

That summer of 1932, Charley went over to the Cobscook Falls and brought two horses back to the farm to ride: Lady (twenty-two years old) and the "colt," Miss Lou, who was nine. Charley rode every day. Margaret wrote, "He thinks I am going to ride Lady, but she is a frisky old dame." However, it was not long before she reported that she was riding.

For Sandy's first birthday on 7 July there was a party at the grandparents' house in West Pembroke. Henry and Lydia arrived by car from Boston, and Hilda Salter and her little son, Charley Ralph, were also there. The whole family went to St. Stephen, New Brunswick, to meet their train. Margaret was quite free to go on expeditions, as she had not only Maymie to look after Sandy, but Mrs. Cook to take care of the house.

Especially in the early days in Maine in the 1930s, family members spent a lot of time fishing in both salt and fresh water. Lee Frost, a childhood friend of Charley's, took the extended family off Eastport and Campobello Island with the small fleet that was fishing for pollock and haddock. The locals were amused at the visitors' excitement when a pod of whales arrived to do their own fishing, diving under the boats. Henry Mahon was an avid freshwater fisherman, much more so than Charley, but they all were charter members of the Dennys River Salmon Club. Boyden Lake produced pickerel, perch, and trout. One day the family stopped at a small store in Dennysville Station after trout fishing, asking for cold drinks. He had a drink of his own concoction on ice, so we all drank merrily. Charley was well launched into his fifth glass when the old fellow said, "Some say that them that's not used to it, it acts as a kind of physic." Golf was also available at Calais. Dr. and Mrs. Herbert Everett's house in St. Stephen was a frequent stop. Margaret had followed Herbert and Miriam as they courted, skating on a pond in St. Andrews, twenty-five years earlier.

In August Charley, Margaret, and Linda left Schooner Cove for Boston. Charley and Henry Mahon played golf, and the women shopped. Linda stayed in Boston for a week before returning to West Pembroke to be with Sandy, while Margaret and Charley went to Toronto to prepare for their forthcoming trip to the XIVth International Physiological Congress in Rome. On the way to Québec, where they were to sail on 20 August 1932 on the *Empress of Britain*, they stopped in Montréal. There Charley met with Dr. John Tait, the Edinburgh-educated professor of physiology at McGill University, at the Windsor Hotel to set the physiology exam for the Royal College of Physicians and Surgeons of Canada. In Québec, Uncle Bruce Macleod, on his rounds as an inspector for the Bank of Nova Scotia, had a car and took Margaret and Charley for a drive and to "Spencerwood," the lieutenant-governor's residence. Then Bruce had dinner on board the *Empress* with the Bests.

They found good seats on board to watch for the arrival of the delegates returning to Britain from the British Empire Economic Conference in Ottawa: British Prime Minister Stanley Baldwin, Dominion Secretary James Henry Thomas, Chancellor of the Exchequer Neville Chamberlain, and their wives, escorted by Canadian Prime Minister R.B. Bennett and Sir Edward Beatty, chairman of the Canadian Pacific Railway. From the lounge of the ship, the Britons made farewell speeches to the people of Canada. Linda Mahon heard the whole thing in Pembroke; people in that part of Maine listened often to Canadian radio and still watch Canadian television.

The voyage to Europe was great fun. The weather was good, and Margaret and Charley spent a lot of time on the top deck playing tennis and quoits.

Charley had met Mr. Chamberlain before, with Sir Henry Dale, and he had a conversation with him on the ship. Margaret noted, "Mrs. Baldwin was much taller than I expected, with enormous hats perched on her pompadour. Every evening, she wore a lace dress — black one evening, red the next, grey the next, and she marched in and out of the dining room some considerable distance ahead of Mr. Baldwin."

After just over five days, they arrived at Cherbourg where they took a train to Paris. The travellers stayed at the Bon Lafontaine, Rue des Saint-Pères, on the Left Bank. They greatly enjoyed an apéritif, made of vermouth, cassis, and soda, at the Dome Restaurant, Rue Montparnasse. They bought posters from the Thomas Cook travel office, which graced the walls of the Schooner Cove farm house in Maine for many years.

The train trip to Rome was "a long and fatiguing journey — exceedingly rough and uncomfortable." However, it was their first trip to the Mediterranean and Margaret remarked on everything that she saw from the train — the yellow and pale blue stucco houses, the blue of the sea, olive trees, tunnels, the leaning Tower of Pisa. At Pisa, Count Dino Grandi, who had been foreign minister of Italy under Mussolini, and was, at this point, the recently appointed ambassador to London (a post that he held until 1939), got on the train and sat down next to Margaret — "a powerful-looking man and quite fine looking too, with a small black beard." She added, "Two soldiers (officers) brought his luggage on board and we heard someone say it was Grandi. He went out to stand in the corridor once and a fussy old man got on the train and came and sat in Grandi's seat. A youth across from us leaned forward and told him that seat was taken. The old chap appeared to say (in Italian) that he didn't give a damn, and sat on. Grandi heard him, and looking in, he smiled at me."

The Bests stayed in Rome at the Hotel Vittoria, Via Marche. They had special tickets for the official opening of the congress at the Hall of the Caesars at the Campidoglio, so they were sitting in the front row. "Pretty soon, in came Mussolini and various other people. He strode in and seated himself under a statue of Caesar and folded his arms, his jaw thrust out, and he really looked a very powerful and imposing person." A.V. Hill gave the opening address, looking entirely the scholar. Apparently, as he told the Bests over lunch, Mussolini told him afterwards that he had understood his talk. Best and Earle McHenry gave a paper on 12 August 1932 on "the inactivation of histamine." Other University of Toronto scientists who presented papers included W.R. Campbell, Velyien Henderson, Laurence Irving, Samuel Soskin, and Norman Taylor.

As Margaret was wearing a sleeveless dress, Charley went into St. Peter's Basilica first and then loaned Margaret his jacket. The most beautiful thing there in her opinion was Michelangelo's *Pièta*. The Vatican Picture Gallery was closed, but not the Vatican Museum. Margaret loved the animal statuary, *Hermès*, "the wonderful Laocoön group," and the Sistine Chapel in the Vatican, with Michelangelo's ceiling — "very tiring to see but wonderful — the Sibyls, the head of Adam were particularly fine."

The same day, the Bests had lunch with Dr. René and Mme Thérèse Gayet of Paris at the Grande Ristorante Rosetta, Piazza del Pantheon. Margaret was fascinated by the building and its garden, and the bronzes, *Boy with the Thorn in his Foot* and *Romulus and Remus*.

A.V. Hill and J.J.R. Macleod were the guests of Prince Doria at his palace. The prince was a graduate of Cambridge and was married to a Scot. He asked his houseguests to invite a few people to see his art collection. Hill invited the Bests and the Adrians. The Bests thought the prince "a very delightful person." Margaret added, "He asked me if I was a physiologist and when I replied, 'No, my husband is,' Dr. Hill said, 'Mrs. Best encourages physiology.'" Margaret thought the Velázquez portrait of Pope Innocent X — "truly remarkable." However, her Presbyterian background was evident when she wrote about the bones of a saint in a casket with one end of glass "and a little blind that could be run up so one could see the bones; it hardly seems decent." Margaret also noted "a very amusing portrait of the Prince himself as a little baby boy in blue and white." She concluded, "The palace is said to be the most magnificent private home in the world."

On 3 September, Norman and Isabel Taylor and Alan and Daphne Drury gave an eighth anniversary dinner for Margaret and Charley at Alfredo's on the Via Della Scroba. Alfredo was famous for his *fettuccine al burro*. Margaret thought it "a most delectable dish and he comes to the table himself and with many magic flourishes mixes the great lumps of butter and the quantities of grated cheese with the piping hot noodles." Norman Taylor, a colleague at the University of Toronto, had co-authored with Best a physiology text, *The Human Body*, which had just been published.

In September 1932 the Bests returned to Toronto where Charles Best reached another milestone in his scientific career. Choline was a compound known by chemists for nearly a century, but its function was unknown. In 1932 Best, James Hershey, and Elinor Huntsman discovered choline to be an important new dietary factor. The research on choline came out of the observation from the time of the discovery of insulin in 1921 that depancreatized dogs, even when administered insulin for long periods, became sick and died. The livers were found to be enlarged and

141

yellow, which was thought to have been caused by the lack of pancreatic enzymes. It was found that if raw beef pancreas was included in a diet of lean meat and sugar the dogs did not develop fatty livers. In 1927 James Hershey, a young man in the insulin testing laboratory at the University of Toronot, hypothesized that failure in fat metabolism rather than a failure in digestion might be responsible for the fatty livers in depancreatized dogs. He added egg yolks "lecithin" to the diet of depancreatized dogs that had developed liver dysfunction. A year later their livers were found to be normal and Hershey concluded that pancreatic enzymes were not essential to life in depancreatized dogs.

Hershey worked for another year with Samuel Soskin, who was working for his PhD in physiology. In 1930 Hershey and Soskin reported to Best, who had recently taken over as professor of physiology from J.J.R. MacLeod, that lecithin alleviated signs of liver dysfunction in depancreatized dogs. Best wrote to Sir Henry Dale, "I am getting very much interested in some work on lecithin. As you perhaps remember, Hershey demonstrated that some component of crude lecithin was capable of alleviating a certain condition which develops in depancreatized animals. As an extension of this work we have been able to show, by recent experiments, that crude and purified lecithin are capable of preventing the deposition of fat in the livers of normal rats receiving a diet high in fat."[347]

In 1931 Mary Elinor Huntsman came as a graduate student to work with Best and Hershey to try and find the factors involved in the production and cure of fatty livers in rats. In a few weeks in 1932 Best, Hershey, and Huntsman demonstrated that the inclusion of lecithin in the diet reduced the fat content of the livers. Within a month they then identified choline as the actual constituent of the lecithin molecule. During the next seven years many researchers in the departments of physiology and in the school of hygiene worked on the problem of fatty liver.[348]

Choline was considered a "lipotropic" (fat changing) factor and the term was first coined, at the suggestion of Dr. Norman B. Taylor, by Best, Huntsman, and Ridout in 1935. Best and his colleagues went on to show that choline deficiency could be reduced in a variety of animal species by dietary manipulation and that, under controlled conditions, choline could prevent the development of cirrhosis of the liver.[349] By far the most complete account of Best's work on choline was that of Dr. W. Stanley Hartroft,[350] a distinguished biochemist who spent several years at the Best Institute in Toronto, served as director of research at Toronto's Hospital for

Sick Children, and held several American posts.

Best's research on heparin, histamine, and choline brought additional attention to his work. On 9 March 1933, Sir Norman Walker, a distinguished dermatologist who was president of the Royal College of Physicians of Edinburgh and of the General Medical Council, wrote to Best on behalf of the Curators of Patronage of the University of Edinburgh to ask if he was interested in the chair of physiology there. Best would succeed Sir Edward Sharpey-Schäfer, one of the founders of endocrinology, who had held the post since 1899 when he had succeeded Sir William Rutherford. It was indeed a tempting offer. Walker, however, did not avoid the problems in the department, which included lack of space and equipment. The salary offered was £1400, but this might have been more as the University Court had approved an increase "up to a maximum of £1600 if necessary."[351] Best, at thirty-four years old, was amazed and honoured that this prestigious post had been offered him. But he was not blind to the negative aspects of the position. Best replied, "I wish to consider the proposition with great care before coming to any decision ... You will perhaps understand that I could not be happy teaching physiology unless facilities for investigation of a variety of physiological problems were available. These facilities are available to a rather extraordinary degree in Toronto."[352] After a further exchange of letters, Best wrote: "After very careful consideration, I have decided that the amount of teaching which would be necessary in Edinburgh, and the prolonged period which would be required for reorganization of the department, render it inadvisable for me to consider changing from Toronto to Edinburgh at this time. I may say, also, that the fact that I have persuaded four or five young men to commit themselves to a career in physiology, has influenced my decision. It is unlikely that facilities for the work of these people would be available in Toronto if I leave ... In withdrawing my name from consideration, I realize very fully that I may never again have such a tempting possibility presented to me."[353]

An interesting result of this offer was the realization by the Board of the University of Toronto how valued Best was by such a prestigious university as Edinburgh. They suddenly saw they might lose him and passed a resolution, moved by Colonel Gooderham, seconded by Dr. H.B. Anderson:

> Resolved: That the Board learns with great satisfaction that the historic Chair of Physiology in the University of Edinburgh has been offered to Dr. C.H. Best, the

Professor of Physiology in this University. The holders of this Chair have been among the most distinguished physiologists in the world. That the offer should have come to Dr. Best is a great tribute to his past achievements and to the assured hopes of further discoveries in his field of scientific research. The Governors keenly appreciate his loyalty to this University in deciding to stay here. They trust that Dr. Best will find in Toronto the fullest opportunity for his activities and that he will make this University one of the great centres of physiological study and research.[354]

There was another baby in the extended family. Charley's sister, Hilda, had had a little girl, Joan, on 27 October 1932, who was still too small to attend 1933 Christmas dinner at 226 Rosedale Heights Drive. There were fourteen there, including Hilda and Ralph Salter, Hilda and Charley's cousins Cyril and Isabelle Hallam, Uncle Bruce Macleod, Ruth and Vin Price and Vin's father and mother. Their favourite after-dinner entertainment was charades and "each family acted the title of a book. The Prices did *The Vanished Pomp of Yesterday* excellently." Hilda's small son, Charley Ralph, "was such a good boy. At about 10 o'clock Charley brought Sandy down dressed in his little white suit... he was very sleepy." Sandy received several toy animals including a "horse hauling a milk cart from the two Solandt boys."

Margaret and Charley left for New York on Boxing Day, where they sailed on the SS *New York* of the Hamburg Line for Southampton, England. Commodore Kruse obviously took a shine to Margaret and called her his mascot. In London, they had a busy time. The Dales, Lawrences, Drummonds, Channons, and Lovatt Evans were among the old friends they visited. Margaret and Charley loved the theatre and they saw many plays: *Nymph Errant*[355] with Gertrude Lawrence, *Music in the Air*[356] with Mary Ellis, *The Old Folks at Home* with Marie Tempest, *Reunion in Vienna* with Lynn Fontanne and Alfred Lunt. *The Sleeping Clergyman* by James Bridie, a Glasgow doctor, was enjoyed partly because of references to the Medical Research Council.

Margaret visited the art galleries and did some shopping, finding an old Sheffield candelabra that she had been looking for and a Sheraton knife box. They often ate at many of their favourite restaurants. Charley gave a series of three lectures at University College for Professor Lovatt

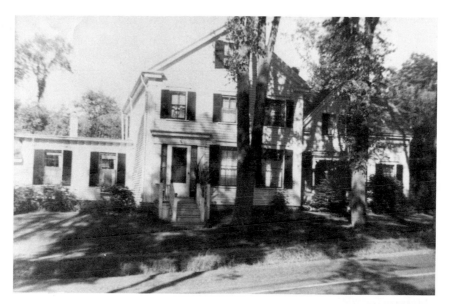

Above: The home and office of Dr. Herbert H. Best,
where Charles H. Best was born, in West Pembroke, Maine.

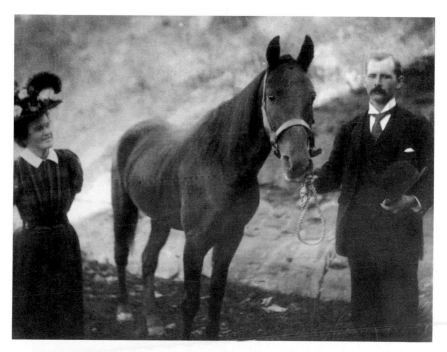

Herbert and Lulu Best with Lady Gardiner, their first horse, c. 1897.

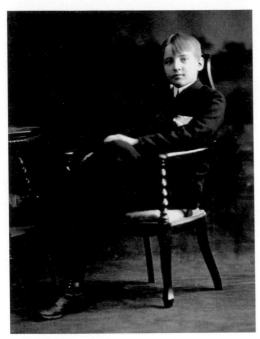

Charles Best at
12 years of age.
Eastport, Maine, 1911.

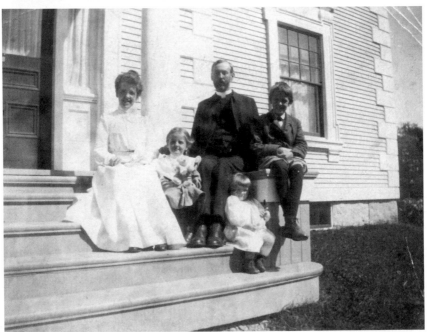

The Rev. A.W. Mahon and Flora Mahon, with Henry, Margaret, and
Emma Linda, on the steps of the manse of Greenock Presbyterian
Church, St. Andrews-by-the-Sea, New Brunswick, 1907.

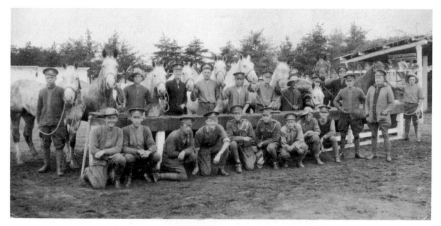

Charles H. Best (rear, third from left)
Camp Petawawa, Ontario. 70th Battery of the Horse Artillery, 1918.

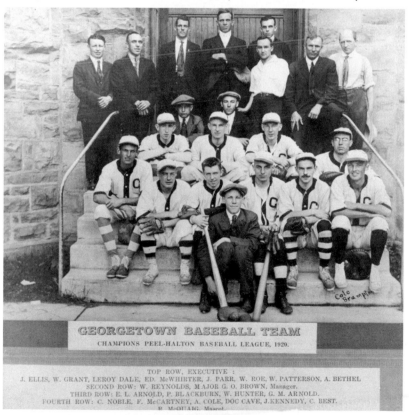

GEORGETOWN BASEBALL TEAM
CHAMPIONS PEEL-HALTON BASEBALL LEAGUE, 1920.

TOP ROW, EXECUTIVE :
J. ELLIS, W. GRANT, LEROY DALE, ED. McWHIRTER, J. PARR, W. ROE, W. PATTERSON, A. BETHEL
SECOND ROW: W. REYNOLDS, MAJOR G. O. BROWN, Manager.
THIRD ROW: E. L. ARNOLD, P. BLACKBURN, W. HUNTER, G. M. ARNOLD.
FOURTH ROW: C. NOBLE, F. McCARTNEY, A. COLE, DOC CAVE, J. KENNEDY, C. BEST,
R. McQUAIG, Mascot.

Georgetown Baseball Team
Champions, Peel-Halton League, 1920
Clark Noble, front row, far left; Charley Best, front row, far right.

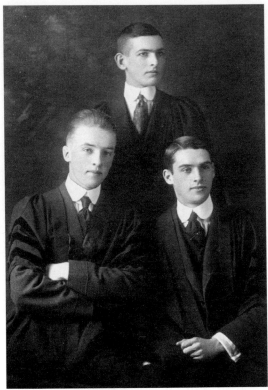

Graduation portrait: Charles H. Best, E. Clark Noble, and Henry Marsh. University College, University of Toronto, 1921.

Sgt. Charles H. Best at Niagara Camp. The Governor General's Horse Guards, June 1921.

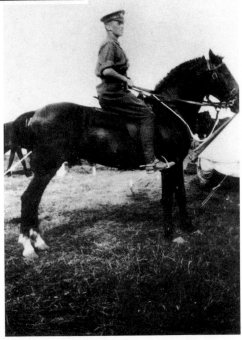

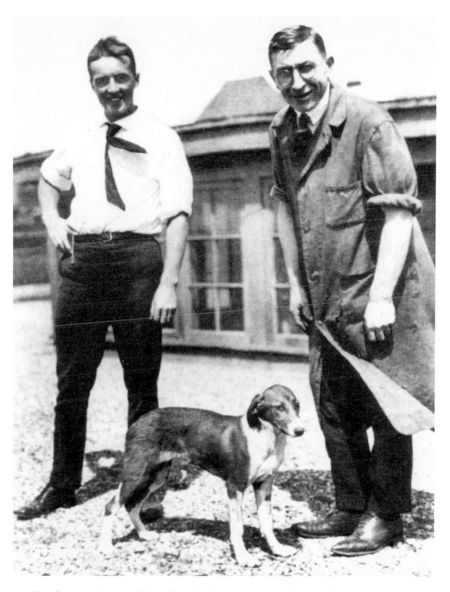

Charles H. Best and Frederick G. Banting with Dog No. 408 on the roof of the Medical Building, University of Toronto, August 1921. Photo taken by Henry Mahon.

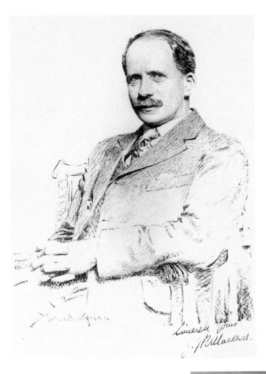

Professor John James
Rickard (J.J.R.) Macleod
by Joshua Smith,
1924.

Dr. Joseph A. Gilchrist, the
first MD to receive insulin,
c. 1930.

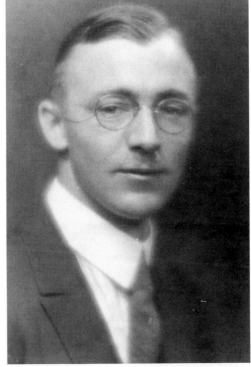

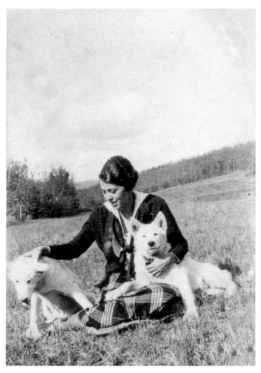

Lydia and Henry Mahon
with Razz and Jazz
Dawson City, Yukon, 1922.

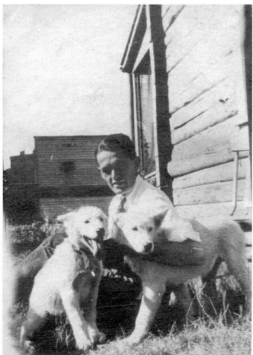

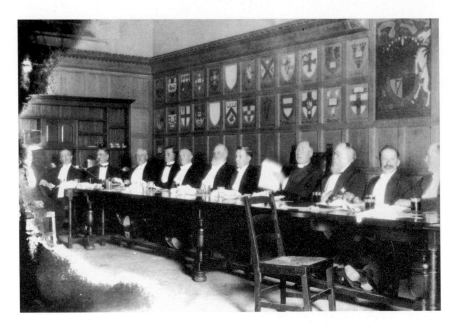

Banquet in the Great Hall of Hart House, University of Toronto,
26 November 1923, in honour F.G. Banting and J.J.R. Macleod,
jointly awarded the Nobel Prize for Physiology or Medicine.

Left to right: J.G. FitzGerald, Albert Gooderham, Dean Alexander Primrose,
W.F. Nickle, C.H. Best, Sir William Mulock, F.G. Banting, Canon H.J.
Cody, Sir Edmund Walker, J.J.R. Macleod, Sir Robert Falconer.

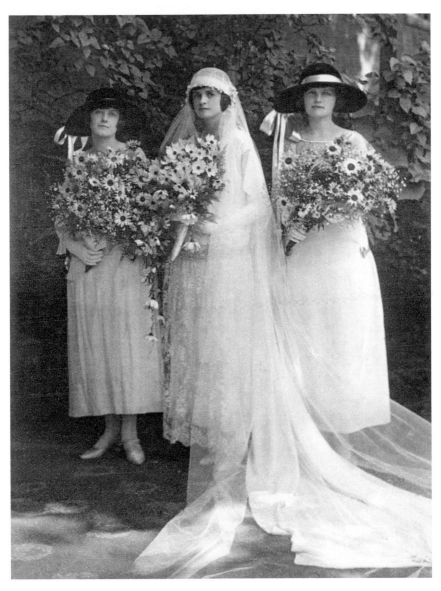

Margaret Mahon, in the garden of her parents' home, 370 Brunswick
Avenue, Toronto, on the day of her wedding, with her sister, Linda,
and future sister-in-law, Hilda Best, 3 September 1924.

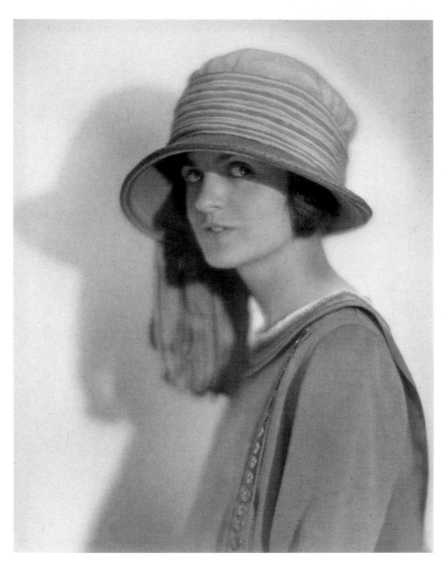

Margaret Mahon Best, in her going-away outfit, or "vamp" costume,
3 September 1924.

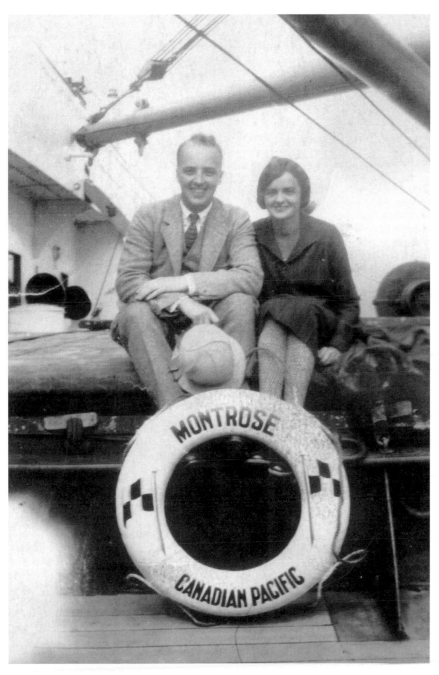

Margaret and Charles Best, on the first of their overseas trips together, on board the CPR liner *Montrose* from Montréal to Southampton, July 1925.

The 25th of this month Marion,
Miss Faums and I leave for
Alaska — where we expect to
spend two or three weeks and
then go to Victoria to the Can. Med. Ass.
    The new Public Health Bld is
almost ready for roofing. It looks
great. Fitz is as pleased as "Punch"
and wears a smile not unlike
the historic gentleman.
    I must get to
work Charlie

    as ever
    Fred

Cartoon of F.G. FitzGerald as "Punch" by Fred Banting in letter to
Charley Best, 13 May 1926.

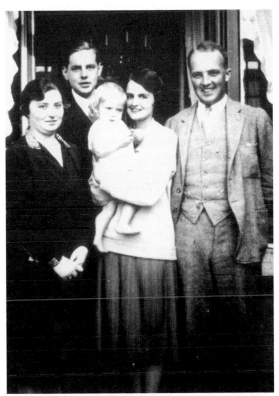

Dr. Joseph P. and
Marguerite Hoet, and
Margaret and Charles
Best, with Joseph J.
Hoet, Antwerp, 1926.

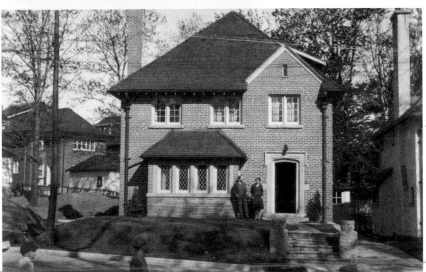

Margaret and Charles Best at the door of their first house,
purchased with his share of Banting's Nobel Prize award,
226 Rosedale Heights Drive, Toronto, 1927.

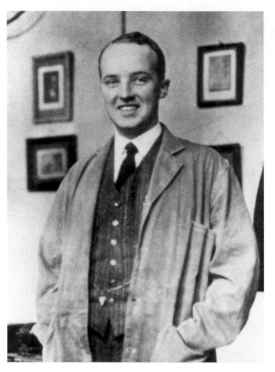

Charles H. Best in Sir
William Bayliss' laboratory
at University College,
London, taken by
Professor A.V. Hill, 1928.

E. Linda Mahon, c. 1930.

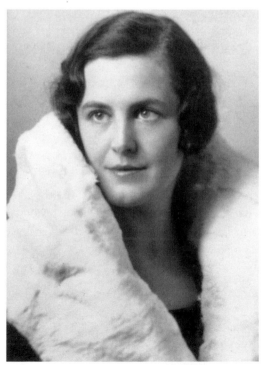

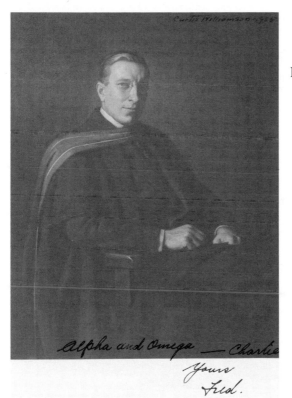

Portrait of
Frederick G. Banting
by Curtis Williamson.
Hanging in the Banting
Institute, University of
Toronto, inscribed,
"Alpha and Omega —
Charlie, Yours Fred."

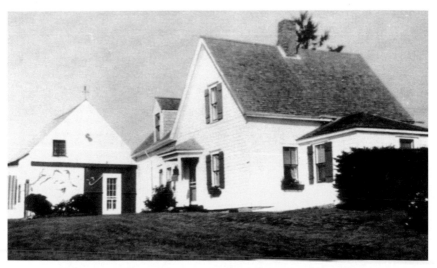

Schooner Cove Farm, summer home of the Bests,
West Pembroke, Maine.

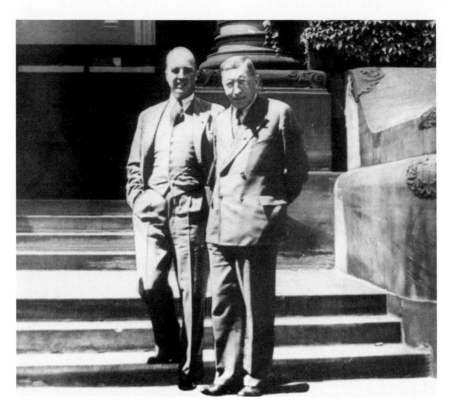

Charles H. Best and Sir Frederick G. Banting,
CMA meetings, Victoria, British Columbia, 1936.

Evans on the subject of liver and carbohydrate metabolism. He also spoke at St. Mary's Hospital and in Cambridge for Professor Joseph Barcroft.

The return trip was on the *Georgic* of the White Star Line, landing in Boston on 3 February 1934. On the ship, the Bests met a man named Auerbach. Margaret commented, "I was quite interested in him because, although Charley had met various German scientific Jews who have had to leave the country, he was the first Jew I had met who had to leave Germany."

With the arrival of their second son, Henry Bruce Macleod, on 9 October 1934, the Bests and Linda Mahon moved from 226 Rosedale Heights to a bigger house at 78 Old Forest Hill Road. The realtor, Chambers and Meredith, listed the property at $37,000. They bought it for $33,500.[357] Although university salaries were not large, Charles Best was receiving a decent salary at a time when many people, because of the Depression, were settling for whatever they could get. It was a good time to buy, but not a good time to sell. The Bests were lucky enough to be able to buy a new house, without having to take what would likely have been a loss on their old house, which they kept, and rented out to tenants. The newspaper advertisement for 78 Old Forest Hill described a "solid, red brick, very good-looking house with much inside charm," six bedrooms, three bathrooms, and so on. There was a third floor that the nanny, Mrs. Cook, occupied, and which the boys moved into when they were older. Half of the basement provided a study and washroom for Charley. The house also had a large garden.

The kidnapping and murder of Charles Lindbergh Jr. on 1 March 1932 had horrified Margaret, as it had the rest of the world. The Lindbergh baby was just a year older than Sandy and Margaret Best feared a similar tragedy in her family. The result was that she did not permit her young sons to climb fences to play in the gardens of neighbouring children or allow them to go back and forth to school alone until they were much older. Margaret did not drive and therefore, while the children were young, she walked many miles taking the boys to and from various music lessons and appointments.

In 1935, however, Margaret was criticized for making the trip to Leningrad for the XVth International Physiological Congress when she had a ten-month-old baby and a three year old. Her priorities were clear — she belonged with Charley — and their trip to the USSR, which rarely opened its gates to visitors, provided them with memories that lasted for the rest of their lives. Also, few children were better looked after. Linda

Mahon worked at the lab, but she lived with the family and was free to take as much time as she wanted to be at home. There were also a nurse and a housekeeper to care for the children and the house. Friends such as Jessie Ridout often stayed with Linda, and Roy Simpson, the paediatrician, was available at very short notice. Worries about what other people thought did not prevent Margaret from enjoying herself.

The opening ceremonies in Leningrad took place in "the Uritsky Palace, formerly the meeting place of the Duma and of the Provisional Government of 1917."[358] There were simultaneous translation services for Russian, English, French, and German. A speech by eighty-six-year-old Ivan Pavlov, Nobel laureate in 1904 for his work on conditioned reflexes, was the highlight of the congress. Aleksandr Karpinskii, president of the Academy of Sciences, aged ninety-one, also spoke, as did Gregorii Kaminskii, the young commissar of health, and several other government officials. Dr. Walter B. Cannon, the Harvard physiologist who in 1932 published *The Wisdom of the Body*,[359] gave the main address, *a pièce de résistance* which John Fulton of Yale described as "bold, forceful, beautifully written and delivered."[360]

Don and Omond Solandt, both brilliant students, and later colleagues, of Best, attended the conference. Omond Solandt later told a story about Fred Banting, sitting above the Bests in a steeply raked lecture hall in Leningrad, rolling up small pieces of paper and aiming them at Best until he attracted his attention. Best had not known that Banting would be in Russia.

Solandt always appreciated the opportunity to attend this congress. "It was an outstanding example of Charley's generosity and thoughtfulness. He talked Don and myself into going and facilitated our registration, but the main thing was everywhere we went, he made sure we met all the big shots. We went with him twice to Pavlov's lab."[361] Best had learned from Dale and Hill in London ten years earlier how valuable such contacts were to young scientists.

The Bests visited a daycare facility where parents could leave their small children while they were at work — though there were nursery schools at the time in the West, a daycare facility of this nature was something unheard of in the 1930s. The youngsters seemed very happy, and their needs were very well taken care of, with even a doctor in attendance. A tour of the "Peterhof," the summer residence of the Tsars, contrasted with visits to a very secular marriage bureau and a similar divorce bureau also on the schedule.

Comments about the hotel were generally very negative. Margaret described the table linen as "unusually dirty and certainly threadbare." The waiters looked "like very grubby street cleaners, and the service was the slowest I have ever seen." Yet their own laundry was done beautifully and returned quickly. They were served "what appears to be chicken cutlets — the chicken really high and each with a claw stuck into the cutlet." Breakfast consisted of "a large slice of stale fruitcake." The tea was always good, but the "coffee was abominable, not really coffee at all." Bread, butter, and jam were good, but the Bests refused the omelettes, "because several people happened on bad eggs."

"Leningrad was a very depressing place, to my mind. It must have been at one time one of the most beautiful cities in Europe … There really are fine buildings one after the other, and all seem to belong to the same beautiful scheme. But they look — many of them — so very shabby now that one longs to have seen the city in the old days of the Tsars. The Winter Palace is over-ornate, but the Admiralty all yellow and white and simple in design with its golden needle spire is one of the most satisfying of buildings." Margaret was fascinated by what she saw but uneasy. "We were very glad to have visited Russia and were very glad to get away." They appreciated even more the next few days in Helsingfors, Finland, which they enjoyed immensely before returning to Toronto and their normal routine.

In late February 1936, en route to the annual meeting of the American Physiological Society in Washington, Margaret and Charley went to Boston, staying at 2 Prescott Street in Cambridge with Henry and Lydia Mahon. Best went to the Joslin Clinic and the Deaconess Hospital to see Dr. Elliott P. Joslin and other diabetic specialists. One afternoon they went out to Hamilton, near Dr. Joslin's farm, to see a pony that they might buy for Sandy. "Smokey" was part Shetland. They liked him and thought $125 a fair price.

From Boston the Bests went to New Haven, Connecticut, staying at the Yale Faculty Club. Best spent a month lecturing at Yale on respiration, metabolism, and ductless glands to the students in Physiology 100 for which he was paid a fee of $1,000. John Fulton, a physiologist and medical historian, and his wife, Lucia, were their hosts. Their host told Margaret that younger scientists were greatly stimulated by Best's presence. The Fultons entertained Margaret and Charley and Margaret and Harry Botterell at dinner.

Botterell was at Yale for a year after studying in London and before returning to Toronto, where he later became professor of neurosurgery. In

1962, he was named dean of medicine at Queen's University in Kingston. In the Fultons' dining room was a bookcase that had belonged to Sir William Osler, given to Dr. Fulton by Lady Osler. Margaret was reading Stephen Graham's book, *The Tsar of Freedom — Alexander II,* and she enjoyed her conversation with Dr. Ross Granville Harrison, sterling professor of biology at Yale. His father spent many years in Russia as a railway engineer and had kept interesting diaries of his experiences there.

In Philadelphia, Dr. Det Bronk, director of the Johnson Foundation and professor of biophysics at the University of Pennsylvania, invited Hugh Long, Herbert Evans, and Best to his labs. The next stop was Baltimore and Johns Hopkins University. On 25 March 1936, the Bests went on to Washington for the forty-eighth annual meeting of the American Physiological Society. It was Margaret's second visit to Washington — the first had been eleven years earlier for her first medical meetings. Margaret and Linda went on a tour of Arlington National Cemetery, the Curtis Mansion, and Mount Vernon. The next day they went to the White House. Margaret would have liked more time in the Library of Congress and also the Smithsonian Institution.

The Bests and Linda drove back to Toronto through flooded areas of Pennsylvania. Charley wanted to stop at Northumberland where Joseph Priestley, the English-born discoverer of oxygen, had lived when he moved to the United States in 1794 as a result of religious persecution (he was a Unitarian.) The house contained some of his furniture and scientific equipment. "Charley was tremendously interested in it all."

In late June 1936, Charley was in Victoria for the meetings of the Canadian Medical Association where he, Fred Banting, and Bert Collip were presented the first medals of the F.N.G. Starr Award, "representing the highest award that lies within the power of the CMA to bestow."[362] On Charley's return to Toronto the family left for Maine at the beginning of July.

The temperature had been 105 degrees Fahrenheit — the highest temperature ever recorded in Toronto — so they decided to leave in the evening, when it was a bit cooler, and they drove as far as Trenton. Mrs. Mills was along to help with the children. The next night, at the Waterbury Inn in Vermont, was somewhat cooler. Sandy was so tired that he said, "I wish I had never left home. I wish Mummy and I had stayed home." When he was tucked in bed, he said, "Why have I this not-at-homeness feeling?" They drove on the next day to Pembroke. Dr. Herbert Best was at home in the village; Lulu Best, with Berla Clark and Winnie

Leighton from neighbouring farms, was at Schooner Cove Farm to welcome them. The house had changed very much with the partition between the two parlours removed and the old wood shed made into a kitchen.

Bruce Macleod soon arrived. He had found Toronto too hot, even when he stayed in Charley's basement study, and so he had taken the train to St. Stephen, New Brunswick. Smokey, Sandy's new pony, and Gold Star, Margaret's gelding five-gaited[363] saddle horse, had arrived from Oxford, Massachusetts, and so Bruce gave Sandy, who had just turned five, his first riding lesson. Smokey was not an easy mount, but within a few minutes they were galloping. Sandy said, "My Smokey went terrific fast around the house." Sandy certainly inherited his father's natural ability on horseback, as indeed did his own children in later years. Margaret's first ride on Gold Star was not so great. Margaret was not brought up to ride, as was her brother Henry, but tried to please Charley, who had bought Gold Star to encourage her. Though perhaps not a natural rider, she clearly had an affection for the horse; in her diary, she called Gold Star "a darling old thing."

Margaret was obviously worried about Sandy and Smokey. On his second day, he went up to Mariner Leighton's farm, got a dozen eggs in a bag and, predictably, delivered them home scrambled. "He trots and canters all over the place, but it must be stopped. I am afraid he might take it into his head to go up to town." Sandy's father and grandfather were totally unconcerned; Sandy reminded them of themselves at the same age.

Everyone was very curious about the Quoddy Tidal Power Plant project at Pleasant Point. The purpose was to harness the powerful high tides of Passama-Quoddy Bay to produce electricity. The family went to look and saw that very nice houses had been put up for the workers on the project. In the middle of the Depression such construction was significant. Dexter Cooper, the designer, was living in the house in Eastport where Dr. Herbert Best had had his hospital.

Henry and Lydia Mahon drove up from Boston. One fine day, the adult Bests, the Mahons, and Linda took a lunch and went to West Quoddy Light, the lighthouse painted with wide circular stripes of red and white, a favourite spot, looking out to Grand Manan Island. The stones on the beach were all worn smooth from being rolled up by the waves and then rolling down again.

After lunch the Bests and Mahons went the short distance to Lubec, a very attractive little fishing village, from where it was a short ride on a two-car ferry (later a bridge) to Campobello Island. A Royal Canadian Mounted Police officer informed them that the Roosevelts were on the Island. The president of the United States, Franklin Delano Roosevelt, and his wife, Eleanor, and their family had a summer house there. Stopping at Herring Cove, they found the Roosevelt family, including the president's eighty-four-year-old mother, Sara Delano Roosevelt, and three of their sons, the eldest, James, with his wife, Betsey Cushing, Franklin, and John. Eleanor Roosevelt invited the visitors to lunch. Charley was about to explain that they had just eaten when Margaret accepted with alacrity. Charley talked to Dr. Ross McIntire, the president's doctor, and they all had a chat with FDR. He had been coming to Campobello since he was two, fifty-two years earlier. Realizing where Schooner Cove Farm was, he said, "I don't know what Quoddy [tidal power project] will do to you people." The Quoddy tidal power plant was a pet project of FDR, providing employment during the Depression. It was also an election year and Roosevelt was coming to the end of his first term as president that summer. After lunch, the Roosevelt boys, McIntire, Best, and Henry Mahon played baseball on the beach against the cabinet of the government of New Brunswick, who had arrived by boat to meet FDR. This was an international sporting event that is not recorded in the history of baseball.

The Bests returned to Quoddy Village a few days later and were shown around by some of the medical people on the project. Dr. and Mrs. Francis Benedict were visiting at the same time. They had retired to Machiasport, Maine, not far from West Pembroke, and the Bests and the Benedicts visited each other regularly. He had recommended Banting for the Nobel Prize in 1923, but there is no record of his ever divulging this to Charley Best.[364]

There had been 5,000 men working on the Quoddy power project the previous winter, and 1,200 were still there. The upcoming 1936 presidential elections would probably decide what would be done. Certainly, given the economy of the 1930s, a project of this size was very important from a political point of view. Due to the location, there had been talk of a plan that would cross the Canadian border. Margaret noted, "If the international plan ever went through, it is likely that Passamaquoddy Bay would be the high basin and Cobscook Bay low. But, if they should continue just with the American dam, Cobscook would be high water all the time at the cottage." She concluded, "Naturally, we prefer our tides." In later years, after the Quoddy tidal power project had long been abandoned, Margaret and Charley said that if it had continued they probably would have moved to Nova Scotia, although they would have regretted leaving his parents in West Pembroke.

Herbert Best rode every day with Sandy while the other adults in the family went for a trip to Nova Scotia — Margaret's first visit to Halifax. Before returning to Ontario, Margaret and Linda went up to visit the Mariner Leightons and the Albert Leightons. Margaret said that Mr. Mariner had tears in his eyes when he said that he would miss Sandy. He said, "He does what I tell him." Margaret wondered if Sandy ever asked for things. "No, he only asked once and that was yesterday when he wanted my chicken coop" — an original request, certainly. Grampy and Grammy Best came down to Schooner Cove Farm to say goodbye. The little boy had made two old men very happy that summer.

There were always visitors to the University of Toronto's laboratories. In the autumn of 1936, soon after the Bests returned from the east coast, their dear friend Dr. Robin Lawrence arrived in Toronto for the first time. The Harley Street diabetic specialist was a severe diabetic himself. Another English visitor, Sir Joseph Barcroft, professor of physiology at Cambridge, had a weekend in Toronto after participating in the Harvey Tercentenary Celebrations at Harvard on behalf of the Royal Society.

For Margaret and Charley the autumn was also beset by health problems. Dr. Cecil Rae removed Margaret's tonsils on a Monday at the Toronto General Hospital; she went home on the Thursday and had nurses for several days. Rae said that it was evident that Margaret had had quinsy more than once. Margaret told how she had had a bad abscess in her throat when she had scarlet fever as a child, and he said that it was all part of the same condition. Charley was having problems with a duodenal ulcer. He virtually stopped smoking and drinking but had put on a lot of weight. Pepper was banned from cooking, along with pork and anything fried.

Throughout the 1930s Charles Best became very involved, with Norman B. Taylor, in writing physiology textbooks. Taylor graduated in medicine from Toronto in 1908 and received his FRCP and his FRCS (Edinburgh) in 1912. He joined the department of physiology in 1919 and was a demonstrator to Best's class in 1920, becoming a full professor in 1931. After leaving Toronto, he was professor of the history of medicine at the University of Western Ontario from 1948 to 1957.

The most important of their texts was *The Physiological Basis of Medical Practice — A Text in Applied Physiology*, published by the Williams and Wilkins Company of Baltimore, which went through eight editions between 1937 and 1966. This large tome, the eighth edition running to 1,793 pages, was translated into Spanish (five editions), Portuguese and Italian (each two editions), and one edition each in Polish and Romanian. In the preface to the first edition, the authors stated, "We have endeavoured to write a book which will be sure to link the laboratory and the clinic, and which will therefore promote continuity of physiological teaching throughout the pre-clinical and clinical years of the undergraduate course."

They gave special thanks to Professors J.K.W. Ferguson, E.T. Waters, C.B. Weld, and A.M. Wynne for their assistance. In the seventh edition in 1961, Best and Taylor wrote, "We ourselves now marvel at the intrepid not to say reckless spirit in which this book was conceived and its first edition written. Though we are not abject in our apology we fully realize and regret the insufficiency of the last edition. There are disconcerting gaps between its text and the more recent advances in physiology and related branches in scientific medicine which made us acutely aware of calling upon others for help."

The seventh edition lists twenty-eight contributors, and the eighth, forty-nine. Unfortunately, the sales figures have disappeared through the sale and merger of various publishing companies. Four further editions appeared between 1973 and 1991, with American editors and contributors. There was no connection with Canada or the University of Toronto, except for the title.

The other two texts by Best and Taylor were *The Human Body* and *The Living Body.* The first was published by Henry Holt and Company of New York in 1932 and revised in 1948 and 1956. It was based on "a course of lectures in elementary physiology given to public health nurses, hospital administrators, and undergraduates in household science, physiotherapy, and occupational therapy at the University of Toronto." *The Living Body* was first published by Henry Holt in 1938 and revised in 1944 and 1952. In the first edition, the authors "assumed that the reader has had some instruction in physics and chemistry," but "no such assumption has been made with regard to anatomy and histology. Though this book has been written primarily for the usual college course in human physiology, we have also had in mind its use as a text in nursing schools as well as the physiological instruction of dental and agricultural students."

Years later, Best reminisced about *The Physiological Basis,* widely identified as "Best and Taylor:"

We had a very friendly relationship in this — a great deal of work was done by Taylor, but he seemed to be delighted to be associated with me ... Our arrangement of 70% to Taylor and 30% to me seemed to be very happy from his point of view, and I was quite content. There was never a ripple until the book began to gain in popularity and the royalties went up, and then Taylor began to feel that he should have a higher percentage. I felt that the book's sales were due in part to my research activities; he felt that they were due, much more, to his ability to write down physiological facts. I would grant that he did that very well. He, actually, became very possessive about it, very proud of it, and it was a big source of income for him relative to his university salary.[365]

On 21 April 1937, Charley and Margaret Best left Toronto for the American Physiological Society's meetings in Memphis, Tennessee, and then the California Academy of Medicine in San Francisco. Best was constantly in demand, giving eight lectures at the University of California in San Francisco, at the California Academy of Medicine, to the medical students at Stanford University, and at the Scripps Clinic in La Jolla.

They took the overnight train from Palo Alto to Los Angeles where they were met early on Sunday 9 May 1937, by Dr. Elmer Belt at Glendale Station, near Hollywood. The Belts were "perfectly delightful people" and extremely hospitable to the Bests. Dr. Belt was a urologist with many patients and friends amongst the movie people of Hollywood, including Frederick March and his wife, stage actress Florence Elridge; Jeanette MacDonald; Harold Lloyd; Eddie Cantor; and many other Hollywood personalities of the period. The Belts took the Bests for a drive through Beverly Hills to see the houses of many movie stars. Although today interest in the lives of film stars is often more cynical, in the twenties and thirties people were fascinated by the glamour, fame and wealth of movie stars. Charley and Margaret, longtime avid filmgoers, were no exception and were intrigued to have a behind-the-scenes glimpse of Hollywood.

"This is an amazing place," wrote Margaret. "Street after street lined with beautiful homes and lovely gardens. Then on the hillside, too, are some of the finest places." They saw "Pickfair," the fabled home of Hollywood's former "Royal Couple," the Canadian actress Mary Pickford and Douglas Fairbanks Sr. Since their divorce the previous year the house had been put up for sale.

Then they saw Frederick March's house. One of the most respected actors of stage and screen, Frederick March, like Laurence Olivier, made films to allow him to work in the theatre. The Marches built a house in Beverly Hills where they lived when he was filming; but their true allegiance was to New England, close to the New York theatres.[366] Next came the sumptuous Mediterranean-style mansion of Western star Tom Mix. Largely because of the horses and the riding, Charley loved cowboy movies so they were interested to see the house where Mix used to ride up the front steps and into the entrance hall on his wonder horse, Tony.[367]

Later they visited Harold Lloyd's immense white stucco house, with a red tile roof, and acres of landscaped grounds, "a nine-hole golf course, an artificial waterfall and river, an old mill-wheel, formal gardens, olive trees and cypress trees, and a perfectly lovely swimming pool made of turquoise tiles." Harold Lloyd was "shorter than I expected and looks quite different without his horn-rimmed spectacles. He talked to Charley about the great things he had done in the medical world and was altogether very charming." Lloyd's two children, little Harold, "about the age of Sandy," and Gloria were also there. Gloria had a delightful small-scale thatched playhouse surrounded by a tiny walled garden with a wrought iron gate.

Dr. Belt also arranged one of the highlights of the trip to California, a tour of the studios. On Thursday, May 13, they first visited the sets of five films at MGM, including *Saratoga,* where they met two of the stars, Walter Pidgeon, "a handsome big fellow" from Saint John, New Brunswick, and Clark Gable. Both actors talked with Charley about playing medical parts in pictures and then getting hundreds of letters afterwards from the "men in white" criticizing their performance. When Margaret was photographed with Gable she said, "I will certainly be envied by the women in Toronto." Another set that they visited was *Firefly* with Jeanette MacDonald and Allan Jones, "both of whom have fine voices." It was the only film they made together. Macdonald "had become so disenchanted with Nelson Eddy stealing all the scenes from her that she asked Louis B. Mayer for a new leading man. Ironically, in *Firefly,* she again played second fiddle. Allan Jones, singing *The Donkey Serenade,* was the hit of the picture. It made him a very big star."[368] Margaret had noticed their makeup was brown with gold flecks, which, on film, gave them gorgeous complexions. Then came *You'll be Married by Noon* with Florence

154

Rice and Robert Young, whom Charley liked best of all the actors they met. They were shooting a courtroom scene and Margaret noticed that the magistrate's chair was sitting on boards on what appeared to be egg crates. Only the part captured by the camera was important. Charley was fascinated by the artifice and ingenuity of the special effects. The legendary head of MGM, Louis B. Mayer, who had invited them to his office, was unavailable as he was negotiating with striking technicians.

Dr. Belt took the Bests to a broadcast by Eddie Cantor. Cantor was very hospitable and "very nice, but oh, how his eyes pop!" Margaret described Bobby Breen, a young boy from Toronto who was on the show, as "a little brat — so ingratiating, with his head on one side and a sweet smile, he said, 'Now don't give me an injection, Dr. Best.' He had been well primed." Deanna Durbin from Winnipeg was part of the same broadcast. Margaret found her "a darling. Only 14, but she has a lovely voice and no mannerisms."

Later Eddie Cantor took the Bests to lunch at the Twentieth Century Fox studio restaurant "filled with actors and actresses in their stage costumes." Margaret wrote, "Eddie is absolutely wild on the subject of Hitler and the treatment of his people. He is a Russian Jew himself." She enjoyed one of Cantor's anecdotes. He told them how kind the Prince of Wales was to him a few years earlier in London. When they first met in New York the Prince had asked Eddie to come and see him. Eddie had replied that he would like to go around the palace, but he would take his meals out so as not trouble the Prince's Mother with the cooking. "Imagine the nerve!" said Margaret. "It went over big with Edward."

After lunch they met Darryl Zanuck, the head of the Twentieth Century Fox studio — "quite young, short, thin, very tanned, with peculiar teeth, very far apart. He was smoking the biggest cigar I have ever seen." Cantor said that Zanuck was the main reason for the success of the Fox Studios and was able to foresee better than anyone else what was going to please the public. The well-known journalist Walter Winchell, inventor of the newspaper gossip column, came along in his car which had a "'smart' New York licence plate, 2 W."

Back at their hotel, Dr. Belt gave Margaret a little book of Sir William Osler's that she had admired. It was *Science and Immortality*, the Ingersoll Lecture for 1904. The author wrote, "To keep his mind sweet, the modern scientific man should be saturated with the Bible and Plato, with Homer, Shakespeare, and Milton; to see life through their eyes may enable him to strike a balance between the rational and the emotional, which is the most serious difficulty of the intellectual life."[369] Before leaving the next day, Margaret received a book on California from Dr. and Mrs. Belt, inscribed "for the wholly delightful Margaret Best."

Five days after the Bests returned to Toronto, Sir Henry and Lady Dale arrived for the annual meetings of the Royal Society of Canada. Little Henry Best met his godfather for the first time. Sir Henry, Charles Best's greatest mentor, had been knighted in 1932. It was on this visit that he recited some of Hilaire Belloc's *Cautionary Tales* and also sang Sir Charles Parry's setting of *Jerusalem* with the words by William Blake. The little boy never forgot either. Both Henry Mahon and Henry Dale considered themselves his godfathers — a heavy responsibility for a small boy. The Bests entertained the Dales at York Downs Golf Club, where Charley played regularly for many years with three of his closest friends, Don Fraser, Alex MacDonald, and David Scott.

A few days later, Margaret awoke with a pain "in the middle of my pinny." By that night, Ray Farquharson arrived and then Gordon Murray. At 1:00 a.m., Charley took Margaret to the Toronto General Hospital. At 2:00 a.m., Murray operated on her appendix, and by 3:00, she was back in her hospital room. There were several medical men at the operation, but Murray was in charge. Margaret was in hospital for eight days before being taken home by ambulance. Gordon Murray dictated a very limited diet — warm water and consommé — for four days, then cream soup and custard for two days, before solid food. There were nurses on duty. At home, Sandy whispered, "You left me in the middle of the night, Mummy."

On 7 July 1937, Sandy's sixth birthday and his uncle Bruce's sixty-sixth, the family left for Maine. Don Fraser, always a devoted friend, was at the house early to see them off. There were seven passengers in the 1935 Chrysler Imperial which Charley had bought at an estate sale: the four Bests, Linda, and two helpers, Mary, the cook, and Maria to look after the children.

On a family excursion to Indian Island, New Brunswick, the smallest in the Grand Manan archipelago, Charley made fish chowder, at which he was very expert, over a fire on the beach — fish (often haddock), salt pork, butter, then milk at the last minute. When asked over the years by reporters for a favourite recipe, that is what he usually gave. Margaret much admired an old house built by the Chaffey family. They met an old man who said that he had been to Pembroke over forty years earlier to see Dr. Herbert Best about some ailment. Charley told him that Dr. Best was his father. The old fellow replied, "Your uncle is the one who should buy this old house. He is just lousy with money." Charley, puzzled, asked, "Which of my uncles would that be?" "Oh, the one who made the diabetes cure. Didn't he give you any money?" "No," said Charley, "He did not." The old man was perplexed. "But surely he gave you a job."

This conversation illustrated three frequent misconceptions — first of all, the assumption that the co-discoverer of insulin was much older than the youthful-looking Charley; secondly, that insulin was a "cure" for diabetes, and third, that whoever discovered it must be very wealthy. Many people who were much better schooled than this man were under the same misapprehensions. Best and his colleagues never got a penny for insulin, though, of course, the fame and scientific respect they received greatly enhanced their professional careers.

Sandy continued to ride Smokey that summer and started to ride Gold Star. Charley tried to get young Henry started on the pony — he enjoyed it but was not a natural like his brother. At high tide, Charley often rowed up through the quiet falls in the boat that his friend Arthur Mahar had made. Arthur had rowed it from his home, down through the falls, and into Schooner Cove. When Charley asked him how much he owed him, Arthur replied that the boat was twelve feet long, and so he figured that $12 would be fine. Margaret christened it *The Sand Piper*.

Margaret, Charley, and Linda were off for a combined lecture tour and family lore visit to Nova Scotia. At the farm, Sandy was keeping everybody busy. After dinner one evening, he tried to rally his remaining troops saying, "Come now, I'll get the pickaxe and you can dig a well." He always worked very hard himself, but he also pressed anyone near into service. These were life-long traits.

Herbert Best was not rushing from patient to patient as much and sometimes stayed at the cottage at Leighton's Point, down beyond the farm. This summer he started to teach his grandsons about the heavens. He would arrive unexpectedly, insist that Sandy and Henry get out of bed and join him. He would then lie down on a blanket on the grass, with a small boy on each side, and point out the constellations.

Charley was very particular about water and milk. He insisted that the milk from Albert Leighton's be boiled before the children could drink it, but this upset his father, who knew which farmers ran a clean operation. Charley persisted. At this same period Charley was invited to visit a new dairy and inspect the pasteurization process. Everything went well until the end of the production line, where a man in soiled overalls was seated, licking his thumb each time he took a paper stopper out of a box and stuck it into the neck of the bottle. The manager, unconcerned, explained that the automatic capping machine had not arrived as yet.

The Best family still has the tattered copy of the 1936 edition of Ruth Webb Lee's *Handbook of Early American Pressed Glass Patterns* that Margaret bought in 1937 and uses her pieces of pressed glass, to which many more have been added. On her top shelf, Mrs. Mariner Leighton had six plain goblets of Continental pattern that had belonged to her mother-in-law. She asked her husband if he would mind selling them to Margaret. He turned away. Mrs. Mariner explained, "He can't tell you until he spits" — he chewed tobacco. Mariner said that he would sell the glasses: "They stay right there on the shelf. She washes them twice a year and puts them back." Pressed glass can still be bought reasonably. Nova Scotia glass that was produced for a limited period in the 1880s and 1890s is a special attraction — buyouts and closures by firms in Montréal and Toronto stripped the Maritimes of their production and the glass workers in Trenton, Nova Scotia, broke the moulds so that no one else could use them.

In the summer of 1937 there was a serious polio epidemic in Toronto; over 1,000 cases had been reported in Ontario, and there were several cases in New Brunswick. Charley had to return to his lab for the beginning of the academic year but he decided to leave the family in Maine. Early in September he and his mother left West Pembroke for Toronto. Lulu Best was going to Coboconk where Hilda and her children were staying at the Salters' cottage. Charley reported that Dr. Defries, at the Connaught Lab, was "up to his neck in the polio work." Although there seemed to be some abatement in the epidemic, there were still lots of cases. In spite of being busy at the lab, being entertained for meals by their friends, and playing golf with Bruce Macleod, he missed the family and was "very much fed up with the empty house."[370]

By 19 September, Charley thought it safe for the children to return to Toronto, and he drove east and joined them. A frequent excursion was to walk down the hill from the house to the cove at low tide and dig clams on the mud flats. The boys soon learned to know where the clams were hiding. They boiled the crop in seawater over driftwood until the clams opened, then dipped them in melted butter. Any that were left over they rolled in cornmeal and fried or used in chowder for another meal. When the gill net was picked in the early morning before the gulls stole the catch, the smelts and herring were rolled in cornmeal and then fried.

Charley took Margaret and Linda to Boston for a few days. On the way, they bought a schooner weather vane for the farm. Margaret got a copy of Robert P. Tristram Coffin's *Kennebec: Cradle of Americans* (1937); the Bests were to show great interest in this Maine writer. Each trip down this coast they stopped at old haunts and made a point of exploring new peninsulas, bays, and harbours. They admired the architecture — there were many fine examples of wooden homes and churches built in a more prosperous era. On this trip, Margaret noted the grand old colonial houses with lookouts and widow's walks at Portsmouth in New Hampshire, at that state's very narrow threshold on the sea.

Charley had a thorough examination by Drs. Elliott Joslin and Leland McKittrick, a vascular surgeon at the Deaconess Hospital in Boston, whose judgment Joslin valued highly.[371] As well as checking his duodenal ulcer, they found symptoms of an infected appendix, but decided that it was quite safe for Charley to carry on with his travels. Dr. Joslin followed up with a letter insisting on more tests. He also wrote of a recent flight to Detroit and back. "Flying really is wonderful, and so much more relaxing than an automobile. Think of it."[372] In his reply, Best said, "With regard to your comments on flying, I would really enjoy it very much. I am afraid, however, that it would be impossible to obtain Margaret's consent to this means of locomotion. I imagine she thinks the danger of flying is greater than that of more carefully controlled motoring."[373] Charley had flown for the first time in 1933 in New Haven, with Dr. John Fulton of Yale. Dr. Richard Light, the expert on Africa, was the pilot. Margaret did not take her first flight until 1949.

The trip back to Toronto was lovely, with the autumn colours, cooler temperatures, and less traffic than at the height of the tourist season. In Toronto, the polio scare was not completely over. Charley accepted some social invitations, but Margaret refused. "I don't like to ask Mary and Maria to stay at home if I won't stay myself."

Following up on the consultation in Boston, once back in Toronto Charley saw Drs. Roscoe Graham and Ray Farquharson, and they decided to take his appendix out at the Toronto General. There was some question that his appendix trouble might be bad for his ulcer. The operation took place in early November, and it was unusually lengthy, but finally Dr. Farquharson called Margaret to say that all was well. She was surprised, as she thought that it would just be starting; Charley had purposely given her the wrong time.

He was in the hospital for five days — rather tiring, with up to fourteen visitors a day. Margaret took down the J.E.H. MacDonald[374] sketch, *Lake O'Hara,* circa 1920, that Charley had recently given her, and hung it in the hospital room. Margaret wrote, "I wish we had one of his of the Algoma country." This came later. While recuperating from the operation in late 1937 Charley started painting. "Charley began to paint as soon as he was able to sit up. He copied the MacDonald and the A.Y. Jackson. He certainly gets a lot of pleasure out of painting." The Jackson must have been *Fox River, Gaspé,* done in April 1936. Charley's first attempts were two small watercolours of the Albert Leighton house and the barn at Schooner Cove, dated by Margaret as July 1936. They show little of the originality and sense of colour of his later works in oil. Best did a small copy — so marked — of Banting's *Church at St-Fidèle,* dated "about 1930," the original had been a gift from the artist.

Several artists tried to teach Charley how to paint, but he was independent. By the mid-1940s, he was painting quite a lot, largely in Maine. Schooner Cove appeared on canvas from every angle and in all types of weather and every time of day. Charley made his own frames from split-cedar fence rails or whatever came to hand.

Fred Banting is much better known as an artist. In Québec and in the Arctic he painted with A.Y. Jackson who obviously influenced his style.[375] A.Y. said that Banting "liked the artist's freedom from responsibility, of which he had had just a little too much as director of a big research laboratory. He wanted to get away where no one knew him, but the name 'Banting' had become almost a household word all over the world. When people would ask him if he was '*Dr.* Banting,' he would say, 'No, he's my cousin,' or 'He's my brother.'"[376] Best also liked to get away from the limelight, but he was not as uncomfortable with his celebrity as Banting.

December 1937 saw another trip to Boston and New York. Charley, as usual, spent time with Dr. Joslin and his diabetic specialists. He lectured after a dinner at the St. Botolph Club,[377] arranged by Dr. Reginald Fitz, to a group of forty surgeons, and he addressed the Harvard Medical Society on his work with heparin. Margaret visited Mrs. Joslin, some of the Macleod relatives, and the Mahons.

In New York, Margaret and Charley visited Dr. and Mrs. William Thalhimer. He was a colleague of Charley's, and the two couples had become good friends since their London days. He was now director of the Human Serum Division of the Public Health Institute of the City of New York. He had worked with CHB in Toronto and in 1938, they had published a paper with D.Y. Solandt, *Experimental Exchange Transfusion Using Purified Heparin.*[378]

Next to insulin, the greatest contribution to medicine where Charles Best was a major player was the purification of heparin. Best greatly respected the work of Jay McLean, the discoverer of heparin in 1916. McLean, of Johns Hopkins University, was delighted that Best was carrying on his work in Toronto and sent him all his papers. Best also appreciated the contributions of Professor W.H. Howell, also of Johns Hopkins, with whom McLean had worked.[379]

From 1933 to 1936 Best organized a team of researchers, both basic and clinical, to first purify and then use heparin clinically. Arthur Charles, an organic chemist, worked with D.A. Scott at the Connaught Labs on the development and purification of heparin. Professor W.E. Gallie, Head of the Department of Surgery, suggested to Best that they could co-operate clinically in the research. Gallie nominated the surgeon Dr. Gordon Murray to examine the possible use of heparin in surgery. This research resulted in a key paper on the subject in 1937.[380]

By 1937 heparin had been shown to have a clinical application in the prevention of thrombosis. A year later it had also been used experimentally in blood transfusions. At that period, however, the great advances in heart surgery of the second half of the twentieth century were yet to take place. Fifty years later, W.G. Bigelow, a top Canadian cardiac surgeon, revealed the history of heparin and the extent of its application and significance: "Besides heart surgery and the artificial kidney there are many procedures that require heparin: one-third of a million coronary arterial dilations (angioplasties); at least two million cardiac and vascular diagnostic studies; the surgical repair of arteries and the treatment of phlebitis; and a vast number of hospital and experimental laboratory techniques."[381]

Bigelow, like Best, had great praise for the contributions of Jay McLean.[382] In No. 53 of his *Selected Papers*, "Preparation of Heparin and its Use with First Clinical Cases," Best quoted at length from letters he had received from McLean in 1940. Bigelow observed: "The priceless knowledge and future benefits of heparin remained locked up for many years. Then Charles Best, a physiologist and a genius with clear and unerring perception, recognized the immense potential of safe heparin. His vision extended beyond its value in research to imagine the use of heparin in clinical medicine (the care of patients)."[383]

Dr. Gordon Murray explored the application of heparin in surgery. Murray examined damaged sections of arteries or veins with the naked eye and under the microscope, and Best examined the effect of heparin in preventing platelets from collecting on an injured blood vessel's lining, which could have formed a clot.

In a close parallel with the experiments leading to insulin's discovery, "Best demonstrated blood flowing out of a heparinized animal, through a glass tube, and back into the animal without obstruction from platelets and blood clots. This was dramatically recorded on movie film by photographing through a microscope" which Bigelow remembered seeing as a student in 1935. "To be able to see cells in action was a whole new thrilling adventure." According to Best, "the experimental evidence of the prevention of thrombus formation initiated by platelet agglutination (sticking) was completely satisfactory before attempts were made [as of 1935] to apply solutions of purified heparin to clinical problems."[384]

Bigelow observed: "The obviously unique feature of the heparin story is the contrast in personalities of the two famous principals, Best and Murray. It would be difficult to imagine a successful team of long standing with greater differences in character. I recall Best, my professor of physiology, as quiet and charming. He was both relaxed and dignified. During a discussion, his softly spoken, but weighty comments were offered with no attempts to ensure that they were heard or understood. Consequently, students had to pay close attention to hear everything he said. Best's great forte was his unusual ability to lead a team to work together successfully. How fortunate that he had this quality, because a great deal of cooperation was necessary in the process of refining heparin. Scientists and graduate students came from all over the world to work with him at the University of Toronto." His colleagues in this work included Arthur Charles, David Scott, Louis Jaques, William Thalhimer, D.Y. Solandt, D.L. MacLean, and Campbell Cowan. "Best had a wide influence. He prepared the minds of a large percentage of the future chairmen of physiology, biochemistry, and pharmacology departments, as well as research institutes in English Canada. Each person knew that his efforts would be recognized. Best would not 'steal the show,' as illustrated by the five Charles and Scott heparin articles ... Best's name does not appear in those articles in the list of authors, although the idea, the resource and the overall direction came from him."[385]

In 1999, Dr. Shelley McKellar completed her PhD thesis on Gordon Murray at the University of Toronto. This work illuminated the relationship between Murray and Best, who did not share a close working or personal relationship. The two were also "different types of researchers and men; in time, these differences became apparent to everyone on the team and a rift began to grow. According to Jaques, Murray refused 'to gloss over the failures and inabilities of other people. Best was a remarkable scientist-politician [and] for Murray this attitude was anathema.'"[386] Whatever the differences in their personalities, there was certainly a professional respect between the two; Best trusted Gordon Murray to operate on Margaret's appendix in June 1937.

A dramatic footnote to the heparin story was that of Helen Chute, a medical graduate of the University of Alberta. She remembered with emotion the birth of her first child, Judy, on 18 June 1941, only a few days after her husband, Laurie, who was one of Best's prize graduate students, had left for overseas military service. Helen's legs gradually turned black as a result of disseminated intravascular clotting — a potentially fatal condition. On learning of the situation, Charles Best came to see her and said, "I will make enough heparin for you. You are one of the family." He made and brought the necessary amount to the Toronto General Hospital each day for three weeks which Helen always considered had saved her life. After a month and a half in hospital Helen went home: "For a long time now I have wanted to tell you how much I appreciated your coming to see me in the hospital and to say thank you for your kindness to Laurie and me in giving me the heparin. I felt so much better after you had been in. I had been so lonely and frightened, I really think I started on the road to recovery from that day. I am now doing very well and have been home a week. I should love to introduce our Judy to you and Mrs. Best some day before I leave for the west in September. Laurie joins me in saying thank you though the very words seem inadequate."[387] Captain A.L. Chute also wrote gratefully to Best from England. "I am more in debt to you than I can ever hope to repay. I know from Helen's letters that for a time at least she was in great terror and I know that your kindness and reassurance had much to do with her recovery. As for the heparin I can only thank Devine Providence that she was in Toronto and that we were fortunate enough not to be born too soon. I appreciate too your generosity in making the heparin available."[388] It was an event that neither of them ever forgot.

Early in 1938, Margaret and Charley Best left Toronto for Eli Lilly and Company in Indianapolis, where they stayed with Dr. and Mrs.

G.H.A. Clowes. Margaret's first comment in her diary was that their hosts had added to their collection of works by Old Masters. The collection now included a Frans Hals self-portrait, from which a special medal had recently been struck; a small Rembrandt of an old man; three Holbeins; two Gainsboroughs; two Reynolds; a Goya; and an El Greco. Ironically, the ability of the Clowes to purchase Old Masters was partly because of insulin. The only time Henry Best ever heard his father express what might be called envy was when he talked of several art collections of which he knew, including that of the Clowes. Charley wished that he could have made it possible for Margaret to indulge her love of art by collecting paintings that interested her.

While Best made a rush trip to Dallas in March 1938, where he spoke six times in one day, word came that he had been elected a Fellow of the Royal Society of London. Professor Macleod had kept his word from 1931 and had nominated Best. Margaret said, "It is a great thing. We are all so happy about it. I met Charley at the train with the good news." Letters of congratulations came from Dr. Frank Lee Pyman, director of research with Boots Pure Drug Company Ltd. of Nottingham, England; Dr. Charles Lovatt Evans; and Dr. John Mellanby, professor of physiology at Oxford. Cables arrived from Sir Patrick Laidlaw and Sir Henry Dale. A cable from Lady Mellanby said simply, "Hurrah!" For Best the Fellowship in the Royal Society was always to remain the most important scientific recognition that he received.

On 27 May 1938, Margaret and Charley Best left Toronto by train for Québec on their way to England for Charley's induction as a Fellow of the Royal Society. Both sons were asleep when they left the house, which was just as well, "as Sandy has taken to sobbing when Charley has gone away the last time or two." They had a rough crossing on the *Empress of Australia*. Margaret came down with the flu. They were travelling tourist for the first time, to save money, and found it fine except for the meals; Margaret did not like the three worms that she found in her salad. Don and Barbara Solandt and their baby daughter, Barrie, were on the same ship.

At the Kenilworth Hotel in London, Margaret recovered in a few days. The Dales, Robin and Anne Lawrence, and others sent flowers to her room. Robin Lawrence was discussing plans for the two couples to tour the châteaux country of France, taking his Packard car.

Charley was very busy. He gave a speech to the staff of St. George's Hospital. On 9 June, he gave the Stephen Paget Lecture at the London

School of Hygiene, for the Research Defence Society, founded by Paget, which supported the use of animals in medical research. There were apparently several anti-vivisectionists there, but they did not disrupt the proceedings. Sir Edward Mellanby and A.V. Hill were on the platform. Various people such as Lady Mellanby came from the lecture to tell Margaret how well it had gone. The next evening Robin Lawrence had a dinner for Charley at the Royal Automobile Club. Charley was delighted that his old friend and mentor from the Connaught Labs, Dr. J.G. FitzGerald, was there.

Margaret said, "We have so many invitations that we don't know what to do with them." They had lunch at the Canadian high commission with Vincent and Alice Massey on 13 June. The Dales were there, as well as Alice Massey's sister and her husband; First Secretary Lester Pearson and his wife, Maryon; and Dr. Arthur Ellis, a Toronto medical graduate and later professor of medicine at London, and his wife. Margaret and Charley spent Saturday evening with Robin and Anna Lawrence and young Rob, Charley's godson.

Next day Charley gave a lecture at University College, London, on "Heparin and Thrombosis." Sir Henry Dale moved the vote of thanks. Margaret was happy that the lectures had gone well. The Bests went to John and Elizabeth Beattie's in Hampstead for dinner. Dr. Beattie was the director of research for the Royal College of Surgeons. Margaret wrote, "Charley is the limit. I think he is wonderful to do so many things. He is off right now to have a French lesson at Hugo's on Oxford Street. This is the third he has had since we arrived." The impetus for improving his French at this stage was the upcoming trip to France with the Lawrences. He had various teachers in Toronto over the years, and used Berlitz records, but his French never developed beyond a fairly rudimentary stage — possibly because his attempts were too sporadic, interrupted by lecture tours or other duties.

Charles Best at the age of thirty-nine became a Fellow of the Royal Society on the evening of 16 June 1938. The other person inducted was Sigmund Freud (as a foreign member), but he was not present. A Nobel laureate Sir William Henry Bragg, head of the Royal Institution, was president. He showed the Bests portraits of previous presidents, including the founder, King Charles II, and also "a great book" with signatures of all fellows. Sir Frank Edward Smith, a physicist, and A.V. Hill were the current secretaries. Margaret recorded, "Then, the little ceremony took place. Charley went up and signed his name in the great book and Sir William shook hands with him." He dined with the other fellows at the Athenaeum Club, just opposite, on Carlton Terrace. He was surrounded by old friends. Sir Joseph Barcroft sat on one side of him, Sir Henry Dale on the other, and Sir Edward Mellanby across the table.

Margaret noted that Dale said on one occasion during this visit, "There are two kinds of scientists: those who explore and do new work and those who carry along in some field discovered by others. He said that Charley is very much an explorer." Margaret added, "Lady Mellanby assured me the other day that, in the scientific world, after her husband comes Charley, as far as she is concerned." May Mellanby, a scientist in her own right, left no doubt about her likes and dislikes. Sir Edward and Lady Mellanby were an unusual and productive research team, first in Cambridge, Sheffield and then in London, on rickets, Vitamin A, and many other topics. Sir Edward was Secretary of the Medical Research Council from 1933 to 1949. Lady Mellanby also carried on her own independent research projects.[389]

The Bests were pleased to accept a second invitation from the Canadian high commissioner, Vincent Massey, and his wife, Alice. At the dinner, "Mrs. Massey remembered that we were going to the châteaux country and she ran off from her many guests to find two books for us on that part of France. She insists that we must keep them. Both Mr. and Mrs. Massey are awfully nice." The Bests and the Lawrences left in Robin's Packard for a week in France. It was a delightful trip. They enjoyed the sights, the food and wine, and each other's company.

The Dales had a sherry party, where the Bests met Lady Marjorie Pentland, daughter of Lord Aberdeen, who was governor general of Canada from 1893 to 1898. Lady Pentland told how her family, when travelling by train in Canada, took horses with them and rode at various points along the way. They also met for the first time Alexander Todd, "very Scotch and very nice," newly appointed professor of chemistry at Manchester. He was married to Alison, daughter of Sir Henry and Lady Dale. Like his father-in-law, Todd went on to receive the Nobel Prize, the Order of Merit, and the presidency of the Royal Society. He was elevated to the House of Lords as Lord Todd of Trumpington. Years later, when Lord Todd was chancellor of Strathclyde University in Glasgow, the students named the campus pub "The Lord Todd" which he considered the most unusual honour he had received. On visits to the pub he delighted in going behind the bar and serving drinks.

Boots Pharmaceutical Company hosted a lunch for the Bests in a private room at the Savoy Hotel in the Strand. This was not the first time that

Boots had entertained the Bests. The host was supposed to be Lord Trent of Nottingham of the Boot family, but he was officiating at the Agricultural Show in Cardiff. Dr. Frank Pyman, the scientific director, was host in his stead. Boots was one of the British firms producing insulin. The company hoped to entice Best to become its director of research.

Before they left home Alison Dale Todd had written to Charley congratulating him on his Fellowship in the Royal Society. She had said that she looked forward to seeing him and Margaret in London: "I'm sure the excitement and Mr. Hitler's antics will have subsided by then and things will be normal again."[390] She was not alone in this vain hope. Though everyone was concerned about what Hitler was up to in Europe, there was still the hope that it would be resolved peacefully. When the Bests were in London, just before Hitler showed his hand by seizing Czechoslovakia in the late summer, everyone was uneasy about the rise of fascism in Europe. Understandably, it was still hoped that war would be avoided.

Margaret and Charley had dinner one July evening with Charles and Laura Lovatt Evans at a favourite restaurant, the Criterion, and saw Robert Sherwood's *Idiot's Delight*, with Raymond Massey. Margaret described it as "quite dreadful in the background of war, especially now when there has been so much talk of war. The play had its light side too, and Raymond Massey was really very fine." This was the only mention Margaret made of international politics during the visit to Britain and France. As events turned out, this was to be Margaret's last trip across the Atlantic until after the war in 1947.

Just before their departure, Lady Dale gave Margaret and Charley a George II silver mug for Henry from his godfather. It was made in London, probably by the silversmith Thomas Moore, in 1748, just when Henry's Best ancestors arrived in Canada.

After a short stay in Toronto, the family left on 21 July 1938 for Maine. Sandy travelled better than ever before. "He was so interested in making a census of the animals he saw on the way that he had no time to be car sick. 'How many chickens are there? People! People! Stop talking and tell me — how many chickens!?'"

That summer saw a lot of basic changes to Schooner Cove. The house, covered in cedar shingles like most houses in the area, was painted white, and there were green shutters added. Two artists, Lucy Jarvis and her friend, Helen Weld, spent several weeks in the area. They had a tent and also used the Bests' cottage at Leighton Point. The Bests met them through the Saint

John artist, Jack Humphrey, several of whose paintings they owned. Lucy was from Toronto and had studied there and in Boston. Helen was from Lowell, Massachusetts. Lucy did many children's portraits, and that summer, she also did a pastel portrait of Margaret with Blarney, the Kerry Blue terrier. After Helen died in 1996, a sketchbook turned up entitled, "Grand Manan and Eastport, 1938." It contained sketches of various places on Grand Manan, with which the Bests were familiar, and several scenes of the buildings at Schooner Cove Farm, one of the village of West Pembroke, and two of Lulu Best's cottage at Leighton Point. One particularly delightful drawing was simply entitled "Sandy" with only a straw hat on the ground, a rake leaning against a shingled wall, and a bunch of carrots. Sandy Best at seven was already an enthusiastic gardener. The portrait of Margaret by Lucy Jarvis was framed and hung in the dining room at 78 Old Forest Hill Road. "The pose is awfully nice, I think, and the colours (pastel) are lovely. And Blarney is perfectly sweet!"

Margaret and Charley's fourteenth anniversary was 3 September 1938. A.G. Huntsman of the University of Toronto and of the Marine Laboratory in St. Andrews that later bore his name, and his wife, Florence, and John Satterly, the brilliant and eccentric professor of physics at Toronto, and his wife, May, arrived unexpectedly for the occasion. Ruth and Vin Price of Toronto came from their farm at Dipper Harbour, New Brunswick, and also Dr. Hugh Farris from Saint John. Herbert and Lulu Best, Lucy Jarvis, and Helen Weld were also there. "Mrs. Best made me a bride's cake and a bridegroom's cake for Charley. There were nine of us for dinner. We had baked beans and pickles, hot rolls and brown bread, pumpkin pie and coffee and the bride's cake." The baked beans are an East Coast specialty, made with salt pork and molasses in a crock at the back of the oven in a wood stove. "After dinner, Mrs. Best played the old organ and Dr. Best sang *Dalhousie*. We had a very gay time. Sandy and Henry came down and had a bit of the cake."

In the autumn the normal routine resumed in Toronto. In December, the Bests went to Pittsburgh. Charley was very busy at the Mellon Institute. Margaret was delighted when it was arranged that she could see the Carnegie International Show of pictures, even though it had closed two days earlier. "I can't think why there is no Canadian exhibit. There were German, French, Polish, Italian, etc., but the British section appeared to be entirely English." There were no paintings from Canada or other Commonwealth countries. There was also the Stephen Foster Memorial "which houses Mr. J.K. Lilly's fine collection of Foster memorabilia." Both Margaret and Charley loved Foster's music. In the Best home, Charley regularly requested such favorites as "Oh Susannah," "Beautiful Dreamer," "Old Folks at Home" and "Come Where My Love Lies Dreaming." Charley liked to sing; Margaret was not musical, but Linda had a good voice. Sandy played well and had quite a good voice; Henry played badly and had the best voice.

Christmas 1938 was "a bit dreary." Sandy was in bed with the flu and measles. Charley and Gordon Murray were called to New York to administer heparin to a Mr. Arthur Schulte who was very ill with a thrombosis. Charley arrived back Christmas morning, bringing some measles serum with him from New York to give to Henry, hoping that he would avoid getting a bad case, and it worked. Margaret added, "It took Jessie Ridout, Linda and me to hold Henry while Charley gave him the injection. He is a little tiger on such an occasion."

Charles Best won a very special honour in early 1939 from the University of Toronto, the Charles Mickle Prize, for his work on histaminase, choline, and heparin. Sir Frederick Banting, Sir Henry Dale, Ivan Pavlov, Sir Thomas Lewis, Edward and May Mellanby, and George Minot were earlier winners. Best had won the Ellen Mickle Prize on his graduation in medicine in 1925 and was the only person to have won both. Margaret was very proud, but she added that the Fellowship in the Royal Society was "the nicest thing of all to Charley's way of thinking."

Early in the new year, the Best family enjoyed one of many happy days at the Connaught Labs Farm with Neil and Hollie McKinnon, and their three daughters, Barbara, Ann, and Jane. Charley rode "Priest," the favourite of all the horses he ever owned. Priest was a large gelding, seventeen and a half hands, that Brigadier General Denis Draper, CMG, DSO, chief of the Toronto police force, had given him. On one occasion, Priest probably saved Charley's life when he refused to canter between two trees. After several refusals, Charley dismounted and found a wire strung across the two trees that only the horse had seen.

On one trip to New York, Best, looking for funding, met with the Millbank Foundation. Jeremiah Millbank, an investment banker in New York, founded in 1917 the Institute for the Crippled and Disabled — the first U.S. rehabilitation centre. Best also saw Arthur Schulte whom he and Gordon Murray had rushed down to see at Christmas. Schulte was president of Dunhill International, a tobacco manufacturer, and may have made a grateful donation to their research funds.

Yale University in New Haven, Connecticut, also seemed very interested in Charles Best's work and had invited him to lecture several times during the 1930s. In 1939, he lectured on "Heparin and Thrombosis." While in New Haven Margaret was invited to the Boston Symphony with Serge Koussevitzky conducting, the fourth time that she had heard this orchestra. She heard Sergei Prokofiev's *Peter and the Wolf,* first performed in Moscow in 1936, and she wished that Sandy had been there.

From New Haven, Margaret and Charley went to Boston where they again stayed with the Joslins at 81 Bay State Road. Charley lectured on recent work on diabetes in the Sanders Theater in Memorial Hall at Harvard. Some 1,200 doctors, medical students, and others attended. Margaret loyally wrote, "You could have heard a pin drop at any moment — many took notes."

In Toronto the Bests went to a rally in Maple Leaf Gardens on 15 March 1939 to support both Fred Banting and Vin Price who were involved in the Leadership League. The Leadership League was a "militant and vigilant organization" that intended to "clean up the old political tools," which "are neither broken nor worn out; they are just dirty." Dr. Herbert Bruce, chairman of the League's Citizens' Advisory Committee, spoke, as did founder C. George McCullagh, publisher of the Toronto *Globe and Mail.* Fred Banting, the vice-president, was on the platform but did not speak. Margaret remarked, "Fred is looking awfully well." McCullagh exhorted the public: "Join this League of yours, not regarding it as a new party or as the enemy of the old ones; not turning from your old political allegiance, but working through it and through this League to clean and reshape the old parties so that they shall honestly and truly serve the people."[391] These concerns took a back seat as world events rapidly unfolded in the next few months.

At eight years of age, Sandy was old enough to go to concerts. Dressed in a grey flannel suit and Stewart tartan tie (he had insisted on wearing a "family" tie: his great-grandmother was Sarah Ann Stewart) he very much enjoyed the Toronto Symphony. A child prodigy played a Schumann piano concerto and Sandy was impressed. He knew the *Romanian Rhapsodies* by Georges Enesco from records. He was disappointed that the conductor did not, "throw his little stick up in the air and catch it." A few days later, Sandy was taken to see the colour film *The Mikado* made by the D'Oyly Carte Company and the London Symphony Orchestra. His mother read him the libretto and the names of the characters beforehand.

This was typical of the care that Margaret took with Sandy and Henry, to make sure that they got the most out of any performance.

That spring, Sandy played Schubert's *Slumber Song* in the first of many piano recitals. He had been in bed again with bronchitis, and Henry with the croup, "a most alarming attack — terrible coughing, like a dog barking. We steamed the room for many hours." Both boys later remembered the blinds closed, the steam rising, and sometimes the wallpaper hanging loose from the walls.

Many scientists and others, particularly those who were Jewish, were attempting to flee Europe. A.V. Hill and Henry Dale were prominent in the movement to help as many of their persecuted colleagues as possible. Otto Loewi had shared the Nobel Prize with Dale in 1936 for their work on acetylcholine. He had fled Austria in 1938 for England and later the United States. On 11 May 1939, Sir Henry wrote to Best thanking him for agreeing to take Loewi's son Guido to work in his laboratory: "I should like you to know that I have found his reaction to the conditions which were sprung on him at the Anschluss better than that of the vast majority of young exiles. He tells me that he learnt to ride well, and care for horses, during his service with the Austrian artillery. He has pleasant manners, and a very humble sense of his lack of any expert qualification for the kind of work you may be able to give him; but I am sure that you will find him ready to do anything you ask."[392] Guido was to be part of the Best household for many years.

There was great excitement over the visit of King George VI and Queen Elizabeth to Toronto, the first visit of a reigning British monarch to Canada. The Bests watched the royal railway car pass on the line at the bottom of the Salters' garden on 22 May 1939. Margaret, Charley, and Linda went down to the university to see the royal couple there. In the evening, they took the boys and Uncle Bruce to Jessie Ridout's family home on Parkside Drive to see the royal visitors drive by. "The Queen looked very happy and sweet each time, but the King was very solemn."

Shortly after the Royal Visit, Aunt Lillie Hallam, sister of Charley's father, died in Toronto on Friday 26 May 1939. Herbert Best had come up from Maine to see his sister before she died. She and her husband, the Reverend W.T.T. Hallam, had been most supportive of Charley when he first came to Toronto in 1915. He had stayed with them until they moved in 1922 to Saskatchewan where Hallam became Bishop of Saskatoon.

In early July of 1939, the Bests went to Maine without Linda Mahon, who had taken a trip to the west. Mr. Albert[393] had built a new chimney in the farm house from old bricks. For Sandy's eighth birthday party at the cottage on 7 July 1939, Lulu Best had a supper of haddock and strawberries. His presents included Howard Pyle's *Robin Hood*, Arthur Ransome's *Old Peter's Russian Tales*, and Ruskin's *King of the Golden River*. Blarney, Margaret's Kerry Blue terrier, arrived by train and was picked up at St. Stephen. The round of supper parties, deep-sea fishing, clam digging in their own cove, golf, and welcoming relatives and friends kept everybody busy. Charley worked several hours every day on articles or revising chapters of one of his physiology texts. The Mahons arrived from Cambridge, Massachusetts, and Henry took up his usual pursuit of the salmon in the Dennys River. Sandy was now allowed to saddle and unsaddle his pony; Great-Uncle Bruce Macleod rode with him.

That summer too, Sandy learned to milk a cow from Mr. Mariner, and, from his father, how to shingle a roof, and Blarney, the terrier, spoiled an attempt to have a broody hen hatch eggs by chasing her down into the pasture. Several evenings were spent at the cottage watching falling stars and the seals and listening to the tide.

Dr. R.D. Defries, director of the Connaught Laboratories, wanted Best in Toronto when U.S. Surgeon General Thomas Parran was visiting in connection with the Rockefeller Foundation, and so Charley made a quick trip to Toronto and back. News of two honours reached him in Maine — the Baly Medal of the Royal College of Physicians in London, for the most distinguished work over the past two years in physiology, the purification of heparin, and an invitation for the summer of 1940 to deliver the John Mallet Purser Lecture at Trinity College Dublin.

On 2 August, Margaret wrote in her diary, "We are in a most distressing state of suspense — worse than last September. If war comes it will be ghastly. Charley is supposed to speak before the New Brunswick Medical Association but he really longs to get back to the lab where he has vitally important work to do" — especially the production of heparin, and the blood plasma project which Best had initiated earlier that year in the departments of physiology and physiological hygiene. Undoubtedly, he wanted to be closer to the centre of activity, whatever happened.

However, the Bests waited for a few more days. Dr. and Mrs. Francis Benedict and Dr. and Mrs. Best came for supper. The Newcombs, cousins of Charley's, came from Nova Scotia. Uncle Bruce took back to Toronto ninety-five jars of jelly — raspberry, apple, and cranberry — as well as many jars of pickles, all made in Schooner Cove Farm's kitchen. Charley addressed the New Brunswick Medical Association on diabetic research at its meeting in St. Andrews. His father attended, as did new acquaintances and many old friends, including Senator Cairine Wilson and some of her family and Dean Del Leighton of Harvard.

The Bests left West Pembroke on 31 August, 1939. Then Margaret wrote, "On Friday, September 1st, the war began by Germany bombing cities in Poland. We got that news as we sat at Firhurst Manor, on the north-eastern shore of Lake Ontario, having lunch." Henry Best, almost five, clearly remembered the adults listening intently to the car radio and being very serious.

On the third, Margaret and Charley's wedding anniversary, the family went to St. Andrew's Church in Toronto. Margaret wrote: "Shortly before 6 o'clock this morning, over there, England declared war on Germany. At noon today, France declared war on Germany." They had dinner at York Downs with Linda, Uncle Bruce, and Jessie Ridout, and went to the Canadian National Exhibition to see movies of the royal tour — the most patriotic thing they could think of to do. They had heard that morning about the sinking of the *Athenia*, but first reports were that most of the passengers had been saved. Charles Best started war work immediately. On 4 September, Margaret wrote, "It is all too horrible. Linda and Charley have worked almost all day at the lab. This is officially a holiday, but no one feels in a holiday mood." On 9 September, Margaret wrote, "The war news is very grave. Poland is having a bad time. Canada's part at the moment seems to be to supply Air Force men."

In early October, the war was obviously on everybody's mind, but there was no idea of how long it would last. Margaret wrote, "The distressing war situation continues. We wonder when things will be happy and peaceful again. Poland is gone now." Already a number of their friends were in uniform, like Dr. Cec Rae who was to go overseas in January 1940 as colonel of the first hospital unit from Canada. Dr. Rae became a brigadier and deputy director of Medical Services, 2nd Canadian Corps. Major Neil McKinnon of the Connaught Labs, professor of epidemiology, set up the lab for the 15th General Hospital Unit (for the Toronto General Hospital), Colonel "Mac" MacFarlane, a consulting surgeon with the same unit and later a brigadier, and several other friends, left for overseas.

The old Grace Hospital had become a military facility, and the blood donor service that Best started at the School of Hygiene was to move there. Drs. Laurie Chute, Robert Defries, Don Fraser, Reginald Haist, Jack

Magladery, Jessie Ridout, and Don Solandt made major contributions to the success of the project. Lorena Wellwood, Linda Mahon, Roy Sproat, and Hugh Aird were all involved in the blood work. Dr. William Thalhimer and Sophronia Myron from New York were working in Toronto at the time and contributed to the early stages of the work. The serum was prepared at the Connaught Laboratories and freeze-dried — a process that took seventy hours. When blood was needed, sterilized water was added to the dried serum. Over two million donations were received and dried, with most of them shipped to England.[394]

Too little has been written about the blood donor service and the preparation of plasma to be sent overseas. Professor Richard W. Kapp, of Ryerson Polytechnic University in Toronto, published two articles that help fill the gap. Of Charles Best's involvement Kapp wrote, "At his disposal was not only a cache of first-rate scientists, but also an excellent production facility. He maintained as well valuable links with the English, American and other Canadian centres working on blood substitutes." Kapp commented, "But surely the development of blood banking in Canada (where Best's part was decisive) ranks with the discovery of insulin in terms of lives saved!"[395]

While waiting for donors to arrive, staff members, many of whom expected soon to don uniform, quizzed each other on sections of the manual *Corporal to Field Officer* by Lieutenant-Colonel R.J.S. Langford.[396] The book covered organization and administration, duties, military law, map reading, marches, infantry in battle, protection, attack, and bugle calls.

Very early in the war in October 1939, Best wrote a long memo to his close friend A.V. Hill, Biological Secretary of the Royal Society, who was working with the Society's Physical Secretary and the Ministry of Labour to co-ordinate scientific manpower. The Connaught Laboratories were already supplying Professor John Beattie, director of laboratories for Britain's Royal College of Surgeons, with "a large quantity of heparin for use in the prevention of blood clotting during transfusion and in the securing of blood for the blood banks which had been set up." Connaught also sent heparin to Professor Ronald Christie for research into blood clotting, a seemingly prominent abnormality in many cases of phosgene gas poisoning.[397]

First, work commenced to prepare for Beattie a trial lot of blood serum. It was expected to use serum in clinical studies at Toronto's Hospital for Sick Children in cases of shock without haemorrhage. Best wrote, "Shock caused by wounds and histamine shock are to be investigated again. Recent studies at the Mayo Clinic have suggested that histaminase, an enzyme which I discovered in 1928, may be of use in preventing the effects of histamine intoxication. Whether or not histamine is actually liberated in shock, and whether or not histaminase counteracts these effects is still quite undecided. The whole staff is being gradually diverted from peace-time activities to those of more importance under our present condition."[398] To prepare for wartime conditions Best was attending lectures on military topics at the University Avenue Armouries every Tuesday and Thursday evening.

On 16 November 1939, Best wrote to Dale about linking British and Canadian war research. Best had thought that perhaps through Canada's National Research Council (NRC) and Britain's Medical Research Council (MRC), he and Fred Banting might go to England to help co-ordinate medical research, but that was off for the time being. "We have had a rather unsettled time giving up all our peace-time researches and trying to find some worthwhile military problems. I think we have been rather successful in some cases but it will take a long while to make sure. I had a very welcome letter from A.V. Hill and have sent back assurances that so far as my own laboratories go, any co-operative enterprises will be most heartily welcomed. A general liaison will be effected through the committee of the NRC which will go to England before very long to consult with the Medical Research Council."[399]

On 18 November, Dale wrote to Best with a standing invitation to stay with them and base himself at the NIMR, which was the only medical or scientific establishment in the London area not yet completely evacuated. The institute no longer had "any natural lighting or ventilation. Window darkening has also much altered the aspect of our corridors, etc., but the laboratories retain all their normal equipment and facilities, and we are an active and going concern."

Dale was resuming work on histamine shock started in the First World War and a project in concentrating blood plasma. He had heard earlier from John Beattie that Best was "accelerating the production of heparin for Britain's practical needs, and encouraged him to use, in this instance to the full, the help that the Connaught Laboratories can give, instead of trying, under emergency conditions, to get a manufacture hastily established" in Britain.

Best was wondering whether he should go to London. Dale stated, "If I thought that you would waste your time, or that the national and empire needs for the war would best be served by your staying where you are, I should say so quite frankly. I feel, on the contrary, that, if you can arrange to come, and if from all points of view it seems to you and your advisers the right thing to do, I believe that it would give important help to present activities here and in Canada. It will, of course, be a very great pleasure to see Banting, if and when he comes; but I believe that you could more easily advance the interest of the particular set of problems with which I am in contact, and in which you and I have common interests."[400] Sir Henry hoped that Best would come and stay with them in London, assuring Margaret that Charley would have "the same immediate access as we have to the Institute, with its air raid shelter and precautions." He closed with a further request for heparin for his own lab.

Margaret and Charley watched with sadness what was happening in Finland. They had happy memories of Finland after their trip to the Soviet Union in 1935. "The war goes on in such a depressing way. Finland has suffered so terribly. The Russians are battling away against Viborg." On Margaret's birthday, 30 November, Charley took her to the Royal York for lunch. They bought a paper telling of the Soviet bombing of Helsingfors (Helsinki) and other Finnish cities. "We loved Helsingfors and Viborg when we were over there in 1935, and we had a very depressed lunch."

Two days before Christmas 1939, Best wrote to Sir Henry Dale confirming that the heparin he requested had been sent. "I feel sure that you will have seen Banting before this and will have discussed with him the most suitable way in which a liaison between research workers in England and Canada can be effected. It will, of course, be of the utmost interest to me to hear what Banting has to say about the whole situation when he returns. It is obvious that if the MRC and the Royal Society group in England, and our own authorities, feel that any one of us would be useful as a liaison officer in England, whoever is selected will be only too glad to discharge that duty to the best of his ability." Charley accepted the Dale's offer of hospitality if he should be sent over to England during the war.[401]

In November Sir Henry had mentioned that their daughter Alison "has given us our first grandchild a week ago — Alexander Henry, who will be called 'Sandy,' to distinguish him from his father Alex [Todd], and also, of course, out of respect, for the distinguished young man who already bears that name." Charley replied that their two boys were intrigued to learn that a little boy in England was called "Sandy Henry."

Sandy continued at Forest Hill School, but Henry moved to Windy Ridge, a school set up by Dr. Bill Blatz of the university's Institute of Child

Study. Some university people sent their children there to support a colleague; others, because it was the fashionable thing to do. It was actually a good place for creative youngsters. Also, there had been fifty-four children in Henry's class in the public school system, compared to twenty at his new school.

Meanwhile, Margaret, who for some time had wanted to have Charley's portrait painted, asked Charles Comfort to do it. She very much liked his portrait of fellow artist Carl Schaefer, and Comfort agreed to paint Charley in watercolour. Apparently it was supposed to be kept a secret until it was finished. She confided to her diary, "It is to be my picture since I have arranged it all and I am going to pay for it myself. I long to have it turn out well." Later in December, she noted, "On Saturday Mr. Comfort came over with Charley's portrait. I had seen it in the studio on Thursday for the first time. It is very startling but I think very good. I have sent him a cheque — $159 with framing."

By mid-February, 1940, Best was growing impatient with the lack of decisions from Ottawa concerning his role in wartime research, and was proposing to take some colleagues to London on his own. "As a matter of fact," he wrote Dale, "I have not received a single word of enquiry or command from any official source in Canada and incidentally none from Banting since he left here. I realize that it is absolutely necessary for him to make recommendations or suggestions through the Department of National Defence here and there is perhaps some good reason for the delay. The arrangement which would suit me best if I am to be sent to England, would be to be given the opportunity and responsibility of organizing a small group from my own department and taking them over to work with you and your group."[402] Five days later, Best informed Sir Henry that Canadian scientists doing war research would probably receive army positions. He thought that he would have been ill-suited for the research on gas warfare that had been suggested for him. "I am greatly interested in the possibility that a Canadian Research Unit may be organized in Britain for the new hospital to be financed by the Canadian Red Cross."[403]

In his next letter, Sir Henry wrote that he had seen Banting, who thought that if Best went to England, he should concentrate on gas defence. Dale, however, disagreeing with this suggestion, urged Best to carry on with the heparin and blood serum projects: "The major medical problem of modern warfare is, after all, still the treatment of mechanical injuries and their results [i.e. haemorrhage and shock], and I am sure that you ought not be diverted from it."[404]

In addition to the lab, Best was busy lecturing and attending meetings in Minneapolis, the Mayo Clinic in Rochester, Minnesota, and the American Physiological Society in New Orleans. At the beginning of April 1940, he was in Montréal, staying with the Wilder Penfields to deliver the annual Hughlings Jackson Memorial Lecture on "Factors Affecting the Formation and Liberation of Insulin."[405]

A few days later in Toronto, Charley gave the lecture for his Charles Mickle Fellowship on "Blood Clotting, Thrombosis and the Action of Heparin." The lecture hall in the medical building was overflowing. Margaret took Sandy to hear his father speak for the first time. Sandy told people later that "his daddy was one of the greatest doctors in the world." In the evening the dean of medicine, Dr. Gallie, and his wife gave a dinner party in honour of the occasion where Sir Frederick and Lady Banting were amongst the guests. This was Margaret's first mention of Banting's second wife, Henrietta Ball, a graduate student at the University of Toronto, whom he had married the previous summer.

At the same time twelve physicians from across the United States met in Cleveland, Ohio, to establish the American Diabetes Association (ADA). Charles Best was not of this group, but several of its members were to become valued colleagues and close friends, particularly George Anderson of Brooklyn, Joseph Beardwood of Philadelphia, Cecil Striker of Cincinnati, the first president, and Frederick Williams of New York. Their names appear frequently in Charley's correspondence and in Margaret's diaries. Banting and Best were both made honorary presidents of the association.

Later in April Margaret, Charley, and Linda spent a night that they would never forget. They had seen Tallulah Bankhead years before in London in *The Green Hat*. Now they saw her in Toronto in *The Little Foxes*.[406] Several nights later, Ruth and Vin Price called to say that the actress was at their house for a party after the performance, and would they please join them. Margaret wrote that, "she was thin and slinky" when they had seen her in London. "Now she is many years older and quite fat. She is a most extraordinary person — with her deep voice and her husky laugh. She wears her hair to her shoulders and flings it about. She wore a red silk dress and nothing else, as far as one could tell — a more unconfined figure I have never seen. Tallulah is a rather extraordinary mixture — rather crude but very witty at times. It does us good to meet people so entirely different."

Dr. Yngve Zotterman of Stockholm was visiting Toronto. The Bests first knew the Zottermans in London in the 1920s, where both men were studying. He was in a highly agitated state, as his wife and three children were in Sweden, and the Germans had just invaded Denmark and Norway.

Early in May, Herbert and Lulu Best stayed with their daughter Hilda and had a happy visit with all the grandchildren. But it was to be Lulu's last trip to Toronto. Later that month, A.V. Hill stayed with the Bests. Aside from scientific matters, there was time for a discussion about education at dinner with guests Roscoe Graham, an abdominal surgeon, and Dr. H.B. van Wyck, chair of the department of obstetrics and gynecology at the University of Toronto. "We had a fine talk about education and what is best to do for our children. Roscoe feels, and rightly, I think, that on the other side there is a fine sense of values. We have a materialistic people in North America: the successful man with us is the man who makes lots of money. How can we impress on our children that money is not the goal? That the important thing is to become really cultivated, civilized people — to have resources within ourselves. We talked of the value of say, Latin, which is rather frowned upon now because it has no particular use in life later on. It is excellent discipline for the mind. As A.V. suggested, it also 'helps one to express oneself more clearly.'"

Hill thought that medical men in particular needed cultivated minds because of their contacts with so many in the community. Van Wyck graduated in classics before studying medicine and he had formed a string quartet with his own children. Hill sent his sons to an English "public" school in Highgate, but as day boys, so that they could meet and get to know many interesting people who visited their home. This discussion confirmed Margaret and Charley's ideas about the education of their own boys — music, literature, and nature were equally important to them.

Sandy and Henry were delighted to have the avuncular Englishman in the house. Unsure what to call him, the boys accepted his suggestion of "Uncle Hill." Henry was charmed by the thought that he now had an "Uncle Hill" and an "Uncle Dale." A.V., who was also the Member of Parliament for Cambridge, told Sandy a secret that he was to tell no one "because it might get to the Germans."

Everybody wanted to help the war effort. Margaret and a number of other women joined a Red Cross group to knit socks for servicemen. At one point she wrote, "The war news is so depressing. However, I don't write much about that in my diary." War guests evacuated from Britain started to arrive in Toronto. Mavis Carr Gunther, daughter of Francis and Hilda Carr, old London friends, came with her three children. Her husband had been an air raid warden and had asked a man to put out his lighter or torch; the man said that he would not take orders from a German and shot and killed Gunther. Two Le Gros Clark children, whose father was professor of anatomy at Oxford, had a letter from their father to Best; they ended up staying with Dr. Eric Linell, professor of neuropathology. The Bests expected Robin Lawrence's three sons, Rob, Adam, and Dan, to stay with them in Toronto, but they went instead to the country, away from London. Margaret commented, "The strain in England must be ghastly. It is bad enough here."

Later in the summer while the Bests were in Maine, two women and four children lived in their home. Mrs. Hugh Anthony Clegg settled in with Jane and Nicholas; she was born in France of Russian parentage, and her husband was editor of the *British Medical Journal*. Dr. Margaret Mitford brought Timothy and Terence; her husband, also Terence, taught at St. Andrews University in Scotland and her father, P.T. Herring, was professor of physiology and dean of science there. The wife of Henry Gilding, professor of physiology at Birmingham, arrived in Toronto with her four children. She was expecting another baby, so Best made arrangements for Dr. Don Low to look after her and promised to deal with the hospital expenses. A Mrs. Black, a cousin of Lady Mellanby's, came with her two children; her husband was in Hong Kong. Many people housed and helped the "war guests."

Margaret and Charley went to New York in early May 1940 when Charley spoke to the New York State Medical Association. Cousins Bill Macleod and Lorne Newcomb were there. Lulu Best had written to Lorne to tell him about the meetings. Drs. Billy Thalhimer and Keith Cannan were also in evidence. Margaret noted that the medical association paid for a room at the Waldorf Astoria for two nights, and then they moved to the Seymour. Even in New York there were reminders of the war. The Bests saw the liner *Queen Elizabeth*, painted grey for her wartime duties as a troop ship, lying in dock there.

They saw Robert Sherwood's *There Shall Be No Night* with Alfred Lunt and Lynn Fontanne, which was about a Finnish doctor who had won the Nobel Prize and his Armenian wife. Margaret noted, "The tears ran down my face and as a rule, I am not openly moved at the theatre." The man sitting next to Margaret was obviously pro-Nazi. He "kept saying, 'damned propaganda,' but on the whole, the feeling in the audience was very anti-Nazi. There were several bursts of applause. Lynn Fontanne was so exquisitely right as the wife. She wore a tomato red dress with a white frill at the neck. She is years older, we hear, than Alfred Lunt, but they make a wonderful team."

They also saw *Romeo and Juliet* with Vivien Leigh and Laurence Olivier. "She was perfectly lovely as Juliet — young and fresh, but I think Olivier was quite disappointing as Romeo." Margaret attended a show of Sir Jacob Epstein's sculptures: "Some of the heads were really exciting, but the gigantic Adam was terrific."

At home in Toronto Sandy and Henry were playing on the third floor, imitating someone in a story who slid downstairs on a tea tray. Sandy hit his head on a radiator and required three stitches. The next day, Sandy, Henry, and Henry's best friend, Tony Rolph, were in the garden. Henry fell backwards over Blarney, the terrier, who was eating a bone, and, not surprisingly, the dog bit him. He required eighteen stitches and, untypically, sat up and watched the procedure. During this same period, Linda Mahon had a bout of Ménière's disease that destroyed the hearing in her right ear. Yet Sandy and Henry later thought that when they were doing something they were not supposed to, she still heard better than most people!

Loving Maine and the sea, and anxious to keep up ties with the east coast, Margaret and Charley chose not to send their boys to summer camp, except in 1940. Sandy's friend, Ian Fraser, younger son of Don and Mary, had already been to the Farm Camp near Port Stanley on Lake Erie and had liked it. So Sandy joined Ian there for three weeks in July. Henry would gladly have gone too. Sandy liked camp but never went back.

After camp, the family drove off to Maine and the war guests moved in to the house. On 11 August, Herbert and Lulu Best went down to the farm for dinner. Lulu complained of a cramp in her hip. The next night, she stayed at her beloved cottage at the point. She wanted everyone to have breakfast on the verandah there on the Tuesday morning. Lulu sat at one end of the table, and Herbert at the other. Charley, Margaret, Linda, Sandy, Henry, Jessie Ridout, and Lorena Wellwood were all there. "We had pancakes and maple syrup and the men had bacon and eggs and we were all quite gay. Lorena and Jessie did all the running around and when the service was considered slow, Linda and Charley hit their glasses with spoons and called for speed."

The next day, back in the village, Mrs. Best was complaining that her hip was very sore, but she was arranging for a church supper. Margaret wrote, "She still looked very well. She had had so many troubles and pains in the past that it was very confusing to know what was the trouble."

Learning of Lulu's distress, several doctors, including Charles Armstrong of Robbinston, Norman Cobb of Calais, Herbert Everett of St. Stephen, and Clifford Harvey of Boston (possibly on holiday in the area), all drove to West Pembroke. They were unsure but decided to operate. Lulu was afraid to go to the Chipman Hospital in St. Stephen, New Brunswick, her husband's preferred facility, because she was concerned that, as she was not a naturalized American, she might not be allowed back over the border to Pembroke. However, they went to St. Stephen. She was made as comfortable as possible on the back seat of the big Chrysler; Dr. Best sat on one of the jump seats, and Margaret and Charley were in the front. The trip was only thirty miles but seemed a lot further.

Dr. Harvey operated, and Charley said that it was done "beautifully." It was a gangrenous appendix. She came through the operation pretty well and spoke to Margaret several times, but later she had a stroke. Her blood pressure was very high. "When Dr. Best knew that she would not get better, he longed to have her at home." On Monday August 19, their daughter Hilda arrived in St. Stephen and in the afternoon brought her mother back to Pembroke. She died shortly after seven o'clock that evening. "It is a tremendous loss for us all. The boys loved their Grammy dearly, and always wanted to go down to the cottage to visit her. Dr. Best feels that he has lost everything." Indeed, he was never well after that.

At Lulu's church, people came with bunches of flowers from their gardens. Rev. Mr. Williamson, "was restrained, and made a really touching little talk about Mrs. Best — her love of the wind and the waves and the trees at the point — her kindness to others. He didn't orate at all." A kind friend deeded a plot to Dr. Best in the corner of the cemetery against a fence, under an oak tree and with a view of the tide down below. "It is a beautiful place and Dr. Best is very happy about it." Her impressive memorial is a large Celtic cross, chosen by her daughter Hilda.

The family was concerned about Dr. Best, and who would keep house for him. Shortly after the funeral, Herbert Best had a heart attack and was confined to bed. Dr. Hugh Farris of Saint John, Charley's old friend, motored over to see him. In the months that followed, Herbert Best started to take large doses of belladonna or some other drug. Dr. Armstrong and other practitioners attempted to have his supplies cut off, but it was very difficult to do so.

When the family returned to Toronto in early September, faithful friends and colleagues Dr. Jessie Ridout and Lorena Wellwood were at the house with food and other supplies. Lorena Wellwood was a sorority sister of Margaret's. She was a teacher and worked at the university at one point. Jessie Ridout never called Charley anything but "Dr. Best" or "the Professor." She first worked with him in 1922 in the Connaught labs and again in 1927, completed her PhD with him in 1939 with a thesis, which came out of the work on choline, entitled "Certain Factors Controlling the Deposition of Liver Fat." She continued to do research into liver problems. As years passed, she became more and more involved in editing papers and other projects where she was working directly with "the Professor." She was very close to Linda Mahon and they did many things together. When the Bests were away, it was usually Jessie who stayed with Linda. Jessie never lived far away from the Bests' home.

For Henry's sixth birthday on 9 October 1940, Margaret, at Sandy's suggestion, cooked a duck. Margaret wrote, "I find that I am quite a good cook when it is necessary." But it was not a favourite task. She was looking for a cook and had already found a nurse-housemaid in Ruth Milnes, just sixteen years old. Dr. Herbert Best came to Toronto with Hilda and stayed for two weeks. He talked to his grandchildren about their grandmother. After a short time back home in Maine, he returned to Toronto, not happy anywhere.

Visitors to Toronto that October were Sir Evelyn and Lady Wrench. He was the founder of the English Speaking Union; she was the sister of Sir Alan Brooke, the general in charge of the defence of England. Charley moved the vote of thanks to Sir Evelyn after his speech about the "totalitarian states" and recounted a story that Mavis Carr Gunther had told him: "My mother and father go into an air raid shelter every night. They all lie down except the cook who sits bolt upright. She says it is too much like mixed bathing." That was about as *risqué* as CHB's stories ever got. "Mr. B.K. Sandwell was at the meeting and he asked Charley afterward if he could use the story in *Saturday Night*," the magazine of which he was managing editor. "It appeared a week or two ago in one of the editorials headed, 'Bomb Shelter Etiquette.'"

That autumn Charley examined candidates for the Royal College of Surgeons of Canada, along with Dr. J.C.B. Grant, head of anatomy at Toronto, and Professor Beecher Weld, head of physiology at Dalhousie in Halifax. He was also travelling again to Ottawa to try to clarify his role in the war effort. After the war Surgeon Commodore Archie McCallum wrote: "About mid-summer of 1940 the Medical Director General had a personal visit from the Professor of Physiology of the University of Toronto and his associate, offering facilities of that Department and of the Banting-Best Institute of Medical Research in whatever capacity the naval service might see fit to apply it in solving any of the problems confronted by the medical branch. This offer was gladly accepted and within two or three months the RCN Medical Research Division was in full operation."[407] The minister of naval affairs, the Hon. Angus L. Macdonald agreed to the formation of the Royal Canadian Naval Medical Research Division, which Best was to direct.

Charles Best had no idea at this stage what problems might be confronted by the medical branch of the navy. As has been seen in his correspondence with Dale, he thought for some time that he could make his best contribution by organizing a group from his department who could work with scientists in England producing heparin and blood serum.

From 19 May to 11 August 1940, Fred Banting kept a diary. Both he and Charley despaired of Canada and Britain's leaders. Banting wrote, "Our government is headed by a senile fossil of a vintage that would do credit to whisky."[408] Banting was attempting to get the necessary equipment for research on aeronautical problems. He was known to change his opinion about people. This was the case with Charley, but from his diary we see that he was also very critical of Ed Hall, one of his own protegés. Banting was impatient and sarcastic with Best's insistence on the need for blood plasma. "I also saw Best. He is rather a sorry figure. … He wants a group of people taken into the non-permanent militia so that they can wear uniforms to draw blood for serum."[409]

Banting had confidence in himself: "What I do feel is the responsibility of being right in my judgment as to what should be done and my judgment as to the best men to carry it through to effective completion and practical utility."[410] Four days later, Banting gave vent to his feelings about Canada and his reactions to war: "As a Canadian, I am deeply concerned with what Canada is doing. My life I consecrate to my Country, to my King, to the British Empire. I hold back nothing — because I believe in the cause that is Britain's. There are hundreds of thousands of my fellow Canadians who feel as I do. I am not pleased to be kept at home while others are in peril." He had served overseas in the Great War. "I would that it were my lot to again serve my country as the Medical Officer of a

Battalion. There is no one who has more abject terror of shells, bombs, bullets and death or destruction in any form than I have. But surpassing this fear is the privilege of service to the wounded, to those that fight, to the forces in the field, to comrades in arms."[411]

These are not the thoughts of the insensitive man that Banting is sometimes portrayed to be. It is worth noting that whatever his opinion of Best at this stage in their careers, they shared many of the same sentiments, hopes, and frustrations.

Charles and Margaret Best liked the results of the November 1940 U.S. vote, with Franklin Delano Roosevelt elected for a third term, although many of their American friends would disagree. During the previous summer when they were in Maine, at a dinner at the home of Henry and Jean Ganong Eaton in Calais, a guest had delivered a stinging attack on the president. Margaret was so upset that she left the party, and she and Charley drove back to West Pembroke. Henry Eaton came to Schooner Cove Farm the next day to apologize for his guest's behaviour. The Bests felt that they knew Roosevelt, and they believed that Americans should not be isolationist.

In the fall Charley considered looking for a small property in the country not too far from Toronto. He and Margaret wanted an outlet for themselves and the boys, and they loved nature. On Thanksgiving weekend in 1940, Margaret and Charley went to see a property described to them by J.A. Willoughby, who had a well-known real estate firm and owned the Georgetown Golf Club, where Charley and Clark Noble had worked as students.

They decided to buy the farm, which was not far from Georgetown, at the edge of the village of Stewarttown. "There are almost 96 acres in all — largish house on the Stewarttown Road (the 7th Line of Esquesing Township) and dilapidated barns — a good many acres of flat fields on top, then the crest of the hill and the lovely hillside and river valley — the west branch of the Credit. We have seen that hillside for twenty years from the golf course … I love the place." As snow fell, the family took skis and hauled supplies across the fields on a toboggan. By 25 January 1941, they had purchased the farm, in Margaret's name, for $5,250. They sold sixteen acres, including the ten-room house and the barns, all in bad shape, leaving eighty acres for themselves.

Charley's schedule was getting busier than ever. On 23 November 1940, the Bests left for Boston and New York. In Boston, Henry and Lydia

Mahon took them to see some small houses that would give them some ideas of what to build on their new farm property. In New York, Cousin Bill Macleod, realizing that they would have very little American currency because of wartime exchange regulations, gave Margaret money so that she could shop. Margaret did some shopping and saw Shakespeare's *Twelfth Night*[412] with Helen Hayes and Maurice Evans.

The big event was on Thursday 28 November 1940, when Charles Best gave the Harvey Lecture on heparin to the New York Academy of Medicine. Dr. Herbert Gasser, director of the Rockefeller Institute, introduced Best. Gasser was to win the Nobel Prize in 1943, and become a Fellow of the Royal Society in 1946. Like Best, "Gasser had worked in London with Dale and A.V. Hill and had never forgotten their inspiration."[413] The evening was a resounding success. Every seat was filled, and many people were standing — the largest audience to date at the Academy. Margaret was delighted "I have never heard Charley speak better."

Dr. Gasser and the Rockefeller Foundation were soon to play a crucial role in Best's work. While officials in Ottawa were still dragging their feet, at a meeting on 1 November 1940, Best had been nominated as one of the six scientific directors of the International Health Division of the Rockefeller Foundation to serve from 1 January 1941 to 31 December 1943.[414] He was the first physiologist on the IHD and the second Canadian; the only previous Canadian had been Dr. J.G. FitzGerald of the Connaught Labs, who had helped Best obtain a fellowship from the Foundation when he went to London in 1925. Charles Best, the new scientific director, as his first assignment early in 1941, was asked to undertake a nutrition survey in the southern United States.

By becoming a director himself Best saw that there was a great opportunity to involve the Rockefeller Foundation in research to help the war effort. Already there was a proposal for a Rockefeller Foundation Commission in Europe with a base in Lisbon.[415] A few weeks before the Bests' visit to New York, Wilbur Sawyer, secretary of the board of scientific directors of the IHD, wrote to a staff member, Dr. Hugh H. Smith, saying that it seemed "probable that there would be advantage in having a staff member in London ... Rapid changes are occurring ... You are of course fully aware of the risks which all of us take when we go into the warring areas of Europe." Sawyer saw an opportunity for "our assistance in the public health field in Great Britain."[416] Shortly afterwards Smith went to London to become the representative of the Rockefeller Foundation Health Commission in England.

Slowly Canadian officials were working on the needs of the different armed services. After New York, just before Christmas 1940, Best went to Ottawa to discuss what research was needed to help the Navy.

On his return before Christmas Charley found everyone had been ill in bed. Drs. Ray Farquharson and Staunton Wishart gave Linda a new drug for an ear infection — sulphathiazole. Wishart was consultant in oto-laryngology to the Hospital for Sick Children and Women's College Hospital, as well as being a member of St. Andrew's Church. Henry had a fever of 104; his room was steamed, and he had a mustard poultice on his chest. Charley and Margaret both came down with high fevers. Margaret had "chills and fever and my heart did queer things." Charley "was in a delightfully gay frame of mind, joking and laughing. I was sunk in the depths and begged him not to be so silly." Sandy felt so awful that he said to the nurse looking after the family, "I don't think I can stand it any longer. I'll have to kill myself."

On his way to spend Christmas with his family, Herbert Best had a coronary on the train between Montréal and Toronto. An ambulance met him and took him to the Salters. On Christmas Day, the Bests went to see Grandfather, and he was up and around to talk to the children. The next day he had another attack and, still at Hilda's, was confined to a hospital bed and had a nurse in attendance. "He has always been such an energetic person that it is a great hardship for him to lie still."

Early in 1941, Best wrote Henry Dale to congratulate him on his election as president of the Royal Society and told him of his own recent election as a director of the International Health Department of the Rockefeller Foundation. "Life here [in Canada] has been one continuous struggle for the opportunity and authority to do the things that obviously needed doing. We are making progress. I can not leave the Canadian Serum Project for the next few weeks and I am anxious to make a short nutrition survey for the IHD in the U.S."[417] — the first IHD assignment mentioned earlier. In addition, Best told Dale that Canada's National Research Council had made it possible for him to go to England and he hoped that "things will straighten out here so that I may be enabled to per-form this duty."[418] Sir Henry replied that, indeed, the dried serum should claim priority, and that "a resumption of German bombing of England would remind people of its crucial role in the war."[419]

For the nutrition survey at the end of January 1941, Best took along Dr. E.W. McHenry, a colleague from the School of Hygiene. They spent two weeks in the southern United States reviewing projects of special interest to the IHD.[420] Although this study seemed irrelevant to the wartime situation, Best felt obliged to undertake it. This experience, however, led to other important and totally relevant initiatives in Britain and Canada during the next several years.

On his return at the beginning of February Charley found everyone sick again. Then, when Sandy was pulling Henry in the toboggan in the garden, the younger boy crashed into the apple tree and broke his radius. Taken into the house, he fainted. His father took him to the hospital, where Dr. R.I. Harris set his arm. Ruth Milnes, the nurse, had abdominal pains and was admitted to hospital for several days but Dr. Gordon Murray decided that she did not need to have her appendix removed.

In February 1941, Charles Best became director of the Canadian Red Cross Blood Donor Service, and he gave a speech at the annual meeting of the Red Cross in Toronto's Eaton Auditorium, with over 1,600 people present. Ontario Lieutenant-Governor Albert Matthews presented buttons to people who had given three donations. Margaret was pleased to see Don and Mary Fraser's son, young Donnie, go up for his button and added that Charley had donated blood seven times.

Banting was very unhappy with Best in early 1941. Charles Best's ambition possibly irritated Banting. Best was ambitious, for himself, for his family, for his colleagues, for his students, for the University of Toronto, for Canada. He felt Canada was not pulling its weight in the war effort and was frustrated by the lack of opportunity to pursue needed research for the Navy. When finally the NRC provided him with the funds to go to Britain to work on medical problems with Sir Henry Dale and his colleagues, Best could not leave immediately. Banting decided to go himself. A medical officer of the National Research Council who was with Banting when he took the telephone call confirming his flight remembered that Banting remarked on the hazards of the trip and said: "If they ever give that chair of mine to that son of a bitch, Best, I'll roll over in my grave."[421]

Dean C.J. Mackenzie of the National Research Council wrote to General A.G.L. McNaughton in England on 11 February 1941, "Sir Frederick Banting has just come in to my office, and told me that he is leaving for England tomorrow by bomber plane, and I am dashing off this note which he has agreed to take. Banting has been feeling for some time that someone should go to England and get first-hand information concerning medical problems. Dr. Best has been wanting to go and we finally made arrangements but he then decided that he had other work to do so Banting is going. He is bucked up about the prospects of flying."[422]

As we saw above, Best had written to Sir Henry Dale on 6 January 1941 that he could not leave for England for several weeks because of the blood serum project and the Rockefeller survey. Best wrote Dale again on 17 January saying that his plans to go to England had to be changed partly because the blood serum project had suddenly "blossomed into fuller life" with an injection of finances from the Dominion Government to organize the project across Canada. In addition he was deterred from going by a domestic situation: "my father who came to Toronto at Christmas time has had two attacks of coronary thrombosis. He has been extremely ill but seems to be improving gradually."[423] Surely by that time Banting and Mackenzie were aware of the importance of the blood serum for the war effort, even if they did not know the important implications of the Rockefeller nutrition survey.

On 21 February 1941, word came that the plane that was taking Sir Frederick Banting to Britain on a war mission was missing. The Bests had guests for Sunday supper "when the messages began to come for Charley and he was at the telephone most of the evening. At that time, of course, we hoped that they might be found alive … On Monday afternoon we heard that the plane was found and for a short time we hoped that Fred was safe. But that evening word came that he was dead. Poor Henrietta Banting has gone through a ghastly time. Her sister came at once from Montreal, and her mother, Mrs. Ball, came from Newcastle, N.B. Charley went several times to the house and did everything he could to help them. Mary MacDonald and I went over on Monday of this week and saw Mrs. Ball and Henrie's sister, but Henrie was with Dr. Duncan Graham, talking about the military details of the funeral." The impressive military funeral was held on 4 March at the University of Toronto's Convocation Hall. "Charley was one of the honorary pall bearers. The flowers were very beautiful. Convocation Hall was filled and many people really mourned his loss."

Contrary to what has been alleged, Banting had not undertaken the trip to Britain as a joy ride to see his pals in the U.K. in 1941. C.J. Mackenzie wrote on 5 March 1941 to General McNaughton, "Banting did not leave on the plane in any sense of adventure. He did not go to England for personal reasons … He felt that the times were critical and that he should be there. He felt that, as he was head of aviation research, he should have all the experiences that the pilot and airmen had."[424]

John Bryden, in his very informative volume *Deadly Allies*, commented on one of Banting's contributions, a memo written in early January 1941, on bacteriological warfare. "It is a historic document ... Banting had written what turns out to be the blueprint for bacteriological warfare research for the next two decades."[425] In fact, Banting made great contributions in the fields of gas and bacteriological warfare, as well as to aviation medical research. Mackenzie told the War Technical and Scientific Development Committee, "When the time arrives to make known the details of Canada's war activities, it will be realized that Sir Frederick's work on insulin, great as it was, has been surpassed by the work which he has done since the outbreak of hostilities."[426] His team consisted of Drs. Robert Defries, Donald Fraser, Ronald Hare, and James Craigie of the Connaught Laboratories. Drs. Dudley Irwin and Colin Lucas had been studying the effects of toxic compounds and mustard gas in Banting's own department.[427]

For Margaret and Charley in many ways the thirties had been the best years of their lives. As professor and head of the departments of physiological hygiene and physiology, and associate director of the Connaught Laboratories, Best had fine facilities and financial resources for research available to him. He and his colleagues were recognized for the purification of the anticoagulant heparin and their discoveries of histaminase and the dietary role of choline. He was in demand as a lecturer not only in Canada, but also in both Britain and the United States.

On the personal front Margaret and Charley had lost three loving parents in a decade, but had the joy of the birth of their two sons. Idyllic summers at Schooner Cove balanced their hectic lives in Toronto. The outbreak of war and Banting's death changed their lives dramatically.

Quite aside from what Banting's tragic death meant to his family, it devastated Canada's scientific community. The nation had lost one of its heroes. For Charles Best, the loss was personal, and it marked a turning point in his career. Also, the fact that he might well have been on this flight was something that neither he nor Margaret ever forgot.

Chapter Five

Margaret's War, Charley's War, 1941–1946

The death of Charles Best's colleague and friend was profoundly to change his professional and personal life. Their relationship had not always been easy; both were men determined to have their own way, but they were staunchly loyal to each other during the insulin debates. Fred's much-publicized divorce from Marion in 1932 cooled their friendship somewhat, especially as both Margaret and Linda were very fond of Marion. Best, forty-two when Banting died, now took on increased responsibilities as director of the department that bore both their names. And, as the surviving co-discoverer of insulin, he started to receive more honours than he otherwise would have.

The most immediate concern was to see what research should be undertaken by the Royal Canadian Naval Medical Division. "The 'keel' of this division was laid in the autumn of 1940."[428] Years later, Best remembered, "The Royal Canadian Naval Medical Research Division was formed one evening in Ottawa at the home of the Hon. Angus L. Macdonald, minister of naval affairs.[429] Fred Banting went along to support me. The Minister and his wife gave us a warm welcome and as we 'spun our yarns' he became increasingly enthusiastic about the contributions which a medical research unit might make to the Navy. He promised me his active support and was as good as his word. Fred Banting was pleased that he had been able to help me 'launch a new craft.' When we went back to the Chateau Laurier we talked well into the night. That proved to be the last evening that Fred and I spent together."[430]

The day after Fred Banting's funeral, Charles Best and Don Solandt, neither yet in uniform, were off on a round of naval and Rockefeller meetings in Halifax and New York to try to chart the direction of their wartime research. "Charley had a most interesting trip. Halifax was quite thrilling. However, we must not talk about these things. They are highly important and confidential."[431] Margaret preserved Best's passes to HMC Dockyard Halifax in her scrapbook. The first pass was issued on 7 March 1941, for entry "at any time"; the second, in September 1941, was for a shorter period, as security was getting stricter.[432] On one visit, Best spoke at the launching of the Red Cross Blood Donor Service for Nova Scotia, with Lieutenant-Governor Frederick Francis Mathers and Premier Stirling MacMillan in attendance. Best was introduced as a direct descendant of a founder of Halifax, a fact that helped him throughout his wartime visits to the province.

Wilbur Sawyer, secretary to the board of the Rockefeller Institute of Medical Research and director of the IHD, noted Best and Solandt's visit to New York. Best spoke of Banting's death, a memorial for him, funding for the Banting and Best Department of Medical Research, and a possible institute of physiology, an early mention of the future Charles H. Best Institute. "It looks as if Dr. Best might have to give up his work in the Connaught Laboratories and the School of Hygiene on account of the new duties which have fallen on him as a result of Dr. Banting's death." Don Solandt joined them. Sawyer was glad to meet Solandt, "who makes a good impression."[433]

At a meeting of the International Health Division on 14 March 1941, Best gave a short report on nutrition studies in places in the U.S. that he had visited in January and February with Dr. McHenry. He reviewed the projects that were of special interest to the IHD and submitted their suggestions and recommendations.[434] At this same meeting, "it was reported that, under authority granted by the Scientific Directors on March 14, 1941, and on the recommendation of Sir Wilson Jameson, Chief Medical Officer of the British Ministry of Health, and Dr. Hugh H. Smith, representative of the Rockefeller Foundation Health Commission in England, the Director had approved an annual budget of £3,450 for a survey of nutrition in England under war-time conditions. Other contributors are the Medical Research Council and the Nuffield Trust."[435] While politicians and officials in Ottawa were still undecided how to make good use of Best and his colleagues, within months of his election as a Scientific Director of the IHD, he was already involved in initiatives of the Rockefeller Foundation that were to help the war effort.

Herbert Best was never at peace with himself after Lulu's death. He moved back and forth between Pembroke and Toronto. He criticized Charley for enlisting when he did not have to and pointed out that Ralph Salter had not. He wrote dismal letters to Charley, and also to Margaret, who finally lost patience. When Charley was away she wrote to him about his father, "His only chance for happiness now is to begin thinking of other people — and that right quickly. Isn't it wicked?"[436]

Hilda Salter did everything that she could to help. In May 1941, she and her younger child, Joan, went to stay in Pembroke, and Margaret noted that his granddaughter's presence "must have been a tremendous help in avoiding those emotional upsets of your father's." Later Margaret reported on another letter from Pembroke. "He talks principally of the monument. It will take him all summer he says to see about it and that his sole purpose now is to keep your mother's memory alive."[437] When their grandfather was in Toronto Sandy and Henry visited him at the Salters' regularly. Margaret had no patience with her father-in-law's worries, believing that the only concern of everybody in the family should be the safety of Charley Best. Herbert Best's heart trouble was less severe, but Margaret described his depression as "alarming," and added, "He is really pathetic."

Margaret was reading the boys W.H. Drummond's poem *Leetle Bateese* (practically unknown today and considered politically incorrect, which is a pity, as Drummond was very appreciative of Québec culture.) Margaret was always on the lookout for books for Sandy, a voracious reader. Miss Smith, chief of the children's section of the public library on St George Street, told her, "You haven't changed. You are just like you were when you were a little girl." Margaret recalled, "When I was at Harbord Collegiate I was president of a club which met in a boardroom at the College Street Library. I think Miss Smith was the moving spirit. She asked about my father. She said, 'I will never forget him nor the way he used to look at you.'"

When Charley was home, they used every possible occasion to go to the farm at Stewarttown. Margaret described walking in over the fields, and down through the old-growth pines on the hillside, and the raindrops bouncing in the frying pan while bacon was cooking. They saw the large pileated woodpecker, which left "great, long, nasty holes" in dying pine trees. Cattle that were pastured on the property had made a path along the top of a hill. Margaret remarked, "Henry likes to walk along it. I think he feels very brave and venturesome." One day, Sandy pulled up all the surveyor's stakes and marked groundhog holes with them. Margaret was scouring antique shops around Toronto for old pine for the farm. Mrs. Paterson's store in Agincourt, near Toronto, and the Johns on Bloor Street were two favourite places.

On the evening of 25 April 1941, Margaret and Charley attended a "Salute to Britain" at Convocation Hall and then went for coffee at the

HoneyDew Restaurant at Yonge and St. Clair. Afterwards they stopped to buy a newspaper — "on the front page we saw Charley's picture and the announcement. The darling, he deserves the best in the world! Nothing could ever be too good for him." The early edition of the *Globe and Mail* announced Best's appointment as professor and director of the Banting and Best Department of Medical Research as of 1 July 1941, succeeding Fred Banting. He also continued as head of physiology but, to Dr. FitzGerald's great regret, resigned as head of physiological hygiene and as associate director of the Connaught Laboratories, although he remained at Connaught as an honorary consultant. To his university salary of $6,000 per year as head of physiology was added $5,000 as director of the Banting and Best. He also received an annual $400 honorarium during the six years that he was attached to the Rockefeller Foundation.[438] "I am so happy that Charley is pleased and the phone has rung so often, people calling to tell us how wonderful it is."

Not everyone was happy about Best's appointment to succeed Banting. Sadie Gairns, Banting's devoted and capable assistant, reacted very negatively. Did Banting roll over in his grave? Gairns suggested that her late idol would not want Best as his successor, and resigned from the university. Both Margaret and Linda were convinced that Gairns had wanted to marry Banting. Gairns was very aware of Charley and Linda's advice to Fred: not to consider such a move under any circumstances. They felt she was temperamentally and culturally unsuitable for the volatile and artistic Fred.

Banting's death had been a great shock to Charles Best. He was uneasy about succeeding Banting as director of the Banting and Best Department of Medical Research. He was aware of opposition from some of Banting's friends and resistance in the department from his former colleagues. Banting, who did not like administration, had a different style from Best who was "hands-on," involved in administration and planning, and carrying out scientific experiments. As Best gained more confidence in himself and in his colleagues at the BBDMR, he became less insecure.

Dr. Colin C. Lucas, a distinguished biochemist, saw Best at work in his new post and may have helped him adjust. Lucas had started working with Banting in the mid-1930s and had acted as a trusted researcher and administrator in the department. He was a key figure in the early production of penicillin in Canada. He commented in his diaries, "With the death of Banting, many army uniforms disappeared from the lab to be replaced by naval attire on many of the new personnel that Dr. Best brought with him ... At that time, he was sometimes a bit pompous and condescending, which infuriated many." Then, one day, "he began a pointless eulogy of the infinite wisdom of medical men, as compared with other lesser forms of scientific personnel. I suggested that that had never been true, except in detective stories, and that future advances in medicine would largely be made by chemists, physicists, bacteriologists, geneticists and biologists. Suddenly, for no apparent reason, he flew into a rage. He was practically shouting and had two cigarettes going he was so upset. He said no one in his department would ever get promotions or a raise in pay unless he had an M.D."[439]

Best believed a medical doctor might see more readily how scientific research could be applied to human health. The emphasis was that the department was one of *medical* research. Best himself attached great importance to getting his own MD in 1922–25. To carry on in medical research, which was his intent, he himself could have gone straight to a PhD or DSc instead of doing the MD first. His father and Fred Banting, however, were both medical doctors and important examples and role models. Years later Laurie Chute confirmed why Best thought being a medical doctor was important when doing medical research. Chute wrote: "Like all true physicians he always sought for the application of his scientific discoveries to the relief of human suffering."[440]

Best and Lucas got off to a bad start. "In those days," Lucas added, "Dr. Best had the reputation of retaining only yes-men, and I had been warned of this. Dr. Banting had been the opposite — he used to say, 'The only reason I pay you good money is because I think you know more about some things than I do. When I ask what you think of something, I don't want you to tell me what you think I think, I want you to have the spunk to disagree if you honestly do not agree.' Several times after our big blow-up, Dr. Best had asked for my opinion on research programs and I had told him what I thought, which obviously annoyed him greatly. One day I said to him, 'Why do you ask me what I think if you really don't want to know? When I say what I think, and try to justify it, you don't have to accept it. I may be completely wrong. You are the boss. What you decide is what happens. I try to be helpful, even if I may be a bit dull-witted at times.' This seemed to strike a note he had not heard before. From that day we became very close friends. We could argue amicably about anything — and often did."[441]

On 11 May, a telegram arrived for Best from W.R. Franks, another member of the department. "Congratulations. Look after my people. Work going well." It was signed, "Franks." Bill Franks was already heavily involved in military projects, including his famous invention of a flying suit. He and Banting had been close friends: Banting was godfather to the Franks' twin sons, Bill and Hugh.

The first cabin built at the farm consisted of a large room, a kitchen, and a sleeping porch. The Bests had not had a dog since they gave away Blarney after he bit Henry, but now they got one for the farm. Allen Snowdon, president of Brading Breweries and master of the first pack of beagle hounds in Canada — the Don Valley Beagles — provided Rambler, son of Relish, for Sandy. The dog had been no asset to the pack as he had refused to follow the others and went off on his own. He was very shy, but Sandy held him on his knees in the car on the way to the farm, and from then on Rambler was his dog.

Rambler lived nearby during the week with Walter Lunan, who was good to the dog. For years, Lunan would watch for the Bests' car returning to Toronto, and he would be waiting at the gate. He always dressed in black and had a lugubrious message — at the beginning of July, with midsummer just past, he would greet the family with, "The nights are closing in."

When visitors came to see the Bests, Rambler would run into the woods, and he would reappear as soon as the strange car left. On one occasion when the family was eating outside, Rambler scooted down the lane with a plate and its contents balanced in his mouth, the knife and fork protruding from each side. "When he thought he was far enough away, he put down the plate, looked around to see if he had been followed, and devoured the food."

Margaret seemed almost deliberately to avoid mention of the war. The radio and the newspapers kept everyone posted. The Best house received the *Globe and Mail* in the morning and the *Toronto Telegram* in the afternoon. She did mention, however, the Rudolf Hess affair and his arrival in Scotland piloting a single engine plane.

At the end of the academic year, Margaret went to Forest Hill School and asked how Sandy had done. His teacher replied that she was not allowed to say, and then added, "Anyway, he is at the top of his class." Margaret, always competitive for herself and her family, pressed her for more details and a comparison with another very able boy. The teacher said that the boy was "a very clever child too. He can learn what is in a book, but he doesn't add anything to it or bring anything to it himself as Sandy does." Margaret wrote to Charley, who was in New York: "He has been moved this morning into the second seat in the best arithmetic row. He changed places with Harry Meredith. I am urging him to get Chuck Wheeler out of his first place but he tells me that no one can beat Chuck at arithmetic."[442]

Sandy was almost nine. He was starting to paint, and he was also developing an interest in animals. On one occasion when he was ill, Charley had lent him his painting kit and Sandy did a picture of the King's Plate horse race. He had never seen a race, but the result was very good. He had certainly looked at many horses in the flesh. On the day of the race, he studied the racing pages and asked everyone in the family to wager twenty-five cents. He listened to the radio, heard that his horse had won, and cheerfully collected his winnings. Uncle Bruce Macleod, who was an expert on horseflesh, was very impressed.

When Charley was away, the purpose and vitality seemed to go out of family activities. His initiative and desire to try new things were missing. Because Margaret could not drive, she had to get someone to take her out to the farm, where she made decisions about the house that she would rather have left to Charley. Knotty pine had not yet become fashionable, but she chose it, and it was relatively cheap to cover the interior walls. Margaret found that linseed oil toned the wood yellow, so she decided on white, clear shellac. She and the boys sanded the walls by hand between coats.

Margaret complained about the difficulty of getting things done at the farm when Charley was not there. Some form of refrigeration was needed, and also the well drillers were taking their time. When the well was finished, it lacked a pump, and, at a depth of 180 feet, it was expensive. Charley was suspicious of well drillers and wondered whether it was really necessary to go so deep. He wrote from Halifax, "We must not make Stewarttown a burden. It is really a wonderful diversion and we are not going to invest great sums there."[443] The Georgetown Lumber Co. made bunk beds, a dining room table, and a bench to Margaret's design. Friends contributed various items; Jessie Ridout gave a large blue Royal Doulton basin and ewer set that still sees good use. Many visitors enjoyed the farm. The tradition of everyone working started early, and the visitors found themselves planting and weeding. They never came a second time in fancy clothes.

One Sunday in early May 1941, thirty friends arrived at the farm for a visit. The next day, Charley, Don Solandt, and Campbell Cowan, none yet

197

in uniform, left for Halifax; they were to be gone two weeks. Dr. Donald Y. Solandt was the elder brother of Omond, and both worked closely with Best. His short but brilliant career deserves more attention than it has received. After completing medical and research studies in Toronto and a PhD with A.V. Hill in London, he succeeded Best as professor and head of physiological hygiene in 1941 and became a full professor of physiology. In later years, his great interest was in biophysics. He and Best published twenty papers together on choline, heparin, histamine, and shock. He became a surgeon commander in the RCNVR as second-in-command to Best and was largely responsible for the development of red lighting for night use by British, Canadian, and American naval and air forces.

Campbell Cowan was a Scottish engineer who was indispensable to many of Best's university and navy projects. He constructed the mechanical heart used by Drs. A.L. Chute, George Clowes, and R.A. Mustard in their research. Cowan published papers with Best on heparin.

Not all of Charley's speeches were to scientific audiences. In late May 1941, he spoke on the blood serum work at the opening meeting and banquet of the Georgetown Golf Club. Old friends such as J.A. and Florence Willoughby, whom he had known since he worked building the course in 1920, were there. He lost no chance to encourage support for the Red Cross blood donor program.

Charley was back and forth to Ottawa and Halifax. On 25 June 1941, Margaret recorded, "In order to facilitate his work in Halifax he now has a naval ranking, Surgeon Lieutenant Commander."[444] She added that in Halifax, Charley and his colleagues had been "doing very confidential work."

Margaret went with Charley on a short trip to Ottawa on NRC business. The Château Laurier Hotel in Ottawa became a familiar stopping place for the Bests. One person they came to know well in the capital was C.J. Mackenzie, who in 1939 had left the University of Saskatchewan, where he was dean of engineering, to become head of the National Research Council (NRC). He was born and brought up in St. Stephen, New Brunswick, before going to Dalhousie University in Halifax to study engineering. As a young man, he knew the Rev. A.W. Mahon, Margaret's father. As she always did in Ottawa or elsewhere, Margaret went to the art gallery and had a "beautiful time."

They saw Captain H.E. "Rastus" Reid, who was apparently involved in projects with both the RCAF and the RCN. Captain Reid became a Vice Admiral and chief of naval staff in 1946. They also saw Senator

Cairine Wilson, who had recently taken part in a big Women's Rally about war work at Maple Leaf Gardens in Toronto. Dr. Duncan Graham was involved in the same meetings in Ottawa as Charley. Margaret paid a second visit to Mr. Macdonald at the Public Archives, who provided further assistance in her study of early days in Nova Scotia.

From Ottawa, the Bests and Don and Barbara Solandt made a trip to Callander, near North Bay, Ontario, where Charley called on Dr. Allan Roy Dafoe, who was physician to the Dionne quintuplets. His brother, Dr. William Dafoe, a Toronto obstetrician and friend of the Bests, had suggested the visit and had helped his brother in many ways, including the writing of some of his articles.[445] The four went into the doctor's simple home on the main street. "The rooms are decorated with pictures of the quintuplets. Dr. Dafoe has diabetes and he has just spent two months in the Toronto General Hospital. He had to have an operation. 'Two months in jail,' he said."

Dafoe arranged for them to see the quints. "They have a log house, or hospital, stained brown, with light green trimming around the windows. There is a high fence and gates and policemen." At the door, they were met by Doreen, the nurse in charge. "She is a very smart, attractive girl who speaks English without an accent. We went into the little office room and she brought the little girls in there to meet us. They were very sweet and natural, not pretty, but lively and charming. They came over one by one to shake hands and curtsy, Annette, Yvonne, Marie, Cécile and Emilie. They are just past seven years now. They were all dressed alike in jade green Chinese silk dresses, patterned with tiny fish. The dresses were bought for the Quints from the Chinese relief organization in New York. Later on, Doreen showed us the little beanie hats and the parasols to go with them. First of all, two of them worked the Victrola for us. They put on *The Blue Danube*. Then I called Annette to come and see the snapshots I had in my bag of Sandy and Henry. So, of course, they all came running and clustered around. Charley said they all looked priceless from behind, all craning to see the pictures. They didn't speak a word of English."

Charles Best had great faith in the abilities of his own children, and Margaret recited the parable of the talents to them. "Play your piece," was often the order from Charley. Sandy could play several piano pieces well, but Henry rarely had even one that he could play presentably. Henry was more proficient and more willing to sing. His father called for a song on almost any occasion, in harmony if possible, and spirituals and Stephen

Foster songs were favourites. He and Linda would join in, while Margaret was hesitant, as she had trouble keeping a tune. Gospel hymns were also popular, as they reminded Charley of his mother and father singing at home or in the Church Hall in West Pembroke.

In mid-June 1941, Margaret and Charley went to New York. He had important meetings with the Rockefeller Foundation. During this same period the IHD made grants in Canada, including aid to the University of Toronto School of Hygiene in developing field training facilities for public health personnel, "to meet the present critical shortage of health officers, sanitary engineers, and public nurses. Calls to military service duty have depleted the staffs of the provincial and local organizations [and are depriving] the civil population ... of essential health protection ... There is a provincial law requiring pasteurization, but practically all the employees in ... enforcement are away on war duty. Unless substitutes can be promptly recruited, there will be a real danger of milk-borne epidemics."[446] Halifax was also on the agenda. The civil authorities in Nova Scotia requested aid "in improving the health organization in the Halifax area, controlling epidemics, and meeting other health problems related to the war. Dr. Charles H. Best was asked to comment. He stated emphatically that such aid to the civil authorities would be welcomed not only by them but by the army and navy medical personnel as the latter were greatly concerned by the possibility that conditions in civilian areas endanger the health of the armed forces."[447]

The Bests also spent some time with Dr. Andrew Rhodes, head of the Memorial Hospital. The Bests took the Rhodes to see Ethel Barrymore in *The Corn Is Green*.[448] "She was marvellous," wrote Margaret, "a Welsh school teacher who encourages a mine boy and makes a great success of him as a scholar." The next day, they saw Clarence Day's *Life with Father*, starring Howard Lindsay. "It was grand. I have never been at a play where the humour was better sustained all through."

Canadians were being encouraged to raise money for the war. The *Toronto Telegram*'s War Aid Fund publicized children's efforts. Sandy, his friend Jimmy Wood, and Henry put on several skits caricaturing Hitler and Goering. Sandy issued instructions to the audience. "You will all sing 'God Save the King,'" he said, and added, "You might think it is the end but it isn't the end yet." They sent about thirteen dollars to the fund and got their picture in the paper.

Sir Lawrence Bragg and Dr. Charles Galton Darwin were in Toronto in late July 1941. Sir Lawrence and his father, Sir William, were joint

Nobel laureates in physics in 1914 for their work on x-rays and crystal structures, and Sir William was president of the Royal Society in 1938 when Charles Best became a fellow. Sir Lawrence had just received a letter from his wife; she had reproved their little girl for something that she had done and received the reply, "I really don't know what Daddy ever saw in you." Margaret found this cheeky, but smart. Darwin was director of the National Physical Laboratory and grandson of Charles Darwin, author of *The Origin of Species.* In 1941, the younger Darwin was seconded to Washington for a year as first director of the mission that became the British Central Scientific Office, set up to improve liaison between the British and American scientific war efforts.[449]

On 4 August 1941, the four Bests, Linda, and Ruth Milnes left Toronto for Halifax. Leaving the family at Allison Farms, Morrisburg, on the St. Lawrence River, Margaret and Charley went to Ottawa, where he had a meeting on "shock." Margaret was obviously unsure of all his roles at this stage, so she asked him and noted the answers in her diary. In Ottawa, he was a member of the NRC's Associate Committee of Medical Research, which Bert Collip chaired. Best himself was chair of the NRC's subcommittee on naval medical research and sat on the NRC's aviation committee, chaired by Dr. Duncan Graham, and on the NRC's subcommittee on shock, which Collip chaired. Surgeon Commander Archie McCallum, based in Ottawa, was the senior naval doctor.

Charles Best often mixed business with pleasure. On this trip to Nova Scotia in 1941, he had meetings in Ottawa and Montréal, and then he met several people in Fredericton, with an eye to starting a Red Cross blood donor program in New Brunswick. The rest of the family joined Uncle Bruce Macleod at the home of his old friend Will Van Wort. Margaret and Mrs. Van Wort visited a neighbour who had the finest collection of pressed glass that Margaret had ever seen. Uncle Bruce had phoned Charley to warn against a long stay in Fredericton because of the number of cases of polio, so the Bests went to Saint John and took the *Princess Hélène* across the Bay of Fundy to Digby, Nova Scotia. They were interested to see a destroyer and a corvette in Saint John harbour. The narrow entry to the Annapolis Basin through Digby Gut is always exciting to pass through. Charley told Sandy and Henry that a narrow passage in the house in West Pembroke was called "Digby Gut."

They followed the "French Shore" from Digby to Yarmouth, noting the oxen and the busy boat-building yards. Along the south shore of Nova

Scotia through Bridgewater and Lunenburg, they came to Chester where Charley had been fortunate to find a cottage, given the many families of service personnel wanting accommodation near Halifax. Charley was off on naval business. Margaret paid several visits to the Crown Land Office in Halifax looking for Mahon family papers, staying with Beecher and Cathie Weld. He had worked at the Connaught Labs in the mid-twenties and was now head of physiology at Dalhousie University.

Don Solandt and Jimmy Campbell came to join Best, and Dr. Alex MacDonald was expected. The first two were involved in work on night vision and emergency rations. James Campbell, PhD, was a somewhat taciturn Scot who became a lieutenant commander in the navy. In peacetime, he made important contributions in diabetes research. When Campbell was promoted to full professor of physiology at Toronto, he wrote to CHB in 1962 "In all my academic life you have been my mentor, my support, my guide and a great source of strength. You have had to criticise me frequently, and I want you to know that I have valued this greatly, because it has been honest and deserved and an aid to development."[450]

Alex MacDonald was an ophthalmologist and a close personal friend who helped on night vision. Margaret was unsure as to what she should say to people about Charley's work. When Dr. Robert Wodehouse, deputy minister in the Department of Pensions and National Health, was visiting Chester, he asked what Charley was doing — "Is it diet for the navy?" She hesitated, and he said, "Oh yes, I can see you are not going to tell me." "So I said if I told secrets to anyone I would certainly tell them to him."

One fine afternoon Margaret arranged for Captain David Stevens, the famous boat designer and builder, to take the family and several guests for a sail in his sloop, and they went to Oak Island for a picnic, where they examined the shafts and the machinery being used to dig for Captain Kidd's buried treasure. Stevens let Henry take the tiller for a while, a real thrill for a six year old.

As the Bests left Chester for Halifax, they drove by the harbour and could see three large tuna lying on the wharf. In Halifax, Charley told the family that he had seen a wonderful convoy of ships file out of the harbour the previous day. He and Margaret took the boys to the Citadel and to the 240-acre Common, which the legislative assembly had set aside in 1763 on a motion by three members, including their great-great-great-great-great-grandfather, William Best. They saw St. Paul's, the oldest Anglican church in Canada, where the same William Best had been the mason in charge of building the foundations in 1750 and where he was a member of the first vestry and a warden.

The family called on cousin Arthur Mahon, the provincial liquor commissioner, at his office. He said to Margaret, "You were holding out on me, not telling me what a distinguished husband you have." His daughter, Margaret, had come home and asked, "Is it possible that that could be Dr. Charles Best, whom I once heard lecture?" For the rest of the war, whenever Charley Best went to Halifax there was a bottle of Seagram's Crown Royal delivered to him. Mahon must have stashed several cases in his office and always seemed to know when his cousin's husband was in town.

The Bests and the Welds had a picnic at Point Pleasant Park. At first, the harbour was shrouded in fog but then it lifted a little, and everyone saw seven corvettes and a destroyer steaming in and an armed merchant vessel at anchor. Margaret started to describe what Charley and Don Solandt had been doing a few days previously off Pictou Harbour, but stopped herself. "I really must not write about it at all in my diary."

The Bests went next to Truro, where Margaret's father had attended Normal School and where, when he was young, his father had taken him to the Armouries to hear Joseph Howe and Charles Tupper debate Confederation. Charley drove Margaret to the home of Judge Robert S. McLellan, who took her to his office at the courthouse. "The old gentleman leaned on a cane and took my arm. As we came out of his office, he stopped before an open door — the Marriage Registry Office — and he called out, 'Can you issue us a marriage license?' The man in the office laughed and replied, 'We only have one or two left.' So I said, 'Well, one or two will be plenty for us!'" In a very short time, the judge had found the wills for Margaret's great-grandfather, her grandfather, and two great-uncles, as well as documents about disputed estates.

In Amherst, the Bests visited Bruce Macleod's friend Garnet Chapman, chief of personnel at the Canadian Car Company, which was building Ansons — twin-engined aircraft for the British Commonwealth Air Training Plan. The Bests visited the factory where they saw the first Anson built entirely in Canada. They also saw damaged planes being repaired, and the excited boys were allowed to sit in a cockpit.

Linda and the boys stayed in a house next to the Chapmans that belonged to an elderly woman. The next morning, Charley gave Sandy a five-dollar bill, a two-dollar bill, and a one-dollar bill to pay her for the stay. He and Henry knocked on the door of her room and found her sitting up in bed in a red nightgown. Sandy asked how much they owed her, and she replied, "Four dollars, I think." The ten-year-old businessman said, "I have five dollars, two dollars, and one dollar, so I think I had better give you three dollars." Later, he told his parents, "You know, three dollars was plenty, and I knew she would not get out of bed to get me change for the five dollars."

From Amherst, the Bests drove over the lovely Tantramar Marsh area, known for its excellent hay at one time shipped to Kentucky to feed race horses. Driving through Moncton where Uncle Joe Mahon had had his bottling business, they stopped in Saint John to see their old friend Dr. Hugh Farris, and spent the night with the Vin and Ruth Price at their summer home in Dipper Harbour.

The days of easy access to the United States were over, at least temporarily. In Calais, Maine, the adults were fingerprinted. At the farmhouse at Schooner Cove, they found a fire in the kitchen stove, a crock of baked beans in the oven, brown bread, a pie in the warming oven, and a tin of doughnuts, courtesy of their neighbour, Delia Leighton. They ate their noon meal down at the "big beach" towards the point. Victor Mahar's fishing boat, anchored in Schooner Cove, provided smelts, herring, and mackerel, all to cook over a driftwood fire.

There was a new colt that summer, the last that Herbert Best had bred. He and Leavitt Hatch, who owned one of the two general stores in West Pembroke, had brought in a stallion to service their mares. This time it was Rip Hanover, one of the famous Hanover strain of standardbreds, and Grandfather had named Miss Lou's foal "Lou Hanover." He was "full of beans" and raced around the pasture, kicking up his heels and nipping anyone who came close. The whole family delighted in watching the new arrival. Smokey "looked like an old witch" to some, but Sandy had good bareback rides on him.

There was no flower or vegetable garden that year, as it had been uncertain whether the family would get east at all, but the neighbours brought vegetables. There were some raspberries, and Mrs. Mariner Leighton did some up, both jelly and jam, for Toronto. Dr. Herbert Best arrived back from visiting Hilda and her family in Ontario and came down to the farm for supper. Margaret remarked that he "enjoyed himself in spite of himself! When he talked about the colt he was quite cheerful. He is doing quite a lot of medical practice." Margaret saw the new moon, a good omen for her wherever she was in the world. Three days was a short stay, but a very happy one.

The trip home took them through Maine, New Hampshire, Vermont, New York, and across the Roosevelt Bridge to Canada. Margaret wrote, "In the evening, we drove on and it was glorious — Sandy loved the evening drives best of all. He was scintillating in the evening, telling stories and singing."

On 3 September, Margaret and Charley's seventeenth anniversary, the family went out to Stewarttown, inviting the Salters and the Prices. Margaret unpacked the wood figures carved by André Bourgault that she had purchased in St-Jean-Port-Joli, Québec, and the wrought-iron candlesticks made by Arthur Smith in Chester, Nova Scotia. Charley served "Cuba Libres — the Navy drink — coca cola with a good dash of rum."

One Sunday on the way back from Stewarttown, the family stopped at the Upper Canada College Camp at Norval. In 1920, when Margaret and Charley became engaged there, Clark Noble's family had owned the property. Now, they met Alan Stephen, headmaster of UCC's Prep School, where Sandy was a student. Sandy's interest in horticulture and agriculture, which were to be his life's work, was developing. The family was eating his potatoes, carrots, tomatoes, and cucumbers grown at the farm.

Linda Mahon had been Charley's personal secretary in the Department of Physiological Hygiene since 1927. She was not only Margaret's sister but had lived with the Bests since her mother died in 1932. She eventually set a record by being on staff at the university for fifty-four years. The roles were quite clear: Margaret was the queen bee at home and in public, and Linda was in charge at the university. Her brother-in-law was "Dr. Best" there and "Charley" at home.

In 1941, Freda Herbert from Georgetown, a long-time friend of the Mahons', started working for Charley at the lab. She looked after the budgets and the accounts and frequently visited the Best house. Her mother continued to live in Georgetown, and, after her mother's death, Freda retired there. Freda was devoted to the Best family but maintained her independence. Many researchers remember her as the person who could untangle complicated files and find money for crucial expenditures. Freda was the only person who had the courage to beard "The Professor" in his den and tell him that he was paying Linda Mahon far too little. Linda was concerned about charges of nepotism and never asked for a raise. During the family's time in Maine each summer, Linda worked on university tasks each morning, but still had herself put on unpaid leave for the weeks that she was away from Toronto.

Charles Best received his first honorary degree — a DSc from Chicago — as part of its fiftieth-anniversary celebrations on 29 September 1941. He gave a lecture on choline. The banquet took place at the Palmer House Hotel. Harold H. Swift, chairman of the university's board of trustees since 1922, and vice-chairman of Swift's Packers, presided. Robert Maynard Hutchins, the university's charismatic and controversial president, and John D. Rockefeller, Jr., whose family gave the money to found the institution, both spoke. Dr. A.J. Carlson, emeritus professor of physiology at Chicago (and the man who discouraged Ernest L. Scott years earlier in his research into pancreatic extracts[451]) and his wife took the Bests to the banquet. "We talked about the Russian Congress in 1935. He teased me a great deal about leaving my eight-month-old baby to go to that congress, but when we were coming home he said, 'I forgive you. You carry your children's pictures with you.' He took a good look at the pictures and when he said goodnight he said, 'I now know all the Best family so far.' Dr. Carlson still speaks with a foreign accent — Swedish. He was very complimentary about Charley's speech — 'It took a genius,' he said, 'to deliver such a speech.' *Time* devoted a cover and a long article to Carlson last winter."

The Bests were entertained by the Max Epsteins. He was a university trustee and had been chairman of the U.S. Draft Board in the First World War. They had a magnificent collection of old masters — Rembrandt, Frans Hals, etc.

On the Sunday morning, Charley dressed in his scarlet and gold DSc gown from London for a church service. Margaret watched as the procession entered the university chapel — "more like a cathedral than a chapel." Charley looked, "like an archbishop sitting up in the chancel, among many dark gowns." Afterwards, Dr. Walter Palmer, one of their hosts and a professor of medicine, took the Bests to their home so that Charley could have a glass of milk, as his ulcer had been causing him some trouble.

After lunch, the university's dignitaries received the guests. Margaret noted, "Hutchins is quite a character — handsome, tall, just over forty, the son of a Presbyterian clergyman. It seems to me that he has his tongue in his cheek a good deal of the time. He has a very ready tongue. Mrs. Hutchins — Maude — is tall, dark, arty — long black hair to her shoulders, very sunburned and very uninterested in faculty wives and university affairs in general. She is a sculptress and prefers to go on with her own work."

Robert Millikan, the 1923 Nobel-prize physicist from California, and Dr. Ernest Lawrence, who won the same award in 1939, were new friends whose company the Bests enjoyed. Lawrence told a story about the absent-minded Niels Bohr, the celebrated Danish atomic physicist. "He was counting his luggage in the station. Twice he counted his bags to nine — looking very puzzled. Then he counted again, and with a beaming smile pointed to himself — ten — Ja!"

The convocation was on Monday morning. Margaret was pleased by the many comments about Charley's London gown. His new Chicago hood was maroon with yellow velvet bindings. Others honoured were Dr. Amado Alonso of Buenos Aires, a philologist; Dr. Evarts Graham of Washington University in St Louis, a specialist in the techniques of modern surgery; Dr. Carlos Monge of Lima, a pioneer in the physiology of life at high altitudes; and Dr. Thomas Rivers of the Rockefeller Institute, an expert in infectious diseases.

In New York after Chicago, Charley spoke at a ceremony of the Academy of Medicine in memory of Fred Banting, but "nearly melted" in the stiflingly hot hall. Elliott Joslin also spoke and read the telegram that he had received from Banting at the time the Nobel Prize was awarded in 1923, when Best was lecturing at Harvard. "Dr. Joslin said that discovering Charley in the early days was one of the greatest things Dr. Banting had done. Dr. Joslin talked about the clinical work on diabetes. Then Charley gave his address on the 'experimental work.'"

Sawyer of the Rockefeller Foundation noted in his diary on 3 October 1941 that Best had come to New York to deliver a lecture at the Academy of Medicine. The next day Best went to the Rockefeller Foundation to discuss his proposed trip to England. "Best expects to be leaving Toronto on about the following Wednesday, October 8, and with transportation supplied by the Navy will go to Iceland. From there he hopes to proceed to England and during this time there he would like to visit the activities in which the IHD is interested. He will also have various other scientific matters to discuss. WAS [Sawyer] invited him to make the visit in England as a Scientific Director, and to visit the activities in which we are interested and discuss with HHS [Hugh H. Smith] any plans for the future. Best stated that he expected that his transportation to England would all be furnished by the Navy without charge to him. He will get in touch with HHS as soon as he arrives in England and WAS will ask the latter to supply him with funds for his expenses in that country. If it should prove necessary or advisable to return by Clipper at the end of his visit, air clipper service via neutral Portugal was a possible means of travel between Europe and North American during the war. WAS [Sawyer] agreed to recommend that the expenses involved be included as part of his travel expenses as SD [scientific director] and that he could also similarly charge any additional expenses for the trip to England not provided by the British authorities."[452] In short, the Rockefeller Foundation was providing the help that Best had hoped for the allies' war effort.

On the subject of the war, while in New York, the Bests saw *The Watch on the Rhine* — "terribly moving" — by Lillian Hellman, a story of a family of refugees from Germany, in which she suggested that the United States would soon have to join the war.

On 8 October, Charley and Don Solandt left Toronto, as Margaret said, "indefinite as to time and place." She and Linda were knitting Charley a black pullover sweater, and Lorena was making black socks. "Charley looks so handsome in his uniform — with his gold braid and red — surgeon lieutenant commander. Two wide gold stripes and a narrow one in between, and red between the gold. He had two ribbons, one for service in World War I and the other the King George V Jubilee Medal."

Most of Charley's letters were very cheery and positive, but his first on 9 October 1941 was not a happy one. "Margaret Dearest, It was one of the hardest things I have ever had to do to leave you last evening. I know that it was even more difficult for you, but I hope you are feeling better to-day." He realized the toll on Margaret but could do nothing about it. The memory of Banting's flight must still have been vivid for him, but he was not going to refuse the tasks that came his way. Also, something that Margaret could never understand, he enjoyed the adventure, the fellowship with other officers and, indeed, the danger. Especially after frustrating months of waiting he appreciated the chance to be on active service. He was not always able to write about what he was doing or whom he was seeing, but he did his best to make his letters interesting. Charley called home as often as he could, and Margaret wrote him every few days.[453] From Ottawa, he and Don Solandt went to Montréal for a day of meetings, and then, with Campbell Cowan and Jimmy Campbell, to Halifax.

Margaret's letters were not happy or encouraging. She, Linda, and the boys were all ill for extended periods. Margaret believed that her situation was worse than anyone else's, and her hair went grey almost overnight. Some letters between them were in code about when he would return, mostly about "sending bottles of insulin to Weld." In October 1941, Best knew that he was going overseas, and Margaret suspected as much. In

Halifax, Charley went to see the Arthur Mahon cousins and mentioned repeatedly the hospitality of Beecher and Cathie Weld. He wrote and phoned his father regularly, but not with any happy response. He talked of the clothing that he had been issued, including a duffle coat (it is still in regular use sixty years later.) Parcels arrived from St. John's, Newfoundland for both Barbara Solandt and Margaret, and letters as well. Margaret's parcel contained sealskin gloves. Barbara interpreted her letters as saying that the men were on their way to Iceland and England, and Margaret, hopefully, that they were returning to Halifax.

Then on 8 November, Barbara had a wire *sans origine* from Don, and on the ninth Margaret received one from Reykjavik. On 19 November, two letters arrived on paper headed "St-Laurent," which was the destroyer HMCS *St-Laurent*, captained by Lieutenant-Commander Herbert Rayner, later a vice admiral and the chief of the naval staff from 1960.

In the first letter from the *St-Laurent*, Charley said he had not been seasick and emphasized the problem of censorship. "My thoughts are with you a hundred times a day and trust that everything will be finished up in good time so that you and I may get on with our plans."[454] The second letter gave a little more news. "We have been able to find a number of very interesting problems and there will be plenty to carry on with in the laboratory."[455] One evening, he reported that in the absence of a duty doctor he had "sewed up a cut over a man's eye." It had been many years since CHB had done anything of the sort.

On 8 December 1941, following the bombing of Pearl Harbour, the United States entered the war. On 12 December, a telegram announced, "Henry's cable received. Arrangements postponed slightly — dearest love." Margaret complained, "The navy is a difficult branch to be in." A cable on 18 December asked her to return fourteen bottles of insulin to Beecher Weld — i.e. code that meant that Charley would not be home for Christmas. On 22 December: "Return five additional bottles of insulin. Well. Dearest love."

Margaret was frantic with worry for Charley's safety. "I don't know whether the nights or the days are the worst to be dreaded now. If I sleep for more than two hours at a time I am doing well." The boys missed their father too. Probably their mother's worries were obvious to them. One evening Margaret heard a sound in Sandy's room and found him in the dark sobbing, "I do miss Daddy." However, they all helped pack ditty bags for the sailors. Each one contained "two knitted garments and all sorts of other things — cigarettes, tobacco, playing cards, flashlights, mouth organs, tinned goods, hard candy, gum, etc." By Christmas 1941, the family had delivered five bags to the Navy League.

Dr. Herbert Best continued to be a trial for his daughter-in-law. He wondered why Charley had joined the forces at his age, saying that he had no need to put himself in danger. In early November, Margaret had written, "We have had three letters from Dr. Best, all in a row — very nice ones. A letter came to the office after Charley had left which was too trying, so I wrote a carefully worded reply — calculated to put an end to such letters. I really think it has worked, for the time being, anyway. I said I thought he should write his reminiscences for the boys' sake, since he had so many interesting cases. It has done as I had hoped." When she received a reply, she immediately wrote to Charley, "A better tone, Charley, than any letter we had from him since your mother died. Reference at the end to sunsets and sunrise. You would never believe it. Not a word that wouldn't publish well."[456] What did Margaret mean by that? At this stage, it was unlikely that she had in mind to publish her diaries or memoirs but she certainly wanted her father-in-law to write pleasant letters.

Later Best wrote for the NRC quite a detailed eight-page report of his trip in 1941. On 8 October 1941 in Ottawa: "Discussed all phases of Franks' suit. He had done a grand job and should be rewarded in any way that is possible." Wing Commander W.R. Franks' invention of a flying suit enabled pilots to withstand heightened G-forces and prevent blackouts. He was, indeed, "a true pioneer of aviation medicine."[457] Further on, Best wrote: "Had many sessions with [RCN Chief of Medical Staff, Surgeon Captain Archie] McCallum — most satisfactory. Many plans for our further work. Arranged to be put on Active Service (Temp.) Attested and received uniform allowance in Halifax." Best was put on temporary service first on 16 June 1941, then again with added duties on 15 October of the same year.

"Went to Montreal on Saturday morning — Collip took us for lunch. Saw Penfield's set up for seasickness work. Nearly ready to go." The next move had been to Halifax to deal with the Red Cross blood donor service. Best had a good discussion with Captain Harold Grant, later chief of naval staff, about a new hospital.[458]

On this trip Best and Solandt did further tests on red lighting. They "recruited a group of young destroyer commanders to act as experimental subjects. The results were dramatically favourable and the officers were extremely enthusiastic."[459] Surgeon Commander David Johnstone, chief medical officer in Halifax, discussed with the visitors various research projects being carried out locally.[460]

"Left Halifax, 8:30 p.m. Monday, October 20, Furness-Withey, *Fort Amherst.*" The party included Eddy Amos,[461] Don Solandt, Campbell Cowan, and Jim Campbell. "Good passage — free [of submarines or icebergs ?] — 3 days." In St John's, Newfoundland, Best saw chief medical officer, Surgeon Commander A.L. Anderson, who showed him his setup. "Has made the most of his facilities. He has difficulty getting things. Has a fairly good supply of our [blood] serum. It saved four lives, burn cases, from a RN corvette." Best's insistence on carrying on with the blood serum work was being increasingly vindicated.

En route to Iceland at the end of October on the destroyer *St Laurent:* "Will never forget the rolling in that Sick Bay. Scores of bottles — had my hot cocoa in the medicine rack, 6" away from hammock. First night the cords at foot gave way when I moved. Tied them with 2 half hitches. One night Don's cough bothered him. We turned on the light and had available the whole pharmaceutical repertoire of the RCN — a little tinctura benzine, a tablet of soda bicarb, and a little milk of magnesia, etc. etc."

Best noted all the areas that needed immediate improvements: "Should be much more blood serum on board. Also distilled water. We must devise an outfit for giving serum. Complete survey of red lights made. Ordinary ship's lighting leaves much to be desired. There should be memo's re fruit juices, canned milk, etc. going out to all ships in the RCN. The supply of a good vitamin pill has not as yet been tackled. Fresh water problem — non-thirst creating compressed food. Canteen sells $400 worth of chocolate bars per month."[462]

In Reykjavík at the beginning of November Best spent a lot of time with Surgeon Captain Fitzroy Williams, fleet medical officer of the British Home Fleet, talking about the incidence of tuberculosis, the danger of fumes in closed spaces, improvements in diet, colour-vision tests, and many other topics. Professor Niels Dungal, professor of anatomy and past rector of the University of Reykjavík, explained that he was happy with the British presence in Iceland but noted that the Germans had gone "all out" before the war to make things easy for Icelanders — scholarships, honours, visits, public works, and so on. The Germans had paved roads, and the unfinished aqueduct was also German. They had realized the strategic importance of the island.[463] "Situation becoming acute — no workmen available — well paid in

British pounds but nowhere to spend them — better with U.S. and Canadian dollars."[464]

One night, "a storm came up and the order was given to hoist all boats. We protested as we were anxious to get back to the depot ship *Hekla.* They agreed to send us and it was the most exciting trip I ever had in a small boat. We were landed safely, however, on the *Hekla's* ladder."

Vice-Admiral Sir John Tovey sent orders that Best and Solandt were to proceed as his guests on the British light cruiser *Sheffield,* commanded by Captain Arthur Wellesley Clark. Best was concerned because Don Solandt had had two gastric hemorrhages, but he was able to continue the trip. "I bunked on a small bed — about 6″ off the deck. For the nine nights on the *Sheffield* as during the twelve on the destroyer, I slept in my clothes with a life-belt on. The weather was rough and the *Sheffield* had a tremendous roll." *Sheffield* received a signal from headquarters "to patrol between the Faroe Islands and Iceland and be on the lookout for the battleship *Von Tirpitz* which had recently completed her trials in the Baltic and made an appearance at Kiel. One night Captain Clark, speaking over the ship's radio to the crew, stimulated us all by saying, 'This may be *Sheffield's* great opportunity. What a wonderful Christmas box the *Von Tirpitz* would be! Keep a sharp lookout.'"[465]

Captain Ford, senior engineer of the battleship *King George V,* pointed out the buckling of deck and side plates produced by firing sixteen three-inch guns at point-blank range — i.e. with no elevation — at the German dreadnaught *Bismarck.* Earlier in the year in May of 1941, the *Sheffield* had been in battle in the North Sea. Paul McLaughlin of Toronto had been the first member of the *Sheffield's* crew to spot the *Bismarck* in the Denmark Strait. "The *Bismarck* sighted the British ship once and bracketed her with the first two volleys. There were a number of casualties on the *Sheffield* and the ward-room was well marked with shrapnel. The picture of the Duchess of Kent, who christened the ship, was hanging over the electric grate. Curiously enough the mat on both sides of the Duchess's picture was carried away, leaving her silhouetted as it were. The picture was re-framed without repairing the mat."[466]

Best referred very favourably to a fellow passenger, Captain Eds, the major of the Marines who had been in charge of the British landing parties in Norway. The chief intelligence officer, whom Eds blamed for a major share of the catastrophe, was Peter Fleming. In the Hart-Davis's biography of Fleming, there is no mention of Captain Eds in the pages about what was identified as "No. 10 Military Mission to find out who was in occupation of the port of Namsos,"[467] north of Trondheim.

The senior medical officer of the *Sheffield* Best said was "lamentably ignorant of medical matters," but his "two juniors were keen and up-to-date. There had been no testing of night lookouts. There was no supply of blood serum for transfusions. The diet was far from adequate. Every morning on the *Sheffield* we were awakened by the call, 'Heave ho, heave ho, wakey, wakey, lash up and stow.' We had 'Action Stations' on the *Sheffield* at about 2 a.m. Each time we thought it might be the *Tirpitz*, but fortunately turned out not to be." The eleven days they spent on the *Sheffield* contributed significantly to Best's understanding of what would be his immediate naval research priorities.

They left her at anchor in Scapa Flow in the Orkney Islands "at just sunrise and the picture of the sun coming over the hills and shining on the vast number of anchored balloons, made a startling picture. The battleship *Duke of York* was lying at anchor near the *Sheffield* and another battleship which we took to be the *Nelson* came in escorted by destroyers while we were there."

A small steamer took Best and Solandt to a landing near Thurso, from where they went by train to Inverness. In 1928 Margaret and Charley had found Inverness "a rather bleak and uninteresting town," but Charley described it in 1941 as "really one of the most attractive small cities which I have ever seen."[468] From Inverness, the two Canadian officers sat up on the train for one night and most of a second before arriving at Euston Station in London where they were based for the first three weeks of December. They tried several hotels before finding a room on the top floor of the Dorchester. That evening, Omond Solandt, Jack Magladery, and Robin Lawrence met them for dinner, and H.G. Wells, the writer and president of the British Diabetic Association, joined them.[469]

Charley Best then moved to stay with Sir Henry and Lady Dale at Mount Vernon House. Unlike Margaret, who complained about her lot in Toronto, Lady Dale carried on cheerfully throughout the London blitz. Best wrote admiringly of her, "The bombing attacks, through all of which she had remained in London, had had no obvious effect on her and she was just her very wonderful self. Sir Henry was much thinner but he was as dynamic as ever and I had many long conversations which substantiated my previous opinion that his grasp on all aspects of medical research was broader than any one else with whom I had ever had contact. Sir Henry facilitated a great many things for us. He arranged introductions to

213

Lord Hankey and we were able to push ahead with a number of medical problems through that channel."[470]

Hankey was a member of the war cabinet and, most importantly, chair of its Technical Personnel Committee from 1941 to 1952. "He was very keen and helpful. He sent us to the Admiralty to see Cheshire and Dudley" — Deputy Chief Scientific Officer Dr. Ralph W. Cheshire and Surgeon Vice Admiral Sheldon Francis Dudley, FRS, medical director general of the Royal Navy. The two men studied their data, "and to make a long story short, the Royal Navy adopted red lighting."[471]

Working in close cooperation with the British were the representatives of International Health Division of the Rockefeller Foundation, Henry O'Brien and virologist Hugh Smith, who were especially helpful. Best spent two nights at Smith's flat on Curzon Street in Mayfair when air raids hampered return to Hampstead. Dr. Wilbur Sawyer, director of the IHD, had set up the contacts before Best left Canada: "During your visit, Dr. Smith will assist you in planning your trips to inspect work in which the [IHD] is interested, and will help you make the necessary contacts."[472]

A.N. Drury of Britain's MRC was chair of its Blood Depot Committee and of its Blood Transfusion Research Committee. He invited Best to give a talk to his colleagues on the work being done in Canada. Best discussed research matters with various Canadians including Colonel Harry Botterell, head of No. 1 Neurological Unit, just after he had removed a bullet from a man's brain; Colonel Milton Brown, in charge of preventive medicine; and Brigadier "Mac" MacFarlane, consulting surgeon, Canadian Army Overseas. Lieutenant-Colonel Ian Macdonald, officer-in-charge of medicine at No. 9 Canadian General Hospital, and Lieutenant-Colonel Don MacLean, in charge of hygiene, and several others hosted meetings. Lieutenant-General A.G.L. McNaughton, commander of the Canadian Corps Overseas, spent considerable time consulting with Best at military headquarters in British Columbia House.

Best's account of problems discussed in England is short but informative.[473] Sir Edward Mellanby, secretary of the Medical Research Council (MRC), arranged for visits to Lulworth, the tank research centre on the Dorset coast; to Porton, the gas and bacteriological warfare research station near Salisbury; and, to Farnborough, the aeronautical research centre in Hampshire. At RAF Farnborough, "two problems were — finding the relationship between altitude and intensity of German search lights; and the study of drugs which would decrease the incidence of refusals to make parachute jumps. These researches required complete courage." Next, "We had a grand day at Porton — the Gas School — with [Charles] Lovatt Evans, [John Henry] Gaddum, and the Naval Commander who was actually in charge of the Laboratories. We saw a big show there with most of the brass hats in attendance. Progressive and defensive devices were exhibited and the whole performance was efficiently conducted." At Lulworth, "where Omond Solandt and Laurie Chute were working, had a most profitable day watching tank demonstrations of all kinds. Mellanby arrived for the show and we caught a glimpse of what must actually happen in tank battles."

At Cambridge, Professor George Macaulay Trevelyan, the eminent historian and master of Trinity College, put them up. "He gave us the Judges' chambers and we will never forget the great beds and the most comfortable surroundings. Mrs. Trevelyan was most hospitable and we had tea with her on two occasions. We dined in Hall one evening and the main point of discussion seemed to be whether the wines would last for six or eight more years of war. We had a morning with Sir Joseph Barcroft, retired professor of physiology and now head of the Agricultural Research Council Unit in Animal Physiology, Professor Douglas Adrian, the current professor of physiology, and Sir Charles Sherrington, retired professor of physiology at Oxford, on the drying processes and other nutritional problems of war interest."

The IHD of the Rockefeller Foundation had just made a practical contribution to the research. "Nutrition work in England has been a part of the Health Commission's program since October 1, 1941, when a grant was made for the Oxford Nutrition Survey, which is carried on in cooperation with the Ministry of Health and under the general direction of Sir Wilson Jameson, the Chief Medical Officer. The purpose of this work is to test, develop, and apply all reasonable methods of assessing the state of human nutrition, and to provide training in their use. This is being accomplished by the study of groups representing different age, professional, and economic levels, patients from hospitals, and persons who submit to experimentally induced deficiencies. Special subjects which have been under investigation are the effect of vitamin feeding in a factory group, the relation between nutrition and TNT poisoning, the effects of yeast feeding in children, fluorosis, and the results of an experimental deficiency of vitamin A."[474]

In Oxford, Best and Solandt stayed at Magdalen College, where Best was amused by "a grand old Admiral who had rooms next to those which I was given. The old lad got up early in the morning and took a cold bath, which was more than I felt like doing." The Canadians visited the lab of Professor Rudolph Peters, the distinguished head of biochemistry, and learned something of his work on neutralizing leucocytes.

Back in London, they met with Brigadier-General Thomas William Richardson, deputy director of supplies and transport at the War Office, and Dr. Charles Seymour Wright, a Toronto graduate and director of scientific research at the Admiralty. Best had several sessions at the Athenaeum with Sir Wilson Jameson, Britain's chief medical officer of health. A note preserved in MMB's scrapbook informed Best that Lieutenant-General Alexander Hood, director general of the army's medical services, also wanted to see him at the War Office.[475]

After learning an enormous amount concerning the actual conditions on board ships and what research was going on in Britain, by 19 December 1941, Best and Solandt had completed their tour of duty. Looking for a passage back to Canada, they took the train to Glasgow. But as there was a wait of a few days they went to Edinburgh to see Ivan de Burgh Daly, who was working on decompression chambers, and Guy Marrian, working on chemical warfare.

Back in Glasgow, Surgeon Rear Admiral John McNee, emeritus professor of medicine and consultant in medicine to the Royal Navy, and his staff were very informative about the problem of immersion foot, a condition frequently seen in survivors whose feet have been exposed for long periods of time to dampness and cold in the North Atlantic.[476] The visitors spent an evening with Stan Graham, a cousin of Dr. Roscoe Graham of Toronto who was professor of pediatrics at Glasgow, and his wife, Grace.

On 22 December, Henry Dale and Douglas Adrian, who were to visit research establishments in Canada and the United States, joined Best and Solandt in Glasgow. After some delay, all four boarded the Norwegian liner *Bergensfjord*, which used to run between Bergen and New York, and shared a very small cabin. "The Captain was named Velle and one day, another passenger, Captain Conolly Abel Smith, asked me to go up to the bridge to meet the captain of the ship. He was a stalwart Norwegian who looked in perfect health. As I was about to salute him on the bridge, he said 'No, I wish to salute you. I take 70 units of insulin every day of my life.' Another time, the principal medical officer, Dr. Kidd, came into the cabin where Dale, Adrian, Solandt and I were reclining. He asked if any of us knew biochemistry. Dale replied that none of us knew very much but that he had better try me if he had a problem. I went out with him and

216

we found a boy — an American lad who had been in Londonderry — in diabetic coma. There was no doubt about the diagnosis and with the administration of insulin his recovery was completely satisfactory."

"We were a very small convoy — the *Bergensfjord* and the *Morton Bay*. We had several thousand British Air Force lads coming out from England to take part of their training in Canada. The *Morton Bay* had several thousand German prisoners and we felt like advertising this latter fact to the submarines." The voyage experienced no submarine scares and the only aircraft were Catalinas on escort duty from Canada. For most of the ten-day voyage, there was an escort of two destroyers. The ship's menu for New Year's Eve 1941, was very generous — fillet of plaice for lunch and fillet of flounder for dinner.

Meantime in Toronto Christmas Day was sunny and mild, with no snow. Barbara Solandt and her daughters, Barrie and Sandra, came for dinner, and other callers kept Margaret busy. Dr. Herbert Best came with Hilda and her son Charley Ralph for a visit. Ruth and Vin Price stayed until after midnight. Margaret commented, "and so we got through the day."

Charley arrived in Halifax on New Year's Day, 1942, and he said, "I was very glad to see the familiar landmarks as we approached the harbour — Sambro Light, Chebucto Head and the reflections of the lights of Halifax certainly looked very good at that time." On arrival in Halifax, Charles Best invited some of his fellow passengers and some Haligonians to the Hotel Nova Scotian for dinner. After experiencing the scarcity of food in Britain he was "rather ashamed of the meal. Not because it was poor but because there was so very much food served. A great deal more than any of us could eat — though I will admit that some of the Englishmen did phenomenally well "[477]

"Many of the scientific discussions held during this trip proved stimulating for our further work in the Research Unit in Toronto. The work on immersion foot which we saw in Scotland stimulated a great deal of that which was subsequently carried out in Canada. Similarly in the studies on nutrition several important leads were obtained."[478] Later, Best described this whole experience as "the most exciting trip of the war."[479]

The *Globe and Mail* reported on 3 January 1942, "Dr. C.H. Best, in Silent Service, Keeps Tongue-Tied Tradition." The story read, "Previously he talked enthusiastically of his work in blood transfusion, but now the genial doctor had nothing to say. Looking down at his uniform rather self-consciously, he explained his silence, saying, 'I'm in the service now, you know,' and refused to be drawn out. Even questions on his work — usually a sure bait — failed to open him up. 'We'd better not say anything about that,' he said, adding, 'It would be just as well if I didn't say anything about my trip to England either.' But he was as friendly as ever."[480]

Then the *Globe and Mail* published on 9 January 1942 a short item, "New Physiology School of Research under Dr. C.H. Best To Be Opened." President Cody announced that the university's board of governors had made this decision. It took another eleven years for the building to materialize.

For Margaret Best, Fred Banting's death had brought the danger of war too close. Charley could have been on that plane. She believed that her burden of worry was greater than that of most people. Although he did not tell her ahead of his overseas trips, she knew that they would happen. What kept her sanity was that she felt responsible for the boys and for Linda, although the latter was much more an asset than a responsibility. Margaret's diaries are full of details of Charley's trips, of visits to the farm, of the boys' activities, of her own doings, and of frequent illnesses. She was certainly relieved when Charley came home from overseas. "I have been so tense and anxious all the time, and now it is hard to relax and to realize he is really home again — safe and sound."

After his return, Best spent a week in New York and Washington. The Rockefeller Foundation's annual report for 1941 contained a section about the IHD's activities: "The year 1941 brought about a considerable shift in International Health Division activities, not away from its fundamental programme of public health, but rather in the direction of emphasis on problems of immediate interest in wartime and on work in such geographical areas as still open."[481] In New York on 26 February 1942 Best reported on his experiences in wartime Britain to Wilbur Sawyer, director of the IHD. Sawyer noted that Best was "in his uniform as Surgeon Lieutenant Commander of the British Navy." To many Americans, there was no difference between the Royal Navy and the Royal Canadian Navy.

"This was the first time he had been in New York since his visit to England. He says he was well taken care of by HHS [Hugh Smith] and O'B [A.M. O'Brien] and had a good impression of the work."[482] In mid-March, he was in New York again for a meeting of the Rockefeller Foundation. "Dr. Charles H. Best gave a brief description of the results of nutrition experiments in which he had been engaged. In addition, he reported his observations of the Oxford Nutrition Survey made during a recent visit to England. He stated that the project had adequate support, excellent laboratory accommodations, and a well-trained staff. The opportunity to render a real service to a nation of people living on a restricted diet is a stimulus to the work, and the study should provide information of great value."[483] A note in the IHD's newsletter of 1 April 1942 stated that Drs. Parran, Rivers, and Best, "appeared at the meeting in full uniform for the first time since the United States entered the war."[484]

A Georgia O'Keeffe exhibit had just ended, but photographer Alfred Stieglitz, owner of the gallery and O'Keeffe's husband, persuaded his wife to show Charley her canvasses, flower pictures, and scenes from New Mexico, which he liked very much. Unfortunately he did not buy a painting. He may not have wanted to choose one without Margaret, or he may have thought it too extravagant a purchase.

Best went on to Washington, DC, to represent Canada at a meeting of the American National Research Committee. Irvine Page, director of the Lilly Laboratory for Clinical Research at Indianapolis City Hospital, took him to a party at the house of controversial columnist Drew Pearson, where he had a long talk with Jimmy Cromwell, recently American minister in Ottawa.

Sir Henry Dale stayed with the Bests for a few days in late January 1942. Sir Henry and his godson Henry sang while Sandy accompanied them on the violin. The Bests planned a party for the war guests whom Sir Henry knew and for their guardians. There were thirty people in all, some children as old as sixteen. Lady Banting (Fred's second wife, Henrietta) was one of the guardians. Arriving at the house with Sir Henry, Margaret found that Henry Best had decorated the living room with all the clay ashtrays and animals that he had made in school. "I admired it all greatly and left many of them about, but some had to be put away to make room for teacups."

Worse was to come! "Then I ran downstairs to see that the study and little bathroom were in good shape. Sandy had employed his time roasting a pumpkin in the furnace. It did not turn out as well as he had expected, so he had tried to dispose of the remains. The drains were plugged in the little bathroom and there were charred remains of pumpkin everywhere. I had to scrub the floor, while Charley plunged long things up and down in the drains. I hope Sir Henry could not hear the remarks I was making through the pipes in his bathroom. One of the mildest was that I could wring Sandy's neck."

The Canadian Club invited Dale as its guest, and Sir Henry spoke on "Science and the War." Margaret listened on the radio; "Sir Henry made several references to Charley, and each time there was applause." Dr. Robert Defries, director of the Connaught Laboratories, Dr. Duncan Graham, professor of medicine, and President and Mrs. Cody all entertained the visitor.

Douglas Adrian of Cambridge, who had come over on the *Bergensfjord* with Sir Henry, Charley, and Don Solandt, came to town as well. During the war, the Adrians' twin children lived with the Detlev Bronks near Philadelphia. A few years later, Charley was offered the chair of physiology to succeed Adrian, who became master of Trinity College.

In early March, both Margaret and Sandy were in bed for a week. Sulphanilamide and other sulpha drugs were a great help, even though they did cause dizziness and stomach upsets. Later in the month, Dr. Silverthorne came and said that Sandy had bronchial pneumonia. He prescribed sulphadiazine and mustard poultices. Sandy sent a message to Margaret via Henry. "Come and take this thing off at once or I'll be flying away to the pearly gates."

On 2 April, Margaret headed to Boston to join Charley, who was at the meetings of the American Physiological Society. A young boy on the same train was going home after his year at Appleby College in Oakville. He had dozens of illustrations of birds with him and showed them all to her. Then he asked, "You wouldn't be interested in snakes?" Margaret replied, "No, very definitely," and he replied, "I was afraid you wouldn't." Lydia Mahon met Margaret at the Boston South Station to tell her that Charley was quite ill with strep throat. He had a fever of 103 degrees Fahrenheit and was quite irrational. A doctor had prescribed sulphadiazine, and that seemed to work. Miss Mack, a nurse from the Massachusetts General Hospital, had taken charge. On the day before Margaret had arrived, Mack had said, "I hope she isn't the excitable kind." Henry Mahon thought the nurse's zeal a bit excessive; she insisted on giving public announcements of her patient's condition in every detail.

Charley recovered quickly, and the Bests took the train to New York. Billy Thalhimer, always helpful, had tickets for Noël Coward's play *Blithe Spirit*,[485] with Clifton Webb as the husband and Peggy Wood as one of the wives. "It was a most improbable but amusing play." Captain Abel Smith, RN, who was on the *Bergensfjord* with Charley, came to have breakfast with the Bests — apparently Charley liked Abel Smith very much.

Margaret and Charley also saw George Gershwin's *Porgy and Bess*,[486] with Todd Duncan and Anne Brown, which they enjoyed immensely. Margaret went to the Museum of Modern Art to see the Théodore Rousseau exhibition. "I think he has had a good deal of effect on more recent painters. I used to dislike him heartily, but I must say that I quite enjoyed the jungles this time." From Toronto they received a nonsense verse from Linda, one of many that she wrote:

> Just a line
> As you rove
> All here fine
> Checked the stove
> Latched the milkbox
> Shot the bolts
> Damped the furnace
> Covered the colts
> As you feared
> Results more dire
> I also checked the humidifier
> Trust this brings
> You up to date
> And so to bed
> As it is late.[487]

In Toronto, Sandy was working hard at both the piano and violin. He was proud to be concertmaster of UCC's Prep School Orchestra. Charley tried to get to his older son's piano recital with the rest of the family, but he had to chair a meeting of the shock committee at the Toronto General Hospital. Sandy was also enjoying painting. Margaret consulted John Hall, the art teacher at UCC, about art supplies for the summer, such as coloured chalk and crayons. Hall said that he wanted Sandy to start using oils: "He said he hardly knew how to describe the quality Sandy has, perhaps sensibility was the word. He said he had had boys who could draw better, more readily, but in all his teaching of art only Sandy and one other boy had this quality. Sandy had a feeling for line, for colour, for tone." He indeed had great talent as an artist. His pastel portraits, watercolour landscapes, and botanical illustrations were beautifully executed. His style could be meticulous or wildly impressionistic. He later became the first undergraduate to have a one-man show in the university's Hart House Art Gallery.

Margaret was getting to know Charley's naval colleagues. She noted "I am beginning to know the Navy." One evening, the Bests had Surgeon Lieutenant Commander Ed Amos of Halifax and Dr. Bert Collip to dinner. Surgeon Lieutenant Commander Don Solandt was a frequent visitor as was Dr. Norman Taylor. In mid-June, Margaret noted that his wife, Isabel, had died suddenly.

Archie McCallum and his wife became good friends. Margaret described Arabelle McCallum as "a Mackenzie from Cape Breton Island — a dentist and a character." Their daughter, Barbara Jane, was "very bright." Years later, Dr. Barbara McCallum Blake reminisced, "I remember your father with great fondness. He visited our house in Ottawa from time to time, showed considerable interest in my high school curriculum, criticized the far-left propaganda of my history teacher and told me frequently that I would never be as good looking as my mother!"[488]

The Best children's doctor, Roy Simpson, loved horses, and when he could no longer ride, Charley bought from him a gelding called Peter for Sandy's eleventh birthday present on 7 July 1942. The horse was always known thereafter as "Peter Simpson Best." When Roy Simpson died in February 1945, Best arranged for his son, Able Seaman Jack Simpson, to come home to Toronto for the funeral. Jack recalled that he came out of Union Station to find a staff car and driver and a surgeon captain to meet him. He did not know whether to salute or to embrace his "Uncle Charley."

On every possible occasion the Bests went to their farm at Stewarttown. Charley worked on his papers and then joined the rest of the family in working in the garden or tramping through the valley. A wood-devouring Quebec heater, installed in the larger room, allowed the family to stay overnight even in the coldest weather. Friends visited — some, like Neil McKinnon's wife, Hollie, and her three girls, had their husband and father overseas. Once, when Sandy walked into Georgetown by himself, Charley asked him why he had done it. His son replied, "You can't expect me to keep a diary if I don't have experiences." Bruce Macleod often joined them. He declared war on the groundhogs one day and, loading his shotgun, he drove his Cadillac over the fields and managed to get it mired.

Identification of wildflowers and birds fascinated Margaret and Sandy. Purple, yellow, and white violets, columbine, anemones, Robin's plantain, bladder campion, moneywort, partridge berry, and cinquefoil were on the list that Sandy kept, and also a lovely Turk's Cap lily near the bank of the river. Many birds flew into the garden in Toronto and at the farm, but a brightly plumaged cardinal was apparently a new sight.

The farm provided much-needed respite, but the war was never far from their minds. A meeting of the Royal Society of Canada included a special session in Convocation Hall on postwar reconstruction. Dr. Wilder Penfield of Montréal, whom Margaret met for the first time, spoke about the future of medicine. B.K. Sandwell, editor of *Saturday Night* magazine, treated the economic aspects, and physics professor John K. Robertson of Queen's University speculated about the role of scientists.

Margaret's schedule did not permit her to use many of her series tickets to the Toronto Symphony, but she did hear Artur Rubenstein and also Joseph Szigeti, the Hungarian violinist, who played a Brahms concerto — "marvellous." She continued to read widely. *Edna St. Vincent Millay and Her Times* (1936), by Elizabeth Atkins, led to some of Millay's books, *King's Henchmen, The Prince Marries the Page, Fatal Interview,* and her love sonnets, some of which she found very beautiful. She also read *Sonnets from the Portuguese,* by Elizabeth Barrett Browning; Christina Rossetti's love sonnets, including *Monna Innominata;* and a book about Rainer Maria Rilke and two volumes of his poetry. Recalling that Sandy had enjoyed poems by Robert Frost, and regretting that his school schedule left little time for them to read together, she read to him *The Purple Grackles,* a poem by Amy Lowell.

Charley Best enjoyed his naval service, even though it took him away from Toronto constantly. He liked the activity, even if he deplored the snail's pace of the bureaucracy. He was aware of Margaret's fears and tried to do what he could to have the family together. One day in early June 1942, he phoned from Halifax and said that he wanted Margaret, Linda, and the boys to take the train east. He called again from Charlottetown and advised them against taking the day coach to Montréal because it would have so many troops — but Margaret wanted to save money. The train was a new experience for Henry, and Sandy had been on one only as a baby. "The soldiers were so nice — wanted to buy ginger ale for the boys — and one, a mechanic, took the boys out to the back of the car where there was some fresh air. Then, we had a tank driver friend and also an Air Force boy. They were all so helpful. We loaned them our magazines and altogether we had a fine day."

In Montréal, the travellers had dinner at the Windsor Hotel and then boarded the sleeper for McAdam Junction in New Brunswick.

Charley came through to McAdam on the Saint John train, and then they all took the short ride to St. Stephen, where Ralph Ayres met them with Grandfather Best's car.

The first sight of Schooner Cove and the white farmhouse always thrilled them. The raspberries were ripe and delicious. The Charles Armstrongs from Robbinston came to supper and the two Charleys hitched Smokey to the buggy. The Bests sent a wire to Henry and Lydia Mahon to join them from Boston but had a reply that Henry, almost forty-five, had offered his services as a liaison officer in the air force and had just reported to Washington, DC. Mrs. Armstrong, Margaret, and Sandy walked down the road with grass in the middle that led to Leighton's Point and went into the woods to collect flowers. Margaret wrote that she did this every day of their visit, just as she and Sandy had done at the farm in Stewarttown. They identified 110 species in that season.

On three occasions, the family rowed up to Long Cove, the next cove up the tide from Schooner Cove, and saw various birds and three mink. "We went up through the falls at high tide, the only time I have ever done that. Then we came back down when the tide had just begun to run again, and that was exciting as there were little whirlpools. We had lunch on a beach near there — a fire and cooked our chops and potatoes and Henry poured his tomato juice on my yellow cashmere sweater. Such a boy to spill!"

One evening, Dr. Herbert and Miriam Mowat Everett and Uncle Bruce Macleod arrived from St. Stephen. Mrs. Mariner Leighton made baked beans and brown bread, rolls, and raspberry pies. There was lots of singing, and Sandy picked out the tunes on his grandmother's piano. Charley and Bruce rode Miss Lou. Henry was improving. "Today he took Smokey by himself up to Mrs. Mariner's and then over to the Albert's. He has not taken to the riding as young as Sandy did. Sandy could do the same thing the summer he was five, but he seemed to be a born rider. Henry is seven now, will be eight in October. Other years, Smokey has just bucked Henry off."

There were fewer day trips than usual that summer, but a run to Eastport was obligatory to get fresh haddock at Rhea's Fish Market and have an ice cream soda at the counter of Havey and Wilson's. The Grand Manan boat was painted grey as camouflage. There was no word of the Quoddy Tidal Project. The buildings were now a youth training camp, and a small airport was being built nearby. Back home the haddock was cooked over a driftwood fire at Leighton Point.

One day, the Bests went to the next village to the east, Dennysville, to visit Charley's adopted aunt, Anna Lincoln, and her sister-in-law, Tishie Brown. Anna Lincoln was eighty-six and in very good form. Anna presented Margaret with a treasured leather-bound book *The Flora of Dennysville* containing over one hundred original botanical illustrations by her late husband, Dr. Arthur Talbot Lincoln. When Charley was young, he loved to visit the Lincolns in their big, beautiful, old yellow house, just where the Dennys River met the tide. This time Tishie Brown gave the boys a full tour. Sandy played a Brahms waltz on the piano, delighting the elderly ladies.

Everyone picked raspberries, and there were plenty to go around, including a twelve-quart pail for Mrs. Mariner to make jelly and jam. The day before they left the idea had been to take another trip in the rowboat, but instead, Charley and the boys built a tide fence so that the horses could not get around into Mariner Leighton's pasture at low tide. Three generations of the Albert Leighton family came to say goodbye. On 3 August, the whole family took the train from St. Stephen to McAdam and from there to Montréal where Charley had a meeting. Margaret took their sons in a *calèche* to the Château de Ramezay in "Vieux Montréal." She shopped at the Canadian Handicraft Shop, and they all went to the Café Martin for lunch.

As soon as they were back in Toronto, a message arrived from Hilda that Dr. Herbert Best was not well, so Charley and Margaret headed for Coboconk, Ontario, and the Salters' island. He had been unwell ever since he had had a heart attack shortly after Lulu's death in August 1940. He then had several more in Toronto at Christmas. After that his health deteriorated rapidly. At the Salters' cottage Grandfather was up and down from bed and deeply depressed. Margaret thought that it was good for Charley to see for himself how his father was. "It is a beautiful spot and if he isn't happy with Hilda he won't be happy anywhere." Depression was not understood by those who had not experienced the condition.

Dr. Herbert Best died on 20 August 1942. Charley had gone up again to the Salters' cottage two days before he died. Hilda and Charley went to Pembroke for the funeral. Margaret wrote, "Poor Dr. Best. He was never happy since Mrs. Best died two years and a day before he did." Charley said that the flowers were beautiful and the service was simple. The Herbert Everetts from St. Stephen, the Henry Eatons from Calais, the Charles Armstrongs from Robbinston, and the Francis Benedicts from Machiasport were among the mourners. A bit later a lawyer wanted Charley, who was in

Halifax, to sign a document permitting him to collect unpaid fees. Charley managed to get a car and drove directly to West Pembroke. He spent all night burning his father's books in the kitchen stove as he knew his father would never have harassed his patients for payment.

At the beginning of September, Henry had his tonsils taken out by Dr. Charles S. MacDougall at the Hospital for Sick Children on College Street, Toronto. Charley insisted on taking him home immediately after the operation. Dr. Alan Brown, the well-known chief of the hospital, followed Charley, who was carrying Henry down the hall, and exclaimed, "Charley, think of the reputation of my hospital." The reply was, "I brought him in here for one thing but I don't want him to pick up several others."

Margaret was meeting more of Charley's naval colleagues. Black-bearded Surgeon Lieutenant Jack Parker and his wife both hailed from the Annapolis Valley of Nova Scotia. Surgeon Lieutenant Edward Sellers and his wife, both from Winnipeg, came out to the farm for supper. Dr. Sellers, later a senior academic at the University of Toronto, made himself popular with Sandy by taking a picture of Rambler, the beagle, with no people in it.

Henry Mahon was now in England, a captain in the U.S. Army air force, doing liaison work between the American Twelfth Air Force and the British Air Ministry. Margaret was horrified, "I think it is most upsetting for Lydia — for us all." Charley tried to help by sending wires to Henry, suggesting people to contact, and to the Mellanbys, the Dales and Milton Brown, asking them to get in touch with his brother-in-law.

Margaret was always anxious about the boys, and, as she did not drive, she walked to Windy Ridge School on Balmoral Avenue every afternoon at three to bring Henry home. Her public contribution to the war effort was her membership on the committee for the Navy League Tag Day, and she spent the day on the corner of King and Yonge streets from 7:30 a.m., as well as making ditty bags. While Margaret was at the Tag Day, Captain McCallum called twice, wanting to take the boys to a rugby game, but the housekeeper would not let them go without their mother's permission.

Charley Best was away at the end of September to Trenton, Ottawa, Montréal, and Halifax. Later he, with Alex MacDonald and other eye specialists, were off to Halifax again to work on lighting for ships. Margaret was happy when he returned home. "It is good to have Charley home again. We don't see much of him, but at least he is here."

Charley, sometimes with Margaret, made many trips to Ottawa, Montréal, Halifax, and to the United States for naval or Rockefeller business. On 28 September 1942, he wrote, "Margaret dearest, I had a very productive session in Ottawa. Archie and I visited the Admiral and everything went well with the plans for the new ventures. The Admiral was most enthusiastic about our researches and wants to be the first guinea pig for the contacts [contact lenses]."[489] Admiral Percy Nelles was chief of naval staff from 1933 to 1943. In Montréal Charley mentioned having dinner with Bert Collip and visiting the Wilder Penfields.

Margaret went to New York with Charley on 16 December to meetings of the Rockefeller Foundation. There, Margaret met Dr. and Mrs. Wilbur Sawyer and Admiral Thomas Parran. They got tickets for Maxwell Anderson's *The Eve of St. Mark* at the Martin Beck Theatre and enjoyed it. Another evening, they went to see the Lunts in *The Pirate*. "They were excellent as they always are. Lynn Fontanne looked really beautiful. Alfred Lunt had a swashbuckling part to play. The stage settings were great fun. The scene of the play was the West Indies." The next evening, the Bests went to see Tallulah Bankhead in Thornton Wilder's *The Skin of Our Teeth*,[490] which she described as "extraordinary. She has lost many pounds since we saw her at Ruth and Vin's."

Christmas was very different in 1942. Charley came home from a short trip on the twenty-fourth. On Christmas Day, the family went to St. Andrew's Presbyterian Church. All the visitors to their home appreciated a brass-bound keg of rye whiskey that Samuel Bronfman, president of Seagrams, had sent to Charley. Margaret and Charley went to see Professor Edgar McInnis and his wife, Lorene. Edgar was an old friend from the days when he was at Oxford and the Bests were in London. He later dedicated his *History of Canada* to Charley because his wife was a diabetic.[491] Lieutenant-Governor Albert Matthews had asked him to be an honorary aide-de-camp, and he attended the New Year's Day levee. The papers announced Charley's promotion to surgeon commander. "Now he is a brass hat. We are very proud."

Henry developed the mumps. "He looks perfectly ridiculous — his darling little face is such a queer shape." A nurse came in to look after him during the day; Linda was at the lab but would be at home at night. Margaret, therefore, was able to accompany Charley on 3 January 1943 on a trip to Halifax where he had naval business and was to give the convocation address at Dalhousie University. The train to the Maritimes was crowded with servicemen. Surgeon Captain McCallum and two other naval officers joined the Bests in their compartment, where they had whisky from flasks filled from Charley's special keg, and pemmican,[492] part of the U.S. emergency rations, which they liked. "It tasted awfully good. There was coconut in it and raisins and quite a high fat content." Best and his colleagues were working on emergency rations for life rafts.

In their hotel room in Halifax on the evening of 4 January, Margaret wrote in her diary as Charley talked to the chief of police in the lobby. "When we got off the train we carried my zipper bag. The porter took Charley's big, brown bag off and my large bag and hat box. The red cap put the three bags on the big wagon and we walked on to the station. In a few minutes, the wagon came along minus Charley's big, brown leather bag. The red cap said that one of a party of three drunken sailors had taken the bag off saying it was his. They were on the train this afternoon and were awfully drunk. I would know all three of them again if I saw them. Charley's lecture for tomorrow night is in the bag, his beautiful scarlet robe for his DSc degree from London University, the hood and velvet hat, his flannel dressing gown and leather slippers, and several new books."

Later on Margaret added, "The Navy police located the sailors on an English destroyer in the harbour. Charley picked them out of a group and so did the red cap. The red cap said it was one of them who took the bag off the truck, but he didn't know which one. They admitted that they were standing by the truck and one said he took his own bag off. They were only located on Friday and the bag had been stolen on Monday night. They all swore they did not take the bag. Charley said they looked quite decent fellows when they were sober." Margaret recalled that Charley's bag had been bought in London, and she went over again in detail its contents and added, "The police were going to search the destroyer on Saturday. I don't think we will ever recover the bag. They had plenty of time all week to dispose of it."

From their hotel room in the Nova Scotian Hotel, Margaret saw several fairmiles and destroyers steam in, and she got on board a destroyer that she did not identify. The medical officer in charge at Halifax, David Johnstone, had been promoted to surgeon captain, as had A.L. Anderson, his opposite number at St. John's. Margaret met them for the first time and renewed acquaintance with Archie McCallum and Surgeon-Commanders Eddy Amos and Donald Webster. The medical service was beginning to pile up in ranks — there were now several surgeon captains, and there would be more.

Best gave his convocation address. He remembered enough of what he had prepared to make notes, and he spoke from those. Archie McCallum was on the platform, and Surgeon Lieutenant Commanders Dave Mitchell and Wallace Graham from Toronto were in the audience. The Bests enjoyed talking to Carlton Stanley, president of the university and a classicist, and his wife. She was a daughter of Dr. William J. Alexander, professor of English at Dalhousie and later at the University of Toronto.

The next day the Naval Hospital was opened. Rear Admiral Leonard Murray, commander of the east coast, and his wife entertained at an "attractive but meagre" lunch. "Mrs. Murray has brassy hair, horn-rimmed spectacles and a very certain manner. The Admiral is perfect — reddish hair, good looking, sideburns and blue, blue eyes. I think he came originally from New Glasgow." After the opening, the Bests went to a reception on board the destroyer *Hamilton* with Commander N.V. Clark at the helm. Margaret met Commander Rayner, who had commanded the *St-Laurent* when Charley was aboard her the previous year. Margaret wrote, "I think I like him best of all the new people I met." She sympathized with him about his wife, who lived out in Bedford with four small children and no help, so she could never get away to events such as this reception.

When Margaret returned to Toronto she received news of Henry Mahon in North Africa. Because of censorship, he could not pinpoint where he was, but there were clues. He talked about Algerian money, of lots of dates to eat, and of being in a city in Allied hands, probably Oran or Algiers. Lydia sent a copy that she had received of a commendation of Harry's service (most of his American colleagues called him Harry) by Brigadier General Delmar H. Denton, commanding the Twelfth Air Force Service Command, "Captain Mahon quickly grasped the problems and rendered invaluable service. He was responsible for maintaining liaison with important sources and sending valuable information on to this theatre."[493]

Dr. Joslin arrived from Boston to give the second Banting Memorial Lecture. He stayed with the Bests and arrived laden with biscuits, dates, prunes, candy, and tea from S.S. Pierce, the wonderful purveyors of fine foods in Boston. The whole family went to the opening of the exhibition of Fred Banting's paintings at the University of Toronto's Hart House. "It was awfully good and there were an amazing number of pictures. Some of them were very good." The canvas that Banting had given to Best, "Church at Ste-Fidèle," was reproduced on the cover of the catalogue. This was painted in 1930 at St-Fidèle de Mont-Murray, on the north shore of the St. Lawrence, a few miles east of La Malbaie.

Best went to New York in early March 1943 for a meeting of the Rockefeller IHD. Drs. Parran and Reed were replaced as scientific directors by Drs. Eugene L. Bishop and Harry S. Mustard. Charles Best was elected chairman of the scientific directors of the IHD for the year. From New York, Charley sent a telegram dated 5 March to Margaret. "Elected chairman IHD succeeding Tom Parran."[494]

For relaxation, Charley read books about the navy, including Lieutenant Nicholas Monsarrat, RNVR, *H.M. Corvette* (1943). Monsarrat had commanded a corvette in the North Atlantic in 1940 and 1941. On 16 March, CHB wrote from Halifax. "Yesterday was a very busy day. We were busy with 'ships' from morning until late afternoon, a very interesting and profitable day. In the late afternoon I gave a lecture to officers who are completing their course for 'commands' of ships, 'Practical Aspects of Naval Medical Research.'"[495]

Uncle Henry wrote again, probably from Algiers, sending a photo of himself studying maps with the caption, "Deep in Thought in North Africa." He had recently been promoted major. News from him was sparse, but he did talk of an Arab maid who "pads around in her bare feet with a veil over her face." Laurie Chute was home on sick leave from North Africa and told Charley of some very exciting experiences there.

Early in April 1943, Charley had an enjoyable trip to Roanoke, Virginia. He and Rear Admiral Luther Sheldon, Jr., assistant chief of the Bureau of Medicine and Surgery, Navy Department, in Washington, DC, spoke at a meeting held at the Gill Ear, Eye and Throat Hospital. Best liked the admiral very much and sympathized with him over his recent loss of a son on active service. Best conducted a clinic on "Physiology in War Medical Research" and gave the evening address on "The Story of Insulin." After the meeting, the two men went to the Gill Hospital's place in the hills and fished for trout. From there they went back to Washington, and, after meetings, Charley went to the admiral's home for dinner. Later that month, Best went to Philadelphia to a meeting of the American Philosophical Society, founded by Benjamin Franklin. There he presented a miniature of Sir Isaac Newton on behalf of the Royal Society of London.

Arriving back from the United States, Charley immediately took the family to the farm. He wanted to burn over a twelve-acre field to get rid of the weeds. Everyone carried pails of water and cedar branches to douse the flames around fence posts and power poles. Margaret found the whole exercise "most alarming," although "the boys quite enjoyed it."

Weekends at the farm were very busy that spring, as they prepared the garden and burned branches pruned from the fruit trees. The family enjoyed the wildflowers in the valley and the daffodils that were naturalized at the top of the hill, as well as the hyacinths and dwarf irises in the rock garden. Field glasses helped to identify the white-breasted nuthatches, wrens, savannah sparrows, and meadowlarks.

On 26 May 1943, the Bests went to the meetings of Royal Society of Canada in Hamilton. A services programme included speeches by Best, Archie McCallum, Brigadier Jonathan Campbell Meakins, deputy director general of the Royal Canadian Army Medical Corps, and Air Commodore J.W. Tice of the Air Medical Service.

On 8 June 1943, the Bests received a telegram from Colonel Willis O'Connor, principal aide-de-camp to the governor general, inviting them to a state dinner at Rideau Hall in honour of Madame Chiang Kai-shek, American-educated wife of the president of Nationalist China, who was trying to raise support for her husband's forces. "His Excellency, the Earl of Athlone, Princess Alice, and Madame Chiang Kai-shek appeared. They circled the room. I shook hands with Madame Chiang and shook hands and curtsied to the Earl of Athlone and Princess Alice. Madame Chiang was lovely — tiny, with gorgeous dark eyes. She wore a long fitted black lace dress, high at the neck and little cap sleeves. She had two ropes of jade beads, diamond and jade earrings and bracelet and jade rings. She looked very beautiful. His Excellency took Madame Chiang in to dinner. Prime Minister King took Princess Alice. Mr. Spinney[496] took me in and I had the prime minister on my left hand. The table looked lovely — white cloth and great silver bowls of red carnations. The ladies removed their long white gloves after we sat down. Princess Alice flung hers, I noticed, with abandon on the table in front of her. She is a very pretty woman. King was a most genial neighbour. He and I had a very pleasant time. He was a great friend of Wilfred Campbell, the poet.[497] We talked of the way in which history is taught in the schools today. It would seem that each generation is unhappy with the way history is taught, either wanting to go back to a previous era or forward to a new approach."

"After the meal, Charley had a long talk with Madame Chiang. She is tired and when she gets very nervous, she develops a rash on her arms and body. She consulted Charley on what she should do. She told him that President Roosevelt had given her some advice. He told her that when she was about to write a lecture or an article and felt tense, she was to throw

down her pen, get up and walk about the room saying, 'To Hell with it!'"
Later Margaret was sent for "to sit with Princess Alice for a time. Lemonade
and water was passed in the late evening, and then Madame Chiang and
the Athlones bade us goodnight, handshakes, curtseying again, and shortly
after, we all went away."

When Madame Chiang addressed a joint session of Parliament the
next morning, Margaret listened to her on a loud-speaker installed outside
the Commons chamber. "She is undoubtedly an amazing woman. I was a
little disappointed in her speech. She seemed to be interpreting British
parliamentary history to us and the history of Canada, and the relationship of the French and the English. I think her speech should have been
more about China." Margaret then went to have lunch with Senator
Cairine Wilson and several other women in government. Charley had a
day of naval meetings before they returned to Toronto.

The *Toronto Star* on 21 June 1943, printed photos of some of the
sponsors of a "Salute to Russia" gathering. Included, along with Charles
Best, were R.Y. Eaton, former president of T. Eaton Co.; Norman
Mackenzie, president of the University of New Brunswick; Dr. R.C.
Wallace, principal of Queen's University; and Sir Edmund Wyly Grier,
past president of the Royal Canadian Academy. Years later, with the advent
of the Cold War, the RCMP questioned Best about his involvement in the
"Salute to Russia," but, of course, in 1943, Russia was a staunch ally.

In late June 1943, Charles Best set out for Ottawa and the east coast.
In the meantime, Margaret and the boys went to the farm and worked in
the garden, readied the house in town for the summer by rolling up the
rugs and packing the silver off to the bank, and packed their bags to join
Charley in Nova Scotia. On 1 July 1943, the *Globe and Mail* had Charley's
picture on the front page announcing his promotion to acting surgeon
captain. "It is a very high naval rank and we are so proud."

On 7 July, Margaret, Linda, and the boys took the train to Montréal en
route to Nova Scotia, and ate the lunch that they had taken with them.
Linda Mahon also wrote a diary for part of the holiday. She told of Margaret
and Sandy's recognizing various wildflowers from the train "and crying out,
'Look at the False Solomon's Seal!' and, 'Oh, look at the Viper's bugloss,' and
other such names fell so glibly from their lips." "When we were leaving the
diner," wrote Linda, "Sandy whispered to me, 'Perhaps people will think we
are distinguished botanists.'"[498] Sandy was twelve years old. (Eventually he
did become a distinguished botanist and an expert on lilies.)

At Baddeck on Cape Breton Island, James Fraser, owner of the Baddeck Hotel, met them. He installed them in little cabins in the apple orchard. Margaret took the family out looking for wildflowers, finding wild lupin, wild iris, purple vetch, Labrador tea, and many other varieties. Charley arrived the next day with a cold, "which he probably picked up from Ed Sellers with whom he had been rooming in Halifax." Margaret never gave up trying to trace the genealogy of a cold or other ailment. Charley discovered a sloop called *The Surf* that was available and a not very busy petty officer to sail it, so the family enjoyed several outings. "Even I have learned a little, for instance, that the three longer words go together: starboard, right and green; then, you have port, left and red."

Shortly after Charley arrived, Mrs. Macmillan, the doctor's wife, came to fetch him because her husband was away and Casey Baldwin's wife, Kathleen, had had a car accident. She was taken to the hospital in Sydney. In 1908, F.W. "Casey" Baldwin, who was born and educated in Ontario, became the first British subject to fly an airplane when he made the first American public flight in Hammondsport, New York. Alexander Graham Bell, who had a summer home near Baddeck, had conducted his experiments with flying machines at Baddeck before the Wright brothers flew in 1903. Baldwin and J.A.D. McCurdy, a native of Baddeck who made the first successful flight in Canada when he piloted the *Silver Dart* over the ice of the Bras d'Or Lakes in 1909, were at the same time colleagues and rivals.

On two occasions, the Bests were invited to the Baldwins' house. He had been in charge of the Graham Bell Laboratories and worked on hydrofoils and other developments used in naval and aerial warfare. In 1943, both of Baldwin's sons were away in the navy. He was very kind and considerate to the Bests. Linda thought that he looked a little like Sir Walter Scott. He wanted to take the boys sailing, and he gave Margaret some kapok to make a life preserver for Henry.

While the Bests were in Baddeck, Gilbert Grosvenor, editor of *National Geographic* magazine, and his wife, Elsie, Alexander Graham Bell's daughter, arrived. A few days later, the Bests visited them at "Beinn Bhreagh" (Beautiful Mountain), which had been the Bells' summer home. "Sandy said it was one of the most nervous luncheons he was ever at. He had Henry sitting beside him and Henry took second helpings of everything that was passed. Henry had a thoroughly good time. Afterwards, Sandy and Henry both played on the old grand piano that Graham Bell played on so often. Mr. Grosvenor was in grand cheer. He loaned a bird book and a flower book and a chart of these waters, and he gave me a copy of James D. Gillis' life of Angus McAskill, *The Cape Breton Giant: A Truthful Memoir.*[499] His grandson took the Bests up the hill to the Bells' grave, marked by a great rock.

Charley Best spoke at the Baddeck Court House to the local Red Cross Society about the blood serum work. "He wore his uniform and his talk was grand and he looked perfect." Casey Baldwin moved the vote of thanks. Surgeon Captain A.L. Anderson and his wife, Gilbert and Elsie Grosvenor, and all the guests from the hotel were there. As Margaret said, "It was quite a meeting."

One day, the Bests borrowed a car and went off to Margaree and to Chéticamp, on the west coast of the island. They stopped at Mrs. Mariner Smith's well-known hotel, where several people they knew stayed when they were fishing on the Margaree River. Margaret and Linda were delighted with the weaving and handicrafts of the Acadian women in the area.

Prime Minister Winston Churchill and President Franklin Roosevelt held their historic meeting in Québec City from 19 to 24 August 1943, to plan for the Normandy landings, operations in Southeast Asia, and the Italian campaign. The University of London wanted to present Roosevelt with an honorary LLD. Their Chancellor, the Earl of Athlone, was the governor general of Canada and in Ottawa. His chief aide-de-camp, Colonel Willis O'Connor, sent a message to Charles Best asking him to come to Ottawa as the University of London had chosen him to present Roosevelt for his degree on 25 August.

There was a small luncheon at Rideau Hall before the ceremony. Among the American guests were Harry Hopkins, FDR's closest adviser, and Admiral Ross McIntire, the president's doctor. The Canadians present included Prime Minister King, Colonel J.L. Ralston, Angus L. Macdonald, Major General Leo R. La Flèche, C.G. Power, and Louis St. Laurent, all senior cabinet ministers, except for La Flèche, who was deputy minister of national defence.

Having lost his London DSc gown in Halifax, Charley borrowed one from Professor John Satterley, a brilliant and eccentric professor of physics at Toronto. Charley's short speech of presentation had arrived from the University of London. It contained a quotation that he did not recognize, so he called Professor W.J. Alexander, who had taught both Margaret and Charley at University College, and asked him. The elderly scholar replied, "Best, I am eighty-eight, of course I won't know." Then Charley called his old friend Edgar McInnis, who recognized it as a passage from Robert Browning. After the ceremony, the governor general asked the source of the quote, and Charley was able to tell him. He was pleased that he had done his homework.[500]

In reply to a Admiral McIntire, Best wrote to FDR recalling their meeting on Campobello Island on 29 August 1936 and attaching a copy of the citation, which also included a passage from the New Testament Philippians, 4:8: "Finally, brethren, whatsoever things *are* true, whatsoever things *are* honest, whatsoever things *are* just, whatsoever things *are* pure, whatsoever things *are* lovely, whatsoever things *are* of good report; if *there be* any virtue, and if *there be* any praise, think on these things." The president replied mentioning the citation and regretting the fact that, due to the war, it was the first year that his cottage on Campobello had not been opened.[501]

The farm at Stewarttown was still a Mecca for the family. In the autumn of 1943, Margaret and various helpers made pickles from the produce from the garden, chili sauce, and mustard beans, as well as tomato marmalade and apple and chokecherry jelly. They had Peter Simpson Best to ride, fences to fix, and wildflowers and birds to identify — ruby-crowned kinglets, chickadees, song sparrows, white-crowned sparrows, and myrtle warblers. Sandy learned a lot from Mr. Beckett, the Scottish gardener. When Charley was away, Margaret, Linda, and the boys would walk into Georgetown to shop. Mamie Moyer, whose husband, Harold, ran an apple orchard nearby, was an expert weaver who encouraged Margaret's interest in that craft.

The boys continued their music lessons. Sandy started in October taking violin lessons with Harry Adaskin, a founding member of the Hart House String Quartet at the University of Toronto. In December, he heard Mrs. Adaskin discussing what she was going to give her husband for Christmas. After his lesson, Sandy said, "I'm very low on funds, Mr. Adaskin, so I am not sending you a Christmas present but I am sending you a card."

The house at 78 Old Forest Hill Road had a problem with damp, and sometimes floods, in the basement room that served as Charley's study. It was a very pleasant spot with a fireplace, but regularly the water rose, rugs would be floating, and Charley's desk and Grandmother Mahon's piano had high-water marks.

On Tuesday, 19 October 1943, Charley left Toronto for Montréal. Margaret suspected that he was probably going overseas, and she was very uneasy. Two days later, he called, and when he was told that the weather in Toronto was lovely, "he said he wished it was lovely where they were going. Then in the evening he phoned me again. On Friday morning, there was no call so I knew they were off. On Saturday morning at seven minutes to eleven, the telegraph office phoned me a cable from Charley from Glasgow to say that they had had a fine trip. So that was a quick way of crossing the ocean. I have no idea how many hours they took." Charley had just made his first flight across the Atlantic. Fully aware of how anxious Margaret would have been, because of Banting's fate, Charley had not mentioned he was going by plane. After his return in mid-November, Margaret noted, "Charley has been talking into the dictaphone telling about his trip. I want to have it all typed out to keep."

In his account, Best told of flying from Montréal in one of three Liberator bombers with RAF crews. Other passengers included Sir Henry Tizard, scientific adviser to the British Air Ministry, who was largely responsible for adoption of radar for air defence; Professor Ezer Griffiths from Oxford, a physicist; and Commander J.L. Little, chief of Canadian medical intelligence.

> We flew at an altitude of 9 or 10 thousand feet and oxygen was unnecessary. The plane was reasonably warm and the mattresses on which we lay were comfortable. There were no seats. There were eleven of us on the plane. The only one whom I had known before, except my travelling companion Lew Little, was Professor Griffiths. An Australian Wing commander, Mason by name, was the next one along and we got to know him fairly well during the trip. Sandwiches and coffee were available all the time ... It was an eleven hour flight.[502]

In London on Wednesday, 3 November, "I spent the morning with Professor Alexander Fleming and Professor Almroth Wright. I was anxious to talk about penicillin to Fleming but Professor Wright, who was getting pretty old [eighty-two] was always interrupting to talk about our work on heparin. Fleming gave me a preparation of penicillin in a watch glass. This was part of the original culture which he had used in the discovery of penicillin."

On 4 November, the Royal Society Club met. "There were about thirty members and six guests," including Field Marshal Jan Smuts, the seventy-three-year-old prime minister of South Africa; Niels Bohr, the Danish Nobel laureate in physics in 1922; Lord Keynes, the eminent economist; and Professor E.N. Allott, a pathologist who became president of the Section of Experimental Medicine of the Royal Society of Medicine in 1944. After the dinner, all the guests were asked to speak. "Smuts was far the best of the lot. He emphasized the fact that England did not always put forward their own case strongly enough. The Mediterranean campaign was 90 percent the result of British effort and was second to none in importance in the war. He spoke enthusiastically about the increase in the use of science in the war."

Bohr "spoke of the situation in Denmark. It was quite good while they were the model occupied country but much worse recently as a result of some Axis sabotage. About 1,000 Danes had escaped to Sweden when the Germans took over the control. The Swedes were most helpful. Krogh, he said, was still in Copenhagen but I learned later that Krogh went to Lund shortly after that time."

Keynes talked about the will to understand each other, that is, the financial groups in the United States and Great Britain, and Allott believed "that England and the United States got along much better when a third party was present ... I spoke very briefly of the presentation of the miniature of Newton to the American Philosophical Society which I had carried out on behalf of The Royal Society. I also described very briefly the presentation of the degree from the University of London to President Roosevelt."

After the banquet, in a bomb shelter during a raid, Smuts invited Best to South Africa, and wanted him to report on nutritional problems in his country. "I was tremendously impressed with his knowledge of scientific affairs and his affability." In London, Best also met Brigadier Basil Schonland, the South African director of Operational Research at the War Office. "Omond Solandt succeeded him a little later."

The next day brought meetings with Sir Thomas Lewis, the heart specialist, and the Bests' old friend Dr. Francis Carr. At noon, Dr. A.M. O'Brien of Rockefeller invited Best and Lew Little to the Athenaeum with John Winant, the U.S. ambassador. "We had a fine talk about a great many different problems. Winant was very enthusiastic about the benevolent dictator of Portugal and I later bought a book on Salazar and read it most carefully. There is no doubt that he's an interesting bird."[503] Best was not as impressed with Salazar as the ambassador.

While he was in London Best missed a Rockefeller IHD meeting in New York when it was recorded that, "Dr. Best, Dr. Maxcy, and Dr. Rivers were overseas on missions connected with military activities."[504] At the same meeting, grants totalling $39,250 were made to the School of Hygiene and the School of Nursing of the University of Toronto.[505]

Surgeon Lieutenant-Commander J.L. "Lew" Little accompanied Best to almost all his meetings in Britain. A general practitioner from Guelph, he was director of the Canadian Medical Intelligence Division. Along with liaison officers in Washington and London, he collected and studied information about health conditions in all theatres of war. Such activity forewarned the commanders in Italy of the typhus fever epidemic in Naples in 1943, and surveys of Japanese territory proved to be very accurate and enabled medical planning for operations in the Ryukyu Islands and elsewhere.[506] The ten years that Dr. Little had spent in the Far East was very good preparation for this part of his work.

On the evening of 5 November the Royal Society of Medicine gave a reception for Best. "Sir Henry Cardy had arranged to invite not only my friends, Robin Lawrence and a number of the Canadian Naval officers, and F.G. Young of St Thomas's Hospital, but also the medical representatives of almost all of the occupied countries who had exile governments in England. I had long talks with the Greek medical officer, with the Dutch, Czech, Belgian and French. In insulin supply, the Greeks had been very badly off for a time, but received Canadian insulin shortly after the German occupation. In Holland and Czechoslovakia and Belgium, there was a great lack of the material, and as one of the medical officers put it: 'It is very hard to have our children thrust back before the insulin era.' I have developed this information into lectures and have used the data several times before medical audiences."

On 9 November, there was a meeting on penicillin at the Royal Society of Medicine, with Robin Lawrence in the chair, and both Dr. Fleming and Dr. Florey[507] taking part. The next two days were "largely filled with straight Naval work. Lew Little and I attended a meeting of the Personnel Naval Research Committee and marvelled at [Edward] Mellanby's efficiency in handling the meeting and at his rather uncompromising attitude on some occasions."[508]

While Charley was overseas, Lydia Mahon was visiting in Toronto and distracted Margaret by taking her out for lunch. The next day, the Upper Canada College Cadet Corps took part in a church parade in support of the Victory Loan Scheme. Sandy mislaid his white gloves, and ended up wearing his father's kid-leather evening gloves — Margaret remarked, "Preserve me from crises like that."

"Charley came home on Saturday last, November 20th. I had a phone call from him on Friday. It came through at 10 to 2 on Friday afternoon, from New York. I was so thrilled. I had been looking for it every minute. Charley had come back on the *Queen Elizabeth* … We all went down to meet the New York train on Saturday morning. Jessie drove the Cadillac. The train was due at 8 o'clock and we all got up at 6:30, but we had been awake most of the night, excitement and not wanting to be late. Charley looked tired and had a bad cold. It was a joy to have him back again. Charley and I talked most of the night, Saturday night."

After their return to Canada, Lew Little wrote to Charley:

> I suddenly realized that I hadn't properly said "thank you" for the good fellowship we had together over the past month. It was more than a trip together. It gave me an insight into your mind and method of achievement. I'm so convinced that you can do big things for this country and the world. I only wish you keep your health and vigor and your quest for improving the health of that sorry figure Genus homo sapiens.
>
> Then too it was good to meet your friends yonder! Robin, A.V. Hill, Mellanby, Parry, Barcroft, Beattie, Young, Winant, McNee, Graham and the others. I'm convinced though that you have a spark that none of them can outdim. The spark that impressed me most was your intense interest in folks as folks, and not mere physiological nerve-muscle preparations. You are as great a friend as you are a physiologist and that's putting a high standard. I'm with you through thick and thin. I hope to see more of you from time to time. Sometimes I'll take the liberty of taking you to the mat but only if I think you are not keeping up your own high standards for yourself. Don't burn out for the best things are still ahead for you.[509] I speak as a seer.

A good resumé of the activities of Charles Best and his colleagues during the Second World War is given in Chapter 59 of Best's *Selected Papers,* entitled, "The Division of Naval Medical Research, Royal Canadian Navy." Here, he mentioned the main research projects undertaken and the people who were involved. Aside from the report submitted to the NRC by Best and Solandt after their 1941 trip to Britain already mentioned, there was another Progress Report submitted by Best and Solandt to Captain McCallum, dated 12 May 1943, dealing with night vision, hearing, immersion foot, and shock, among other subjects.[510]

One topic that precipitated considerable debate, particularly between scientists at the University of Toronto and at McGill University in Montréal, concerned the most effective seasickness remedy, and taking a patent. C.J. Mackenzie wrote in his diary: "I have never seen anything like the fuss that is being kicked up all over the world, requests for the formula, etc. It is a first-class hoax … I would not want to be in Charlie Best's place."[511] The final formula for the seasickness pills is given as 0.1 mg of hyoscine and 0.3 mg of hyoscyamine, combined with 120 mg of the thiobarbiturate V-12.[512]

Best recounted in a draft report entitled "Medical Research in the Royal Canadian Navy," the story of a young captain who, while reading a chart under red lighting, was called to the bridge to find that they were "proceeding at right angles through a large convoy." His night vision was not decreased "as it would have been by ordinary illumination, and he was able to evaluate the situation immediately and to give orders which averted a collision." Red bridge lighting was adopted on the ships of the Royal and the Royal Canadian navies in November 1941.[513] A portable laboratory kit became available in early 1943 for use by medical officers of both navies ashore and afloat.[514]

In a briefing to the Defence Medical Research Advisory Committee, Rear Admiral E. P Tisdall said, "In 1939, Dr. Charles Best arrived in Halifax, and in a series of simple demonstrations to rather sceptical and tradition-bound officers, soon changed all that. Among his triumphs were, the provision of ruby lighting inside ships to prevent night blindness, a motion sickness remedy for poor sailors, and the development of excellent survival equipment and protective clothing. For these alone the Navy owes him much."[515]

In Toronto in early December 1943, Best gave a lecture to the Royal Canadian Institute in Convocation Hall. The packed room heard him speak on the blood serum work and also on a new topic, penicillin. He was able to tell of his meetings with Fleming and Florey in England. Best gave another public speech as the special guest on 3 December at the Art Gallery of Toronto in connection with a loan exhibition of paintings from

Canada and the United States to raise money for the Navy League and its work with merchant seamen. Best went to Baltimore for the launching of a 10,000-ton Liberty ship named the S.S. *Frederick Banting*. Lady Banting performed the honours.[516]

Ten days before the launch in Baltimore CHB had been in New York to chair his last meeting of the scientific directors of the IHD on 10 December 1943, just before he completed his three-year term. At the December meeting of the scientific directors, it was reported that the trustees of the foundation had elected Drs. Thomas Parran and Wilton Halverson to succeed Best and Rivers. "Dr. T.M. Rivers and Dr. C.H. Best gave brief accounts of their recent visits overseas."[517] John D. Rockefeller, Jr. thanked Best for his three years of service to the IHD in a letter dated 19 January 1944.

Margaret commented on the end of Charley's appointment with the Rockefeller Foundation. "One has to retire then. He has enjoyed it enormously. He said that many said they hoped he would be back on again after a year off." However, Margaret was not entirely happy. "His appointment certainly came at a poor time for me. In normal times, I could have gone to New York with Charley when he was attending those meetings."

Christmas 1943 was fairly quiet. Margaret was busy shopping for the children of English friends who were war guests. Henry received *The Oxford Book of Carols,* from which everybody sang. There were gifts of pine furniture for the cabin, subscriptions to *National Geographic, Canadian Nature, Natural History Magazine, Popular Science, New Yorker, Mademoiselle, Atlantic Monthly,* and *Vogue,* and Margaret bought a small oil of a northern forest scene by John Hall for Charley and Sandy, for which she paid thirty-five dollars.

Between Christmas and New Year's Day, Charley learned that he was being made a Commander of the Order of the British Empire (CBE), in the King's New Year's Honours List. The citation read, "Outstanding contribution in the field of Medical Research and particularly on behalf of the Armed Forces of Canada and the United Nations."

On 24 January 1944, Lieutenant-Governor and Mrs. Albert Matthews received in honour of Lord Halifax, who spoke to the Board of Trade. Halifax had been Viceroy of India from 1926 to 1931, foreign secretary from 1938 to 1940, and was the UK ambassador to the United States from 1941 to 1946. Margaret Best noted "that Lord Halifax made his famous speech … suggesting a very close co-operation of members of the British Commonwealth of Nations, after the war. It has caused a enormous amount of controversy." Prime Minister King "was simply dumbfounded and stated that, 'I am perfectly sure that Canada will not tolerate any centralized Imperialism on foreign policy.'"[518]

Margaret and Charley spent a weekend as house guests at Rideau Hall in January 1944. The other house guests were Field Marshal Sir John Dill and Lady Dill and Mrs. Basil Price of Montréal. Dill was UK representative to the chiefs of staff in Washington. Mrs. Price was the wife of Major General Basil Price, head of the Overseas Canadian Red Cross, previously commanding the Third Canadian Division.

Princess Alice poured whisky or lemonade for them. She told Margaret that the furniture at the Citadel in Québec was "obscene." When Churchill came to Ottawa he stayed at Rideau Hall. "Princess Alice told Margaret that Mr. Churchill had our rooms when he stayed with them. He carried on telephone conferences with London from that sitting room and he sucked his cigars and wandered out in the hall in a big dressing gown and he kept awful hours. 'He slept in that bed,' said the vicereine, pointing to the far one in the big bedroom. 'Then I know which one I am going to sleep in,' I said. She gave me a poke, and she chuckled, 'Don't tell your husband until the morning.'"

On the Sunday morning, the vice-regal couple walked to church. "The aides told Charley to keep out of the corridors at ten to 11 – zero hour – or he would find himself gathered up willy-nilly and taken to church." Margaret found Lord Athlone hard to talk to "because he mumbles," and she was amused at his refusal to eat the chocolate cake offered at tea. "No, it is no good any more." "Charley said that he consulted him about his health. When I asked Charley what seemed to be his trouble, Charley said, 'bowels.'" Margaret concluded, "It was a very pleasant weekend. Princess Alice is a perfectly charming little lady who keeps her eye all the time on the comfort and happiness of her guests." Charles Best was certainly the most junior of the military guests. There was no special foreign visitor. The Bests had been invited by the Athlones because they liked them and enjoyed their company.

From Ottawa, Charley went to Halifax, and Margaret to Toronto. Charley, Don Solandt, and Ed Sellers took the train to Boston and then returned to Halifax on a tank-landing ship, doing experiments on seasickness for three days and two nights. Margaret wrote to Charley in Halifax on 3 February 1944 that she had been to Laing's Art Gallery to see the

J.E.H. Macdonald and Tom Thomson paintings on view. "They have half a dozen Macdonalds that they never had before ($75 each) and three or four Thomsons. They are $200. I am anxious for you to see them. They are really lovely — both."[519]

Margaret kept close tabs on the boys' school results. Sandy's exams were delayed because of a quarantine for scarlet fever. He got 87 percent in geometry, 91 percent in French, 86 percent in history — top of his class in the last two. He stood fifth overall, but his parents were pleased because there was a lot of competition. Henry was now at UCC in form 3 of the prep school. To his chagrin his mother always compared his report card with Sandy's at the same stage. At Christmas, Henry stood second in his class. Form Master Earl Elliott told Henry that he might have stood first if his handwriting were better. By Easter, he was down to fifth. However, by the end of the year, Henry and his friend, Tony Rolph, had tied for first place.

On 6 March, Margaret left with Charley for Washington. She spent a day at the National Gallery of Art, a new building of Tennessee marble. Andrew Mellon gave the building, and a collection of paintings, to the nation. Margaret described the building in detail, and then the paintings. Both she and Charley went to see the impressive new Jefferson Memorial, a replica of the third president's home, Monticello, with a standing statue of the American hero inside. One evening, they went to see the film *Madame Curie* about the Polish-born double Nobel laureate Maria Sklodowska-Curie, starring Greer Garson and Walter Pidgeon. "I liked it fairly well. It was to me a very serious, earnest, sad picture."

In late March, the Athlones entertained five hundred guests including the Bests at the Royal York Hotel. "We had an awfully good time, seeing many old friends. Princess Alice looked very beautiful in a sparkling white gown, pearls and great blue stones hanging on the front of her bodice, gorgeous. Her white hair was blue in tint. She is really very lovely. As the long line-up went through to be received, I took her hand and curtsied and she smiled so sweetly and said, 'We will see you later.'"

After "God Save the King," the Athlones stopped to shake hands with President Cody and his wife, with Boris Hambourg, the well-known cellist and impresario, and Mrs. Hambourg, and with the Bests. "I curtsied to both of them. Princess Alice said to me, 'You are much more rested now,' meaning than when I was in Ottawa, and I answered that I was. They are really very sweet, and then off they went with Vera Grenfell [Princess Alice's lady-in-waiting] waving goodbye to Charley and me."

The Bests, with Linda, went to Rideau Hall again in late April so that Charley could receive the CBE from the governor general. At the ceremony, "Everyone was affected when a widow or mother of the recipient received the medal, especially when a little girl went up to accept her late father's decoration." Willa Magee Walker, head of the Women's Air Force, received the MBE. Her family and the Mahons were friends in St. Andrews; her husband, the novelist David Walker, was a prisoner of war. Dr. Duncan Graham, professor of medicine at Toronto and prominent in the NRC, also received the CBE. Wing Commander Bill Franks received the OBE for his work on the Franks flying suit.

Margaret in her diary referred to D-Day, the landing of the Allies on the coast of Normandy on 6 June 1944, an event "we have all been looking forward to and dreading too." It seemed the beginning of the end, but there was the inevitable toll in casualties. Charley, however, was safe in North America, with no more overseas duty in sight. Henry Mahon also was safe in Washington on sixty-day duty. In Toronto, everything seemed almost normal. Henry, at nine, won the seventy-five-yard dash at his sports day and was happy as he accepted his ribbon from Mrs. Matthews, wife of the lieutenant-governor.

On 15 June, the whole family went to the west coast, where CHB had medical and naval lectures to give. Claude Dolman, who was in charge of the regional branch of the Connaught Laboratories, introduced them to Ira Dilworth, head of the Vancouver office of the Canadian Broadcasting Corporation. Dilworth had edited the books written by the artist Emily Carr, and he arranged for the Bests to visit her in Victoria. Margaret and Charley deposited their sons at the Provincial Museum, having heard that she might not tolerate a visit from a thirteen year old and a nine year old. Margaret admired Carr's work and was looking forward to meeting her.

"We drove to Miss Carr's house on St. Andrew's Street, a little house with a sign on the gate telling visitors to take the left-hand gravelled path to Miss Emily Carr, and another path for her sister. We went around to the left and toward the back was a door saying 'The Studio.' A woman let us in and showed us into the room at the back of the house — the studio." Margaret carefully described Carr. "Her hair was encased in a heavy net. She wore a tan, loosely fitting smock or dress, that hung around her neck. She had bright eyes, but she was miserable with asthma and could hardly speak at first. She got her honey and lemon and some such mixture in a glass and several times took a bit of it with a stopper."

Animals filled her life. "There was a squirrel in a cage. Her pictures stood in racks around the room. She told of her painting trips — living in a caravan, with her dogs, her monkeys, her white rats. She never liked to stay in sportsman's hotels, where those men go who always 'kill things.' She talked about Ira Dilworth and said that she has given to him the manuscripts of her autobiography. It is not to be published until she dies. She thinks it a much better plan to wait. We told her how much we liked 'The Clearing,' the picture that she wants to put at the end of her book." Carr liked to keep her work fresh. "She says she has always liked to experiment — didn't want to get in a rut. When she studied in Paris years ago, her teacher or teachers said they were glad that she wasn't afraid to try out something, even when a picture was almost completed. She said she was very excited, herself, when she went to Toronto years ago and saw the work done by the group there — Group of Seven — trying to do something really different — something Canadian — painting what they saw in Ontario — Georgian Bay, etc., and doing it in a suitable way for the Canadian landscape, not just following the European manner. She said that that made her happy because it was the same thing that she had been trying to do in the West — but she was alone in her effort there. She said that she tired of doing the Indian paintings — totem poles and villages. In a way it was documentary and historical. She had been very much interested in them. But lately she wanted to do her impressions of the trees, the woods, the mountains, etc., and do them in rather a large way, out of doors. So she began doing oil paintings on paper — fairly large, out of doors. Charley pulled out a picture that was a portrait of a woman, 'Oh, put it away,' she said, 'That was a maid I had and I couldn't bear her.' Then she said that she never liked doing portraits. 'It doesn't seem quite decent — prying and probing into other people's personalities.'" Margaret and Charley were thrilled to buy four large paintings and Linda one — oil on paper, for fifty dollars each.

After they returned to Toronto Miss Carr wrote to Charles Best, "I cannot tell you how I enjoyed your visit to my studio. To meet grand people doing grand things is a treat in my hum drum slot in life and gives me a stir. The day after you had been, someone gave me a write up in the paper about you and the letters tacked to your name amazed me but this was not what impressed one. It was the niceness of all three of you that I enjoyed."[520]

The family spent a few days on Bowen Island, courtesy of Ernest Buckerfield, a man with varied business interests such as Union Steamships and Steele Briggs Seeds, and then at a cottage on Lake Edith in Jasper Park on the way back east.

The farm continued to recharge the Bests' batteries. "We were getting more attached to the little cabin and the farm all the time. However, it is not an ideal place in the very hot weather. Once that was past it was lovely. Charley got out when he could and he enjoys the exercise he gets out there." By the autumn of 1944, Henry, almost ten, was doing some real work. Margaret, Linda, and Jessie Ridout did a lot of pickling and preserving and had prepared one hundred jars for the winter, including pickled beets, chow-chow, uncooked pickles in crocks, strawberry jam, and plum jam. At Thanksgiving, there was a rush to get all the vegetables in, and moonlight helped. Later in the month, Sandy was planting bulbs while Charley worked on an oil painting of the woods and the valley called *Wind in the Pines*, which became a Christmas card to raise money for the Canadian Diabetes Association and later was donated by the family to be hung in the foyer of the Charles H. Best Institute.[521]

Sandy's work in watercolours was progressing well. He gave Jessie Ridout a striking study of two kingfishers. Margaret rarely permitted any of Sandy's or Charley's work to be given away. Sandy did a picture of two heavy horses for Margaret and Charley's wedding anniversary on 3 September 1944. The same evening, Margaret, Charley, and Sandy went to Convocation Hall to hear Dr. George C. Vaillant of Philadelphia talk about the Aztecs. "Sandy enjoyed it enormously and took eight pages of notes in the dark." He later showed great interest in Pre-Colombian art and became a collector. At the reception afterwards, "One saw Dr. Vaillant, Mr. Otto Holden (last year's president of the Royal Canadian Institute) and Professor John R. Dymond of the Royal Ontario Museum, and Sandy, seated around a small table, having a delightful talk."

Sandy had great encouragement in his botanical interests. When he was preparing an oral presentation on the sagyz, or Russian dandelion, from which rubber can be made, Margaret's botany professor, George Duff, provided roots, seeds, rubber made from the plant, and slides. One day, Dr. John W. McCubbin, a PhD in chemistry and Sandy's science teacher at UCC, exploded, "My God, Best, I wish you wouldn't ask me so many questions!" "Sandy said that he did not blame him at all — he really did ask a lot of questions." McCubbin later apologized: "Ask me all the questions you like, Best. I was rather tired." "As a sequel Sandy told me that he had loaned Dr. McCubbin his little service magazine that Daddy got him, and that Dr. McCubbin had loaned him a book on molecules! Charley had a good laugh over the whole story. Sandy was home with a little cold on Wednesday of this week, and he was boiling up a brew of some kind of bark over a little lamp and he got me quite nervous. I don't want him doing that when I am not around to watch the fire hazards." Botany and agriculture became Sandy's dominant interests.

Towards the end of 1944 Best's naval responsibilities were gradually winding down. In October, he gave a paper at one session and chaired another at a Hormone Conference held at Mont Tremblant, north of Montréal. He enjoyed a straight medical meeting — he hadn't been at many since he was in the service. Shortly afterwards, Best was back in Montréal as an examiner for the Royal College of Physicians of Canada.

Best heard from his old friend Dr. A.N. Drury, of Britain's Medical Research Council, late in 1944. Drury explained that no further supplies of dried blood serum would be needed after the end of the year. "I need hardly tell you how valuable this supply of Canadian dried serum has been to us. We fulfilled special and urgent demands for D-Day which we could not have done from our own resources. We had a sense of security during the flying bomb period when we never knew when a transfusion depot in Southern England might not only be put out of action but have its serum stocks destroyed."[522] At the beginning of the war Best had thought the blood serum project would be very important for the war effort. Against Banting's wishes, but with the emphatic support of Sir Henry Dale, Best had continued research on blood serum and set up the Red Cross blood banks. By May 1942 the Canadian Red Cross was receiving 3,500 donations of blood per week; over two million donations were received and dried and shipped to England.[523]

On 10 December 1944, the first Nobel prizes in physiology and medicine awarded since 1939 were presented in New York. The American Nobel Anniversary Committee and the American-Scandinavian Foundation invited Charles Best to the special ceremony at the Waldorf-Astoria Hotel. His old friends Herbert Gasser and Joseph Erlanger shared the 1944 prize for their "discoveries concerning the highly differentiated functions of single nerve fibres." Gasser was director of the Rockefeller Institute from 1935 to 1953, including the years when Best was a scientific director of its IHD. He, like Best later, had spent two years as a young man working with Henry Dale and A.V. Hill in London. The 1943 prize went to Dr. Henrik Dam of Denmark, who "discovered Vitamin K, essential to the blood, and without which the body is unable to heal wounds," and to Dr. Edward A. Doisy of the U.S., who "discovered the chemical nature of Vitamin K and made it synthetically."[524]

Visitors came to Toronto from India. Lieutenant General House, head of the medical service, and Colonel S.L. Bhatia had dinner at the University Club with the Bests. They had met the Bhatias at the International Physiological Congress in Stockholm in 1926. Don and Mary Fraser and the Bruno Mendels were the other guests. The Mendels were Jews who had fled Germany in 1933 for Holland, arriving eventually in Canada; he had worked under Frederick Banting, and then under Best, in the Banting and Best Department of Medical Research. The visitors from India went back to the house and wanted to talk to the boys, who were in bed. "Charley said that for once Henry was a bit quiet and shy — the combination of the general and the dark man was too much, even for Henry." Margaret found Bhatia "just as handsome as ever and so nice."

Charley gave a luncheon for Sir Robert Watson-Watt, the Scottish inventor of radar, at the Toronto Club. Guests included President Cody; Dr. Sidney Smith, president elect of the University of Toronto; Dr. Elwood S. Moore, president of the Royal Canadian Institute (RCI); George McCullagh, publisher of the *Globe and Mail*; and Don Fraser. After his lecture, Sir Robert and some sixty other guests moved to the Bests' house. Henry shook hands politely with the honoured guest and assured Sir Robert that he did not need to tell him anything about radar as his daddy had already told him all about it.

On another occasion, Dr. Ronald Hare was host to Sir Alexander Fleming, discoverer of penicillin. Hare had started work at Connaught Labs in 1936, in research on streptococci, and in 1946, he returned to Britain to become professor of bacteriology at the University of London. Sir Alexander was interested to learn that Charles Alexander Best was called "Sandy." Margaret asked him if he thought that it would be too childish a name when her fourteen-year-old son grew up. "Oh, no, it is not childish, it is intimate. His best friends will always call him Sandy." In May 1945, Charley brought home some penicillin pastilles — "round, yellow jelly things" — for Margaret and for Sandy, who both had bad throats. They were the first that the family had seen.

On 12 January 1945, Margaret and Charley left for New York to attend the annual meeting of the American Diabetes Association (ADA) — soon a regular fixture in their lives. As mentioned earlier, on 2 April

1940, twelve American physicians had met in Cleveland, Ohio, to establish the ADA, with Banting and Best, who were not present, as honorary presidents. In 1941, after Banting's death, the ADA set up the Banting Medal for Distinguished Scientific Achievement and the Best Medal for Distinguished Service in the Field of Diabetes in 1974. A memorable event of ADA gatherings for many years was the golf match played by Joe Beardwood of Philadelphia, Charley Best, Art Colwell of Chicago, and Hank Mulholland of Charlottesville, Virginia.

The Bests stayed at the Seymour, by now their regular hotel in New York. Dr. Joslin came to see Margaret, and they talked about the fund that he had set up to help British refugees in Toronto. He suggested that they use any balance for charities such as the University Settlement in Toronto. Margaret and Charley found the play *Harvey*, with Frank J. Fay as Elwood P. Dawd, "extremely amusing in spots," However, "there were things about it that I did not like — neither did Charley. The portrayal of the doctors and attendants at a mental institution would cause great alarm to anyone who had a friend or relative in such an institution." That was probably the intention of Mary Chase, the author. Margaret and Charley, however, took the play as an attack on the medical profession. If Charley knew of such conditions, he preferred to protect Margaret from the unpleasant truth.

In New York, Margaret and Charley each independently bought a bird-feeding station for the boys. While they were away, Linda held a Sunday evening supper party. Henry "swooped down and lighted cigarettes, Sandy sang Latin hymns. I have never head him sing Latin hymns but apparently he felt moved to do so."

The Bests were back in Montréal in March 1945 for CHB to address a French-language scientific gathering. A number of the participants were English-speaking, including Drs. Bert Collip, Robert Noble, and Hans Selyé, all professors of biochemistry at McGill. Charley received an honorarium of $300, which pleased Margaret. After dinner, Charley gave his lecture at the Botanical Gardens. Dr. Paul Dumas presided, and Dr. Henri Gariépy moved the vote of hands. CHB also gave a radio broadcast on the universities after the war.

While in Montréal, the Bests received an unexpected invitation to a ceremony at the Université de Montréal. "It seems that in the state of Vermont a lot of blood was collected and they had no near place to process it. They gave it to Montréal and it has been processed there. Now it is to be sent over for use in France." Margaret and Charley went to "the huge university built

249

on the mountain, with a great tower." The imposing art deco building was designed by the Montreal architect Ernest Cormier. "We went right up to the blood-drying department and Charley was thrust into a group whose pictures were being taken. A bottle or two of serum was being held in front. A very nice speech of welcome was made by the scientific director, Dr. Armand Frappier, for Charley and me, telling that Charley had begun the blood work in Canada in 1939. Then glasses of sherry were passed around and tiny cakes." Frappier was founding director and dean of the Institut de microbiologie et d'hygiène at the Université de Montréal. Mgr. Olivier Maurault, the recteur, was "spare and enormously active and enthusiastic." He took them on "a tour of the building — the house as he calls it. Charley says there are 13 miles of corridors and I can well believe it. The lecture rooms are fine. They have a most beautiful auditorium and a great rotunda, when you enter by the main door. They had planned a reception for Charley and me which took place in a beautiful room. We signed the Visitor's Book of the university and again we were given wine and cakes. The dean made a very gracious speech of welcome, first in French and then in English."

That evening, the Hans Selyés entertained the Bests, Professor David L. Thomson, chairman of biochemistry, and his wife, and Dr. John Browne, professor of medicine, both at McGill. There was no sign of Bert Collip as Selyé and Collip were at daggers drawn: on one occasion the graduate students of one stole the experimental rats of the other, and the two men had parted company in 1938 after several years of disagreement.[525] Each received a separate department to run.

Charles Best delivered the Banting Memorial Lecture in Toronto on 2 March 1945 — "Insulin and Diabetes, in Retrospect and in Prospect." Best paid tribute to Banting: "As I wrote at the time of his death, his chief monument will be in the minds of young men stimulated by his brilliant and fearless career and in the hearts of successive generations of diabetics who owe so much to him." He retraced the contributions of Paul Langerhans, Joseph von Mering, and Oskar Minkowski. "One has a very keen sympathy for these scientific workers who so narrowly missed the goal toward which their own findings had partially paved the way. I have been told many times by German scientists of the meeting at which one of their members made, perhaps with some justification, an impassioned plea for recognition of the priority of Minkowski's work on pancreatic extracts. Minkowski listened attentively and at the end, rose and said very simply, 'I too regret that I did not find insulin.'"[526]

Martin Goldner, of the Jewish Chronic Disease Hospital in Brooklyn, New York, had attended a lecture by Minkowski in Breslau in1923 and wrote to Best attaching an account. He related that Minkowski lifted a small vial to show his students and said, "This is the first insulin to reach our country. It has been sent to me by Dr. Banting and Dr. Best, of Toronto, who have discovered it. It was once my hope that I would be the father of insulin. Now I am happy to accept the designation as its grandfather, which the Toronto scientists have conferred on me so kindly."[527] The University of Toronto's Insulin Committee later helped to rescue Frau Marie Minkowski from Nazi oppression, and she went to live in Argentina with her daughter.

After referring to the various accounts of 1921, CHB mentioned "many interesting sidelights … preserved only as rough notes or as a part of personal correspondence. These will some day be of historical importance, and could provide material for several lectures." What did he have in mind? The Gooderham letters are a plausible answer, and other accounts by the major players. "The first extracts from normal beef pancreas, prepared with the modifications and improvements made by Professor Collip in the procedure which we originally used, had an appreciably longer duration of action than an equivalent amount of the purer insulin now available." Collip's purification methods were crucial but knowledge of insulin's properties "were so meager that, even after treatment of patients had commenced, the secret of securing active material was lost for weeks — which seemed like years! The struggle in the sub-basement of the Medical Building during the winter and spring of 1922 deserves a chapter for itself."

Hans Christian Hagedorn of Copenhagen had developed protamine insulin, and then David Scott and Albert Fisher at the Connaught Labs developed protamine zinc insulin. Best commented, "When your only source of insulin was from dog's pancreas the ducts of which had been tied some 8 or 10 weeks previously, Banting and I visualized herds of cattle upon which this operation had been performed at the appropriate interval before their demise. Indeed, we went as far as obtaining some steers at the country seat of the Connaught Laboratories and after anaesthetizing them we rearranged their internal structure to suit our convenience."[528]

As for the situation in occupied Europe, Best said, "Through the kindness of Sir Henry Tidy, president of the Royal Society of Medicine, London, I was given the opportunity, slightly more than a year ago, to discuss the insulin situation with the medical representatives of the

'Governments in exile' of practically all of the countries which were at that time occupied. The lack of insulin was only one of their many woes, but the Canadian Red Cross had sent insulin to Greece, and supplies were now reaching other countries." His close friend Dr. Joseph P. Hoet had helped obtain insulin for Belgian diabetics.

Best applauded the "scientific accomplishments of our diabetic medical colleagues — the greatest of these is the liver treatment of pernicious anaemia, in the discovery of which Dr. George Minot [a diabetic] was the senior partner. Many diabetics (including the first physician treated with insulin, Dr. Joseph Gilchrist of Toronto) treat the condition which they have learned to control in themselves. My friend Dr. Robin Lawrence has set a fine example during the war, as he did before it, to his fellow members of the British Diabetic Association, the president of which is Mr. H.G. Wells (who writes that he has found diabetes 'an invigorating diathesis')." Prospects revolved around "many physiological and chemical avenues of approach which have not been explored," including "reliable methods for the estimation of insulin in small quantities of blood"; the possibility that "diabetes may be produced by an excess of the secretions of the anterior pituitary or adrenal glands"; and "the development of better diets for diabetics." Penicillin had introduced "a new era of progress in relation to the control of infection in diabetic patients." He was sceptical about administering insulin by mouth. "In the mild or new cases and perhaps in some of the older patients, there is hope that a cure will be discovered. This problem, and the prevention of the disease, are two of the most urgent ones which face workers in this field."

The Bests mourned FDR's death on 12 April 1945. "We all were unutterably sad. He was surely a very great man. I will never forget our meeting him at that picnic on Campobello. And then Charley presented him in Ottawa for his University of London degree. We admired him very much." When he had won his fourth term in November 1944, Margaret had been very glad. "Dewey (the Republican candidate) strikes me as an insignificant little fellow. At all events he hasn't shown so far that he isn't." April 1945 was a dramatic period. "During this week, Mussolini has been done away with by the Italians and the reports are that Hitler is dead too. The atrocities in the German prison camps have been almost unbelievable, but we must believe the worst because all sorts of reliable people have seen the camps and testified to the horrors."

The trips to Halifax were over. On 3 May 1945, Best spoke before the Canadian Club of Ottawa and was entertained by Senator Norman

McLeod Paterson of Fort William, who was very interested in the Red Cross Blood clinics.

On 7 May, when Linda called from the lab to tell Margaret to turn on the radio and listen to the announcement of the end of the war in Europe, Margaret burst into tears. She had taken the worries that war brought very personally, particularly concerning Charley and Henry Mahon. Soon Charley and Linda came home from the lab. Schools were let out. Henry had called home, and his mother told him to stay at school till he was picked up. He was not very happy about this, and less so when he saw his brother, Jimmy Wood, Hugh Rowan, and Harry Sutherland walk by from the upper school heading for the stores in Forest Hill Village, as Harry had twelve dollars in his pocket, and all four boys drank ginger ale and ate tarts and peanuts.

Everybody was very excited. The Bests' reaction was to pack the car and head for the farm. Toronto celebrated the end of the war with few problems. Halifax went wild. Cousin Arthur Mahon, liquor commissioner for Nova Scotia had been in Toronto recently and, when asked if he expected any trouble, had replied, "Not a bit!" He planned to close all stores as quickly and quietly as possible. In fact, they were the first places looted. Many servicemen felt that Haligonians had treated them badly, with high prices and poor accommodation. The tremendous influx had been more than the city could handle, but many people had generously invited those in uniform into their homes.

When the war in the Pacific ended, the Bests were staying at the Johnson farm guest house at Whale Cove, North Head, on the island of Grand Manan, New Brunswick, sixteen miles off the coast of Maine. The family enjoyed the scenery and going out with the men to seine one of the many herring weirs. Charley, Linda, and Sandy painted, with Sandy doing the first of his few excellent pastel portraits, in this case of Howard Primrose Whidden, retired chancellor of McMaster University. Canadians did not have as many men fighting in the Pacific as did the Americans, but on the New Brunswick islands, there was a lot of intermarriage. "August 14th was a big day — V.J. Day [Victory in Japan]. It is so hard to realize that the war is over. How wonderful to look forward to the winter and no war! I think it was about 7 o'clock when the news came over the radio. We had had supper and gone to the village for our mail. The Post Office had not opened. They were sorting mail and we leaned against Gaskill's Store across the road waiting. Then the bells began to ring in the churches and there was a feeling of unreality about it all."

The official holiday took place the next day. "Sandy had pruned some of the apple trees in the Johnson orchard, and he and Charley had hauled the dead branches out into the open. Bonfires are apparently against the law but it had rained heavily and there was no wind." Charley, in his uniform, and Henry visited the fire warden, who told his wife to pull down the blinds on the windows on that side of their house. "So we had a beautiful fire, helped on at first by a liberal supply of kerosene thrown on by Mr. Johnson. We sang songs as we stood about the fire ... It was a very pleasant way to celebrate the end of the war."

On 9 November 1945, at Sidney Smith's installation as president of the University of Toronto, Charley represented the University of London wearing his DSc hood from Chicago — "beautiful, too," but hardly the equal of London's scarlet and gold. Premier George Drew spoke, as did Dr. J.B. Conant, president of Harvard. Margaret was reading "Conant's *General Education in a Free Society* — a splendid thing — comprehensive and well put together." After the installation, Charley went to a banquet at Hart House, and Margaret and Linda took the boys to the Russian ballet with Massine as the star dancer.

That autumn, Margaret Best joined the Champlain Society. Started in 1905, with Sir Edmund Walker as its first president, it published documents and studies in Canadian history. The first six volumes, plus a portfolio of plates, had been the journals of Samuel de Champlain, translated by H.P. Biggar. The society also published the diaries of Simeon Perkins of Liverpool, Nova Scotia, and other volumes on the Maritimes that particularly interested Margaret. Members received a new volume every year, but the earlier volumes rarely came on the market. Luckily Edwin Fickes of Spruce Point House, Annapolis Royal, Nova Scotia, was ready to sell his set to Margaret for $240. Professor Stewart Wallace, chief librarian of the University of Toronto and a member of St Andrew's Presbyterian church, and Miss Julia Jarvis, his trusted and able assistant, were both very active in the society.

Charley received a letter from the Sorbonne in Paris and took it to F.C.A. Jeanneret at University College to help with translating details. The new principal congratulated Best on receiving another honorary degree and added that he was probably the first Canadian to receive the distinction from the Sorbonne. The ceremony was to take place on 15 December, but Best received it *in absentia*.

The IHD's newsletter of 1 January 1946 announced the election on 5 December 1945 of Charles Best as scientific director for 1946–8 by the trustees of the Rockefeller Foundation. Raymond Fosdick, president of the foundation, wrote to Best to congratulate him, apologizing for his tardiness, although "anyway you are a member of the family and I don't know why formality is necessary at all."[529]

One of the few documents that describes the functions and the role of the scientific directors is a memo, approved by the IHD's director, George K. Strode, dated 4 January 1946: "The Scientific Board in practice does not initiate the program of work. The initiative lies with the officers. The Scientific Board may check or curb the program at any point by declining to approve expenditures ... Similarly the Scientific Board takes no initiative in respect of personnel either in determining what additions to personnel may be needed or the individuals for appointment. The Scientific Directors, however, pass on the recommendations of the Director of the Division in respect of both program and personnel. The Scientific Directors understand that they have no administrative or executive functions ... The IHD encourages the Scientific Directors to make visits to the field. The purpose is for the education of the Directors and to increase their understanding of the field situations and operations ... The Scientific Directors serve as a check or a brake on the officers. Since the Directors are specialists the officers would hesitate to place before them any projects which were not well considered."[530]

As a scientific director of the IHD during the war, Best had been able to increase his understanding of conditions on board ship, nutritional needs, and general public health issues in Britain and Canada.

An announcement had been made in January 1942 that the University of Toronto had decided to build a new Physiology School of Research under Dr. C.H. Best. The war intervened and nothing further was heard until April 1946, when Premier George Drew wrote to Colonel Eric Phillips, chairman of the university's board of governors, "that the necessary steps will be taken at once to enable the Province to convey to the University of Toronto the site for the new Physiological Institute, immediately west of the Banting Institute. The university is therefore free to proceed with its plans with the assurance that the land will be available when it is required."[531]

Young researchers were again beginning to travel to study in foreign centres after the war. Dr. and Mrs. Jaime and Rebeca Talesnik arrived from Santiago, Chile, both to work in the Banting and Best Department of

Medical Research. Dr. Tede Eston de Eston came from São Paolo, Brazil. One of Charles Best's colleagues was Dr. Jacob Markowitz. "Marko" had earned a PhD in physiology from Toronto in 1926 with "Contributions on Carbohydrate Metabolism as Influenced by Insulin." He was a brilliant experimental surgeon with a general practice and a part-time appointment in physiology at the university. He had been in the Far East during the war and spent several years in Changi, near Singapore, one of the worst Japanese prison camps, doing operations with the most rudimentary instruments, and wrote a vivid account of his experiences there.[532] Another colleague was Cliff Shorney, whose family owned a well-known optometrist establishment on Bloor Street. He was active in naval research, and the connection continued after the war. He was also an expert photographer and helped the family in that field, particularly Sandy, who liked doing close-ups of flowers.

For a UCC production of *The Mikado*, Sandy had played violin and had designed sets for the second act — a beautiful scene of cherry trees in bloom, lilies, and a mountain behind. "The trees had crooked trunks and the blossoms were pink through to flame shade; the lilies were yellow." Margaret had a small-scale plan of the sets for her scrapbook. On display as well at UCC were paintings by various students; Sandy showed his portrait of Chancellor Whidden, several watercolours of Ste-Adèle in the Laurentians and the farm, and the design for a large canvas of fishermen at Grand Manan, which he never completed.

The seven-passenger Chrysler Imperial had given the family good service for eleven years, but finally Charley decided to get a new car. Prolonged strikes held up a promised Oldsmobile, and when Charley was offered a Chevrolet, he took it. He advertised the Chrysler in the paper and had several bids from taxi drivers. Henry stood wide-eyed beside his father at the front door of their home watching the buyer hand over $300 more than the car had cost in 1935.

A.V. Hill, who had been the Bests' first house guest on Rosedale Heights Drive in 1927, had stayed with them at 78 Old Forest Hill in 1940. Another visit from Uncle Hill delighted the Best boys. The Bests took A.V. to the farm. President Smith gave a luncheon for him at Hart House. Don Solandt had worked with Hill in London, and he and Barbara entertained him. Hill recounted the death of his brother-in-law, John Maynard Keynes, and the funeral in Westminster Abbey, where the Hills accompanied Keynes' ninety-three-year-old father.

During the war many health and nutrition problems had been identified and new inventions and fields of research had been stimulated. The Royal Society of London set up a series of meetings to take place in London, Cambridge, and Oxford in the summer of 1946 to allow scientists to exchange ideas with each other and chart new directions after six years of war. Margaret was not happy to see Charley leave Toronto on 30 May 1946, on his way to the seven-week British Empire Scientific Conference, but it was too expensive for them both to go.

Charley sailed from New York on the *Queen Mary*. "It is a lonesome thing when he goes away." Joseph Hoet had written to say that Monsignor Honoré van Waeyenbergh was travelling to North America in search of funds to rebuild the library of the Université catholique de Louvain, which had been destroyed during the Second World War, as it had been in the First. Charley saw the rector briefly in New York. Margaret and Linda entertained him at home in Toronto, and he often later recalled their hospitality.

Best's letters from England were lively. In London, he saw the Dales, the Lawrences, the Hills, and the Lovatt Evans. On 19 June, he wrote that Frederic Hudd, deputy high commissioner, "told Dean Mackenzie and me that Lord Athlone had called at Canada House and that Queen Mary, his sister, had expressed the wish that the two of us should call to see her."[533] Two days later Charley gave details of the visit, saying that he had polished up his buttons before going to Marlborough House: "Mackenzie, Penfield and I foregathered at Canada House and were sent to Marlborough by car. Marlborough House is a beautiful place. Princess Alice came in to greet us and she looked as beautiful as ever. Her dress was a very deep rose and I would like to see you in the same colour. It was very beautiful. She really is a lovely looking person. We had an animated conversation. Mackenzie was taken in first by Lord Athlone to see Queen Mary, then Wilder and then myself. We had fifteen or twenty minutes. I enjoyed talking to Queen Mary thoroughly. She wore a lovely robin's egg blue — Wilder called it lavender. We talked about insulin, the navy, and many minor things.[534] She was easy to talk to. Lord Athlone stayed with each of us. Queen Mary is of course more dignified than Princess Alice. The latter just throws her head back and laughs when she is really amused."[535] Charley gave Queen Mary the opportunity to say "bring your wife to see me when she comes here" but she did not rise to it.

Then Best went to Cambridge and stayed at Magdalene College, where Sir Henry Tizard was master. On 24 June, he received his third honorary degree[536] as did Mackenzie, Tizard, Professor Basil Schonland of South Africa, and Professor Frank Macfarlane Burnet of Australia. In Cambridge, Charley saw the Verneys, the Todds, the Barcrofts, and the Adrians. He took part in several congress sessions, including those on hormones and nutrition.

The delegates had excellent meals — even while the Bests and others were still sending much-appreciated food packages to British friends. Best dined at several of the Cambridge colleges — Clare, Downing, King's, Magdalene, and Trinity. He had breakfast with Professor Saul Adler from Palestine in an old Tudor room in the college — "charming, a good breakfast as well."[537] Charley got to know Sir Robert Robinson, a chemist and president of the Royal Society — "a fascinating person." At Magdalene, CHB was shown Samuel Pepy's library; "I will read the diary now with unusual zest."[538]

On 1 July, Best chaired a panel on "The Physiological and Psychological Factors Affecting Human Life Under Tropical Conditions and in Industry" that consisted of Adler, Frank Macfarlane Burnet, E.H. Cluver of South Africa, Charles Hercus of New Zealand, Sir Edward Mellanby, and Colonel Sir S.S. Sokhey of India. The panel produced eight recommendations, including one on co-operation between researchers in "physiology, psychology, industrial hygiene, the related aspects of nutrition, and also, representatives from the allied field of tropical animal physiology."[539]

In Oxford one evening, Best had a long talk with Lord Nuffield, the first person to mass produce a cheap car (the Morris) in Britain. In 1943, he established the Nuffield Foundation.[540] The next day, CHB had further discussions with Nuffield and talked with Sir William Goodenough, chairman of Barclay's Bank and a senior Nuffield adviser, and with Lord Cherwell, professor of experimental philosophy at Oxford and one of Churchill's personal advisers.

Charles Best did not often wax philosophical, but on 3 July, he wrote, "I am quite ready to leave Oxford but have had a very profitable and pleasant time here. The discussions today have been good and we are very fortunate in Canada. In other parts of the Empire, disease and malnutrition are widespread and it is not lack of knowledge but the absence of application of what we know which permits these ghastly situations to continue." In the same letter, "This afternoon I spent most of the time at the Institute of Social Medicine. I enjoyed it but one old witch made me mad by being very condescending about Canada. The Mayor of Oxford gave us tea. A rather dull and illiterate person not in the same class with Lady Bragg,"[541] [Sir William's wife and mayor of Cambridge.] A conversation with Schonland led him to reflect, "The situation in South Africa must be very difficult and the Whites have very little future there in my opinion … I think that I have learned a lot. I have changed my mind about many things in research."

Of the proposals emerging from the conference, Charley stated, "I have to draft a resolution regarding the collection of pancreas in all parts of the Empire."[542] Months earlier, Best had written to the NRC asking to have the topic added to the congress's agenda. "Steps should be taken to conserve all of the pancreas available as the indications are that it will be needed for the preparation of insulin for diabetics."[543] The report of the conference stated, "In view of the steady increase in the demand for insulin, the Conference urges that a strong recommendation be made to all the countries of the commonwealth that every effort be made to collect, process, and preserve all available pancreas."[544]

A gathering in London on 5 July celebrated the twenty-fifth anniversary of the discovery of insulin. In appreciation, the British Diabetic Association presented CHB with "a fine, silver box which can be used for cigars! cigarettes! or for better things if you so desire."[545] He wrote to Margaret, "Dale gave a good oration and my talk went as well as I expected. Actually, I was rather inhibited by four hundred diabetics. The importance of the application of insulin, i.e. the tangible evidence of its effect on human beings, created a curious reversal of times in my mind. Dogs are obviously less important than human beings and the presence of so many whose lives had been saved made it almost seem as if they had been treated before the dogs. This slight psychological observation did not seriously interfere with my talk on the early experiments. I was inhibited by Collip's presence but did my best to be absolutely sporting."[546]

"I met a lot of very grateful people yesterday and it gave me a lot of pleasure to see them. It would have been infinitely more pleasant if you had been with me." Charley added that he saw Joseph Hoet for the first time since before the war. "He is the same as ever. He is proceeding with plans to get the whole Best family to Louvain next year. He is wonderfully grateful for insulin. His diabetic boy is the most wonderful of all his children."[547] Joseph went with Charley to see the Dales and to the diabetic meeting, and he spoke at the dinner that evening. Joseph Hoet signed the menu for the dinner held on 5 July at Claridge's Hotel, as did J.B. Collip, Henry Dale, Charles Fletcher, Francis Avery Jones, and Robin Lawrence. "I was quite touched yesterday when Joseph said *au revoir*. He sent his kindest regards to you and Linda and the boys. He said, 'We do not know them but we love them.'"[548]

The day before he left London, Best went for a walk with the man whom he most admired, Sir Henry Dale, in Green Park and the streets around Buckingham Palace. Joseph Hoet and Colonel Margaret Eaton Dunn, daughter of R.Y. Eaton of Toronto and the director general of the Canadian Women's Army Corps (C.W.A.C.), had tea with CHB at the Lawrences' flat. Then, Charley had dinner again with the Dales at the home of Brigadier Charles Kellaway, director-in-chief of the Wellcome Research Foundation — the position that CHB had considered in 1941. From the *Georgic* in Liverpool harbour: "We have a peculiar mixture of brides, service women and service men. The *Georgic* is really a troop ship."[549] For the property at Stewarttown, Charley suggested the name "Landfall Farm" — quite appropriate for a sailor home from the sea.

Chapter Six
World Travellers, 1946–1952

After Banting's death in 1941, Charles Best was completely involved in the war effort. With the end of hostilities, however, everyone's attention turned to reconstruction and the future of research, which required a new agenda. The Royal Society Empire Scientific Conference in 1946 gave leadership and provided great stimulus. Best played a prominent part and was given his third honorary degree (after Chicago in 1941 and Paris in 1945) by Cambridge University. Probably, if Banting had lived he would have been the one to receive some of those honours.

Certainly, Banting would have been the star of the celebrations in 1946 for the twenty-fifth anniversary of the discovery of insulin. On 15 September, people interested in diabetes from many parts of the world converged on Toronto for these celebrations. A photograph taken in front of the Royal Ontario Museum shows many of the better-known delegates, including Joslin, Hagedorn, Lawrence, and Houssay. The sixth annual meeting of the American Diabetes Association (ADA) took place at that time, with Dr. Joseph Barach of Pittsburgh as president and Dr. Cecil Striker of Cincinnati as secretary.

At the opening ceremonies, President Sidney Smith said: "We are not far removed in this Convocation Hall from those meagre and ill-equipped quarters in the Medical School where Dr. Banting and Dr. Best and others worked ... prompted by the idea, 'Service and not self.'"[550] Charles Best was about to speak, and "the whole gathering rose up when he went to the platform. I was glad that the boys were there," wrote Margaret.[551] Dr. Walter Campbell, the clinician at the Toronto General Hospital in charge of the first insulin given to a patient, spoke, as did Dr. Russell Wilder of Rochester, Minnesota, incoming president of the ADA. The last speaker was Dr. Seale Harris, who had recently written a book on Fred Banting.[552] Margaret was somewhat nervous about this speech. "Seale Harris was quite nerve-wracking with all of his references to Fred's sweetheart who turned him down, etc. He depicted early life as quite a hard row to hoe for Fred. I trembled because I knew our turn was coming. Everything was rosy and fine for us — Charley's father was a doctor, his sweetheart, now his wife, was the only one for him, etc." All of this was probably true, but Margaret found it quite unnecessary, particularly with Banting's son Bill and Henrietta, Lady Banting, in the audience.

Of the addresses at the banquet in Hart House, Margaret wrote, "Dr. Cody gave quite a long speech — very fluent, very fine. It was really a funeral oration for Fred Banting. It was not the time for that particular speech." Dr. Barach presented Banting Memorial Medals to Houssay, Hagedorn, Lawrence, and Eugene Opie[553] of the Rockefeller Institute, as well as to the University of Toronto. "Robin Lawrence spoke on the care of diabetics in England in wartime. Robin looks so young and has so charming a manner. He referred to his own diabetes and the fact that he has taken insulin for twenty-four years. He said he had no intention of getting any of those awful things — gangrene, etc., that the doctors talk about. I think he said that he planned to attend the fiftieth anniversary. He was very fluent and clever and witty too." Next came Dr. Hagedorn — "he was practically impossible to understand in a quite long and very scientific speech which he read. Dr. Houssay was difficult to understand too." Dean C.J. Mackenzie reminisced about Banting and how he developed as a writer.

The next day, 16 September, saw the scientific presentations. Best gave the first paper: "The demonstration that an effective antidiabetic hormone could be extracted from the pancreas was essentially complete twenty-five years ago today. Interestingly enough, the last page in the original notebooks which Banting and I kept together records the work which we carried out on September 16, 1921."[554]

The evening after the dinner, Elizabeth and Elliott Joslin, Maria and Hans Christian Hagedorn, and Bea and Roscoe Graham came to the Bests' home for dinner. "Joslin spent a lot of time with the boys, talking about music and pictures and books. Henry helped serve the meal — and very nicely too — except that he was fascinated by a story that Bea was telling and a little inclined to let his attention wander when passing plates." Margaret found that Maria Hagedorn had aged a great deal. "I think she had a pretty grim time throughout the occupation. Her husband was outspoken against the Germans and he was threatened and she was frightened. When the word came that the occupation was over she told me, 'I was all alone in the country. My husband was in the city. I had no one — no one to talk to.'"

Another visitor, Major General Sir Sahib Singh Sokhey, educated in the Punjab and in Edinburgh, was the Director of the Haffkine Institute in Bombay and had been a delegate to the Empire Scientific Conference in London. At a party at the Bests "Sir Sahib said that the money that England took out of India was used to start the Industrial Revolution." Fifteen-year-old Sandy replied, "'Why didn't it start in Holland, for instance, which had Colonies too?' I noticed that there was a slight argument, so Charley stopped that. Sandy loves an argument but he must learn not to be too serious about it with a guest in our own house."

The Bests and the Lawrences went to Buffalo to take the train to Indianapolis for Eli Lilly and Company's celebration of the anniversary; the company had played a crucial part in the development, purification, and production of Insulin since 1922. Lilly's, as always, entertained with grace and flair. Ruth Lilly gave a luncheon for some of the women, including Mrs. J.K. Lilly, Lady Banting, María Hagedorn, and Anne Lawrence. Lady Banting was a medical doctor and sometimes had to choose between the scientific sessions and the women's events. The same evening, there was a large dinner. "Charley said to me that it was a very unusual thing for a big group of scientists to be gathered together like that, all speaking in such whole-hearted commendation of a business firm, a commercial firm. I am sure that Lilly's have been a most honourable, high- principled group." J.K. Lilly, who had built the Stephen Foster Museum in Pittsburgh, arranged for a quartet of singers to perform at the dinner. Margaret told J.K. that she loved Foster's songs, particularly "Jeanie with the Light Brown Hair." It was Lilly who discovered the manuscript of this song. He asked the quartet to turn around and face Margaret, and sing it again for her. She never forgot that evening.

That autumn, Sir Henry and Lady Dale were in North America. Sir Henry received an honorary degree from Princeton University, and they came to Toronto for the meetings of the Canadian Physiological Society. Margaret had not seen Lady Dale since 1938. On Sunday, 27 October 1946, the Bests took the Dales to the farm. Sir Henry told stories, and Margaret got caught up on the news of the Dale family. Driving home, Sir Henry sang Gilbert and Sullivan songs with the boys and then started reciting Hilaire Belloc's *Cautionary Rhymes*. Yehudi Menuhin was in Toronto, and the Dales took Sandy to his concert and afterwards he met the virtuoso. Sir Henry knew many musical people through his brother, Benjamin, a professional musician. The next day the Dales went to the rehearsal of the

Toronto Symphony, and then Lady Dale had lunch with Lady MacMillan, wife of the conductor, Sir Ernest.

Sir Henry and Charley discussed the future. There were certainly great opportunities for Best in Britain and the United States, where he had received several offers. However, Charley felt an obligation and loyalty to the University of Toronto, because he had made his reputation there, but he knew that facilities and funding for research would have to be greatly improved. He also felt loyalty to Canada, partly because of his Maritimes background of which he was very proud, but also because he had served Canada in two world wars.

A few months later Charles Burns, president of Burns Bros. and Denton Limited, investment dealers, took Charley to lunch one day. Burns was a governor of the University of Toronto and married to Norman and Senator Cairine Wilson's daughter Janet. Burns asked Best to make a list of offers he had received from other countries. He told Burns that he had received offers of two positions in the United States to be in charge of the production of insulin and scientific research.

In addition, he had been offered three professorships at three large American and two British universities. Also in Britain two pharmaceutical companies had offered him posts as director of their medical research institutes. Best went on to say that "these positions which have been offered to me and the honours which I have received should be considered as an indication of the continued scientific appreciation of the results of the work which my staff and I have been able to do here in Toronto." Best emphasized his desire if possible to remain in Canada but he feared that, unless the promised research facilities were provided, many young men would seek opportunities elsewhere.[555] Best's priority in the spring of 1947 was to see that the promised facilities were realized.

Both Banting and Macleod had given Beaumont Lectures of the Wayne County Medical Society. In early February 1947 the Bests went to Detroit where Charley gave the twenty-sixth Beaumont Lecture, in two parts — "Diabetes Past, Present and Future," and "The Lipotropic Factors in the Protection of Liver and Kidneys."[556] He also addressed the Physiological Society and the Honor Science Fraternity of Wayne State University.

Best also accepted invitations to receive honorary degrees from Louvain and Liège in Belgium and Oxford in England, all of which he saw not as personal tributes but recognition of the work carried out in his labs. It was not only recognition from abroad, but, perhaps more importantly, it made the work more valued at home. Best also understood well the importance of making and sustaining contacts with scientists and others all over the world. It may not have been called "networking" at that time but by then he had become very expert at it to the benefit of his colleagues and students. Further recognition of Best's scientific contributions were made by his appointment to the Defence Research Board and the National Research Council of Canada.

At the end of the war, the federal cabinet had decided in 1945, after much debate, that "research for the three defence departments should be co-ordinated under a single Director General of Defence Research, that this position should be filled by a civilian with scientific training, and that it would be on the same level as the Chiefs of Staff."[557] Best was a civilian member of the cabinet committee picking a director general. At a meeting chaired by C.D. Howe, Best and NRC President C.J. Mackenzie suggested Charley's former graduate student Colonel Omond Solandt. He was a Canadian recently appointed chief scientific adviser to Admiral Louis Mountbatten, the Supreme Allied Commander in South-East Asia.

Best stated, "The most definite evidence that Colonel Solandt should be seriously considered for the post of Director General of Defence Research is the fact that he has served efficiently for three years as Deputy Director and Director of Operational Research under the British War Office and the British Ministry of Supply. This organization, made up of several hundred of the best scientists in England — physicists, chemists, engineers, biologists and mathematicians — had, as you know, the function of setting up standards of armament, construction of experimental models, scientific testing of prototypes, and the approval of final design prior to production." Best added that Solandt had graduated from the University of Toronto in medicine, "with honours not exceeded by any other student in the history of our School." Solandt spent two years, in 1932–3, working with Best, who said of him, "I have always felt that he has a finer mind and a broader outlook than any other research student of my acquaintance … As you will perceive, I have no hesitation in recommending Colonel O.M. Solandt for any senior position for which his experience and ability qualify him. Actually, I am more concerned that he should choose a broad field in which he will utilize his outstanding abilities than that he should secure some particular position at the present time."[558]

Solandt got the job and wrote to Best: "The main thing is that all the Chiefs of Staff seem enthusiastic so it should be possible to get things done.

I am most grateful to you for your help and support. General Foulkes said that your letter would convince the most skeptical. I think that it is going to be a fairly difficult job but one well worth doing."[559]

On 1 April 1947, Best received a two-year appointment to Canada's new Defence Research Board. Other charter members included the three chiefs of staff — General Charles Foulkes, Air Marshal Robert Leckie, and Vice Admiral Howard Emerson Reid.[560] The first official meeting of the board took place on 15 December 1947. Best was a member of the standing committee on extra-mural research. It "forged the general policy DRB has since followed."[561]

In March 1948, "an informal meeting was held between Dr. C.H. Best, Dr. J.B. Collip of the University of Western Ontario, and Dr. Solandt to discuss the best methods of handling the medical aspects of defence research in peacetime."[562] It set up a committee under Dr. R.F. Farquharson to co-ordinate "all Canadian medical research having military implications and in February of 1951, a Defence Medical Research Co-Ordinating Committee was established."[563] The committee created fifteen medical panels on subjects ranging from anti-coagulants to Arctic medical research. Best was chairman, and J.B. Collip was alternate chairman — evidence that the two could and did work together. The relations between Best and Collip were cordial but they were never close friends. Best could never forget the incident in January 1922 that led to blows between Banting and Collip.[564]

When Best completed his two years on the DRB, Solandt wrote to him, "Very few people in Canada realize how important your contribution to the work of the Board has been. Your part in moulding its work began in 1929 when you first taught me the basic principles of research, which have been the foundation of all my later work. I know that it was you who, in 1945, suggested my name for this job. I am deeply grateful to you, not only for suggesting my name, but also for giving me the training that made it possible for me to do the job, and then helping as a member of the Board to make sure that I got off to a good start. Your sound knowledge of science, and of naval matters, and your world-wide scientific contacts have been of inestimable value in the formative stages of the Board's work."[565]

Within months of his appointment to the DRB, Charles Best became a member of the National Research Council (NRC) of Canada. The NRC has played an important role in science since its foundation in 1916, under Henry Marshall Tory, then president of the University of Alberta.

Tory had also played a role in the insulin debates in 1922–3. He, as president of the NRC from 1923 to 1935, oversaw the building of a national laboratory in Ottawa in 1928. General A.G.L. McNaughton was president from 1935 to 1939, when the NRC provided a crucial contribution to the upcoming war effort. C.J. Mackenzie was president from 1939 until 1952, and E.W.R. Steacie from 1953 to 1962. Best's first formal connection with the council was on its Associate Committee on Medical Research, organized in 1946 under J.B. Collip. Other members included old friends of Best's: Louis Berger from Laval, D.T. Fraser and John Scott from Toronto, and C.B. Weld from Dalhousie. In May 1947, the NRC named Best to its committees on scholarships and the *Canadian Journal of Research*, and to its Russian Committee. Best nominated J.K.W. Ferguson and D.Y. Solandt to the advisory committee.

At the same period in the spring of 1947 the Bests were preparing for their first visit together to Europe since before the war. As throughout the war, the Rockefeller Foundation contributed in many ways, by helping to fund the Best's trip and by making contacts and organizing schedules. George Strode, the new secretary of the IHD, was in Paris in April and he discussed Best's schedule in Europe with Dr. Johannes H. Bauer of the Paris office. Best would be free between 9 and 20 July, and Bauer offered to drive him about Holland. He would also make arrangements for Best's visit of about ten days to Norway and Sweden, "and will if it seems desirable, accompany Best in his visit, though this hardly seems necessary as looked at today."[566] Strode's diary for 24 June reported that Dr. and Mrs. Best had come to have lunch with the IHD group in New York and were sailing at midnight.

On 23 June, Margaret, Charley, and Sandy left Toronto for New York and Europe. Just before their departure, the American consul general in Toronto presented Best with the medal and citation of the Legion of Merit, Degree of Officer. The citation, signed by President Harry S. Truman, read in part, "during the period of active hostilities in World War II, Best rendered exceptionally meritorious service in the field of scientific research and development ... Surgeon Captain Best fostered close cooperation among scientists of Canada and the United States."[567] Best may have been nominated for this honour by the U.S. Embassy in Ottawa or more likely by one of his Rockefeller colleagues such as Admiral Parran.

England and Europe

Charley, Margaret, and Sandy sailed on 24 June 1947 from New York on the *Veendam* of the Holland-America Line bound for Rotterdam. They met a couple from Rotterdam, Jacob and Emmy van Stolk Mees, whom they became very fond of on the journey. The two couples talked of literature, art, and other common interests. Margaret, Sandy, and Emmy Mees read Wordsworth, Robert Frost, Walt Whitman, and Emily Dickinson together. Mrs. Mees did pastel portraits of Margaret and Charley. The one of Margaret was Charley's favourite portrait of her. Margaret wrote "It was a most unusual and touching friendship to develop in a short time!"

During the Bests' short stay in Holland in 1947, Dr. John Logan of the Rockefeller Foundation's IHD and his wife, Dorothy, came to Amsterdam to see Charley. Logan was a Canadian who earned a DSc from Harvard. After service in the American army, he joined the IHD in 1946. He was preparing to move with his family to Cagliari, Sardinia, to take charge of the anti-malarial project there using DDT. On 12 February 1948, John Logan wrote to Charley, attaching photographs taken the previous summer in Holland. "It was indeed a pleasure to have made your acquaintance and from the developments in Public Health Engineering in Holland since you left it is evident that your visit was extremely valuable in stimulating and encouraging this particular phase of Public Health work ... Our all-out campaign for the eradication of *Anopheles labranchiae* from Sardinia gets under way in its final stages on Monday, February 16. Our spray-painting campaign during which every man-built structure on the Island was treated [with DDT] has terminated and we are now engaged in the rather complicated procedure of transferring from one phase of operations to another."[568]

In the Sardinian project, the IHD "tested eighty drugs for therapeutic action against malaria and of those effective against malaria in animals, two were found useful for treating the disease in man."[569] Best used DDT at his farm outside Toronto and explained the Sardinian project to the family.

Because of its connection with causing cancer DDT has been banned in the Western world since the 1970s. In spite of this, one expert stated recently, "While it is true that we don't know every last risk of using DDT, we know very well what the risk of malaria is — and on balance malaria is far, far more deadly than the worst that one could imagine about DDT."[570] Charles Best would have been interested in this continuing debate.

On 7 July 1947, Best received an honorary doctorate from the Université de Louvain. This was a very special occasion because of the family's long connection, both scientific and personal, with the Joseph Hoets, with whom they stayed. Margaret described the university rector's robes as "black with tiny red velvet buttons, wide red sash, red hat on his head and red gloves." Margaret obtained a copy of his speech for her scrapbook. "He referred to his pleasure at seeing the Arms of Louvain University among those decorating the Great Hall of Hart House at the University of Toronto … He went on to talk of Charley and of how they wished to link him up with their faculty of medicine. It was a very touching speech. The rector himself was moved to tears and mopped his eyes. He is extremely eloquent and I think quite sentimental."

The previous year in London at the British Diabetic Association Charley had been astonished and moved by the presence of four hundred diabetics who were the "tangible evidence of the importance of the application of insulin to human beings."[571] Until then he had often met individual diabetics, but never hundreds at one time. In Brussels, the Society for the Protection of the Interests of Diabetics, one of the first (with the Portuguese, British, and the Dutch) lay diabetic societies in the world, organized a meeting at the Palais des Académies. Margaret was startled and touched by the presence of so many diabetics. "I shall never forget the faces of the audience as they looked up with love and admiration in their eyes," When Charley got up to speak, "Right beneath us was a mother and young daughter. The tears ran down the mother's face; their emotion was very touching." The Society had gathered several hundred diabetics in the hall. Best was used to speaking to large groups of doctors, scientists, and students but not to so many diabetics. He was taken aback by their emotional outpouring, which he soon learned to respond to compassionately. After the speeches Margaret was presented with several kinds of orchids and an exquisite, large round centrepiece of Brussels lace. The Queen Mother Elisabeth was present. "She is quite old now but wonderfully slim and young-looking and very quiet and composed in manner — with the most amazing eyes. After the lecture the Queen asked to speak to Charley and to me again. She said she hoped that we could come to lunch with her one day during our visit."

A few days later M. de Streel, the Queen's secretary, greeted the luncheon guests in the entrance hall of Laeken Palace. "Then we went up great stairs and the lady-in-waiting (the Baroness Carton de Wiart) was there to take us along to the Queen's drawing room. It was a very charming room,

269

not large, with pictures and books and a piano. The Queen was quiet rather at first. We all had sherry. The Dorés and the Hoets were there and the wife of the secretary, Madame de Streel who is an American — a Lodge."

Jean Doré, the Canadian ambassador, and his wife attended several of the events, and the Bests were proud to have such excellent representatives of their country. Doré's spoken French was considered "most beautiful and literate" by their Belgian hosts. "It was one of the nicest and really most delightful parties that was given for us. After lunch, the Queen talked to me for a long time in the drawing room, over our coffee. She plays the violin, she sculpts, she weaves, she knows the birds and the flowers. She is bright and lovely in her manner. She wants to visit Canada and I urged her to do so." Her Majesty said to Margaret, "You are interested in exactly the same things that I am interested in." She complimented Margaret on her hats and how she wore them. "Sandy thought she was wonderful and when we all said goodbye Sandy came directly after Monsieur Doré, who kissed her hand. I saw to my amazement Sandy bending low over the Queen's hand and for one minute I thought he was going to kiss it. Later when we asked him about it, he acknowledged that it had crossed his mind that he might kiss her hand but he decided just to bow rather low in shaking hands." The Bests were flattered to have been guests of the Queen Mother and Charley was delighted that Margaret got on so well with her.

On 15 July at Liège, Acting Rector Chevalier Braas conferred an honorary degree on Charles Best, and then people went to a large room where several hundred diabetics had gathered. Thirty children filed by, presenting flowers and each saying, "Thank you for my life." They were all patients of Professor Lucien Brull, dean of medicine. Margaret wrote, "It was very moving and very touching." When the Bests left the university, the car was so surrounded by well-wishers, that "Charley said he did not want to run over any diabetics. They held on to our hands and called out to us and wept and smiled too and were altogether as French as we expect the emotional French to be. Charley, Sandy and I will never forget that occasion."

In London on 18 July, Charley gave the Banting Memorial Lecture at King's College Hospital. Also there was Fred Banting's widow, Henrietta, who had graduated in medicine from the University of Toronto in 1945 and was doing postgraduate work in England. Cousin Mary Scott joined the Bests for lunch at Charley's club, the Athenaeum. The Lawrences took the Bests and Lady Banting to the Ivy Restaurant in Soho. Food was not easy to get, and many things were still strictly rationed; visitors received a few food coupons. Margaret used the candy coupons to buy chocolate to give to friends. She bought jars of jam at Fortnum and Mason's for their own breakfasts. At the National Gallery and the Royal Academy, the staff were gradually bringing out paintings stored for safety during the war. At the British Museum, burial remains from the *Sutton Hoo* Viking ship were on display, along with the fourth-century Mildenhall silver treasures.

The Bests spent almost a week from 21 July at the meetings of the XVIIth International Physiological Congress in Oxford, with Sir Henry Dale as president. There were few spouses at the meetings, as both food and accommodation were scarce. Sir Howard Florey, co-discoverer of penicillin, and Lady Florey entertained them at Lincoln College. "Oxford is the most distressing place in which to move about. The sidewalks are crowded constantly. You are jostled and pushed into the street if you are not careful and the streets are full of motor cars and bicycles. The colleges are so beautiful but I think it is too bad that Oxford has become such a bustling, commercial city."

Lady Dale wanted very much to see Charley Best get his honorary degree, so she came from London. Janet Vaughan, principal of Somerville College, invited her, Margaret, and Sandy to lunch. Of the principal, MMB wrote, "She is quite an imposing and handsome woman … She was very active in science during the war and flew a good deal to the Continent and I think to India — about the blood work.[572] After lunch we walked through the streets — Sir Henry and Janet Vaughan in their gowns — and when we entered the Sheldonian Theatre, it was filled with people. Our reserved seats were in the raised part in the front, facing the audience and there were many old friends holding Oxford degrees."

Sir Richard Livingstone, a classicist and vice-chancellor, entertained the five honourees at lunch at his college, Corpus Christi, and they walked together to the Sheldonian. "Charley said he was the last to arrive at lunch and Dr. Livingstone had begun to introduce him very formally. Professor Best — Dr. Gasser — Dr. Szent-Györgyi — Dr. Houssay — all of whom said, 'Hello Charley,' and Dr. August Krogh of Copenhagen, another old friend who would not go so far as to call Charley by his first name but at all events, an old friend." At that time neither Margaret nor Charley was aware of the role played by Krogh in the nominations for the 1923 Nobel Prize.

"When they arrived at the Sheldonian, the great doors at the very back of the hall were thrown open and the procession came up the centre aisle and sat at the front. Then each one was called separately and came forward to receive the degree … The whole proceeding was in Latin. That was the third honorary degree that Sandy and I had seen Charley receive within a few days, Louvain, Liège, and now Oxford." By that time, Best had been recognized by universities in the United States, Britain, and Europe, but ironically not yet in Canada.

Back in London, the Canadians visited the Dales at the Royal Institution on Albermarle Street. Charley had stayed there with them during the war, and he recalled that one night when there was particularly heavy bombing, Lady Dale said, "Come, Charley, come down with me to the shelter." "Charley told me about it and said he knew that Lady Dale felt responsible to me for his safety. She paid no attention to Sir Henry and another guest (Lord Stamp[573]). Charley was highly amused."

Margaret noted, "We found many disgruntled people in England this year, particularly in the London hotels. At the Park Lane where we stayed, the waiters and maids were constantly fighting in the dining room. I think they are completely fed up with the austerity reign in England and they would no doubt feel much happier and friendlier if they had a few good meals with plenty of meat, butter, sweets, etc."

On 1 August, the Bests boarded a small ship, the *Stella Polaris*, in Newcastle bound for Bergen, Norway. In Oslo, King Haakon VII received Charles Best and decorated him with the Haakon VII Liberty Cross. Dean Gallie of the Faculty of Medicine at the University of Toronto and Dr. T.A. Carson, superintendent of the Christie Street Hospital (where Banting had done the insulin clinical work in 1922), had received the same honour. Toronto had played an important role in training Norwegian airmen during the war. Now in his seventies, the king talked to Charley about the Norwegians who trained in Canada, about medical matters, and about his own experiences when he and his cabinet went to Britain during the war. The Edvard Munch paintings at the National Gallery particularly impressed Margaret and Sandy.

In Copenhagen, on 3 and 4 September, Charley gave lectures for Dr. Hans Christian Hagedorn, for whom he had great admiration for his pioneering work on the development of insulin. Hagedorn took his guests to his country house near Staverby.

Travelling by train through Germany to Holland, the Bests found the scene at each station disconcerting: "During the day we were conscious in every station of people staring into the train — just standing on the platform staring. The heat had been very great all summer and the country was terribly dried up. It must have meant a terrible loss in crops and in food for this winter. The same thing was true everywhere. In Germany, we saw people working in their dried-up gardens, trying to get something from them. We came through Hamburg and Bremen. Those cities about the railway stations and tracks were very largely devastated. They must have been bombed terrifically."

They got off the train at Bentheim at the Dutch border. There was a sign in English in the station. "'You are endangering the lives of children by throwing food from the carriage windows. Keep death off the rails.' I shall never forget the appearance of the people — the set, almost expressionless, faces." These impressions stayed with Margaret Best for a long time. Her first thoughts were for the children, then for the expressionless adults, then of what the German forces had done to other people.

When the Bests reached Amsterdam they were met and entertained by the Dutch, who tried to be as hospitable as possible in spite of the scarcity of everything. "They are having very austere days in Holland as in England. These are days of rigid economy for the Dutch. They suffered during the war and they are suffering over the loss of prestige in the Dutch East Indies." Dr. and Mrs. John Logan of the Rockefeller Foundation joined them in Amsterdam and took them to Leiden where Best visited the Public Health Institute. On the way there they left Sandy off to see bulb growing nurseries where he was presented with very special tulip bulbs. The Bests had been invited by Mr. and Mrs. Mees, with whom they had made friends on board the *Veendam*, to visit them in Rotterdam, but Emmy Mees was very ill. Charley went to see her in hospital, which was pitifully short of medical equipment and personnel. To their great sorrow Emmy Mees died during the night before their departure for Canada next morning on the *Nordam*.

On 22 September 1947, Strode of the Rockefeller Foundation wrote, "Best has just arrived from abroad and reported a very good summer, during which he was able to visit but a few of the IHD interests. With the help of JHB [Bauer], he saw the Institute of Preventative Medicine in Leiden and a few other interests in Holland. In Denmark most of his contacts were with physiologists and other scientific workers. He did not get to the Serum Institute. In Norway and Sweden he of course met the leaders in public health and got a very unfavourable opinion of the Institute of Hygiene in Oslo which seems to be fairly universal. In regard to the Stockholm Institute, he was impressed with Forssman but not with the general setup of the Institute of Public Health, which he considers quite properly too narrow and compartmentalised. GKS [Strode] asked Dr. Best to report on his visits to the Board at the October 31st meeting, at which time we hope to provide 20 or 30 minutes for the purpose."[574]

In September 1947, the National Research Council of Canada appointed Best and Collip to represent it on the board of the Canadian Cancer Institute. In the months that followed, Best missed several NRC meetings as he was travelling, but he attended the Standing Committee on Assisted Researches and on Medical Research. During 1949–50, Best chaired the Associate Committee on Medical Research.

In early December, Henry and Margaret joined Charley in Ottawa to stay at the Château Laurier — a sort of a consolation prize for Henry because he had not gone to Europe. Margaret and Henry went to the Senate to see Cairine Wilson, and at eleven o'clock, they went to the Peace Tower, where Margaret turned a page in the Book of Remembrance. Harry Jackman, Conservative MP for Rosedale, took them for lunch in the Parliamentary Dining Room. That evening, the Bests went to a cocktail party at the home of Dean C.J. Mackenzie and his wife. Omond and Elizabeth Solandt, C.D. Howe, minister of reconstruction and supply, Norman and Cairine Wilson, and Graham Towers, governor of the Bank of Canada and his wife, Mary, were among the guests. Henry, at thirteen, was quickly making his way around the centres of power in Ottawa.

For the next few years, the building of the much anticipated new research facilities at the University of Toronto was the family's highest priority. Best and others made speeches to raise funds for it at various alumni functions. Margaret's diary of 5 March 1948 mentioned "a campaign on to get money for the university. They want it for Charley's new building, among other things. Charley and Mr. Vincent Massey (the chancellor), were entertained at lunch in New York not long ago by Mr. Thomas Watson of the Business Machines [IBM]. Mr. Watson gave Charley as a little memento, a gold pencil with a watch at the end of it and he sent home to me a lipstick, gold also, with a watch in the end — from Cartier's, very lovely." In a speech to potential donors, Best reminisced about the early days of Hart House, built for the university by the Massey family. "I saw both Mr. Raymond Massey and Mr. Vincent Massey play in the little theatre in Hart House, and at that time I thought that Mr. Vincent Massey had equal promise."[575] Both brothers were present.

In the spring the Bests went to Ste-Adèle, Québec, where Charley received the Gold Medal of the Canadian Pharmaceutical Society; the only other recipient had been Sir Alexander Fleming. When Charley got up to speak, he mentioned the white-throated sparrow singing outside the window; he then went on to speak about his work with insulin, heparin, and choline.

For several years, the Bests had been planning to spend some time in Québec in order to learn more French than their school studies had provided, plus something of the architecture and other arts of French Canada. Margaret had been studying Ramsay Traquair's *Old Architecture of Quebec.* Later that summer, while on route to Maine, they stopped at Ilahee Lodge, the camp for diabetic children in Cobourg, Ontario. They went on to Québec City and stayed at the Château Bel Air right on the St Lawrence in the village of Ste-Pétronille on Ile d'Orléans.

Near Miss Queenie Murray's house in the St-Pierre area, on the north side of Ile d'Orléans, the Bests found an ideal place to paint, looking down at a white house with a black roof and a long barn with red doors and beyond to the river and the hills of the north shore. Charley and Linda painted in oils, and Sandy in watercolours, with seven small children looking on, saying, "C'est bien." Henry took a black and white photo of the same scene. The style of each artist was completely different, and seeing all the results together is quite fascinating.

In Québec they visited the Hôpital Général on the St-Charles River, the Séminaire de Québec, and the Ursuline convent, admiring the painting and wood carvings of the Baillargé and Levasseur families and other artists. At their first visit to Barney Kane's Antique Shop on Champlain Street in Québec, Margaret and Charley decided to buy a wooden candelabra from the church at St-Pierre, "$75 — horrors — an awful price but we wanted one and St-Pierre we really love." Henry so enjoyed those days in Quebec in 1948 that he hoped to return and spend longer.

In Maine, there were projects to keep the house and barn in shape — new steps, making curtains, cutting the spruce hedge. The multi-coloured *catalogne* fabric from the Ile d'Orléans was made into cushion covers. The short trip from Eastport to Deer Island was always fun — the ferry consisted of a Cape Islander lobster boat tied to a skow; Grandmother Best had always refused to go on "that tea tray." On Deer Island Charley made a drift wood fire and cooked fresh salmon.

In 1948, visitors from Toronto included Don and Mary Fraser and "Van" and Jean Van Wyck, who had never been to Schooner Cove. They all were taken to the point and to help set and pull the gill net. Everyone dug clams in the mud flats of the cove. Mackerel, haddock, smelts, herring, and clams were on the menu. Blueberries and cranberries were there for the picking. Van, Linda, and Charley painted, the last doing a larger canvas from the sketch that he had made at St- Pierre.

One day the family went to Dennysville to see Aunt Anna Lincoln and her sister-in-law, Tishie Brown. Ninety-two-year-old Mrs. Lincoln made a real stage entrance, coming down the stairs in a black pajama suit with large red flowers, her white hair piled high on her head. She put her arms around Charley and said, "Charley Best, forty-nine years old." It was on this visit that Mrs. Lincoln gave Margaret and Charley two beautiful amethyst tulip vases, Sandwich glass. She talked a lot about her husband's family. When Dr. Arthur's father, Thomas Lincoln, was a young man, John James Audubon came to Maine and named the Lincoln sparrow for him.

Back in Toronto, Dr. Hermann Fischer, son of Emil Fischer, the Nobel Prize-winning organic chemist, and his wife were getting ready to leave for California. The Bests were sorry to see them go. Fischer had joined the Banting and Best Department in 1935 as head of the Sub-Department of Synthetic Chemistry. He and his colleague and successor, Dr. Erich Baer, did "brilliant work on the synthesis of natural compounds of physiological significance." In 1950, Baer synthesized a lecithin that showed therapeutic potential in hyaline membrane disease in babies.[576]

On Thanksgiving weekend 1948, several friends drove out to the farm and, like all visitors, were put to work. They picked one hundred bushels of pepper, or acorn, squash for Loblaw's grocery chain and sixty bushels of carrots for a wholesaler. "Mac" and Marguerite MacFarlane deposited their son, Andy, to help with the vegetables and took Margaret and Charley to see the house that they were having built near Terra Cotta. Ronald Tasker, professor of neurosurgery at the Toronto General Hospital, recalled two visits to the farm. Best was "the squash king of the township, and prided himself on the seemingly overwhelming production of squash. These weekends were very informal, among which [CHB] became a regular farmer working the fields."

Tasker arrived at Best's lab in 1946. "During these years I got to know him extremely well. I was utterly amazed that a junior person like myself should receive so much attention, advice, direction and downright good friendship from a man of his stature." The Banting and Best Department had coffee and tea breaks "in the morning and afternoon, respectively, which your father deemed 'a parade,' and everybody was expected to attend. He would sit at the head of the table and everything under the sun was discussed: personal matters, new research ventures and discoveries, the latest news in the scientific world. Apart from serious matters, he had a puckish sense of humour." One day, Best recounted a wartime experiment "to study the effects of underwater explosions. This required a huge tank of water on the roof of the Banting Institute into which rats were floated in condoms. A small test explosion was then set off. He remembered with glee an occasion in which the explosion propelled a rat in a condom not only out of the tank, but over the wall of the roof of the Banting and onto the sidewalk of College Street below. The ill-fated animal landed at the feet of some distinguished female Toronto resident, and caused a great consternation."[577]

Charley Best was on the road a great deal to Québec, Ottawa, and Chalk River for the DRB, and to New York for meetings of the Rockefeller Foundation. The minutes of the Rockefeller Foundation of 25 October 1948 treated a subject that had already been mentioned in previous years but would be of special interest to Best in 1949. A motion was moved to approve a grant of $18,120 "designated for East Africa — Yellow Fever Investigations — Entebbe, Uganda, to be available during the year 1949."[578]

While they were in New York in late October, Margaret and Charley went to see *A Streetcar Named Desire*[579] by Tennessee Williams, with Jessica Tandy and Marlon Brando. Margaret did not like it as well as *The Glass Menagerie,* and Charley did not like it at all. He rarely enjoyed plays or movies that were negative or unhappy — he felt that there was enough of that in real life.

At the end of November 1948, Charles Best became a commander of the Order of the Crown of Belgium, presented in Toronto by the Baron de Gaiffier d'Hestroy, the Belgian chargé d'affaires. Linda, the boys, and several friends witnessed the ceremony. Margaret found the press photographers somewhat rude. "They have no shame about interrupting conversations." At the end of November, Charley went to Montréal to receive the Award of Merit from Nu Sigma Nu, his own medical fraternity. He spoke about "The Canadian Scene," using slides from paintings by the family and Henry's colour slides. For the University of Toronto Faculty Art Show that autumn, Best entered his large painting of the Ile d'Orléans and another of Henry's Island at Schooner Cove. Sandy loyally said that some of the canvases were "pretty drab and dreary but that Daddy's looked gay and bright."

Charley travelled to New York again on 12 December 1948, to his last meeting of his second term as a scientific director of the Rockefeller Foundation. It was not to be, however, the end of Best's connection with

Rockefeller as they continued to support his work for many years. The day he came back to Toronto, he left for Ottawa, for meetings of the NRC and the DRB. It was also in 1948 that Best became an honorary member of the American Academy of Arts and Sciences, and as a result received for many years its fascinating journal, *Daedalus*, published by Harvard University, with articles on a wide variety of topics by distinguished experts.

There were eighteen for Christmas dinner in 1948. Guido Loewi, who had worked at the lab before the war, was back. He said that the last time he had had Christmas dinner with a family was in 1939 with the Bests. Dr. Shou Shan You and his wife, Rosemary, from China, both worked at the lab. "The Yous brought us a most lovely piece of carved jade, in round shape on a little wooden stand — the carving is of a *chilin* — a mythical animal somewhere between a horse and a deer in appearance. They brought it from China. Dr. Balu from India brought two pieces of carved ivory, one of the Goddess of Learning, Art and Music, and the other a blotter. He had told Linda that he didn't eat meat so she prepared stuffed eggs. He said that his vegetarian ways were 'not for sentimental reasons.'" Charles Vuylsteke, from Joseph Hoet's department in Louvain, and his wife, Elisabeth, were there with their little daughter, Katrine, and they gave the Bests some Brussels lace. Dr. Fritz Gerritzen of Leiden brought paint brushes for Charley and a copy of Saint-Exupéry's *Le Petit Prince* for Margaret. Dr. Stanley Hartroft, also from the lab, and the Vincent Prices, with their daughter, Laurie Anne, made up the party.

The sculptors Frances Loring and Florence Wyle, known as "The Girls,"[580] came for tea in February 1949. Margaret noted, "I had met them only once — when I went for tea to their studio in the little old church. They are great characters and I like Miss Wyle a great deal — little thing with her hair cut like a man — very New England in style." Wyle was allergic to cigarette smoke, and Margaret made certain that there would be no one smoking. "Wyle marched in, in her flat shoes, Basque beret perched on her head — took off her coat and she had a warm sweater underneath and the first thing she said as she advanced into the hall was, 'That's a queer Emily Carr.' It was the pool of light over our chest of drawers. She went on to explain that it was merely different from any that she had seen before." Carr visited their studio once. "She thinks Lawren Harris brought her — and pretty soon Emily fell asleep holding her tiny dog which she had brought with her."

According to Margaret, "Miss Loring had a deep voice like Tallulah Bankhead. She wore a cerise dress and sat in our rose chair. Linda, who was in a bright red suit, kept severely away from Miss Loring and the pink chair." Loring had done a head of Charles Best which just missed being a good likeness. The clay sculpture was never cast; it is part of the collection of the Art Gallery of Ontario. Loring's bust of Fred Banting, however, is excellent and a bronze cast of it stands in the foyer of the university's Medical Sciences Building, along with the very good likeness of Best sculpted by Ruth Lowe Bookman.

On 15 February 1949, Margaret recorded, "Charley got a most exciting cable yesterday from Lord Addison saying that the British government want Charley to succeed Sir Edward Mellanby as secretary of the Medical Research Council. They want him, accompanied by his wife, to come to England, all expenses paid, to discuss it." It was not the first offer from Britain. "There was the chair at Edinburgh, the Burroughs Wellcome offer, the British Drug Houses and the National Institute for Medical Research (Sir Henry's position)."

If Charley had been really interested, Margaret would not have stood in the way. He did ask Sandy and Henry one evening at dinner if they would like to live in London and they were both enthusiastic. The Bests were strongly Canadian, however, and, much as they loved Britain, they really did not want to live there. Margaret noted, "there are several reasons against — one very strong one is that the Charles H. Best Institute here is really going to come, I think."

It was typical of Charley Best that, when Margaret asked if he would like to have a party for his fiftieth birthday, he replied that he would rather go to the farm. He did, however, receive a number of books, including *Human Destiny,* by Pierre Lecomte de Nouy, and Alan Paton's *Cry, the Beloved Country,* (he and Margaret were soon to go to South Africa). Young Donnie Fraser, son of Don and Mary, doing his PhD at the lab, sent a card signed, "From all your children." At the farm, Charley and Henry got to work cutting up old fence posts for the stove.

The year before, the author Louis Bromfield had been in Toronto to speak to the Royal Canadian Institute. Charley went to a lunch that Ralph Salter gave in his honour. The Bests hosted a supper party for him that included Dr. Gunnar Ahlgren of Stockholm, Floyd and Jean Chalmers, Grant and Willa Glassco, Nicholas and Helen Ignatieff, and Paddy and Wilhemina Lewis (all people interested in farming) before Louis spoke to the students at Hart House. Morley Callaghan was at the talk. He had known Bromfield in France.

"Louis told us later that they had a chance to talk about their old friends such as Scott Fitzgerald. Louis said that Zelda was not beautiful. She made him feel uneasy long before she had the nervous breakdowns. She had strange reactions. Scott himself was brilliant but weak. When he drank, he got nasty and was unpleasant to waiters and others who could not talk back. Louis thinks that the legend is greater than the man or his work but that there are very fine bits in his writing — *The Great Gatsby* is probably his best and bits of others are very good." For many years the Bests had been interested in the books of Louis Bromfield, particularly in his farming volumes, *Pleasant Valley* and *Malabar Farm*. Sir Sahib Singh Sokhey was a great friend of Bromfield and he arranged for the Bests to go to Malabar Farm, at Mansfield, Ohio, where they had a fascinating visit.

The previous June Charles Best became president of the American Diabetes Association. When the ADA was formed in April 1940 both Banting and Best, neither of whom was present, had been made honorary presidents. In late March 1949, the ADA was meeting in Jacksonville, Florida, and many old friends, such as Elliott Joslin and Hugh Wilkerson of Boston and Joseph Barach of Pittsburgh were there. Charley spoke five times in two days. Margaret enjoyed the lay meeting, where Joslin and Charley spoke and then answered questions from the audience. Charley was able to take time away from the meetings to go to historic St. Augustine and to see the small Anglican church with a memorial window to Harriet Beecher Stowe, the novelist, who had lived there.

For the first time since the 1920s the spectre of the Nobel Prize arose to haunt Charles Best. Professor B.A. Houssay, who had received the Nobel Prize in 1947 for his discovery of the part played by the hormones of the anterior pituitary in the metabolism of sugar, had fallen afoul of the Peron regime in his native Argentina. He was forced into temporary exile in the United States, where he worked at the Public Health Service Laboratories in Washington, DC and early in March 1948 he had come to Toronto to give the Banting Memorial Lecture. He had just won the 1947 Nobel Prize for his work on the role of pituitary hormones. Best had nominated him to the Nobel Committee in 1943.[581] Houssay surprised Best by nominating him for the 1950 Nobel Prize in Medicine for his work on choline and heparin. Best wrote to Dale "This is very pleasing but I do not expect it will come to anything."[582]

However, unbeknownst to Best, Sir Henry also had been in touch with Gøran Liljestrand of the Nobel Committee and had received a reply dated 9 December 1948. Liljestrand confirmed that only those specifically invited could make nominations, and for the 1950 Prize this consisted of past laureates in physiology and medicine and the ordinary members of the medical faculties in Sheffield, Aberdeen, Cork, Montréal, and Melbourne.[583] Both Dale and Houssay were eligible to make nominations.

Dale kept Best informed and wrote on 16 April 1949: "I shall have the opportunity of confidential talk with Liljestrand ... What I want to find out is whether the committee would be favourably influenced to considering [your work on choline and heparin] by recalling your part in the insulin discovery, and incidentally the blunder they made in bringing Macleod into the award; or whether it would be better to leave that unmentioned." They tend "to favour some single, concrete discovery which can be pinned to the credit of one man, rather than an impressive and mixed output, in which the one man had led and inspired, so that his precise degree of responsibility is not easily judged from the published record."[584]

In late 1949, Houssay informed Best: "I have sent to Stockholm my proposal for the Nobel Prize for Physiology and Medicine be awarded to you in 1950. I mentioned your outstanding work on Dietary Factors in the Protection of the liver and kidney and I hope that my proposal will be successfully accepted. That would be justice."[585]

In his submission he stated: "His principal discoveries have been: Insulin (with Banting); Lipotropic and Antilipotropic Factors; The Prevention and Treatment of Fatty liver and Cirrhosis; The Role of Choline and Related Substances; Kidney Lesion by Deficiency of Choline and Late Hypertension; Histaminase."[586]

Houssay also nominated Dr. Vincent du Vigneaud, professor of biochemistry at Cornell, "because his work on Transmethylation and the Role of Nigration of the Methyl Group in the Body has opened a new field in Biochemistry and has illuminated the work of <u>Best</u> on the lipotropic substances, choline and methionine."[587] Du Vigneaud isolated vitamin H and synthesized oxytocin, for which he received the Nobel Prize for Chemistry in 1955.

Dale reported that he had sent his proposal to Liljestrand, "for the work on choline and 'lipotropic factors.'"[588] Heparin appeared only under the heading "subsidiary evidence." He cited "the work carried out by Professor <u>Best</u> with a succession of assistants and collaborators, which has led him to the very important discovery of the essential part played by the base choline, and by its metabolic precursors methionine and betaine, as so-called 'lipotropic factors,' in the normal, healthy functions of both the liver and the kidneys. This discovery has already proved to be of fundamental importance, both for the understanding of certain pathological processes and of the diseases resulting from them, such as fatty infiltration and cirrhosis of the liver, and circulatory hypertension of renal origin, and, in a more general sense, for the elucidation of previously obscure or uncertain features of the metabolism of fats in the normal animal body — of the transport of these substances from the general depots of the body to the cells of the liver and of their utilization and fate thereafter."[589]

After arguing that Best should have been included in 1923, Sir Henry stated: "Since those earliest days, such further advances, towards the discovery of the nature of insulin and the mode of its action, as have been contributed by any of those who were concerned in any way with the original discovery, have been made by <u>Best</u>, and not by either Banting or MacLeod — both of whom, of course, are now dead." The work for which Dale was now nominating Best, "though essentially different, actually began with observations which were first made in the course of the discovery of insulin and its action." He added, "<u>Best</u> himself remained, with conspicuous dignity, aloof from personal rivalries and contentions, which unfortunately arose among others concerned with the insulin discovery and its public recognition."[590]

Dale mentioned other achievements of Best's, such as heparin and histaminase, not "as a basis, in itself, for an independent claim to the award of a Nobel Prize: I put them forward only as contributing evidence of the outstanding quality of his wide influence on the progress of medical science, and for any reinforcement they may thus give to the strong claim which can be specifically based on his discovery of the vital significance of choline and the allied lipotropic factors, in the normal metabolism of the animal types so far studied in that connexion."[591]

Mario L. De Finis, professor of physiology at the National University of Paraguay in Asunción, also nominated Best for the 1950 Prize for his work on "Dietary factors in the protection of the liver and kidney."[592] Only at the end of 1950 would they know whether these lobbying efforts had succeeded.

The first meeting took place on 2 May 1949 of the Ontario Diabetes Association, a lay group that eventually grew into the Canadian Diabetes Association (CDA). Wally Seccombe was the first chairman, and Ralph Mills drew up the constitution. Best had worked very hard to get this group started. He believed fervently in the value of societies for lay diabetics and described the role of societies in England, Belgium, Holland and the United States. He became honorary president, and at the meeting, he told of the many parts of the world where insulin was not available. Laurie Chute from the Hospital for Sick Children "was most inspiring as he told of the many difficulties for diabetic children — how much help they need." Bob Kerr, head of the department of therapeutics, spoke, as did Gerry Wrenshall, a PhD in atomic physics from Yale and in physiology from Toronto, who was a severe diabetic and worked at the lab. The whole Best family became very involved in the activities of the CDA.

On 17 May 1949, Charles Best received his first Canadian honorary degree from Dalhousie University in Halifax. "After the four hundred MD's were awarded, Dean Grant and President Alexander E. Kerr spoke about Charley. Dean H.G. Grant named the great men of science back over the ages and added Charley's name to the list. They both referred to his and to my connection with Nova Scotia and with Dalhousie — both of our fathers had been there." Charley felt that this indeed was a special honour. It was an appropriate year to receive it in Halifax, two hundred years after the Bests arrived there in 1749.

The return trip to Toronto was unusual and fun. Ontario Lieutenant Governor Ray Lawson was in Halifax to receive an honorary degree from King's College, and he and his wife, Helen, invited the Bests to travel back to Toronto with them on their private railway car. They stopped in Québec to have lunch at the vice regal mansion, Bois de Coulonge (Spencerwood), with Major General Sir Eugène and Lady Fiset. He won a DSO in the Boer War, was the former MP for Rimouski, and served as lieutenant governor of Québec from 1939 to 1950.

Margaret and Charley left Toronto on 1 June for the meetings of the Lay Diabetic Association of New York. There they heard much discussion about diabetics hiding the fact of their condition. Charley spoke at the Lennox Hill Hospital, and there was a question and answer session. Cousin Dr. Bill Macleod was there. Guido Loewi (who had renamed himself Geoffrey Lowe) told the Bests that his father, the Nobel laureate Otto Loewi, by then living in New York, was celebrating his seventy-sixth birthday, and they went to his home to congratulate him. Otto said to his wife, "You didn't tell me that the Bests were coming," and she replied, "No, it is my birthday present to you."

Then, in Atlantic City, Charley finished his very busy year as president of the ADA; Dr. Howard Root of the Joslin Clinic in Boston succeeded him. Margaret remarked that there was a great deal of talk about state medicine and that many people felt very strongly about it. The British experience was not popular in the United States.

Charley arranged for Margaret, Dr. Hugh Farris of Saint John, and himself to see the medical art show. His entries were his *Ile d'Orléans* canvas and *Imaginary Island in Passamaquoddy Bay*. As they did at many meetings in Atlantic City, the Bests took the people from the lab in Toronto out to dinner, this time to Hackney's, a well-known seafood restaurant.

When at home, Charley Best spent the week and usually Saturday morning either at the Department of Physiology or at the Banting and Best, but he almost always took the family to the farm on the weekend where he relished the release and relaxation of physical activity. He loved to have people visit the place and he was proud of it. There were plans that summer to have the people from both departments out for a picnic. Unfortunately, the strawberries were a failure because of lack of rain, and the farm did not have irrigation. No doubt Sandy, who was becoming more and more involved in the farm, would have liked to do something about this but the obvious water supply, the west branch of the Credit River, which flowed through the property, was a long way away from the gardens.

The first lab party for forty-five people went off well, despite the heat. Charley cooked sausages on the outdoor stone fireplace, and there were rolls, salad, and punch. Strawberries were found from a grower who had irrigation, and there was cake to go with them. Some people went for a walk in the valley, and Charley took them on tours with the tractor and wagon. There were guests from China, Holland, India, New Zealand, and the United States.

The same day Charley received a call from Sidney Smith to say that the university's board of governors had decided to provide $1.5 million in order to proceed with his building. As guests arrived at the farm news came that Sandy had not passed into third-year honours math, physics, and chemistry. He was advised to apply for third year in the pass course. Of nine people in the course, four had passed (no one with first class), four, including Sandy, were advised to transfer, and one failed completely. Margaret wrote gloomily, "Professor George Wright seems to take pleasure in failing people. One year he was very proud that he failed his whole honours chemistry course. Charley is trying to help Sandy to decide what to do. It is a thorny problem from several points of view." Sandy had always excelled at everything that he did, and for Charley and Margaret failure was not something they considered either for themselves or for the family. However, Charley never took out his disappointment on his sons if they did not come up to his expectations.

The Bests left on 12 July 1949 for Maine and Schooner Cove Farm. A fishing trip with Captain Elton Chaffey from Chocolate Cove, Deer Island, produced several pollock and the company of a whale and a school of porpoise. Anna Lincoln and Tishie Brown came to visit for the last time. On 8 August began a friendship that brought infinite interest and pleasure to the Best family, especially to Margaret. That was the day, on the introduction of Mary Bogue, an antique dealer in East Machias, they met Lea Reiber, a retired actor, and Walter Sinclair, who had for several years been director of Hart House Theatre. Through them, they met eighty-year-old John Marin, the eminent American artist. They all lived at Cape Split, South Addison, Maine, a rather isolated community sixty miles south of West Pembroke.

Margaret and Charley had admired Marin's watercolours of the Maine coast at the Phillips Gallery in New York and elsewhere, and had read MacKinley Helm's 1948 biography of him.[593] Margaret described him in 1949: "He is rather little and frail with amazing gray hair, almost a cut, and bright eyes." Sandy and Marin talked about music, and both played the piano. John Marin, Jr., and his wife, Grace, ran the American Place Gallery on Madison Avenue, previously run by Alfred Stieglitz, husband of Georgia O'Keefe. "I wish we could get a Marin watercolour from them sometime. I suppose it would cost a great deal." Margaret never did own a Marin; the prices were already too high.

Three weeks later, the new Cape Split friends came for dinner at Schooner Cove Farm. John Marin and Walter Sinclair walked to Leighton Point with Charley. Margaret and the artist went out to wish on the new moon. The day before they left for Toronto, the Bests returned to Cape Split to have dinner with the Marins.

That summer, the Best family set off from Maine for Nova Scotia. There were two reasons for this trip — Charley had been planning for some time to get a boat that he could use to travel the islands and coves of Cobscook Bay, and he and Margaret wanted to show the boys the region of their Best, Fisher, and Mahon forebears. Charley recalled the summer of 1916 when he and another man had sailed a small steamboat hauling freight between Pembroke, Eastport, St. Stephen, St. Andrews, and the islands. He wanted the boys to learn about the tides, the currents, and the fogs of the area. After dinner at Dr. Hugh Farris's house in Saint John, the Bests boarded the *Princess Hélène* to cross the Bay of Fundy, entering the Annapolis Basin by the Digby Gut. From Digby, they drove down St Mary's Bay to Meteghan, Acadian country. Margaret commented on this route, known as "the longest main street in Canada" because of the farms, only one deep, with the houses close together. Spans of oxen were common.

Atlantic Shipyards was the Bests' destination. Charley wanted a typical Cape Island lobster boat, forty feet long. He said that it would be called the *Margaret B*. The people at the boatyard agreed to send on the specifications of the craft with a few modifications to make it suitable for the family's purposes. The boys were delighted with the idea. Margaret did not voice any open reservations, but neither was she enthusiastic. She realized that it had been a long time since Charley had navigated the dangerous waters of Cobscook and Passamaquoddy Bays and that the rest of the family had none of the required skills. Also, though generally healthy, Charley had been plagued of late with some health problems, including persistent and painful neuritis. She also realized that the boys were getting to the age where they would not always be there to help. In any case it was a lovely dream that never came to pass.

On their return to Toronto they started preparations for a very special trip. Honouring General Smut's invitation of 1943, Prime Minister Daniel Malan had invited the Bests to South Africa. This trip was sponsored by the Nuffield Foundation in England. As usual the Rockefeller Foundation also helped with arrangements and contacts. On 27 October Margaret wrote that they were leaving that evening for New York on their way to England and to South Africa. They had an unhurried day in New York. Margaret bought a nylon shirt for Charley with plain cuffs; for some reason, he disliked French cuffs — perhaps thought of them as affected. Dr. Tom Parran accompanied them to the Rockefeller Foundation offices on the fifty-fourth floor of the Rockefeller Center, from where they saw the *Queen Mary* lying in the river. By now, Margaret knew the Rockefeller people — Drs Strode, Parran, Robert Morrison, Hugh Smith, and Logan. John and Dorothy Logan were heading back to Sardinia. Charley got the latest anti-malarial pills recommended by his Rockefeller colleagues.

South Africa

On 29 October 1949, it was misty and mild as the *Queen Mary* steamed out of New York bound for England and Margaret was very happy. A note from Captain Grattidge asked the Bests to sit at his table. On this crossing, they had good companions: Edward Savage Crocker, the American ambassador to Baghdad, who knew Maine well, and his wife; Sir Hartley Shawcross, attorney general of Britain; the Hon. Lionel Berry and his wife, Helen, (he was the eldest son of Viscount Kemsley, owner of *The Times* and other newspapers); Mrs. Rueff, "a beauteous blonde Belgian lady"; and William Donald, deputy chair of the Cunard Line. The Bests liked Donald very much and enjoyed hearing about his family. Also they met General Sir Richard and Lady McCreery — he had commanded the British 8th Army in Italy in 1944 and 1945. "General McCreery is very tall and very thin and is lame. Lady McCreery is very nice."

In London, the Bests stayed at Nuffield Foundation House in Leinster Gardens. In South Africa Best was to study nutritional problems among the black population, assess medical research in universities, and make recommendations to the foundation and the South African government. He went to see Dr. Neil Hamilton Fairley in Harley Street, an expert in the prevention of malaria. Charley knew something about malaria because of the Rockefeller connection and John Logan and the Sardinia project. He went to a physiology meeting at the School of Hygiene at University College on Gower Street, later having lunch with Sir Henry Dale and Dr. Harold Burn.

Margaret described their departure for South Africa on 8 November 1949 from Southampton. "Our plane lay there on the water — a great silvery beauty, a Sunderland called *The City of Edinburgh*, with Captain Carey, our pilot." Charley gave Margaret one and a half grains of Nembutal and took the same himself. He knew that it was going to be a long trip, but it was her first flight, and Margaret did not want to miss anything. "We taxied for miles and then took off. The earth there beneath us when I looked down was like a children's farm set — little houses, fields green and fields ploughed — very lovely really — tiny cattle in the fields. There was a long point to our right and white cliffs — not Dover. The sea was lovely beneath us — shadows of the clouds — whitecaps and clouds themselves all around us." Travelling at two hundred miles per hour, they soon saw the coast of France near Cherbourg.

The plane usually stopped for the night at Augusta in Sicily, but there were strikes there, so they made for Marseilles. Captain Carey flew along the Bay of Biscay and crossed the narrow isthmus between Spain and France, with the Pyrenees on the right and the Cevennes on the left, heading for Marseilles. "It was a glorious sensation flying — even the taking off. Charley said that the sea was really choppy as we taxied across from Southampton and also that the bumps were considerable. He was very pleased with me — I looked down from the very start because I wanted to get every impression and the French country looked lovely from the air — the fields narrower and smaller than the English — the coastline of France very lovely — a band of foam."

After four hours of flying at four thousand feet, they landed, not in Marseilles, but on Lake Marignane near Aix-en-Provence. They drove through low hills with olive trees and small fields to the Hôtel du Roy René. The Bests invited a fellow passenger, a boy of twelve who was going home from boarding school in England to Victoria Falls, to join them for dinner, and they enjoyed talking to him.

The next morning the travellers were up at 6:30 for a long day. Going out to their plane by boat, they took off for Augusta, Sicily, seeing the Alps away to the left. Off Toulon, they saw Corsica and then Sardinia, site of the Rockefeller anti-malaria project. From ten thousand feet, the plane came down to Augusta, northeast of Syracuse, on the east coast of Sicily. "It was very exciting and rough, the last part of the trip. I felt quite sick but managed to look out and see what was happening. Augusta is a very grey-beard looking town — even the tiles on the roofs were gray — not red. We left our passports at the quay with officials and walked to the hotel, which is new and operated by BOAC.[594] It is there that the Italian staff has gone on strike — only a skeleton staff of BOAC people."

The take-off from Augusta "was very bumpy with spiral turn. We went very high — many clouds — they looked somewhat like snow-capped peaks." The travellers could see the stars and Venus very large and bright. On their way to Egypt Charley suggested that Margaret re-read Antoine de Saint-Exupéry's *Le Petit Prince*.

The plane stopped in Alexandria for the night, and the Bests stayed at the San Stefano Hotel, with a view of the sea. The waiters spoke French as well as Arabic; most had white robes and red or embroidered sashes; some wore a red fez, others a white headcloth. Margaret noted every detail of what they had to eat and of people's dress. They had an uneasy, short rest

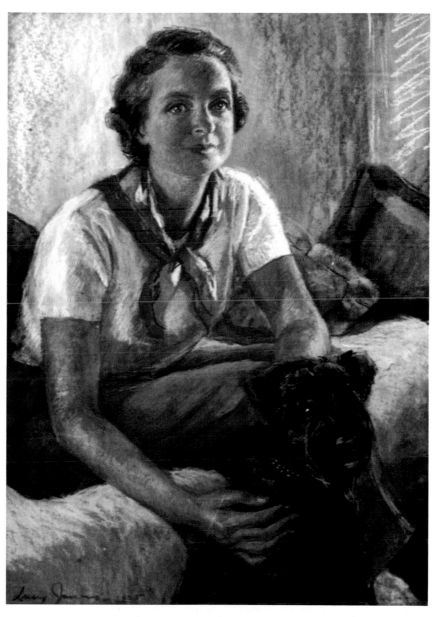

Portrait of Margaret Mahon Best with "Blarney"
by Lucy Jarvis

Schooner Cove Farm, West Pembroke, Maine, 1938
(courtesy of Margaret Cairine Best)

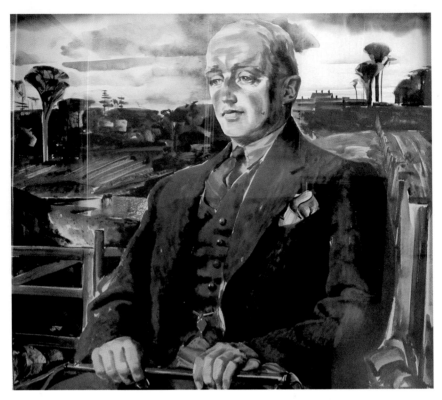

Portrait of Charles Herbert Best
by Charles Comfort, PRCA

Connaught Laboratories Farm, Toronto, 1939

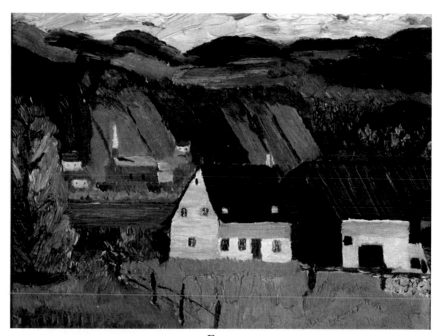

Farm
St-Pierre, Ile d'Orléans, Québec, 1948
by Charles H. Best

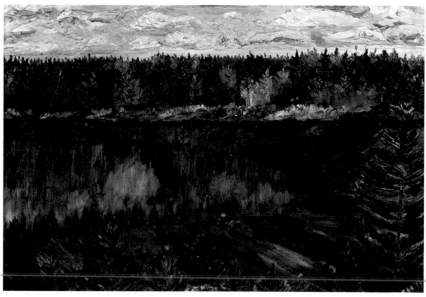

Clam Diggers
Schooner Cove Farm, West Pembroke, Maine, 1951
by Charles H. Best

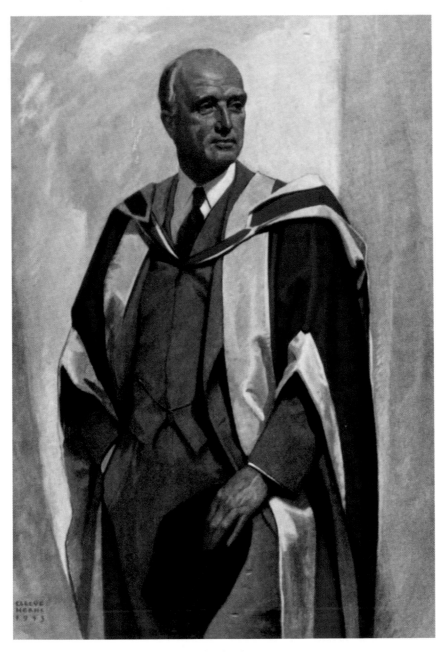

Portrait of Charles H. Best
by Cleeve Horne, RCA

In the foyer of the Best Institute,
University of Toronto, 15 September 1953

before the mosquitoes began to buzz; there were no nets on their beds. By 1:30 they were ready to leave. They flew over the Nile: "There was the river, the narrow green strip on either side and then desert. We saw Wadi Haifa; the houses looked like rectangular outlines, near the border with the Sudan." The plane stopped at Khartoum to re-fuel, the passengers going to a reception centre. There was no time to go into the city but Charley took some pictures. Back in the air, Margaret noted that the White Nile "winds like a silver ribbon through the country." Charley's lips got very blue, and he required oxygen.

They landed at Port Bell on Lake Victoria, in Uganda. Dr. and Mrs. Stuart Kitchen of the Rockefeller Foundation station at Entebbe came and drove the Bests to the Silver Springs Hotel between Port Bell and Kampala. After dinner, the Kitchens took their guests for a drive through Kampala and on to Entebbe, the capital, where they stayed in the compound of the Rockefeller Yellow Fever Research Laboratories. "Charley was very interested in the work being done there." The next morning they could see how enormous Lake Victoria was, and they noted the many flat-topped mountains so common in Africa. The plane landed on the Zambezi River near Victoria Falls. It was very bumpy, and Charley was very nearly sick. "When we came down I was able to say to him, 'You will feel alright very soon.' That was quite an achievement for me to be able to be encouraging Charley."

The flamboyant trees, with their large spreading tops and great clusters of orange-red flowers, like a pea blossom, were "absolutely wonderful. Flamboyant is a good name for them." At this point, the Bests enjoyed meeting their fellow travellers, the Nivens, citrus growers near Port Elizabeth, South Africa. Mrs. Niven was the daughter of the late Sir Percy Fitzpatrick, author of the 1907 novel *Jock of the Bushveld*, the classic South African story of the bull terrier and his adventures. They had time for a short tour of Victoria Falls, noting the "baobab" trees and the statue of Dr. David Livingstone, and they compared what they saw with the Niagara Gorge and Falls. Margaret tried to identify the flowers and noted that "the birds squeak and pipe and whistle but don't really sing." They saw the "Eastern Cataract when we stopped near the War Memorial. There you look directly up the very narrow gorge and see the falls and spray — that is a very lovely sight. I liked that view the best of all." Margaret was stung by something, and Charley gave her anti-malarial pills ahead of schedule.

In a game preserve, the travellers saw their first giraffes, sable antelope, zebras, warthogs, and ostriches in the semi-wild. The bougainvillea and frangipani were in bloom. In the town of Livingstone, Charley went into the hospital and talked to Dr. Cowen. "He said that he had been called to go to the plane once or twice when people thought they had developed kidney disease. He told Charley that the water is chlorinated but they boil all of theirs. They get fresh milk for their children and three times over bring it to the boil and strain it. He gets about forty cases of malaria a day."

The next morning there was less turbulence, and the pilot flew over the falls. Beyond they could see the Salt Lake and the Kalahari Desert. Then slag heaps announced the region of the gold mines. The plane landed on Vaal Dam, and they took the bus into Johannesburg, where they were met by Dr. Sarel Oosthuizen, who, with his artist wife, Juliette, was their host and guide for much of their stay in South Africa, and driven to their home in Pretoria. Oosthuizen was a radiologist and chair of the Committee for Research in the Medical Sciences of the Council for Scientific and Industrial Research (CSIR), following Dr. Basil Schonland. He showed his guests the home of Prime Minister Dr. Daniel F. Malan, the Union Buildings, and the home of Paul Kruger, the great Boer leader.

Everywhere Margaret remarked on the flowers and trees. She made copious notes every day. Once home, she assembled the scrapbook for the trip. On 18 November 1949 Margaret wrote, "Today we are to meet General Jan Christiaan Smuts, I am so thrilled." He lived on a farm near Irene, south of Pretoria, but had an office in the city. He and Charley recalled their meeting in London in an air raid shelter following a meeting at the Royal Society Club in 1943. It was then that he had invited Best to South Africa, and even though he was defeated as prime minister in 1948, he had arranged the Bests' visit. "General Smuts looks very ruddy and fit — very immaculate in appearance and altogether charming." He was just off to London by plane for a celebration for Chaim Weizmann, the first president of Israel. "We talked of wildflowers in South Africa. I told him that I had bought, in London, *A Botanist in Southern Africa* by John Hutchinson of Kew Gardens. He said, 'I know him well. He is in this country now. I went with him around Lake Tanganyika collecting specimens all the time.'"

When Smuts mentioned the wildflowers growing on Table Mountain, Charley told him that Margaret was not too keen to go up there by cable railway. Smuts said, "'Well, don't go up by cable railway — walk. I have never gone up by the cable in my life and I have been up hundreds of times.' He added that the flora at the tip of the cape is quite different from any other. He likes plant life better than animal — no arguments, everything peaceful and beautiful."

Smuts "told us that he had been in Canada in 1930 — saw snow on the ground and was a great admirer of General Sir Arthur Currie, the senior Canadian officer in the First World War and later principal of McGill University. He had written an introduction to a life of Currie."[595]

A few days later, Sarel Oosthuizen took the Bests to meet Prime Minister Malan. "I had an idea that he and General Smuts were bitter enemies but Sarel says no, that they were really quite good friends — enemies politically, but personal friends. They often lunch together. Just the same I wish General Smuts was still the prime minister. Dr. Malan is a very nice, solid sort of man — rather the Paul Kruger type. Dr. Malan told us that he knows Mike Pearson and likes him very much. Sarel told him that Charley now has the title 'Oom Charley,' meaning Uncle Charley. He said, 'You know, he has a great many honorary degrees and honours of all kinds but we have given him a new one.' Dr. Malan mentioned the protea, the national flower, and urged us to be sure to see it in the Cape Province."

When he returned to Toronto, Best gave an illustrated lecture, "A Month on Modern Medical Safari," to his two departments and a few other guests. He talked of the diseases for which one could be inoculated and those for which one could not, including malaria, amoebic dysentery, and bilharzia. Six years in the International Health Division of the Rockefeller Foundation "sharpened my interest in international health ... I was and am especially interested in kwashiorkor [malnutrition due to insufficient protein] which is the most important nutritional disease in the world today." Provision of skim milk could cure this condition, but none was available where it was most needed, despite the huge quantities stored in some countries. Best talked of resulting liver damage and cirrhosis and noted that "a great deal of fundamental information was not available." He concluded, "I have learned a great deal about the present status of these problems in Africa that was not available from the literature. I helped to initiate a dietary survey. We hope to receive soon samples of basal diets which will permit us to help unravel some of the controversial findings of the South African laboratories. There are many pitfalls in this type of experimental work — we have learned the location of some of them and this should be helpful."[596]

Also as a result of the South African trip, the minutes of the Nuffield Foundation's thirty-first meeting reported, "The trustees agreed that action should be taken with a view to implementing the following two suggestions arising out of Professor Best's visit to South Africa:

1. The possibility that, by paying their travel expenses, the Foundation might assist South African postgraduate medical students to work in the University of Toronto under Professor Best's supervision;

2. The desirability of making known to the Foundation's Liaison Committees and in particular to the Canadian Committee, the excellent work and reputation of the Veterinary Research Laboratory at Ondestepoort, South Africa."[597]

At the fifty-third meeting it was recorded that Professor Best was prepared to accept one South African postgraduate student for one year to work in his department.[598] One participant in the program was Robert Metz, who completed his PhD in 1963 with a thesis entitled, "Factors Influencing Urea Synthesis."

The 1950s was a period of great positive activity but also of immense strain for Best, primarily because of difficulties and anxiety about the funding and construction of the new research facility. In July 1949 the board of Governors of U of T had decided to provide $1.5 million in order to proceed with the building. But they had put Best in an awkward position by naming the building after him, while expecting him at the same time to raise the funds needed to complete it. In addition to his normal responsibilities with his two departments, Best had demanding travel and hectic lecture and meeting schedules. On 12 January 1950 he was off to New York for two days at the ADA, then to give the Christian Herter Lecture at the New York University Medical School, to Bellevue Hospital, and to Washington, DC for two days with the United States Public Health Service. A few days later, he was off to Ottawa for the National Research Council and the Defence Research Board.

After the war, Canada agreed with Britain and the United States to share information and research on both offensive and defensive chemical and biological weapons. A board meeting of the DRB on 20 March 1950 decided to establish a "Bacteriological Warfare Review Committee to examine all the Canadian activities in the BW field and to make recommendations as to how DRB's effort could be increased."[599] Best was to be the chair and members included Ray Farquharson, Otto Maass from

McGill, and Joe Doupe of the University of Manitoba. Dr. L.W. Billingsley, a former graduate student of Collip's, was secretary. The chair and secretary visited American BW labs, and Best had discussions with the staff of Porton, the British establishment. The committee's recommendations led to the reopening in 1951 of the Grosse Ile Experimental Station at the old island quarantine station in the St. Lawrence below Québec, and construction in 1953 of a new laboratory in Kingston. Grosse Ile focused on the production of rinderpest vaccine, against a severe disease of cattle and other animals found primarily in Africa. It was produced in conjunction with the Department of Agriculture. The committee found that there were not enough medical bacteriologists in Canada.

The joint projects on weapons research were both chemical and bacteriological and rinderpest and anthrax were on the list. Even as recently as 1988, a government report repeated the oft-repeated assurance that Canada was not "engaged in any research with offensive overtones."[600] Neither chemical nor bacteriological agents were ever used, but Canada participated in research and production. Few people realize that Grosse Ile was once the main source of anthrax for Canada, Britain, and the United States. John Bryden MP explained, "Britain never had the anthrax because it was made in Canada; Canada never had the anthrax because it was made for Britain." In any case, the story is still far from complete. We do know that Banting, Collip, Maass, and Philip Greey, among many others, were involved during the war, and Best in the years that followed. Greey was head of bacteriology at Toronto for over twenty years.

Dr. Clarence MacCharles headed up a section on medical research at DRB headquarters in Ottawa and acted as secretary of the Defence Medical Research Advisory Committee from 1953. As well as working closely with Best, "MacCharley," as he was known, and his wife, Eve, became close friends. Later in 1951, a Defence Research Advisory Committee was established, with Best as chair. He described the duties of this body as "a mechanism for bridging the gap between the [Defence Medical Research] Co-Ordinating Committee and the actual research workers. It will review the medical work being done in each field of defence and advise the Co-Ordinating Committee of the support required."[601]

Starting in 1950, Best's name appeared as a member of the Associate Committee on Dental Research of the National Research Council, a reflection of the work being done on periodontal problems by Dr. William J. Linghorne in the Banting and Best Department of Medical Research. In

293

March 1950, the NRC gave $25,000 research grants to Best, Collip at Western, and J.S.L. Browne at McGill. Wilder Penfield, also at McGill, received $40,000. It made the same allocations in March 1951. In the meantime, Best had been appointed to the council for a second three-year term. During 1951, Charles Best was involved in NRC discussions on the hormone ACTH, cortisone, and growth hormone. In December 1951 and in March 1952, Best, Collip, Browne, and Penfield received further support, and in 1951, Hans Selyé received $8,500. Charles Best's membership on the NRC expired as of 31 March 1953.

Margaret could not stop reading and thinking about Africa. "I can't get away from it. It is so fascinating." On several occasions, the Bests showed their slides to various friends. Among these were Captain and Mrs. Jock de Marbois. He taught German at Upper Canada College, had travelled widely in Africa, and taught his students many interesting things, such as how to play Zulu drums.[602] In early March 1950 it was time for the annual Gilbert and Sullivan production at Upper Canada College. Both Sandy and Henry had been involved in previous years. Sandy had either designed sets or played violin in the orchestra and Henry sang. This was his first year as the tenor lead, "Frederic" in *The Pirates of Penzance*. Faithful family and friends were in the audience. Rose Macdonald, writing in the *Telegram*, particularly mentioned the "Frederic-Mabel duet" — "as charming a bit of acting as might be seen on any amateur stage."[603]

Sir Henry and Lady Dale were in Toronto after a wonderful tour of New Zealand. Sir Henry gave the Fred Tisdale Memorial Lecture.[604] On Sunday there was a party at the farm: Linda made chili con carne and served it in the large bowl that had belonged to Emil Fischer, the Nobel laureate chemist. Sir Henry made side trips to New York and to London, Ontario. Everyone marvelled at the Dales' stamina. The Bests took their guests to a reception given by the lieutenant-governor for Sir Basil Brooke, prime minister of Northern Ireland. Margaret was touched when she introduced the Dales to Lena MacAlpine, a parishioner of St. Andrew's church, who talked to them about the Rev. Mr. Mahon: "We loved him. It was like a benediction to talk to him. You don't find people like that." The two couples went to Kingston, where Sir Henry received an LLD from Queen's on 20 May, and the Dales went on to Montréal to stay with Wilder and Helen Penfield.

It was after this stay in Montréal that Sir Henry told of meeting Dr. C.F. Martin, emeritus dean of medicine at McGill. Martin said to him,

"When Collip discovered insulin," and Dale did not reply, so Martin repeated, "When Collip discovered insulin." Dale said, "I heard you the first time, Dr. Martin." Both McGill and Western Ontario were pro-Collip — understandable, as he had been on faculty at McGill (1928–41), and at Western (1947–61). In 1927, Martin had written to Collip in Edmonton, encouraging him to accept the chair of biochemistry to succeed A.B. McCollum at McGill.[605]

On Saturday 3 June Margaret and Charley drove to Queen's University, Kingston, where he received an honorary LLD. His convocation address, "Medicine in a Restless World" reflected his interest in international medical problems as they prepared for another trip to Europe. They were to sail on 29 June, this time taking Linda and Henry with them. Sandy, almost nineteen, had left at the end of May to spend the summer at the Experimental Farm in Ottawa. On 14 May he sent a fourteen-page memo detailing the tasks that the fifteen-year-old Henry was to do at the farm in the two weeks before he sailed.

> Remember: get more hose. Water strawberries in the evenings. ... Get some more strawberry boxes; I guess Freda can order them in town. I suppose between a hundred and 2 hundred quart boxes ... perhaps you can judge for yourself how many you will need. Remember, you picked between 3-4 hundred quarts the last year I was away.
>
> Concerning the row planting of the vegetables and flowers — better bring the rows closer together than I have them — 3 feet is ample room & 3 feet would probably be o.k. between most of them. ... Just before I come back you should have any empty space there well disced — and either run over it with no cut on the discs or the harrow — so that it is smooth also have a bag of Vigoro on hand. Also have the land down in the orchard cultivated. — I suppose I mentioned before about weeding thoroughly around those young grapes there, mulching them — and perhaps a little water if necessary. ...
>
> Please read and re-read the previous notes that I sent you so you will not forget anything.
>
> See that the spring bulbs are all weeded ... — also put in good stakes between varieties. ... Lully [Linda]

should plant the alyssum seed along the border & water it now and then. ... Please write me a detailed description of how the various things are doing. ...

Henry — remember to plant that extra row of potatoes where I told you. ... A good thing to do, would be to put in good stout stakes between the different varieties [of bulbs] and at the end of the rows. Better do this fairly soon, before the foliage withers and the different types become difficult to distinguish. You can make lots of stakes now. Use the leftover lumber, some of which is hanging in the toolshed. You can make a good number of 2 foot ones and sharpen their ends for row markers. ... This about finishes the spring bulbs. ...

Gladiolus — really as soon as you get out there, you should start cleaning the rest of the glads ... put the smaller ones about 2-3 inches apart in the row and about 3 inches deep; the larger ones 4-5 inches apart and about 4 inches deep. First make your trenches, put in a layer of manure, then some earth on top of that, and then the corms on the level earth; then cover up with earth and firm down on top. ...

Lilies — Mummy knows best what they look like and can do some of the weeding in the rows — you should help her by hoeing out the weeds ... actually, there is usually room between the individual plants in the row for one or two scrapes with the hoe. ... Stakes at the end of rows please. ...

[Grapes, Trees, had similar detailed instructions.]

Vegetables — ... One of the first things you should do as soon as you get out there is to plant some turnips. ...You should plant either 1 or 2 rows ... run the disc over s over the spot where you are going to sow the seed — hoe out any tough weed spots — and finally run over the ground with hardly any curve on the discs — to flatten out the ridges. Then rake over the area by hand so that it is nice and smooth; then get out that ball of string from the toolshed and set up your stakes the proper distance ... and sow your seed. ...

[Near the end] <u>Also,</u> I think Lully will have obtained some white cosmos seed — <u>You should sow that right away.</u>[606]

England and Europe

On 29 June 1950, Margaret, Charley, Linda, and Henry sailed from New York on the *Nieuw Amsterdam* for Southampton. Hugh Barrett, a former student of Best's and chief of Porton Down, the British biological research establishment, met them at the boat with two Humber sedans and government drivers. The twenty-two-mile drive to Salisbury, on the left and very fast around the curves, was exciting for Henry, on his first trip overseas. While Best worked at Porton, the others visited the area. Dr. J.F.B. Stone, a scientist, took them to Stonehenge and all four went to the Farnborough Air Show, where the Canberra jet bomber was the star attraction. London saw a round of museums, art galleries, theatres, including T.S. Eliot's *The Cocktail Party*, with Rex Harrison, and visits with Henry's godfather, Sir Henry Dale, and Lady Dale, as well as the Lawrence family.

On 20 July, the family took the ferry from Dover to Ostende, and the Hoets drove them to their villa at Coq-sur-Mer, seven miles down the coast. There the Bests met Godelieve Brusselmans, known as "Pep," young Jo Hoet's fiancée. (Princess Mathilde of Belgium looks very much as Pep did in 1950.)

Belgium was in turmoil: exiled King Leopold was returning to Brussels, and the Hoets and the Vuylstekes of Gant, where the Bests went next, were very pro-royalist. Shortly afterwards King Leopold abdicated in favour of his son, Prince Beaudouin. Dr. Charles Vuylsteke and his wife and daughter had spent a year in Toronto, where he worked with Drs. A.M. Rappoport and Donald Fraser on "the effects of the ligation of the hepatic artery in dogs."[607]

The Bests were welcomed by the Hoets at their home, Les Conifères, Corbeek-Lo, near Louvain. Dinner at the Brusselmans' home was also a happy affair. Including Pep, there were ten Brusselman children, and, with the six young Hoets and the Canadian guests, it made a large cheerful gathering. Margaret noted, "Pep is a dear, sweet-looking girl — and Jo we love!" When the guests were leaving, Mr. Brusselmans said, "Send Henry over here to learn French. He can spend his time between our house and the Hoets." Though other friends in Europe and elsewhere gave similar invitations, the Bests never did take advantage of these generous offers. This was strange since Margaret and Charley themselves had so benefited from their early experiences overseas in the mid-1920s. Though Charley might have encouraged his sons to spend time learning another language and culture, Margaret would have been afraid to let them go even to such close, responsible friends as the Hoets. Her reaction was puzzling considering the freedom that she herself had had as a teenager.

The Bests and five Hoets went to Silvaplana in Switzerland and hiked for a day near the Bernina Pass. They walked up the Val del Fain to the Strela Pass, everyone helping Margaret gather wildflowers in the snow, rain, and sun. Philippe Hoet, a child diabetic, recalled, "We had walked about twenty-two kilometres. We had done some stiff climbs, and very steep and rough descents. We will never forget that expedition!"[608]

On 12 August 1950, the Bests, Linda, and Pierre Hoet, an excellent travelling companion, left Louvain for the XVIIIth International Physiological Congress in Copenhagen, where they stayed at the Angleterre Hotel. There were many old friends from all parts of the world. Four of Charley's Toronto colleagues, Jim Campbell, Ed Sellers, Stan Hartroft, and Donnie Fraser, were delegates. A highlight was dinner at the Hagedorns' with the Houssays.

Driving through Sweden, the Bests stopped at Uppsala, where Linnaeus, the great eighteenth-century botanist, had taught. A special treat was a visit to Sturefors Slott, the seat of Count and Countess Bielke, friends of the Brusselmans. The Bests enjoyed their spirited hosts, and their castle, built in 1704, was full of treasures, fine pictures, and beautiful furniture. Henry was particularly impressed by the four-poster beds and the tapestries in his and Pierre's bedrooms in the oldest part of the castle.

In Stockholm, Best lectured on "Dietary and Hormonal Control of Fat Metabolism" at the Wenner-Gren Institute, where Dr. Jakob Möllerström was in charge. The next day, the visitors enjoyed lunch with Axel and Marguerite Wenner-Gren.[609] One evening, Henry, aged fifteen, went by boat with Anders Möllerström and his friends to their country home on an island. Henry was disappointed that his parents were not in favour of his staying the night. He was never sure if it was he or the Swedish girls whom they did not trust.

From Stockholm, they travelled north through the Dalecarlia region and around Lake Siljan. The farms and countryside were reminiscent of parts of Canada. On the way south, they visited "Mårbacka," near Sunne, the home of Selma Lagerlöf, author of *The Story of Gösta Berling* and winner of the 1909 Nobel Prize for Literature. In Oslo, Kjell Johansen and Jak Jervell, whom Henry had met at the Lawrences' in London, showed the Canadians the sights. The Viking ships, the Kon-Tiki raft, and Edvard Munch's murals at the university were especially memorable.

From Norway the travellers went to Holland. Conditions in Holland were much improved since they were last there three years earlier. In Amsterdam, a luncheon was given "In honour of Professor C.H. Best of Toronto on the occasion of his nomination as Honorary President of the Netherlands Diabetic Association, September 5, 1950." After lunch, Margaret, Charley, Linda, and Henry had a tour of the canals in a beautiful boat owned by a diabetic, who deposited them right at their hotel, the Amstel. In the evening, 1,200 diabetics and their families gathered to honour the co-discoverer of insulin. "We were given Dutch chocolates and they gave us pictures of tulips to show what the association was sending to Canada as a gift for us. It was a very charming idea and this last spring we have enjoyed our 'Diabetic Tulips.' We came away with our arms filled with flowers and books and candy. They handed us, too, the translation of a little poem written by 'the thankful mother of two diabetic girls in a little town in the Province of Groningen.'" Margaret and Charley had attended several such emotion-charged meetings since their first experiences in 1946 and 1947 in London and Brussels; Henry would never forget this, his first. Many people have had their lives saved by the administration of penicillin or heparin, or by a blood transfusion. But they are not reminded every day as are diabetics when they take insulin.

At the end of the year it was announced that the 1950 Nobel Prize in Physiology and Medicine went to Philip Hench, Edward Kendall of the United States, and Tadeusz Reichstein of Switzerland, for their work on the adrenal hormones. However, Dale soon started preparing a nomination for Best for 1953. "I have been to Stockholm and find that there may be a favourable chance to reinforce last year's proposal, if we act promptly."[610]

Best acknowledged Dale's letter. "It is very good of you to bother with the Stockholm matter. I have heard from Houssay that he saw you. He wrote in his charming way, 'Sir Henry and I remembered you very much together.' We are really struggling to write a comprehensive monograph[611] on the lipotropic agents and are making some progress."[612]

Sir Henry replied, "Thank you for your letter of January 4th and for the reprints duly received. I dealt with the matter immediately, and can now only hope that those concerned may be moved to the right decision. I do not know, in fact, what other claims they are likely to have before them this year."[613]

On 19 January 1951, Best sent Dale news about the new Best Institute; he was hoping that construction would begin in the spring and be finished in eighteen months. War threats (Korea) "make one think very seriously about the plans for boys of seventeen and nineteen." Then, "I can't thank you enough for all the trouble you are taking with regard to the Nobel matter." Despite the efforts that were being put towards his Nobel nomination by Dale and Houssay, Best thought the prize was a long shot. If he hadn't received it for the insulin work, he didn't think he was likely to get it at this stage. He added, "I will not permit my thoughts on these matters to interfere with my peace of mind or my research work."[614]

Charley's meetings at the DRB in Ottawa, with the Macy Foundation in New York, and the United States Public Health Service in Washington, DC, continued to absorb his energies. In early February, Charley and Margaret went to London, Ontario. Dr. and Mrs. Bert Collip gave a luncheon and entertained at their home after the University of Toronto Alumni Dinner where Best spoke to three hundred people on the "Health of the World." Best had always been very focussed on his research work, and in general the work he was involved in was a direct progression from the early work on insulin. Both choline and heparin were projects that had their genesis in diabetes research. Other projects, such as the blood plasma work, first arose as a perceived need to treat wartime injuries; now the blood donor program was required for the civilian population. As he travelled more and more and worked with various foundations, his interests and knowledge widened to include world-wide public health projects, malaria, yellow fever and malnutrition.

For personal, scientific, and political reasons, Professor Bernardo Houssay had urged Best for some time to visit Argentina. The IHD of the Rockefeller Foundation suggested an itinerary to five South American countries. Both Charles Best and H.B. van Wyck were studying Spanish with Linguaphone records. The van Wycks were off to Mexico. On 22 February 1951 Margaret wrote, "We are to leave tonight for New York on the first leg of our trip to South America." The last thing before they left,

Best was present at the unveiling of the bust of Fred Banting by Frances Loring at the Academy of Medicine.

South America

The IHD of the Rockefeller Foundation had arranged for the Bests (after a brief stopover in Panama) to visit Peru, Chile, Argentina, Uruguay, and Brazil. As usual the IHD was helpful in making contacts. In Panama Charley was interested in the Canal Zone, partly because of the malaria and yellow fever that had plagued those involved in the construction of the canal. The arrival in Lima was dramatic as the pilot circled for three hours before they could find a hole in the clouds. Dr. Alberto Hurtado, who had been minister of health under ousted President José Luis Bustamante, had invited them to Lima. In an interview Best, described as "still very youthful looking," stated that the purpose of his trip was to give talks and establish contact with medical representatives in Latin America to exchange ideas concerning current medical problems.[615] Dr. Hurtado, an expert on high altitude sickness, or *siroche*, took Margaret and Charley into the mountains to Rio Blanco on the highest paved road in the world at 11,500 feet. Margaret remarked on the fields of sunflowers, cotton and corn, and the gardens of potatoes, tomatoes, peppers, and lime trees.

On Charley's birthday, 27 February, they went to see Monsieur Emile Vaillancourt, the Canadian ambassador, and Murray Cook, the first secretary, at the Canadian embassy. Instead of honorary degrees, the custom in South America was to give honorary professorships. Best was made an honorary professor of the University of San Marcos, the oldest university in South America, which that year was celebrating its four-hundredth anniversary. He gave several lectures on diabetes and cirrhosis, "illustrated with perfectly coloured slides." Joking with doctors at a reception after the well-received talk Best suggested they should take choline with their pisco to prevent cirrhosis.[616]

The next stop was Santiago, Chile, where Best lectured on heparin and thrombosis, choline and cirrhosis, and insulin. Once more the "luminous colour slides" were remarked on. (Charley found he could not buy colour film in South America.) At the University of Chile Best received the second honorary professorship. Professor Samuel Middleton; Jaime and Rebeca Talesnik, who had both recently been working in Best's department; Dr.

John Janney of the Rockefeller Foundation; Guy Beaudry, the Canadian Chargé d'affaires; Dr. Francisco Mardones Otaiza, the minister of health; and Dr. Hernán Alessandri Rodriguez all entertained the visitors. Margaret had a copy of T.H. Goodspeed's *Plant Hunters in the Andes* to help her identify flowers, and Pál Kelemen's *Baroque and Rococo in Latin America* for architecture. They both enjoyed the School of Fine Arts run by Señor and Señora José Perotti, who also showed them the Museum of Fine Arts.

The Panagra flight across the Andes to Argentina was thrilling. Bernardo Houssay met the plane in Buenos Aires, as did Group Captain F.A. Sampson, military attaché at the Canadian embassy. Dr. Houssay had arranged a very busy program for them. On arrival in Buenos Aires Best said that he hoped that the first society of diabetics in South America would be formed in Argentina.[617] Houssay was out of favour with the Perón government, and a private institute had been established for him. His colleagues included Drs. Luis Leloir and Eduardo Braun Menéndez, and they and their families became very good friends of the Bests, meeting in various parts of the world. Everywhere there were signs, "Perón Cumple, Evita Dignifica" (Perón does what he promises, Evita dignifies everything). When Charley spoke on diabetes, choline, and heparin, as he did in Buenos Aires, Córdoba, Rosario, and La Plata, he left no doubt about his admiration and support for Houssay. On one occasion, when Best lectured to the doctors of the Policlinico San Martín in La Plata, Dr. Virgilio Foglia, a colleague of Houssay who had worked in Montréal, translated his talk into Spanish. While the Bests were in Argentina, Gainza Paz, editor of *La Prensa* and a brother of Señora Leloir, escaped to Uruguay when the government closed the newspaper.

A major event for the Bests was the opening of the Mercedes and Martin Ferreyra Institute in Córdoba, another private institution. The whole Ferreyra family entertained their Canadian visitors, both in Córdoba and at their *estancia* in the Sierras. Dr. Oscar Orías, the director of the new institute, had, like Dr. Houssay, lost his university post because he was not a Perón supporter. Later the Bests visited another estancia seventy miles from Buenos Aires, which belonged to Senor Carlos Duggan, a breeder of shorthorns and Herefords. He was a great fan of the humorous writings of Stephen Leacock. Margaret admired the work of Gomez Cornet, Alfredo Guido, Jorge Larco, Raoul Soldi, and other Argentinian artists in several galleries.

The Bests had received word that President Peron and his wife, Evita, wanted to meet them, which they ignored. They were then summoned to the presidential palace, at which point their friends advised them to leave the country. They had spent a month in the Argentine and enjoyed it immensely. On 4 April, Margaret and Charley went by flying boat across the La Plata River to Montevideo, Uruguay, for a stay of two days. Drs. Roberto Caldeyro and Diamantino Benati were their hosts. Best received his third honorary professorship from the University of Uruguay, where he gave two lectures. Best's wartime work on dried blood serum received much emphasis in newspaper articles. Margaret saw the art gallery where she remarked particularly on the work of Pedro Figari.

The next stop was São Paulo in Brazil. Charley lectured on the discovery of insulin while Margaret was taken to the art museum, where she was especially impressed by the work of Cândido Portinari. She noted the orchids, hibiscus, acacias, poinsettia, and parrot flowers that she saw in bloom. The Bests and Dr. and Mrs. Mauricio Rocha e Silva, senior physiologist at the Instituto Biológio, drove from São Paolo to Rio de Janeiro in a Buick with a driver supplied by Brazilian Traction Light and Power Company, or "The Light" as it was known, a Canadian firm chaired by Henry Borden. Most people had advised them not to travel by car, but Margaret commented, "The drive was fascinating — one of the most interesting things we did in South America." In the small town of Nossa Senhora Aparecida — Our Lady Who Appeared — they went into the church, and Margaret joined the procession to the high altar crowned by a tiny black Virgin. In Rio, Canadian Ambassador James Scott Macdonald and his wife, Ruth, looked after them. While Charley lectured at the Oswaldo Cruz Institute, directed by Dr. Carlos Chagas Filho, Ruth Macdonald took Margaret to buy amethysts and topazes, which she later had set in Toronto. The Macdonalds also drove their guests to Petrópolis, high up in the mountains, where the Rockefeller Foundation had a station headed by Dr. Ottis Causey. By 14 April, the Bests were back in Toronto after their fascinating and unforgettable trip to five South American countries.

Charles Best presented a number of medical graduates for their MD at the 1951 medical convocation at the University of Toronto. He wore his Queen's University hood. One version of the occasion is that he put the red and green poncho that he had bought in Chile over his gown, saying that everyone would think that it was a recently received hood from a South American university, but Margaret did not think that the University of Toronto's sense of humour would extend that far.

In mid-June, Henry received a phone message from a Mr. Bradford of Boston, who was urgently trying to reach Margaret. The family thought that their friend, Eddy Bradford, was calling with bad news about the Mahons. Henry had unsuccessfully tried his uncle's house in South Duxbury, and several of their friends. Soon a call came again from a Mr. Bradford, not their friend Eddy, but of the Little, Brown Publishing Company. "He had heard that I kept a diary, they are most interested, could he come up?" Margaret told him that she and Charley were planning to write a book some day of their experiences. "I said I thought it would chiefly be of interest for our children." She mentioned Maine. "Oh, good," he said, "that would be splendid — we can get together in Maine. Where will you be? ... I could come up from Boston." "The next morning Charley received a telegram from Houghton Mifflin Publishing Company about my diaries — most anxious to do something about it. Well! Well!" Apparently, Dr. Joslin had recently spoken glowingly of Margaret Best's diaries and the two companies were competing to publish them. Nothing ever came of it.

Sandy had not completed his full year, but his father believed that he should have a base of chemistry. He transferred to botany, something that he probably should have done earlier, and launched a new horticulture venture. The farm at Stewarttown was already blossoming with many rare lilies. He went to New York to a meeting of the North American Lily Society, taking some of Miss Isabella Preston's lily seedlings, and they won the Griffith Cup. Margaret was busy too. "I did all sorts of work with the lilies on the weekend, hybridizing like mad and really knowing very little about it. I have kept a record for Sandy of exactly what I did."

Sandy was back in Ottawa at the Central Experimental Farm. The day after his twentieth birthday on 7 July 1951 the rest of the family and Jessie Ridout left for Ottawa to see him. They then left Henry at the University of Western Ontario's Summer School in Trois-Pistoles on the lower St. Lawrence, and went on to Maine. While they were in Maine, a telegram came from Toronto to say that Henry had received three firsts and seven seconds on his senior matriculation at UCC. He had been accepted into the first-year pre-med program at Toronto.

By the end of the war, for reasons that are not entirely clear, Margaret did not want any contact with Charley's sister, Hilda, and her husband, Ralph Salter. The surveyor from Calais was completing plans to divide the Maine property and investigating ownership of the two islands in Schooner Cove, which were joined at low tide. The family called them

Sandy's Island and Henry's Island, but an old chart named them Hawser Island and Cat Island. When it was legally divided, Hilda Best Salter took the point, and Charley, the farm. It had been a difficult matter to settle, but a deed was signed, dated 18 June 1951.

Charley had a man at the Pleasant Point Passamaquoddy Reserve make signs saying "No Hunting or Shooting," but the neighbours reported that as soon as the Bests left all the pheasants were gone. The same thing happened with the clams. Charley often cut spruce or hackmatack trees in order to provide vistas from the house out to the water. Increasingly, he got Sandy and Henry to do this sticky and prickly work. Nasturtiums, sweet peas, and lupins continued to be the most successful flowers. On 3 September the boys had set the gill net in the cove for smelts and herring. There was a tinned whole chicken left in the larder, so Linda roasted that for Margaret and Charley's twenty-seventh anniversary dinner, and Sandy made a cranberry pie, served with whipped cream. Henry regularly made sauce from the yellow transparent and red astrican apples and consumed it with six Mack's cinnamon doughnuts.

When they arrived back in Toronto, "We were very disturbed to find that the estimates for Charley's new building were too high. Some of the members of the Board of Governors were in favour of cutting off the last building on the list and doing the Charles Herbert Best building just as it was planned. Others thought there were alternatives — getting more money or cutting off the fifth floor of the building. Charley is much involved now in plans with President Smith, Mac (MacFarlane, dean of medicine), Eric Haldenby (the architect), etc. I long to have it go properly, it is very important to us all. Charley wants that building and needs it badly." The first Sunday they were back, the MacFarlanes came over from their place at Terra Cotta so that Mac and Charley could discuss the situation.

Best had written to Prime Minister Louis St. Laurent about federal support for building the new institute. On the advice of Omond Solandt, he met with the Hon. Paul Martin, the minister of health, to whom the PM had referred the matter. Martin "told me that they could not give a capital grant towards our building but that he personally would approve an application for the complete furnishings of the building which might amount to from three hundred thousand to four hundred thousand dollars."[618] The Hon. Mackinnon Phillips, the minister of health of Ontario, backed the idea. On 31 October, Best spent an hour with Mr. St. Laurent. "He is an attractive and interesting-looking man with deep black eyes which make an interesting contrast with his white hair … I must say that I thoroughly enjoyed my meeting with Mr. St-Laurent and have a renewed and increased respect for him as a man."[619] Apparently, the discussion covered many topics, including approval of support for the new building. After this meeting Best went to see his old friend Don Cameron, the deputy minister of health, about the funding of the Canadian Diabetes Association. Cameron was very helpful to Best on many issues during the twenty years that he was deputy minister.

That autumn, Sandy began his formal studies in botany, his real love. Henry entered the sixth form at UCC — an experiment for boys who were perhaps too young for university. The idea was for him to take more maths and sciences, although he did not need them. Sandy had had trouble entering university at just sixteen; Henry was almost seventeen. He enjoyed his year, being a prefect, playing on the first soccer team again, singing the tenor lead for the third time in Gilbert and Sullivan's *HMS Pinafore,* and editing the *College Times* — the series of student publications. It would have been more useful for him to spend a year abroad learning another language and another culture.

The boys did not often visit other people's farms or cottages because there was so much to do at their own, but Henry occasionally went to the place near King owned by Ernie and Mary Rolph. Their son, Tony, his oldest friend, was very much involved with his father's dwarf apple orchard and Idaho potato fields. He was one of the few visitors to the Best farm who was not annoyed at the work involved. Margaret asked why each time Henry invited friends out for the weekend, it was always a different group — for some their first visit had warned them to expect too much work.

Dr. and Mrs. Eduardo Braun Menéndez, from Argentina, were in Toronto with their daughter, Finíta, who had had polio. They had been consulting polio experts in Boston. "It seemed so wonderful to have some of the Braun Menéndez family here with us. I really love Maté and Eduardo and Finíta. There was music after dinner — Eduardo, Finíta, Sandy and Henry." Their third son, Rafael, wrote to his parents in Toronto to say he missed them. "Now I know what it is to be an orphan." Eduardo gave a lecture at the university. Charley, Margaret, Eduardo, Maté, and Finíta went to Strawberry Hill, the name now used for the farm. Finíta had asked Sandy to send her one of his paintings, and she would send him one of her musical compositions. When they left Toronto, Eduardo said, "I don't keep a diary, Margaret, but I will keep it all in my heart." Maté added, "It is incredible to me that we have only known each other since March."

Princess Elizabeth and Prince Philip were in Toronto. The Bests went to the state dinner on Saturday, 13 October 1951 Charley was in his tails and silk hat and was wearing his miniatures, which Henry had updated with the American, Belgian, and Norwegian honours, all recently received. There were nine hundred people there. The Bests sat with Sir Ernest and Lady MacMillan. Margaret was interested that Princess Elizabeth removed her long gloves. "I have always disliked gloves turned back at the hands so I took a look to see what she did." Major Reade, an aide-de-camp to the lieutenant-governor, telephoned to say that Prince Philip had particularly wanted to meet "Professor Best." The university received the royal couple in the Great Hall of Hart House. "She was very pale and rather tired looking but very sweet. She had less assurance than one might expect but she has a great deal of dignity. Everyone speaks most highly of Philip also — his good looks and charm." Prince Philip spoke to the Board of Trade, referring to Charles Best by name. "'Indeed one does not have to look very hard for the achievements of Canadian scientists. At the University of Toronto, Professors Banting and Best developed insulin which means life to diabetics.' He went on to mention Dr. Wilder Penfield and the Neurological Institute in Montréal."

Laurie Chute was appointed head of the Sick Children's Hospital and Professor of Pediatrics at the University of Toronto. Replying to Best's note of congratulations Chute wrote, "If there is honour in my appointment much of it is owing to you. No one else inspired or challenged the imagination of a young student like yourself. Your continued interest set my feet in the path which has led to the present goal, for you made it possible for me to go to the 'Children's' in the first place and then to England. Moreover your interest and friendship did not begin and end in the classroom. Despite the very heavy demands on your energy you found time to take a very personal interest in the individual problems of all those with whom you were associated. … when Helen lay ill after Judy's birth it was your generous provision of heparin — which itself would not have been available but for your great vision and effort — that restored her to health. … Since the war your generous support, council and friendship have been one of my most prized possessions. These few words seem most inadequate to express my heartfelt gratitude and my esteem for your high scientific attainments but most of all for your warm and generous friendship."[620]

Best still had very heavy demands on his time and energy. In Indianapolis at an ADA banquet in January 1952, Margaret made a remark to one of the Lilly people that there were far too many meetings — morning, noon, and night — and he repeated it in a speech. Everyone laughed, but nothing changed. During a meeting that evening, Margaret experienced the novelty of television in the lounge of the Columbus Club. "They have television and it is frightful — almost all of the lights are turned out and strange figures were sitting there in great big easy chairs, watching the most stupid programs. I am sure that the programs will improve and there will be many fascinating things to see, but I fear that most of the programs are bunk." She preferred to read *Venture to the Interior*, a story of Nyasaland by Laurens van der Post. The next morning she noticed two ADA council members' wives "breakfasting demurely by themselves. It really was great fun with the men. They are the nicest group. I like every one of them."

The Bests had thought of sending a note to the Clowes and the Lillys before they left Toronto, but Charley decided not to. However, when they arrived in Indianapolis, they ran into G.H.A. Clowes by chance, and he "knew nothing of our coming," and was "quite upset." The next day Ruth Lilly said, "No one tells Eli anything any more since he had retired about what is happening in the company." Margaret decided that the next time they went to Indianapolis, she would write ahead to old friends. The Bests visited the Lillys' country home and their orchid business. At the Clowes' home, Golden Hill, on Spring Hollow Road, Margaret admired the new additions to the wonderful art collection since their last visit.

On they went to New York, where Charley attended a meeting on blood clotting and heparin at the Macy Foundation. Once again, Margaret complained about three sessions in one day. She went to see *Gigi*, Colette's book made into a play. "I enjoyed it immensely. Audrey Hepburn plays Gigi. The scene where the old aunt, a charming coquette, explains to Gigi about jewellery is very good. She brings out her own jewellery case and gives Gigi a lesson. 'What is this Gigi?' 'A diamond,' says Gigi. 'Yes,' replies the elegant old lady, 'and anything smaller than that I would call a chip.' 'And what is this one, Gigi?' asks the Aunt. 'A topaz,' replies Gigi. 'No, certainly not. Never mention topazes again — a woman who receives topazes is a failure. That is a jonquil diamond.'" Sitting in Schraft's the next day, Margaret noticed that a lady at the next table was wearing a lovely aquamarine ring with two rows of small round rubies. After her trip to South America, despite the opinion of Gigi's aunt, Margaret always paid attention to semi-precious stones.

Another evening, the Bests went to the Ziegfeld Theater to see Shaw's *Caesar and Cleopatra,* with Sir Laurence Olivier and Vivien Leigh. "It was magnificent. Charley thought that he had scarcely ever seen anything that he liked so well." Best probably liked theatre better than paintings. He also liked some music but the boys used to say that when he really liked a concert, he fell asleep.

On 9 February 1952, at a meeting of the Royal Canadian Institute (RCI) in Convocation Hall, John Dixon, the president, spoke about the death of King George VI three days earlier. "We stood and had a minute of silence and we sang, 'God Save the Queen.' It was quite moving." Mr. Dixon introduced the speaker. Charles Best's speech, "Medical Research and World Health" reflected his preoccupation with international health problems. "Charley always says that it is more difficult for him to give a non-scientific lecture. He made the subject fascinating and he seemed to talk so easily. He spoke mainly about South America." After Charley finished, "a little black-haired man rose and called out that he wanted to ask some questions about the operations on animals. A woman was posted down below who called up to her pal, 'We want to hear him.' They were quite belligerent. Charley arose again and said that he had never heard a mother of a diabetic child object to the use of a few rats or a dog. He spoke in a kindly way, not at all aggressive. There was tremendous applause from the audience but the outcries were still vocal."

The Bests with Mary and Don Fraser went to Hart House for a university evening. Professor Robert Finch of the French Department at University College played the piano, and Professor Ned Pratt of the English Department at Victoria College read from his unpublished poem on the building of the Canadian Pacific Railway. "There were so many Scotch names and he read the part about the effect of oatmeal on the Scotch." Later, however, Helen Ignatieff found her husband, Nicholas, warden of Hart House, lying unconscious beside their car, apparently having tried to change a tire. The fire department came, and three doctors — Best, Fraser, and MacFarlane — tried to help. Charley said that "he never got a pulse at all." Helen Ignatieff's sister Shelagh, and her husband, Nicholas "Niki" Goldschmidt, soon arrived. "It was really ghastly." Warden Ignatieff's sudden death was an enormous shock to his family and friends. The funeral took place in the Great Hall of Hart House. Henry had asked the warden to write a foreword for the final issue of the UCC *College Times* for 1952, which he had done. A few weeks later, the Bests went to see Menotti's *The Old Maid and the Thief,* put on by the Opera School, with Niki Goldschmidt conducting.

In April, Charley headed to New York with Dr. Hank MacIntosh, chair of physiology at McGill University. MacIntosh, a Cape Bretoner who had studied with Dale in London, was chairman of the organizing committee for the 1953 congress of physiology in Montreal. Charley was to be its president. Margaret could not go as she was very ill with pneumonia, and Ray Farquharson gave her large doses of penicillin. But, by 25 April 1952, she had recovered enough to see the wrecking operations at the site of the new Charles H. Best Institute at Queen's Park Crescent and College Street. "Last week I saw the steam shovel on the very first day that it operated. It has taken a very long time for things to get moving but at last we can be confident that we will really have our building. No honour in the world could give Charley as much pleasure as having that building." A high blue fence went up with a large sign reading, "Charles H. Best Institute, University of Toronto, Mathers and Haldenby, Architects, Hardy Builders." When the building was complete, the sign became a divider in the basement of the Best's house at 105 Woodlawn Avenue West, and much later it was mounted on the back wall of the institute's lecture hall.

One of the most able and interesting people to come to work at the lab was Dr. Aron Rappaport. He and his psychiatrist wife, Rosa, had come through very difficult times in Europe. Both established excellent reputations in Toronto. They were at the Bests for dinner, and when Charley drove them home, he bought a copy of the next morning's *Globe and Mail,* which had Sandy's final results for his BA in botany — a creditable second-class standing. He had never had a course in either botany or biochemistry before but had extensive knowledge of botany. Dr. Klaus Rothfels of the Botany Department told him that he got firsts in his three botany courses. The family wanted to give him a watch as a graduation present, but he said, "No, a watch is such a tyrant." He refused to go to his own ceremony, saying that he would do so when he got his PhD.

Around the World

Margaret and Charley were finishing their shots for the longest trip that they would ever take, travelling east around the world. The baggage allowance had been reduced to sixty-six pounds, which made it very difficult to pack.

On 26 June 1952, Charley and Margaret Best left Toronto for a three-and-a-half month trip to Australia and New Zealand via Britain, Holland, Belgium, Italy, Lebanon, Pakistan, Ceylon, and Singapore. Two Australian scientists, Dr. Victor Coppleson of Sydney and Dr. Ewen Downie of Melbourne, who had both known Best in Canada, were instrumental in inviting them to Australia. They would not be back until mid-October, and Don Clarke, Reg Haist, Frank Monkhouse, and Ed Sellers were at Malton Airport to see them off; these four senior people from Charley's two departments made it possible for him to travel so much. Campbell Cowan looked after the technical side with expertise and judgment. Best was known for preparing people and then leaving them free to proceed on their own.

Perhaps the most unusual member of this team of researchers and administrators was Linda Mahon, Margaret's sister, who, since 1927, had never worked for anyone but her brother-in-law. She was lively, efficient, knew what "Dr. Best" would want done in any given situation, and Linda was well liked and respected. She was also in charge of the home when her sister was away. On her own, she was the life of the party. With Margaret, she was always the "little sister." Margaret was the "queen bee" at home and socially. Linda was the "queen bee" at the university. Amazingly, with the occasional blip, the system worked very well. Amateur psychologists have insisted that Linda was in love with Charley. She was certainly devoted to him, but the situation was never a *ménage à trois*. For Sandy and Henry, "Lully" was a cross between a second mother and a big sister.

In London for only a few days, the Bests saw old friends such as the Dales, the Haydons, the Lawrences, and the Mellanbys. Margaret loved the exhibition of Leonardo da Vinci at Burlington House, and went also to the Tate Gallery and the Victoria and Albert Museum. The evening they arrived, they went to see Peggy Ashcroft in Terence Rattigan's *Deep Blue Sea* — "wonderful acting and a fairly absorbing play, certainly not a jolly one." Margaret went to a matinée of N.C. Hunter's *Waters of the Moon* with Edith Evans, Wendy Hiller, and Sybil Thorndike. "It was very fine acting, really not much of a play. Edith Evans is a whole cast in herself." They both saw Katharine Hepburn in Shaw's *The Millionairess* and Flora Robson in *The Innocents*, a play made from Henry James's *The Turn of the Screw*.

Dr. Fritz Gerritzen and representatives of the Dutch Diabetic Association met them in Amsterdam and drove them to Noordwijk and a room looking out over the North Sea. Dr. Joslin, from Boston, Joseph and Marguerite Hoet, and Charles and Elisabeth Vuylsteke from Belgium joined them for dinner. The next day at Leiden, the university senate received the visitors. Joslin spoke briefly. Charley gave a speech, "Insulin and the Patient," and then Robin Lawrence spoke, with his usual erudition and humour. Willem and Cornelia Dutilh, whom the Bests had befriended on their trip to Europe in 1950, took them to dinner in Rotterdam with their diabetic son, Jan, twenty-four.

Charles Best had decided that he was unable for financial reasons to attend a meeting in June 1949, where "some seventy-five patients and doctors from eleven different countries gathered in Brussels for the first international symposium on diabetes."[621] Subsequently, the International Diabetes Federation was founded at a meeting in Amsterdam in September 1950, with Robin Lawrence as its founding president and Fritz Gerritzen of Leiden as the first secretary. In Leiden in July 1952 Charley spoke to the first meeting of the International Diabetes Federation (IDF) and Jim Campbell and the Wrenshalls represented the lab in Toronto.

Medical students in Leiden who had helped with the congress were invited to a dinner in a small restaurant. By the time the delegates arrived, all the seats inside were taken. Margaret wrote:

> The boys carried tables out under the trees in the middle of the square. We had soup, veal cutlets, vegetables, salad, red wine — many toasts, much singing. Before dinner, Charley took a ride about the square on the back of a little boy's bicycle. A policeman in uniform came, then came the chief of police in a brown suit and smoking a pipe. He drank a glass of wine. Then a photographer came from the local paper. There had never been a dinner party in the local square before. It was quite a party. Eventually we moved into the restaurant for coffee — more singing — Charley led *Alouette* very capably. Robin sang a Highland song and we all joined in the chorus by holding our noses in imitation of bagpipe music. We signed our names on the labels of the wine bottles which the students carried away. When the taxi came to bring Dick and Wilva Connelly and Charley and me back here, the students, boys and girls, formed an archway, holding up the bottles for us to go under.

Margaret and Charley drove with the Hoets to Brussels to have lunch with Queen Mother Elisabeth, who was now a mild diabetic, not on insulin. "The Queen was very welcoming — 75 years old — all in grey or perhaps light beige — two carnations pinned to her dress by a dragonfly pin of diamonds and emeralds — ropes of pearls. She asked at once for Sandy. She said, 'that beautiful boy.' (Since we last saw her, her grandson had become King. They have had a troubled time in Belgium.) When lunch was ready, she put out her hand to me and I walked with her into the dining room. Charley sat on her right hand, Hugh Long[622] on her left."

After lunch, "Queen Elisabeth rose — put out her hand to me again and I walked out of the dining room with her. The French doors were open on to a terrace and we went out there for coffee. Frank Young took a little snuff and gave the Queen some — nobody sneezed. Then Charley got his camera and the photography began. Charley, Hugh and the Queen all snapping pictures."

On 20 July 1952, the Bests flew by Constellation to Rome, on to Beirut and then Karachi, where Kenneth Kirkwood, the very experienced Canadian high commissioner, met them. The travellers were interested to know that he had co-authored the book *Turkey*[623] with Arnold Toynbee. Kirkwood had lived and taught there.

The next short stop was Colombo, Ceylon, where Best's old friend W.A.E. Karunaratne, professor of pathology, and his wife, Benedicta, were their hosts. Charley gave a lecture at the medical school, after Professor Karunaratne introduced him: "Your name is familiar to all of us. Your masterly work, *The Physiological Basis of Medical Practice,* is the invaluable *vade mecum* of every medical man, be he student, practitioner or professor. The entire world honours you today as one of the leading medical men of the age."[624] "The lecture hall was packed to over-flowing. The students got there one and a half hours ahead of time." It was a very long but fascinating day for the Bests visiting the great botanical gardens at Peradenyia and the four-hundred-year-old Temple of the Tooth at Kandy. Before they left, "Dr. K." presented Margaret with a lovely, large topaz which, unlike Gigi's aunt, she was thrilled to receive.

In Singapore, they stayed at Raffles Hotel. Don Armstrong, Canadian trade commissioner, and Malcolm Macdonald, British commissioner general for Southeast Asia, invited the Bests for dinner. Dr. C.J. Poh, who had been in the infamous Japanese Changi prison camp with Charley's colleague Dr. Jacob Markowitz of Toronto, took Margaret and Charley to the site of their ordeal.

Their next destination on 26 July 1952 was Darwin, North Australia, where the district medical officer said that he had heard Dr. Best speak in Johannesburg in 1949 and that as a student he had used Best and Taylor's textbook. In Brisbane, the professor of medicine at the University of Queensland, Alex Murphy, and his wife were their hosts, and Charley lectured several times at the medical school. Dr. and Mrs. J.V. Hynes of the physiology department took the Bests on a drive to Mount D'Aguilar, and Margaret had a wonderful time with her copy of Thistle Harris's *Wild Flowers of Australia*, identifying gerbera, billardiera, waratah, and many more plants. The book is full of her notations. They ate custard apples for the first time — "an amazing flavour, very good." There were articles in several newspapers about Margaret's interest in wild flowers and art. Margaret was also interested in Australian literature and bought books by Clyde Fenton, Elisabeth George, and Henry Handel Richardson. University of Toronto professor Claude Bissell was one of the first to do comparative studies on Australian and Canadian literature, but unfortunately, his important article, "A Common Ancestry: Literature in Australia and Canada," did not come out until later.[625]

In Melbourne Ewen Downie was in charge of the Bests' busy schedule. Downie was dean of the Clinical School of the Royal Prince Alfred Hospital in Melbourne. During the Bests' visit to Australia he hoped he would be able to repay the many kindnesses Charley had shown him on his frequent visits to Canada in 1944 when he was senior medical officer at the Australian Military Mission in Washington, DC.[626] Charley gave several lectures on diabetes, heparin, and choline. Dr. S. W. Cooper, president of the Resident Medical Officers' Club, wrote thanking Charley for his visit. "In Australia we tend to become rather insular in outlook and it is very refreshing to hear the views of overseas visitors. Also, as you may have guessed from the questions put to you after dinner, carbohydrate metabolism is still largely a mystery and your answers helped clear up a number of contentious points."[627] The Bests also saw Sir Macfarlane Burnet, an expert on antibodies and the director of the Hall Institute for Medical Research for many years, and Lady Burnet, whom they had known for some time and who had been in Toronto the previous fall. Margaret and Charley's first real contact with Australian art was at the Melbourne Gallery; particularly the works of William Dobell and Russell Drysdale fascinated them. Later in Sydney, after much thought, the Bests bought a Kenneth Macqueen watercolour landscape with eucalyptus trees, and a very striking and colourful Margaret Preston monotype of a waratah, or "Giant Lily."

The Bests were in Sydney several times over a month where Victor and Enid Coppleson were their hosts. "Cop" had planned much of their Australian trip when he was in Toronto not long before. He was senior surgeon at St. Vincent's Hospital and an orchid grower. Best was interviewed by Ronald McKie of the Sydney *Daily Telegraph* who described him: "Professor Best is a man of great personal charm and good looks. He has an easy informal manner, a soft musical voice, a pink unlined face, amusing blue eyes that must have got him into a lot of trouble in his younger days, and he looks 10 years younger than his 53 years."[628] Best recorded a talk for the Australian Broadcasting Commission entitled "What is most needed in medicine?" He emphasized the importance of the family doctor with a good patient-doctor relationship. But he added: "In Canada, perhaps it's the same here, the public health nurse and the Victorian Order of Nurses make great contributions and undoubtedly help to compensate for the absence of the family doctor ... I wish I knew a great deal more about the Flying Doctor service here in Australia but I hope to learn more about it. ... We should wish to retain the courage and rapidly growing determination of educated people to evolve a sound and durable system which brings good medical care within the reach of all members of the community."[629]

In Sydney, as everywhere, many people were most hospitable and Margaret and Charley were constantly entertained. Dr. Kempson Maddox and his family took the Bests on a "chop picnic." The visitors went to see Dr. David Monk-Adams, a brilliant young man and a severe diabetic who had worked from 1948–50 in Best's lab. Charley lectured to various groups, including the Sydney Hospitallers' Club, where he spoke on "Medical Research in Canada."

Wherever he went in the world Best encouraged the formation of lay diabetic associations and Australia was no exception. The secretary of the Diabetic Association of Australia, Ruby W. Board wrote to Charley: "You are a wizard! Dr. Ingram's letter today promising, at your request, all support for the Diabetic Assoc. was the best news I could have had. Professional opposition is a serious matter. But it is of course your visit which will give the stimulus to the movement that was so much needed. On all sides I have heard appreciation for your lectures."[630]

Two senior interns from the Royal Prince Alfred Hospital, Drs. Richards and Burns, drove the Bests to Canberra, where they stayed at the official residence with Canadian High Commissioner C. Fraser Elliott. Fraser, a distinguished Canadian public servant, and Marjorie Elliott were old friends. On a tour of the capital, the Bests were particularly impressed with the unfinished War Memorial especially commemorating the Gallipoli campaign in the First War.

In Melbourne Charley received an honorary degree and spoke at the Australian Medical Congress. Margaret mentioned the hospitality of Judge Douglas Menzies, a first cousin of the prime minister, and his wife, Helen, whom they had met on the flight to Australia. They enjoyed a drink called "Brandy Crusta" before meals — brandy with maraschino, curaçao, cherry brandy, and lemon juice with the top of the glass frosted with sugar.

On they went to Hobart, Tasmania, where Dr. and Mrs. Bruce Hamilton were their hosts, and to Launceston, where Best gave two lectures. In Adelaide, Brigadier Sir Stanton Hicks, a distinguished physiologist, and Lady Hicks, were their hosts. He had written to Charley on 10 July, "I will post to you a brief survey of the local situation to enable you to prepare those few well-chosen words which make an isolated community feel justified in its own self-esteem!"[631] Charley gave two lectures and they both went to see the Australian pictures at the art gallery. Dr. Hugh Le Messurier was also an artist and gave the Bests a striking portrait of "Menjana," an old chief of the Ngalia tribe, located west and north of Alice Springs.

On 13 September 1952, the Bests flew to Perth, West Australia. Dr. Bruce Hunt, their host and senior physician at the Royal Perth Hospital, was on the plane, as well as Dr. Francis Avery Jones of the Central Middlesex Hospital in London and Surgeon Rear Admiral Sir Gordon Gordon-Taylor, a past president of the Royal Society of Medicine. Charley lectured three times at the university in Perth and to an audience of lay diabetics. On their arrival there the Bests had sent a telegram to Omond Solandt, Canadian Director General of Defence Research, who, with other experts, had just arrived at the Woomera Rocket Range in South Australia to witness atomic tests.

One of the highlights of the whole trip to Australia was travelling 120 miles north of Perth, to Cranmore Park, a sheep station belonging to the Edward Lefroy family. A son, Dr. Dick Lefroy, drove the Bests and Dr. Avery Jones, and everyone helped Margaret gather, identify, and press flowers, including several kinds of orchid, mountain primrose, and "most lovely of all, the blue leschenaultia."[632] That evening, the hosts helped to identify wildflowers, and the next day, the visitors had a tour of the station. Dr. Hunt took the Bests to Fremantle, the port of Perth, to see the wool warehouses and, to Charley's delight, to the trotting races. When they left Bruce Hunt wrote to thank them for coming, "It is a very pleasant thing when people one has revered from afar live up to the mental image — and have nice low tastes like beer and trotting into the bargain. ... Stay as young as you both are now and remember occasionally the wildflowers and Cranmore and some of the people who like you and want to see you again."[633]

Back in Melbourne Margaret came down with influenza and had a fever of 102 Fahrenheit, so their departure for Christchurch, New Zealand, was delayed from 25 to 29 September and the planned schedule there shortened. However, Charley did give two lectures in Auckland, and they both visited its art gallery.

On 7 October 1952, the Bests flew to Fiji and then on to Honolulu. Margaret thought, "Hawaii was absolutely perfect." There were not supposed to be any lectures in Hawaii, but, as so often happened, Best was persuaded to talk to a medical group. Pearl Harbor was a "must" visit. Gladys Muttart of Edmonton, a severe diabetic very active in the Canadian Diabetes Association, owned a florist business in Honolulu, and the manager, Frank Lang, brought ten leis to the airport and danced attention on the visitors. On the beach Margaret and Charley ran into Omond Solandt, who was also returning from Australia. Frank Lang not only packed sprays of orchids ordered by Margaret and Charley for Omond to take back to his wife, Elizabeth, in Canada, but also drove him to the airport. Flying via San Francisco, Margaret and Charley arrived in Toronto on 15 October 1952. It had been a wonderful trip. Charley had given sixty lectures in Australia, and they both had memorable experiences. Charley's five major overseas lecture tours in as many years, and his connection with the Rockefeller and Nuffield Foundations, had increased his awareness, knowledge, and dedication to the cause of world health.

As so often happened after a strenuous trip, Margaret had a relapse of her Australian 'flu and could not be present on 7 November for the laying of the cornerstone of the Charles H. Best Institute — "our building." Ed Sellers recorded the ceremony, so that Margaret could hear the speeches of President Smith, Board Chairman Colonel Eric Phillips, and Charley.

Chapter Seven

Joys and Sorrows, 1953–1964

In September 1953 the XIXth International Physiological Congress was to be held for the first time in Canada in Montréal. As so many distinguished physiologists from around the world would be in the country at that time it was decided that the opening of the Charles H. Best Institute would follow immediately after the congress. Charley wrote to Sir Henry Dale about working with a former student of Dale's, Hank MacIntosh, on preparations for the congress. "It is a great joy to work with Hank MacIntosh and he is a wonderful addition to our Canadian group. Addition is not quite the right word as he is a Canadian product as you well know. Margaret and I stayed over night with Mary and Hank on our way to Quebec city where I was getting an honorary degree from Laval. We had a wonderful time with all the MacIntosh family."[634]

The winter and spring of 1953 saw the Bests frequently away from Toronto. With all his departmental work, arrangements for the congress and construction of the Institute, Best probably accepted more invitations to speak than he should have, but many came from former colleagues and students and were thus difficult to refuse. He also was anxious to keep abreast of new scientific work so that he could share the knowledge with his researchers in Toronto. He believed strongly in keeping in contact with people of similar interests.

On 12 February they went to New York for two days of meetings with the New York Academy of Sciences. At the beginning of April Best travelled to Iowa City, lecturing in Chicago on the way. Later he served for a week as physician-in-chief at the Atlantic City Hospital, meeting doctors and students and giving a lecture each day. At the end of May, he went to New York for the meetings of the American Diabetes Association, where he presented Banting medals to Walter Campbell and Almon Fletcher, the two senior clinicians involved in the early administration of insulin at the Toronto General Hospital.

Cleeve Horne was painting Best's portrait in his magnificent scarlet and gold DSc robes from the University of London for the foyer of the new institute. Laurie Chute, Donnie Fraser, Reg Haist, and Ed Sellers made up the committee that chose the artist. When Henry and Lydia Mahon were in town from Boston, they went to the studio to have a look at the unfinished canvas. "Charley has had many sittings for his portrait, all in the evening. I have gone there too. It is quite thrilling, I think. Cleeve Horne is a clever fellow. It is just about finished."[635]

One evening the Bests went to the Royal Conservatory of Music of Toronto to a concert given by Madame Irene Jessner, who had come to Toronto with Edward Johnson when he had retired as general manager of the Metropolitan Opera in New York. Typically, Charles Best had decided that if Henry's voice was any good at all he should have the best of instruction. Arnold Walter, principal of the conservatory, and Nicholas Goldschmidt, head of the Opera School, had suggested Jessner as a teacher. Despite his heavy course load at the University of Toronto, once a week, Henry rushed back to Hart House to change out of his soccer togs and dash down to the conservatory annex on College Street. The previous student would still be there — Henry liked the little, dark, vivacious girl and thought her voice quite nice. When she emerged they would greet each other — "Hello Henry," "Hello Teresa." She was Teresa Stratas, who launched her dazzling career at New York's Metropolitan Opera in 1959. That was as close as Henry Best would ever get to the Met.

Before the university results were out, Charley asked Henry how he thought he had done in his first pre-med year. Henry had participated in all sorts of activities so said that he thought that he probably had not done too well. Charley went to the meeting of the faculty council where the results would be released, slipped in at the back of the room, took a look at the list, and quickly left. Bob Janes, professor of surgery, went after him and asked why he was leaving. CHB said, "Henry's name is not on the list." "Where did you look?" asked Janes. "From the middle down." "Well, then, come back and start from the top." To his father's pleasure, Henry got first-class honours and stood tenth out of 123 in his year.

On 3 May 1953, the family went to the farm and picked twenty dozen daffodils to sell and to give away. There were many hyacinths and rarer items such as "heavenly blue anemones," primroses, and several new varieties of tulips planted by Sandy. Later that spring three hundred quarts of strawberries were picked and sold. Sandy and Henry went frequently to the farm, and Sandy wanted to visit other bulb growers or look for unusual species, so their father bought them a second-hand Prefect — a British Ford.

Henry had wanted a dog for a long time and decided on a golden retriever. One Sunday he was in King, north of Toronto, at the farm of his friend Tony Rolph, and at the dinner table Mr. Rolph said that they had just received a yellow lab pup as a stud fee. As they already had several dogs, did anyone know of a good home? Henry went home with the pup. In the discussion about a name, his mother suggested "Luke" from *Dr. Luke of the Labrador,* by Norman Duncan, and that was it.

On 3 July 1953, Margaret and Charley were off for the east coast, taking Linda's poodle, Dochet, with them. "Dochet had quite a good day, but it is rather like travelling with a baby." He took exception to a bulldog and tried to jump out of the car to challenge a spaniel. In Montréal, Charley had a meeting with Hank MacIntosh about the upcoming congress; they sat on the lawn at McGill University while the dog was moored to a tree. Harry Sellers, Ed's father, had arranged for the Bests to have a suite at the Ritz during the congress, and they went and looked at it.

Many years earlier, Larry Irving, a colleague in Toronto and a graduate of Bowdoin College in Brunswick, Maine, had given Margaret and Charley a volume of poems by Robert P. Tristram Coffin, professor of English there. In Pennelville, Maine, George and Kitty Anderson introduced the Bests to the poet. Charley's boyhood friend Ronald Bridges had told him that "The Country Doctor" was inspired by tales that he himself had told Coffin about Charley's father. Margaret wrote: "Coffin looks as I expected he would look — big mustache with waxed or pointed tips, blue, blue eyes, a gentle rather roguish air — sometimes puts his hand over his mouth when he laughs (after he makes an audacious remark) as Dr. Best used to do. After dinner he recited his poetry for us. He started, 'This one I finished at five o'clock this afternoon.' Then he recited and said, 'Is it good Kitty? I never know for at least a year.' He recited 'The Country Doctor,' 'The Lullaby,' and several others, no gestures, rather a low, deep and somewhat sad voice, really very impressive and very moving."

While Margaret and Charley were in Maine, the Saturday *Globe and Mail* reported that Sandy had taken the North American Lily Show in Hamilton by storm. As well, there had been a lunch for forty people at the farm. Henry worked day and night, as did Linda and Jessie Ridout. Sandy had stems that ordinarily bloomed over an extended period all out on the same weekend, using the greenhouses at the University of Guelph and the coolers at Calvert's Flower Company in Brampton. At the last minute, Sandy ordered the exhausted Henry to weed an area that displeased him. Henry refused, and the two boys rolled on the ground while their almost always impartial Aunt Linda shouted, "Hit him again, Henry!" The show established Sandy's reputation in the field. Of all the silver cups and trays available, there was only one that he did not win.

Sandy wrote to his parents about his work in the federal election campaign in Halton County. Miss Sybil Bennett, a lawyer and niece of R.B. Bennett, was Conservative candidate for the seat, which had been Liberal for seventeen years. Her campaign chairman had had a serious heart attack after the vote was called. Bennett, sensing that she was not doing well, opted for a totally new approach, with a younger person. Sandy Best was twenty-two and brought in new ideas and boundless energy. Miss Bennett was elected to Parliament for Halton County. Margaret and Charley were puzzled. "I never expected to have a politically-minded child." It is hard to say what politics Charles or Margaret Best had. Like many Ontarians, the Bests usually voted Liberal federally and Conservative provincially. Politics as such did not much interest them.

On 28 August, Charley, Margaret, Henry, and Jessie Ridout drove from Toronto to Montréal. Delegates for the XIXth International Physiological Congress were arriving from all over the world. The opening ceremonies took place in McGill's Currie Gymnasium. Margaret sat in the front row between Lady Dale and Mrs. Bert Collip. The heat was excessive. Bert Collip, president of the Canadian Physiological Society, spoke entirely in French. Charles Best used several languages, to the surprise of those who knew him: English, French (after coaching from Joseph Hoet and from Henry), German, Spanish, and Mohawk, the last as the result of a very short coaching session by Professor Thomas McIlwraith. Margaret recognized the last word of Charley's Indian section as "Wickachee," the name of a favourite restaurant in Calais, Maine. In Gaelic, he thanked Professor Hank MacIntosh, a fluent Gaelic speaker from Cape Breton Island, for his wonderful work chairing the organizing committee.

"In his speech Charley stressed the point that he wished the young people present to get a lot out of the congress. If later they could remember that they had talked to the older and more experienced people and had got to know some of them, it would be helpful. If they could talk a little about their scientific problems with some of the specialists in their lines, it would be a worthwhile congress."[636]

"Mayor Camilien Houde spoke. Between our luncheon party and the opening ceremonies, Charley had gone to his office along with about twenty specially chosen members and had a meeting with the mayor. In his speech at the opening, Houde was telling about the multinational backgrounds of Montréalers, so many French, so many English and so on, down to quite small numbers. One group was three hundred. He said, 'I must mention them all, they are all important. We will have an election soon and they all have votes.'"

At the supper offered by the city of Montréal at the Chalet on Mont-Royal, Margaret wore a corsage made from Sandy's lilies and recorded that Houde said they were to sit down on the steps to eat supper but then he said, "Oh, you must not in your good clothes." "We said it was all right and he said something about 'les perrons.' He went off and came back with a newspaper and he spread it out on the steps. 'You must not sit on my "perron" without something clean to sit on.' As he opened it out, I said, 'I don't want to sit on your picture or my husband's.' 'Oh, you never miss a thing, Mrs. Best,' he said. The Mayor had been made an Indian chief. I asked him what his name is. He says he cannot remember what it is in Indian, but in English it is 'Saviour of Montréal.' He said apologetically, 'They are very, very complimentary.'"

Houde "personally greeted every member of the Congress and especially, every wife." At the garden party Margaret noted that "the water ran out though the whiskey did not." Most of the foreign delegates were "invited to the houses of the local participants, a measure of hospitality long remembered by guests." On an outing to Mont St-Hilaire, "the Swiss and German physiologists ... surprised the locals by scaling the rocky face instead of ambling up the prescribed path winding to the top."[637]

At a special McGill convocation in Molson Stadium, Sir Henry Dale, Dr. Walter Rudolf Hess of Zurich, and Dr. Einar Lundsgaard of Copenhagen, all previous congress presidents, received honorary degrees. Sir Henry spoke for all three. At the congress's closing ceremony on 4 September at the Université de Montréal, Professor Douglas Adrian of Trinity College, Cambridge, president of the Royal Society, received an honorary degree and announced the election of Best as president of the new International Union of Physiological Sciences, to represent the physiological societies from around the world. Dr. Houssay thanked the local organizers for their efforts. Paul-Emile Cardinal Léger officiated at the convocation with Mgr. Olivier Maurault, the *recteur magnificus*. Margaret tried a joke in

French by introducing Henry, 6'3" tall, to the rector saying, "C'est mon petit fils." The rector laughed and replied, "He is not your grandchild."

Following the congress, at the Alpine Inn at Sainte-Marguerite in the Laurentians north of Montréal, a small gathering discussed the future of physiology. Among the participants were Douglas Adrian, Gøran Liljestrand of Stockholm, Rudolph Peters of Oxford, and Hans Hausler of Graz, Austria, whose son, Hans, worked with CHB.

Shortly after the meetings in Montreal, on 15 September 1953, the Charles H. Best Institute of the University of Toronto was officially opened. The main part of the building cost $2.5 million, a large part of which Best had raised himself; the remainder from the Varsity Appeal, the federal and provincial governments, foundations, companies, and individuals in Canada, Britain, and the United States. Robin Lawrence brought from London a DSc gown, hood, and hat as a gift to replace what had been stolen from Charley in Halifax. Many of the guests came directly from the physiology conference in Montreal: the Adrians, Bronks, Dales, Hoets, Joslins, Houssays, Penfields, Peters, and Whitbys. When speaking at a dinner the evening before the official opening, Joseph Hoet said, "'Before discovering insulin, Charley Best discovered Margaret.' When he rose to speak, Sir Henry Dale said, 'That was very good. I wish I had thought of that.'" At a meeting of the CDA later that evening, "Robin was most amusing in his speech, and Joseph was impassioned."

On the day of the opening, Charley and Margaret went to the luncheon given by president Sidney Smith in the Music Room at Hart House for the honorary graduands. "There were about sixty-five people at the luncheon, very official and extremely pleasant." Ray Farquharson introduced the distinguished guests who were to become honorary graduates, and Det Bronk responded. "Ray was splendid. Det made a very serious and wonderful speech. I was quite touched that he included my name. He stood at the end of the table where the president had sat and he turned toward me at one point and spoke of his 'long friendship and warmest feeling for Margaret Best.'" Particularly since 1947 Margaret had accompanied Charley on most of his trips and became endeared to his friends and colleagues.

Honorary degrees went to Detlev Bronk, Bernardo Houssay, Elliott Joslin, Wilder Penfield, and Lionel Whitby. "The whole affair was wonderful — the colourful procession. The president acted as chancellor, Vincent Massey has retired as chancellor, and Dr. Samuel Beatty has not yet been installed. Mac (Dean MacFarlane) presented the men for honorary degrees.

He was very good. Sir Lionel Whitby made the address. Then Sir Henry made his speech, quite long, about the new building, the history of physiology and medical research in Toronto and Charley's scientific history."

Then all the men in their colourful robes marched over to the new building. Lady Dale and Margaret Best were the only women on the platform. Charley's uncle, Bishop Hallam, gave the prayer of dedication. Sir Henry opened the door with a golden key. Dean MacFarlane presented Cleeve Horne's portrait to the subject. From behind the scenes, Reg Haist and Henry Best led the audience in singing "God Save the Queen." "Well, it was all quite perfect!" The institute had taken a long time to build, and it was certainly far from finished. The effort of collecting nearly half of the required funds had exhausted Best, but it was a momentous day.

That evening, "the Great Hall of Hart House was filled." The Hon. Paul Martin, federal minister of health, and his deputy minister, Dr. Donald Cameron (who had both helped fund the furnishing of the building) were among the guests, as also were Walter Campbell, G.H.A. Clowes, Bert Collip, Almon Fletcher, and Eli Lilly. Margaret described the occasion: "A few of us met first in one room and finally walked in. The tables were all full, everyone with a place card and a special place to sit. We sat at the High Table ... I have never been at a great large party that seemed more a friendly and intimate occasion. Over and over again, people have remarked to me since that evening: 'What a perfect party!' Several people spoke and President Smith was the host. Charley made a beautiful speech, introducing each of the special honoured guests and mentioning a good many others too. He said some very touching things about me, that I was 'the centre and inspiration of everything.'"

Robin Lawrence brought a gift from the IDF — "a beautiful silver-topped pad for Charley's desk. Inside the lovely plain sheets of silver it says, 'Thank you for our lives.' It was made in Holland." Joseph Hoet gave Charley a reprint of an article by Louis Pasteur entitled "Le Budget de la science," published in Paris in 1868. It was beautifully bound in tooled leather with a representation of the Hôtel de Ville de Louvain, and bore the inscription, "to Charles Herbert Best." The text could have been written by a scientist of our own day. Pasteur concluded with a quote from a visitor to his research lab in Paris: "I honoured your efforts as I recognized their importance. Now that I know the resources at your disposal, I admire them." These words could have been written about the meagre resources available to Banting and Best at the time of the discovery of insulin.

For the next day, Best had organized a session in the lecture hall of the new institute. Each participant — Adrian, Bronk, Dale, Houssay, Joslin, Penfield, and Whitby — was asked, "Which of your own investigations has given you the most pleasure and satisfaction?" Hoet and Lawrence each gave a short talk apart from this session. In the afternoon, Adrian gave the Banting Memorial Lecture. The opening of the institute was a truly happy occasion, especially since the realization of Best's dream for a first-class research facility had taken a long time and much effort.[638]

Later, all the out-of-town guests went to a party at the farm. Linda, Jessie Ridout, and Freda Herbert had prepared a cold buffet. Sir Henry started the singing, and Pep, young Jo Hoet's wife, and Henry Best, as they did each time they met, sang "Les trois cloches."

As Best had predicted, having well designed facilities in the new Best Institute soon attracted both funding and researchers. Professor E.A. Sellers, who had been in Best's naval research group during the war, directed a major study of external radiation starting in 1951. The Medical Research Committee of Defence Research Board gave $70,000 to establish a radiation unit at the Best Institute and $50,000 to Dr. Sellers to launch the radiation program. The committee built a large facility for the DRB's Medical Laboratories at Downsview, Ontario, in 1953, and Best spent a lot of time there. The first superintendent was Dr. Morley Whillans, formerly professor of pharmacology at Dalhousie, and Sellers succeeded him in 1955.[639]

After the excitement of the opening, the Bests were soon back on a more normal schedule. On 20 September 1953 Charley was off to Princeton, N.J. for meetings of the Macy Foundation. Margaret was making several types of pickles, as well as grape jelly and peach preserves. In mid November, they were both in Boston for meetings of the National Academy of Sciences. It was Det Bronk's last year as president; speaking after the dinner, he said, "If you think Charley Best is deserving of all his honours, you should know Margaret Best." Both Margaret and Charley visited Henry Mahon at the office of the *Harvard Alumni Bulletin* in the lovely, old, pale yellow Wadsworth House on Harvard Square. It had been the home of the early presidents of Harvard. After the meetings the Bests had two days in Duxbury with the Mahons and played some golf.

After the unsuccessful attempt by Sir Henry Dale and Dr. Houssay to have the 1950 Nobel Prize awarded to Best, Sir Henry immediately prepared to nominate him again for 1953. The Nobel Committee received at least one other nomination for Charles Best for the 1953 prize. Otto

Loewi, who had shared the Nobel Prize in 1936 with Dale for their work on nerve impulses and their chemical transmission, wrote Best from New York on 27 January 1953. "The letter is on its way to Stockholm by air."[640] It discussed the work on choline. Stan Hartroft wrote a fifty-four-page document on choline in connection with the 1953 nomination of Best for the Nobel Prize in physiology and medicine.[641]

Sir Henry had written early in 1953: "There has been such an uproar in Stockholm about the award made last November to Waksman [Selman Abraham Waksman of Rutgers University, for the discovery of strepto-mycin], that there is a feeling of expectation that another proposal (not for you) which was running in close competition with his in the Committee, is thought likely to be given some priority of consideration this year. That, however, is mere gossip and rumour; it would be most desirable that such stories of what happens in the Committee should not escape at all. I only say this just to warn you that, as presumably often happens, other considerations than those of the sheer merits of the pro-posals before the Committee may, in a particular year, have a special effect. In any case, they do seem to have dropped a real brick, with resounding effect, in making the award to Waksman, after all that was revealed by his lawsuit in the USA."[642] Apparently, Dr. Albert Schatz, first a doctoral student and then a colleague of Waksman's, settled out of court for a share of the royalties.[643]

Best sent Dale a handwritten note on 5 January 1954: "I am not sure that you will feel that a useful purpose will be served by sending copies of these papers to the Nobel people — but here they are. With the season's greetings, Charley Best."[644]

Dale replied: "I had been jolting my memory from time to time, con-cerning the desirability of writing to you, and asking for a supplementary set of reprints, of your publications for 1953. Now, to-day, I get your pack-age, without having had to write for it; and I am glad indeed to have it. I shall send it forward to Stockholm, and let it take its chance. It is never possible to foresee what may happen there. I always feel sorry for the Members of the Committee, with so many rival claims pressed upon their notice, among which several in each year must probably appear, to differ-ent Members, to be worthy of an award. The only thing to do is to take action, and then forget it."[645]

In the end, the prize for 1953 went to Fritz Lipmann of the United States, for his research on the molecular structure of co-enzyme A, and to

Hans Krebs of the United Kingdom for his work on the nature of metabolic processes.

At the time, Best was not surprised or bothered that he did not receive the Nobel Prize for either 1950 or 1953. Professor Bernardo Houssay and Sir Henry Dale were very keen to nominate him, but he had always known it was long chance. Besides, he was far too busy with preparations for the new Best Institute of which Margaret had said, "no honour in the world could give Charley as much pleasure as having that building."

However, once the excitement and activity of the Physiology Congress in Montreal and the opening of the Best Institute had passed, the adrenalin associated with those events subsided. Although he was thrilled and relieved finally to have the building, it was not yet complete. He had found the task of finding money difficult and stressful: he was a researcher and administrator and, although he was good at procuring research grants, he was not a fundraiser. He was tired and his health deteriorated.

At fifty-five Best realized that it was unlikely that he would make any further major scientific discoveries. His recent nomination for the Nobel Prize for 1953 reminded him that he had never been nominated for the 1923 prize, a fact that he had learned on reading Gøran Liljestrand's article on the Nobel Prize in Physiology or Medicine, which the author presented to him in 1951.[646] Professor Macleod must never have explained to Krogh the part played by Best, both in the initial work with Banting in 1921, and in the subsequent purification, development, and large-scale production of insulin in 1922.

In November 1953 Sir Henry Dale wrote to Best saying that he had heard that, at the opening of the Best Institute, J.B. Collip had been offended by Dales's remarks, which he considered did not give him enough credit for his contribution to making insulin available for the early clinical trials. Dale, wanting "to do everything possible to prevent a reopening of that tiresome old sore," proposed to Best that the published version of his address at the opening of the Best Institute be amended to give more prominence to Collip's role.[647]

Then Sir Henry, who was to give the Banting Memorial Lecture of the American Diabetes Association in San Francisco in June, wrote with an unexpected request to Best about a 1932 letter from A.B. Macallum of McGill that Dale found recently while going through old Royal Society files. In 1932 Macallum had stated to the Royal Society that in 1921–22 Banting and Best "had not carried the matter to the point at which the use of insulin in treating the human patient could be contemplated, and that the real discovery of insulin as a practical remedy was due to Collip. Secondly, the suggestion that Collip, in addition to working out the method for obtaining insulin from the normal pancreas, was also responsible for discovering its hypoglycaemic effect on the normal animal, and therewith making the control of its activity a much more reasonable possibility."

Dale continued, "I would really like to know exactly what the position was, not because it will in any way seriously alter my view concerning the primary and central importance of what you achieved. If, however, I have tended at all to under-estimate the importance of what Collip did, I want to be put right, and I know that I can trust you to give me clear and unprejudiced statement of the position." Dale wanted to be sure he knew fully and exactly what happened, should anyone bring up the subject with him in San Francisco.[648]

Best replied to Sir Henry's request, giving a detailed account of the period at the end of 1921 and beginning of 1922 of the early purification and development of insulin.

> Banting, more than generously, assigned equal credit to me and never assigned credit for the discovery phase to anyone else. There seems, however, to have been some misunderstanding about the situation which brought Dr. J.B. Collip into the group and the relationship of his work to that which Banting and I had done. I may state here that I have the very highest admiration for Collip's ability and would give him a very great deal of credit for the improvement in the methods of purifying insulin and for his prominent part in a number of other advances which were published by the Toronto group at that time, i.e. by Banting, Best, Collip, Macleod, Noble, Hepburn and others. Banting and I had noted hypoglycaemia and had recorded this and the beneficial effects of sugar. We had written out a plan to investigate normal animals, but this was first done by Collip or E.C. Noble — or both. Noble perhaps before, and certainly independently of, Collip studied the lowering of the blood sugar in normal rabbits by insulin.
>
> I would like to make it clear, however, that Collip did not join the group because our work was at a stand-

still. This was not so. Before Collip joined us we had presented our results before the medical faculty and before the Academy of Medicine in Toronto. Scores of Americans asked, "When can these dramatic findings on dogs be tested on human diabetics?" There was, therefore, far more than the usual degree of pressure on us. ...

I can remember Banting's words as if it were yesterday: He said "Charley, this thing is far bigger than we are. I know what you really want to get on with is the work on the respiratory quotients." This was actually so, and we agreed that J.B. Collip should be invited to participate in the purification of insulin and we should give him all the data we had collected. We did that. ...

After some weeks Banting began to get very restless about Collip's activities and his relationship to us. The cause of Banting's restlessness was the accumulating evidence that Prof. Macleod, with support from Collip, was forcing us out of the picture. ... [Banting] spoke to me one day about preparing some potent insulin to give to the first human case of diabetes which was to be treated on the wards of the Toronto General Hospital. Banting's statement to me was: "The insulin which Collip is making may be somewhat freer of impurities than that which you have made and which we have given to depancreatized dogs. ... I think it would be more appropriate, Charley, in view of our work together, if this first case should receive insulin made by your own hands and tested by us on dogs and on ourselves." I had no hesitation in agreeing. ... [Best made the material which they tested on their diabetic dogs and on themselves.] We took this material to the Toronto General Hospital where Dr. Ed Jeffries gave the injection to Leonard Thompson ... [resulting in] "marked reduction in blood sugar and the urine was rendered sugar free." I do not remember how many injections of this material were given but it was soon superseded by Collip's improved extract and the large-scale production of the latter was begun under Collip's direction. ... A few weeks later the report came to us that he [Collip] had lost the secret of making an active preparation. We did not know what to make of this but the Director of the Connaught laboratories was not anxious to have Collip continue under their auspices and he told us that he had terminated Collip's relationship with the Connaught.

I was requested to give up my work on the action of insulin and assume charge of the large-scale production. It was a very trying period because some of the patients who had been rescued, died because of lack of insulin.

About his relationship with Collip Best said: "I may say, in conclusion, that my associations with J.B. Collip were slight until the last war. Since then we have worked closely and harmoniously. I have found him fair and honourable in every way." Best went on to say he did not ever intend to publish this account but that Sir Henry could file it with A.B. Macallum's statement in "an appropriate place."

Best concluded his letter to Sir Henry: "I have to confess that even after all these years the revival of the memory that professor Macleod and later Collip, instead of being grateful for the privilege of helping to develop a great advance, used their superior experience and skill, with considerable success, in the attempt to appropriate some of the credit for a discovery which was not truly theirs, still makes me warm with resentment. I must state, also, that I have only to think of the understanding and fairness of scientific colleagues in many countries who have read our reports carefully, to replace resentment with a much better feeling."[649]

Sir Henry thanked Best for his account, saying that he "had never received or invited a full and frank disclosure from you of the details of memories which I knew must contain incidents which you would not willingly recall. After what happened with Collip, however, and when the sight of Macallum's old letter had recalled these almost forgotten controversies, I thought that I had better know, once and for all, the real truth of the matter. You have given me just what I wanted."[650]

A.V. Hill was in Toronto over New Year's. He went with Charley and the boys to the lieutenant-governor's reception at Queen's Park. He visited his old student Don Solandt and his family and went to Upper Canada College to see John Barcroft, son of Professor Henry Barcroft of London, who was in Canada for two school terms.

Early in the year Best undertook a number of speaking engagements, mostly in the United States. These trips bolstered his self confidence as he felt he still had something to contribute. Furthermore, it provided a change of pace from the pressures of the University of Toronto and the still unfinished Institute for which he was in search of further funding. Charley and Margaret were always given VIP treatment on these trips and they enjoyed seeing many old friends. But Charley often had a gruelling schedule.

The Bests left Toronto for Rochester, Minnesota, on 16 January 1954. On the train, they met someone who was to become a very good friend — Edwin Gates of Niagara Falls, New York. Gates had been a medical student at Harvard when Best went to lecture there in October 1923 and Banting's famous telegram was read saying that he intended to share his Nobel Prize with Best. Gates told them, "That was what really started me off on diabetes. You looked about 16 years old, Dr. Best, and I thought if he can do something like he has done, it must be a very interesting study." So he decided to become a diabetes specialist. The fact that Best *looked* so youthful, even younger than his twenty-four years, may have contributed to his not being nominated for the Nobel Prize. It was hard to believe that anyone so young could have taken part in such an important discovery.

The Hoets were also in Rochester for the refresher course on diabetes at the Mayo Clinic; Joseph was an invited expert on diabetes in pregnancy. There were many old friends from the ADA. Herbert Everett was there from St. Stephen, New Brunswick. Members of the Mayo family were very hospitable. Dr. Donald Balfour, married to Carrie Louise Mayo, was fascinated to hear from Charley about Margaret's diaries. "He wondered whether it would be possible to sit down and recapture a good deal and write it down years later. I think it would be a wonderful thing for him to do." Dr. Ed Bortz said that he had been asked to write about diabetes for lay people. "He had the idea that he might do it in story form, perhaps a love story. He started it on the train. Now I have the name for the heroine, he told me. She will be Margaret. There is to be a baby and George Anderson said, 'Name the baby Sandy.'"

In February and March 1954 the Bests visited Kingston, Ontario, as guests of honour at a charity ball in aid of sick children, and New Orleans, where Charley lectured to the physiology students of Louisiana State University on "Recent Studies with Insulin and Choline." Then they went to Boston. Margaret did not feel well, and Dr. Leo Krall from the Joslin Clinic came to see her. Charley spoke to the research staff of the Deaconess

Hospital, gave a talk in the afternoon on current research projects in Toronto, and in the evening lectured on "Insulin Past and Present" in the Joslin Auditorium to a mixed medical and lay audience in a session chaired by Dr. George Thorn, professor of medicine at Harvard. The next day Best spoke to a group of medical students from Tufts University. After a busy schedule as guests of the Joslin Clinic, the Bests had two days with Henry and Lydia in Duxbury, with lots of golf. Back in Boston, Charley spoke to several hundred medical students at Harvard and gave lectures at the Boston Lying-In Hospital and at the Boston City Hospital. Margaret thought the whole schedule far too heavy.

The next trip was to Atlantic City and New York. Best spoke before the University of Toronto Club of New York about fundraising. The new Institute still required funds for its completion. On 27 April the Bests drove to Rochester, New York, where Charley gave a speech to the members of the AOA (Alpha Omega Alpha) Honor Medical Fraternity, of which he had become a member in 1923. On the way home, after four exhausting months, they went by the farm and picked daffodils.

On Thursday evening, 6 May 1954, Charley was very tired and went to bed right after dinner, which was most unusual for him. On Friday he worked all day. He did not feel well at noon, but thinking that it was trouble from his ulcer, he decided to walk down to the University Club, which he had joined in 1941, and have something very bland for lunch. On the way back to the lab he was in such pain that he had to sit down on the curb several times. When he got back to the office he lay down on his little red couch. A doctor from Cape Town — Hoffmeyer — came to see him, but Linda did not allow him in.

Margaret described what happened later: "We had a lovely dinner. Charley said he was hungry but probably should not be eating a hearty meal. However he enjoyed it. Then he went off to bed as he had the evening before. I packed his bag partly and Henry's bag and had my own bag ready. We were to leave for West Virginia the next day at noon picking Henry up as he finished his last exam. Charley was suffering when midnight approached and he came down to the kitchen with me to have bananas and cream, tea. We came upstairs and he rapidly got worse."

Henry was startled to hear his parents arguing. He investigated and found that his father was refusing to allow a doctor to be called. Henry phoned Dr. Ray Farquharson, but he was away; however, Dr. Ian Macdonald, the chief of Sunnybrook Hospital, came quickly. He gave

CHB an injection, probably codeine, using the only syringe that he had — an old glass one — which had to be boiled. His patient asked him if he had been given water and refused to relax. He received another large dose and lay back on his bed. Macdonald was back twice the next day, and then Farquharson came and stayed several hours, finally deciding that Charley had had a heart attack. During his last exam on the Saturday, Henry fell asleep over the desk in the University Avenue Armouries, but one of his father's graduate students was a proctor and woke him up.

"On Sunday Ray said that we must go to the hospital. It was a heart attack." Margaret wrote, "It was a most shattering experience. Charley was so brave and wonderful. It broke my heart. We had some bad times in the hospital." The nurses in the Toronto General Hospital were excellent. "Henry drove me down each morning at nine o'clock and brought me back each night at ten or ten thirty. I had my lunch and dinner with Charley. It was so wonderful to be able to be right there with him. Every night Mrs. Smith, one of the nurses, phoned me at midnight to tell me whether he was asleep. He was given so much sedative. Then she called me every morning at eight o'clock before she went off."

Some of Charley and Sandy's paintings were hung on the walls of his hospital room. Many cards and all sorts of flowers arrived; Margaret kept a detailed list so that she could thank people. Ray Farquharson and Ian Macdonald were regularly in attendance, as well as Cal Ezrin, Bill Greenwood, and Bob Macmillan. Mac MacFarlane came to visit several times. Campbell Cowan, who was crucial to the running of the Banting and Best Department, was a tower of strength; Henry took him his father's messages and questions about the continuing construction of the Best Institute and returned with answers. On one occasion, a more junior medic was seen backing out of the hospital room; he had asked Best to take dicumarol, the oral form of heparin, and the patient told him angrily that he had no intention of taking rat poison[651] — Charley was getting better. After three weeks in the hospital he went home.

On 19 June Henry drove his parents out to the farm in their new 1953 Nash. Sandy brought another load, including Dochet the poodle. Charley slept much better in the country. Six weeks after his attack, he started to drive the car again, as well as the tractor — Margaret insisted that he use the kitchen steps to reach the tractor seat. Ray Farquharson asked a classmate from 1922, Dr. Claude Williams of Georgetown, to keep an eye on things, and he visited the farm every few days. Margaret wanted to do everything she could to make things easier for Charley, including learning to drive, but, despite her determination, she soon gave up. She really did not like driving.

Sandy's lilies and other flowers at the farm provided continuing pleasure. Sandy Best was now on the lecture circuit himself. Flying for the first time, he had gone to Texas to lecture on lilies to the garden clubs of Dallas to an audience of two hundred. Then he had been in Ottawa to talk to the Horticultural Society and Montréal to address a meeting of garden clubs. As well as working at the farm, Sandy was registered for his MA in botany. At the end of April he took his oral exam and did well. Dr. George Duff, a former professor of his mother's, called it "a hell of a good show."

On 9 July, Charley and Margaret, with Henry driving, left Toronto for Montréal, Quebec City, and Maine. In Montréal they went to see the new wing of Dr. Wilder Penfield's Neurological Institute, under construction. After a short visit to the Jardins Botaniques, they went on to Québec. Dr. Rosaire Gingras, secretary of the Faculty of Medicine, and his wife, Cécile, had kindly offered them the use of their lovely new home on avenue des Gouverneurs, at the edge of the new Cité Universitaire in Ste-Foy. The next day the three travellers had lunch at the Château Frontenac and visited the city. The following day they went to see the new recteur of the Université Laval, Monseigneur Alphonse-Marie Parent, in his office in the old city, who kindly gave them a guest membership in the university club, Le Cercle Universitaire.

Margaret and Charley had hoped to attend a session of Laval's summer school to improve their French, but with Charley's illness they took classes for a few days only. Mgr. Parent arranged for a parking spot near the entrance to the university building and "he gave us a key so that we may go up and down on the lift and walk through the medical section and come out at the summer school without Charley climbing any stairs." The classes were not large. André Vachon, a historian and later director of the Laval University Press, was one of the instructors. Another was Claude Fortin, a medical student. He directed the discussion towards medical topics, and Charley "had a wonderful time." Charley promoted himself to the class that Henry was in to see just how advanced it was.

When they said goodbye to Mgr. Parent, "he put his hands quite close together and said in French that, 'For a very small course we could have a very small diploma.' He laughed at that witticism."

Margaret loved anniversaries and never let members of the family forget them. On 12 July, the thirty-fourth anniversary of their betrothal, the Bests went for a drive around the Ile d'Orléans. At Ste-Pétronille, they stopped at the Château Bel-Air, where they had stayed in 1948. Margaret said, "It was a very pleasant day and I was a happy woman to have my sweetheart well and be able to enjoy life again."

Dr. and Mme Gingras entertained at their country house at Cap Rouge just west of the Quebec Bridge. There was a discussion of words that sound and are spelled alike in French such as *péché* (sin) and *pêcher* (to fish). The Bests met Robert Lesage, the young lawyer who was to marry Andrée Gingras, the daughter of their generous hosts. They were delighted to find a bowl made by the Deichmanns of New Brunswick to leave as a gift for the Gingras. "They have been very kind to us. This house has been the greatest help in having a restful week."

From Québec they drove to Maine. The Bests had crossed the international border from St. Stephen to Calais, or vice versa, hundreds of times. On this occasion, Charley was asked, "Is all this junk your personal effects?" When CHB replied in the affirmative, the response was, "All right, open the trunk and see what falls out." The family always had anecdotes about this crossing that dated back to Dr. Herbert Best who did not believe in the border. He usually drove around and behind the customs house and over the bridge. The officials at both ends knew his car.

That year Margaret had insisted on a phone at Schooner Cove so that she could call a doctor if necessary. Two days after they arrived it was in operation. A sad message came from Toronto that Don Fraser, Sr., had died in Santiago de Chile. "That was more than one could bear." Don and Mary Fraser were as close friends as Charley and Margaret had. The family reminisced about the many good times with these old friends, including those at Schooner Cove.

A new screened porch off the coach house overlooked the cove; the old one next to the small "grandmother's" bedroom off the living room, where Margaret and Charley slept, was to be enclosed to make a dressing room, and Henry laid a new floor. Construction continued. Henry learned how to use cedar shingles. Fred Marshall, who was in charge of the work, had lived in the house for eighteen years and had married Jessie Leighton.

Margaret and Charley went for walks down to the point. In the pasture, rapidly being overrun by spruce and alder, they found some purple-fringed orchids and canadense lilies. Word came from Sandy that some of his own hybrids were blooming for the first time.

Margaret was being very careful about Charley's diet. "We are back on the old ulcer diet of the war days, milk and all the bland things." People kindly offered fresh produce. Harland Brown, who owned one of the two general stores in West Pembroke, arrived with a peck of fresh peas. Charley asked him if he knew where to obtain one of Captain Leighton's pump organs. Harland said that he had one; he would not sell it but would "bring it down here and I will loan it to you indefinitely."

Lea Reiber from Cape Split came for lunch; he and Henry played and sang, and Charley put on a Kathleen Ferrier record — he loved her voice. Lea brought a jacket and a sweater of the late John Marin's that Margaret was proud to wear. He talked about the burial service earlier that year for John Marin and said that MacKinley Helm had given the prayers.

Margaret wrote, "Twelve weeks today since Charley took ill. He looks so much better, brown and well. Schooner Cove is good for him. Last night he slept all night long and no sedatives." The place looked nice — sweet peas and nasturtiums in bloom, and the lawn under control with the help of a new rotary mower. Friends, both local and more distant, visited. Tony Rolph, Henry's friend, arrived in a taxi that he had borrowed in Bethel, Maine — Henry wanted to show him the area. The Det Bronks arrived in their ketch, the *Buccaneer,* and were served a family favourite, a casserole of haddock and scallops.

One evening when Dr. Charles and Cora Armstrong from Robbinston, on the St. Croix River were there, Henry played the Leighton organ and sang "O, Holy Night," "Abide with Me," and "Nearer My God to Thee" — three of his father's favourites. Dr. Armstrong invited Henry to go on rounds with him for a day or two. "On Friday night they came to get him. He stayed with Cora and Charles at their lovely house. On Saturday he did rounds with Charles. I think they saw eleven patients. Henry carried the little black bag and Charles always introduced him as 'Dr. Best.' Henry got quite a thrill out of it. It was kind of Charles to take him. The organist, Mrs. Brooks, came to their little church, Congregational, and practised with Henry." Henry cleaned some of the pump organ's brass reeds with his simple tools, and there were fewer whistles or blank notes. "On Sunday morning, Charley, Linda and I went to Robbinston to church. They have an old Baptist clergyman. He is a clever old man and he had a fine service. He announced that Henry would sing. 'Grandson,' he said, 'of the late Dr. Best of Pembroke.' Henry sang 'Abide with Me' and later 'The Holy City.'"

Several days later George and Peggy Clowes sailed into Schooner Cover on their sloop, *Sirocco*. The son of Dr. G.H.A. Clowes of Lilly's, George and his family spent several years at Best's lab and they were frequent visitors both in Toronto and at the Stewarttown farm. Their home port was Woods Hole on Cape Cod, Massachusetts. Linda and Henry sailed with them to Cutler on a bright and breezy day.

The Bests took the shortest route to St. Andrews, New Brunswick, on the ferry from Robbinston, Maine across the St. Croix River. In St. Andrews their dear friend Senator Cairine Wilson joined them at the Algonquin Hotel for lunch. Charley bought a "forest brown" tweed jacket at the Charlotte County Cottage Craft, and Margaret and Linda both bought material. Charley liked colourful clothes and often wore a St. Andrews tweed jacket and flannels rather than a suit.

At Schooner Cove, among local people who came to call were Carl and Frances Hersey, who had a lovely old house nearby at Byron Lurchin's Cove. He was a Pembroke man who chaired the department of art and archaeology at the University of Rochester, NY. Harold and Mary Blackwood visited. He was a school friend of Charley's, and they reminisced.

On 1 September, the Bests left the farm by the sea and drove down the coast. The previous day Hurricane Carol had killed several people and demolished houses and boats. At Freeport Henry bought a red fedora at L.L. Bean's. In Duxbury, the Mahons' garden was a shambles with the old cherry tree and the locust trees blown down. Henry Mahon borrowed a truck, and he and his nephew took six loads to the dump.

Back in Toronto, Best soon started to go to his office on a regular basis, for administration and to work in his own small lab next to his office. He slowed down somewhat. Since the heart attack he did not sleep as soundly as he used to, and the noise of Dochet and Luke playing tag on the stairs of the four-storey house disturbed him, so Henry closed the two dogs each night in his room, and they slept on his bed. Also as a result of his heart attack, Charley realized he was mortal. In the decades since his work on insulin he had always been very forward-looking and was able to shrug off the fights over recognition that had surrounded the discovery. However, this first encounter with his own mortality forced him to realize that his scope was finite and made him wonder what his legacy would be.

Margaret was determined to do everything in her power to help Charley. She started once more to take driving lessons. "The boys and Linda have not been told. I am to have three more lessons this week. I got along pretty well, was not nervous. At my third lesson he had me park and I am certainly not a natural-born parker. I quite enjoyed driving in the traffic."

In mid-October, Charley represented Cambridge at the centennial of Queen's University Medical School and gave a lecture at Grant Hall. In early November, the Bests went with Reg Haist and Jim Campbell from the lab to Detroit to a meeting on growth hormones at the Henry Ford Hospital. Margaret took the streetcar to the art gallery to see the Orozco murals, Cândido Portinari's canvas of peasants and cattle (she had been intrigued by his work in São Paulo), and several works by John Marin. There was a show of pre-impressionists, impressionists, and post-impressionists. "It was quite interesting but I found that the well-known people, Degas, Renoir, Cézanne, Gauguin, were wonderful and the lesser people were not particularly thrilling."

Don Fraser, Sr., had always sent Margaret flowers on her birthday. She was very touched when Mary Fraser sent her flowers in November 1954, the first birthday after Don died.

On 16 January 1955, the Bests left Toronto for New York and Philadelphia. Margaret went to the twenty-fifth anniversary show at the Museum of Modern Art. "The loveliest one of all was a Cézanne — pine trees and rocks. It has been in my mind ever since Monday, so beautiful. There were some fine Matisse — one lovely open window, little boy at the piano (a very large picture). There were two by Ensor of Ostend in Belgium. They were quite weird."[652]

In Philadelphia, Charley chaired one ADA meeting and gave a paper at another. Dr. Joseph Beardwood, who had been the third president of the ADA, presented Charley with the Reber Medal of the Philadelphia Diabetic Association. Margaret wrote, "Some of the nicest doctors we know belong to the American Diabetes Association." They obviously enjoyed Margaret's company and were very gallant. At the banquet Fred Williams, the president said, "And, this is Margaret Best for whom we all have a great affection and I think we should all stand up to show her."

In Toronto there continued to be many visitors. The dean of medicine had a dinner for Sir Howard Florey, of penicillin fame. The Bests took him to the farm. Margaret recorded that Florey enjoyed the family and the music, adding, "I think he is such a nice man." Alex and Alison (Dale)

Todd were in town. Todd enjoyed particularly talking to Dr. Erich Baer, a fellow chemist, who was head of the Sub-Department of Synthetic Chemistry in Relation to Medical Research at the Best Institute. Dr. Per Hedenius of Stockholm visited the lab. Dr. Bruce Peck, Sr., had succeeded Clowes as scientific director of Lilly's, and he and his wife were in Toronto for a few days. Sir Harold Himsworth, who had become secretary of the Medical Research Council when Charles Best declined the post in 1949, was another visitor to the lab, and the Bests gave a dinner for him at the University Club.

On 30 March 1955, Donald Young Solandt, Charley Best's brilliant student, colleague, fellow naval officer, and friend, died after a long illness. He had taken his PhD with A.V. Hill in London, was awarded the Medal of Freedom by the United States government for his work in the Royal Canadian Navy. He became a full professor of physiology and succeeded Best as head of the Department of Physiological Hygiene in 1941. In his obituary for the Royal Society of Canada, Best wrote: "Dr. Solandt was a man of phenomenally wide interests who had an extensive knowledge of literature, music and natural science as well as his own field. His friendship was a rewarding experience and he will be vividly remembered for his courage, his loyalty, and for the exceptional keenness and adaptability of his mind."[653]

For over a year the Bests had been actively looking for a house in the Annex neighbourhood near the university, where Charley could walk to and from the lab. Also the taxes in Forest Hill Village were getting very heavy and they were finding the house a financial burden. One house that they knew on Walmer Road went for $33,500 before they had a chance to look at it. Another on Prince Arthur was where Dr. J.G. FitzGerald used to live. The price seemed high at $55,000, and probably Margaret did not want to live in the house where their old mentor and friend had died.

Then they were shown 105 Woodlawn Avenue West, overlooking the city from the top of the Avenue Road hill. Eric Haldenby, the architect for the Best Institute, knew the house well. It had been built in 1890 by a well-known architect, Henry B. Gordon, for his own use. For years Brigadier Hamilton Cassels and his wife had lived there. The conservatory on the ground floor would make a good bedroom to avoid stairs. The top floor made an apartment to rent, and there was space for another, smaller flat on the second floor. The asking price was $36,000; the Bests paid $31,250. They already knew the neighbours, Dean Vincent Bladen of graduate studies, Nicholas and Shelagh Goldschmidt (he was director of the Opera School), John and Frances Gray (he was president of Macmillan of Canada), and Bertie and Edith Wilkinson (he was professor of medieval history).

Almost exactly a year after Charley's heart attack, the family moved into the new house on 25 May 1955, their home for the next thirty-three years. To tide them over, Margaret sold her Bank of Nova Scotia stock, left to her by Uncle Bruce Macleod, and Charley borrowed on his life insurance and took out a mortgage. Eventually, they sold 78 Old Forest Hill Road to Howard Phillips, an alderman, lawyer, and son of Nathan Phillips, "the mayor of all the people." The house had originally been listed at $39,500 and then reduced to $37,000. Before leaving the old house, Margaret Best made sure that it was cleaned thoroughly from top to bottom. The new owners and the real estate agents said how unusual it was to find a house in such excellent shape.

The day the Bests moved into their new home, they rented out its third-floor apartment, with its magnificent view over the city, to the heads of nursing at two of Toronto's hospitals. Though not as close as the Annex to the university, Charley now walked regularly to the lab. The Woodlawn house suited them perfectly with kitchen, breakfast room, spacious dining room, and a forty-foot living room, plus Margaret and Charley's bedroom, dressing room, and bathroom, all on the main floor. The taxes were not as high as in Forest Hill and the two apartments provided some income. But they spent a lot on the alterations and it took a while to recoup their finances.

Having had doubts for some time, human anatomy in first-year medicine precipitated Henry's decision: his would-be medical career was coming to an end. He could not deal with the dissecting labs. In February 1955, he had viral pneumonia, and it took him several weeks to recover. He then spent some time working at the new house and transporting books. He did not return to medical school. His classmates were not surprised; they could see it coming. Dr. Farquharson was very understanding. Dean MacFarlane however, summoned him to his office and shouted at him for a half-hour — he did not care what Henry wanted to do, his duty was to carry on in medicine. Charles Best was terribly disappointed as he had dreamt of a third-generation MD, even though he realized that his second son was unlikely to choose a career in medical research. To his great credit, he never took out his feelings on Henry. Two years later, when Henry brought home the diploma for his MA *magna cum laude* in history from Université Laval in Québec, he beamed, looked up, and said, "Well, perhaps you will amount to something after all!"

Henry's reaction to abandoning his medical studies was to get as far away as possible from Toronto. On 30 May 1955, he left by bus for Espanola in north eastern Ontario and then drove forty miles into the woods from Webbwood to work for the KVP (Kalamazoo Vegetable Parchment) Company on its timber limits and on putting out a forest fire near Sable Lake. He bought a 1930 Model A Ford in Copper Cliff for $150 and periodically visited his hospitable Robertson cousins in Sudbury.

Sandy had started to work on his PhD in botany and continued to speak to botanical groups and garden clubs; his favourite topic was "Consider the Lilies." He had now almost reached the top of the lily world. In December 1955, he was in New York for a meeting of the North American Lily Society of which, at twenty-four, he was the vice-president. He stayed for three days at the Park Avenue home of Mrs. Hess, mother-in-law of Jan de Graaf of Oregon, probably the largest lily grower in the world.

In 1955 Pope Pius XII appointed Best to the Pontifical Academy of Sciences. Margaret was listening to a radio report at the farm, and it finished with, "Dr. Best is a Presbyterian." The communication from the Vatican stated that henceforth Professor Best should be addressed as "Excellency." Occasionally the boys would greet their father this way at the breakfast table. His reply was invariably, "How much?" With his new connection to the Vatican, particularly when he knew that an audience contained many Catholics, Charley would assure people that the Pope had the very best medical advice on all matters, including birth control.

Charles Best had always been very proud to belong to the Royal Society of London. In early February 1955, he received a cable asking him to give its Croonian Lecture. Planning for the trip in June commenced immediately. The Croonian Lecture is the Royal Society's premier lecture in the biological sciences. Previous lecturers included Douglas Adrian, Henry Dale, Howard Florey, A.V. Hill, August Krogh, and Joseph Lister. "Charley wore his dark grey suit with waistcoat. The title of his lecture was 'Dietary Factors in the Protection of the Liver, Kidneys, Heart and Other Organs of Experimental Animals: The Lipotropic Agents.'[654] It was a strictly scientific lecture, with few personal comments." The final sentence read, "The rather barren framework which these facts serve to outline is, we trust, made of good steel, but it will be much more attractive when the bricks of future findings are in their proper places." Best considered giving the Croonian Lecture one of the high points of his career.

"Anna Lawrence and I," Margaret wrote, "took the 'tube' and went to Hammersmith to the Lyric Theatre to see *The Lark*, a play by Jean Anouilh, translated by Christopher Fry. Joan of Arc (The Lark) was played by Dorothy Tutin. I had read about *The Lark* in the *New York Times* and it was very good." (Margaret read the *Sunday New York Times* regularly for many years.)

The next day, Margaret went to the Tate Gallery to see the Ben Nicholson show. "It is too abstract for me." However, she did admire Cézanne's *Mont St-Victoire* and Graham Sutherland's portrait of Somerset Maugham. The Wolstenholmes of the Ciba Foundation took the Bests to Glyndbourne to see Rossini's *Le Comte Ory*, and the Lawrences invited them to Claridge's for dinner before going to Regent's Park to see *The Tempest*. The Norman Robertsons gave a dinner for the Bests at the Canadian High Commissioner's residence at 12 Upper Brook Street.

The Bests were both invited to Canadian Club banquets; at the ladies' evening, chaired by Countess Alexander, Margaret was delighted to see Princess Alice again. Other wives of former governors general of Canada present were Lady Tweedsmuir and Viscountess Willingdon. The speakers were the Indian high commissioner, Madame Pandit, sister of Nehru, and Viscountess Astor, the first woman MP. Much to his surprise and delight, Best received fifteen guineas for a BBC broadcast, so he went to Simpson's of Piccadilly, owned by his old friend, Dr. Leonard Simpson, and bought himself a new raincoat.

Many old friends attended the IDF meeting in Cambridge, including the Gerritzens, the Hoets, and the Joslins. At the formal opening, the vice-chancellor, Sir Lionel Whitby, and Robin Lawrence, as president of the IDF, spoke. "Everyone referred to the early work and the Discovery of Insulin by Fred Banting and Charley. In the row behind us sat Sir Henry Dale and Lady Dale, the first time I had seen them since their recent return from America. Dr. Joslin delivered the Banting Memorial Lecture." Joslin hosted a dinner that paired Margaret with Dr. Jacob Poulsen of Copenhagen and Charley with Marguerite Hoet. After dinner Bruce Peck of Lilly's gave a talk about "Diabetes in the Americas." The next day the Whitbys gave a lunch at his college, Downing. By now they were on more familiar terms as Margaret noted that Sir Lionel called, "Hi Margaret!" and gave her a kiss. The congress banquet took place in the Great Hall of Trinity College, of which the recently elevated Lord Adrian was master.

Back in London, the Bests went to Kew Gardens to see the director, Sir Edward Salisbury. He talked of Sir Joseph Banks who had been president of the Royal Society for over forty years. Future presidential terms were thereafter limited to five years. Sir Edward gave his visitors a wonderful tour of the buildings and the gardens. The roses were pretty well past, but the delphiniums and the fuchsia were lovely. Not surprisingly Margaret and Charley were particularly interested in the lilies, Sandy's specialty.

After their return to Canada the Bests left Toronto on 31 July for Maine. Sandy and Dr. Bruce Casselman from the lab came along in their car, helped with the driving, and collected some flowers along the way. On 12 August Charley, Margaret, and Linda set out for Orono and the University of Maine, where CHB was to receive an honorary degree. Maine's commissioner of education presented him for the degree. It was a very special honour for Charles Best from the university of the state where he was born. "Charley's convocation address was splendid — reminiscing and humorous at first and then some good advice. He mentioned Harold Blackwood and how he and Harold missed the train in Calais and walked to Pembroke — how they rowed down the river, landed on Red Island, wrestled all day and rowed home. Charley did not know then that Harold was in the audience but later we found that he and Mary and Cora Armstrong were there. Charley mentioned Styles Bridges, and Ronald."

Soon the Bests drove down the coast again, this time to Bar Harbor, for meetings at the Roscoe B. Jackson Memorial Cancer Laboratory, of which Dr. C.C. Little, previously president of the universities of Maine and Michigan, was the founding director and Charley was a director, a position he enjoyed. Other directors included Dr. Leonard Carmichael, former president of Tufts University and now head of the Smithsonian Institution. Bar Harbor was home to many large summer houses and stores that catered to the "carriage trade." From one of the bookstores Margaret bought the *Selected Poems of Robert P. Tristram Coffin* for Charley. On the way back north, the Bests stopped for a concert at the music school run by Pierre Monteux, retired conductor of the San Francisco Symphony.

In the autumn of 1955, there were lecture trips to London, Ontario for the Canadian Physiological Society, to New York for the New York Diabetes Association and the Nutrition Foundation, and to Detroit where Charley lectured to the Wayne County Medical Association on the "History of Insulin and the Present Position." Margaret bought a copy of Carl Sandburg's *Abraham Lincoln* for Henry, who was writing an essay on

Lincoln in one of his final-year arts courses to which he had transferred on withdrawing from medicine.

The family was participating in Henry's musical activities, particularly the Hart House Orchestra. He was secretary of the music committee of Hart House (his father had been a member of the first "hall committee," and his brother, secretary of the art committee). Dr. Boyd Neel had founded an orchestra in England that bore his name and saw great success. Having become dean of music at Toronto, he started the Hart House Orchestra. There was no other chamber group in Toronto, but the new orchestra, though an artistic success, did not do well at the box office.

Four students formed the Hart House Orchestra Association. The group organized a concert on a Sunday evening at nine o'clock, after evening church services. Everything proceeded quietly until Henry received notice that he was contravening the Lord's Day Act by selling tickets for an event on a Sunday and was liable for prosecution. Warden Joseph McCulley of Hart House was most helpful but was aware of the possible consequences and sent Henry to see President Sidney Smith. The latter phoned Laddie Cassels, the university's lawyer, insisting that he charge a fee for his advice — one dollar. Instead of selling tickets, Cassels advised Henry to sell *memberships* in the Hart House Orchestra Associates with regular meetings every second Thursday at noon, and occasional concerts on Sunday evening. It was obviously a ruse, but all three Toronto newspapers must have had a shortage of news items because the Hart House Orchestra was on every front page. The Lord's Day Alliance capitulated and withdrew its complaint.

At breakfast that morning, Charles Best was reading his *Globe and Mail* and said, "Some student has got himself into a difficult situation." He lowered the paper slowly and looked at Henry. "This isn't you, is it?" As soon as the new associates' membership cards were ready, CHB took a large number and sold them to all his friends. Margaret and Charley Best and Linda Mahon were in the audience for the first concert.

On a regular basis, the Bests had graduate students or visiting faculty members from the Department of Physiology and the Banting and Best Department either to the house in town or to the farm. In early December a group from Chile, England, India, Italy, Mexico, and Pakistan joined several Canadians at 105 Woodlawn for punch from Sandy's large lily-prize bowl, plus turkey, ham, and all that went with them, while Sandy played grandmother Macleod's piano.

On 8 December 1955, Charles and Margaret and Henry Best went to Alliston for the unveiling of a portrait of Frederick Banting at the Banting Memorial School. They took Lillian Hipwell, widow of Fred Banting's first cousin, another Fred, with them. First they went to the farm where Fred Banting was born and where his brother Thompson — a successful potato farmer — lived. They stopped at the drugstore still run by Fred Hipwell's father, aged ninety-three. At the school, Lillian Hipwell unveiled the portrait by Dorothy Stevens, painted from a photograph that Fred Hipwell had taken. Everyone was pleased with it. Charles Best talked about Fred Banting. On the way back in the car Lillian Hipwell reminisced. "The conversation was certainly interesting for Henry to hear. The Hipwells were very, very fond of Fred. Lillian said, 'Fred certainly was not a good judge of women.'"

Henry and Lydia Mahon came up from Boston for Christmas 1955. Margaret was proud to have her brother there; though he was a full colonel in the U.S. air force during the war, he wore with pride his blazer with the crest of the Royal Military College of Canada. The whole family made a rare appearance at St. Andrew's Church and saw a few elderly people who remembered Margaret and Henry Mahon's parents. Henry Best took his Aunt Lydia, an Episcopalian, to Grace Church on the Hill for midnight service. There were several gatherings of friends at the house, and the forty-foot living room, with its large windows overlooking the city, was a wonderful setting.

Charley continued to have health problems. His heart was not bothering him, but his ulcer had reappeared and he was advised to slow down. This, of course, was not easy — he was interested in so many things, and the invitations to speak piled up. The farm was no longer relaxing as it had become increasingly Sandy's flower growing business. He moved out there to live and his parents started to look for another place in the country for themselves.

In early 1956 Dr. John Logothetopoulis and his wife, Ismene, arrived in Toronto from Greece, initially for two or three years. They stayed, however, and he became one of the senior investigators at the Best Institute, known especially for his work on the islets of Langerhans. Logothetopoulis was attracted to Toronto to work with Best. He, in turn, kept in touch with scientists in Athens thus widening the "network" for colleagues in Canada and Greece.

Over the years there had been several films made about the discovery of insulin. In 1954, Leslie McFarlane of the National Film Board of Canada talked to Charles Best at the lab, and Margaret showed him the original manuscript of the first paper and charts and her early scrapbooks.

The working title of the screenplay was *The Seekers*. In 1956 Dr. W.R. Feasby started work on a book and a film about Best. Feasby was an MD who had served as a lieutenant colonel with the Royal Canadian Army Medical Corps. He was the author of the official two-volume history of the Canadian Medical Services during the Second World War.

With improved health, but still bothered by the ulcer, Charley resumed the round of lectures and meetings. The Bests really did enjoy seeing many friends at these annual gatherings. They took the train to New York in late January, 1956, and then flew to Dallas for meetings of the ADA. These meetings regularly had a gathering of lay diabetics with a panel to answer questions — in this instance, Charles Best, Ed Bortz of Philadelphia, Alex Marble of the Joslin Clinic, and Randy Sprague of the Mayo Clinic. In true Texas fashion, Best was made an honorary deputy sheriff of Dallas County and an honorary admiral in the Texas navy. Seated next to Charley at the closing banquet was film star Greer Garson, Academy Award winner for her title role in *Mrs. Miniver*. Margaret remarked on the enormous pear-shaped diamond ring that Garson was wearing. "Greer has good features, interesting eyes and hair like golden straw — she was wearing a full-length coat of silver-blue mink."

In mid-April Best lectured for five days at the Atlantic City Hospital during the meetings of the Federation of American Societies for Experimental Biology. There were, remarkably, twelve papers from Charley's colleagues, which brought great credit to the Best Institute. Margaret was pleased that her trip was paid for as well.

Later in April, the Bests went to Atlantic City for CHB's first meeting as a member of the Association of American Physicians — a select group of 250 people. Between trains in New York they went to the Gallery St-Etienne on West 57th Street to see the work of Käthe Kollwitz. "It was all prints, all black and white. I think she is wonderful — very moving and sad." After Atlantic City the next stop was Sky Top in the Pocono Hills, Pennsylvania, for a meeting of the Nutrition Foundation, where Best gave a lecture. Margaret noted happily that once again her expenses were being covered.

In early June the Bests were in Chicago for the retirement of Dr. Carlos I. Reed as professor of physiology — Best and Bill Feasby were to have lengthy correspondence with him on events surrounding the discovery of insulin. Best lectured to the medical staff and students. The Bests stayed on in Chicago for a meeting of the ADA. Old friends at the gathering included Joseph Hoet from Belgium. Typically, he brought flowers for Margaret.

On their return, Charley and Margaret went with Linda to Stratford, Ontario, where they stayed at a guest house and dined at Knox Presbyterian Church. They saw *Henry V* in the festival's tent; Christopher Plummer played the king — "a wonderful performance. The costuming was magnificent." It was the fourth year for the Stratford Festival in the tent — something that many remembered with nostalgia long after it was gone. They thoroughly enjoyed the visit, seeing many friends in the audience: Charles and Helen Band, Cleeve and Jean Horne, and Roland and Norah Michener.

Both boys were no longer living at home. Sandy was working on his PhD in botany at the University of Toronto, but living at the farm. Henry had left the day after his exams for Val Cartier, Québec to work in a lab at the Canadian Armament Research and Defence Establishment (CARDE). He then became liaison officer between CARDE and the small research establishment on Grosse Ile, the historic quarantine station down the St. Lawrence, where he gained administrative experience and improved his French.

On 2 July 1956, the Bests left Toronto for Montréal and the *Empress of Britain* to Liverpool. Charley was intrigued that a Home for Diabetics at Parksgate, on the estuary of the Dee, was to be named after him. Anna and Robin Lawrence came up from London to join them for the official opening ceremony.

For years, Margaret had wanted to go to Ulster, the home of her Mahon ancestors. She and Charley arrived in Belfast on the "glorious 12th" and saw the Orange Parade. They had their own celebration for their thirty-sixth betrothal day. They went unannounced to the Department of Physiology at Owens College, where they met Dr. Bob Whelan; he and Dr. Jack Smyth, a diabetic specialist, took the visitors to the Public Record Office but could find nothing of family relevance. The next stop was Derry, or Londonderry. CHB had sailed into that harbour on Loch Foyle during the war. Professor Thomas Finnegan, president of Magee University College, helped them locate old records.

For their three days in London, the Bests stayed at the Ciba Foundation House at 41 Portland Place, where the director Dr. Gordon Wolstenholme and his wife Dushanka welcomed them. Best chaired a conference on ageing, and he and Margaret saw the Dales and Eduardo Braun Menéndez, their good friend and host from Buenos Aires. They all enjoyed *Romanoff and Juliet*, written, directed, and starring Peter Ustinov. Charley gave the Addison Lecture at Guy's Hospital; Sir Henry Dale chaired the meeting, but a technician mixed up all the slides. Once again an unexpected fee of twenty-five guineas was welcome.

Margaret and Charley went to the Tate to see a special exhibition of paintings by Wyndham Lewis — who had lived in Toronto — and other Vorticists, Ezra Pound's term. "I have seen the portrait of Edith Sitwell before and I think it is very fascinating. There were portraits of T.S. Eliot, Ezra Pound."

The next stop was Brussels, where Marguerite, Jean, and Philippe Hoet were waiting at the air terminal; Joseph had a tumour, which happily turned out to be benign. Marguerite and the Bests had lunch with Dr. and Mrs. Maurice Delaet; he was president of the Permanent Committee of the Medical Society of Brussels. Each morning Joséphine, the Hoets' housekeeper for over sixty years, would bring breakfast to the Bests' room. St. Margaret's day was 20 July, and the Hoets celebrated it the next day in honour of the two Margarets — Hoet and Best. "I think Charley and I must add St. Margaret's Day to our list of days to celebrate."

Best spoke at a meeting of the Fondation médicale Reine Elisabeth on "L'Insuline, hormone de croissance," first in French for several minutes, then in English — the technician showed someone else's slides. "Charley said that he sometimes had to lecture when his slides were mixed up (as he had in London) but he could not lecture with someone else's." Mgr. van Waeyenbergh, long-time recteur of the University of Louvain, was there as was Queen Elisabeth, who recalled the Bests' visits to Laeken Palace. Later a beautiful medal arrived inscribed "Her Majesty the Queen Elisabeth, Honorary Perpetual President of the Medical Society of Brussels, Professeur Charles H. Best, Hommage et Gratitude, 1956."

The XXth International Physiological Congress took place in Brussels. Best chaired a meeting of the International Union of Physiological Sciences (IUPS) attended by representatives from forty countries; the members decided to meet again in Argentina in 1959. CHB spoke at the congress's closing ceremony and was presented with *Some Apostles of Physiology* (1902), by William Stirling, outlining the progress of physiological study across the centuries.[655] On the front was inscribed, "To the first President of the IUPS, 1953–1956, as a token of friendship," and autographed by C. Heymans, B.A. Houssay, Alex von Muralt, and Maurice de Visscher.[656] In making the presentations, Heymans, president of the congress, "said some very nice things about Charley — that in due time his name would belong with the apostles of physiology. He said that

Charley had laid the firm and strong base for the pyramid into which the International Union of Physiological Sciences would grow ... It is impossible to think of a greater administrative honour coming to a physiologist than to have been the first president of the IUPS."

When the congress was over, Jean and Philippe Hoet drove the visitors from Brussels to "Les Conifères." While watching the young Hoets play tennis, Charley lit his first cigarette in years. The two Margarets started to smoke as well, in the hopes of embarrassing him, and Marie-Noëlle, the youngest of the Hoet children, went off to tell her father. That was the end of Best smoking!

Linda Mahon had forwarded two copies of Sandy's new lily catalogue to his parents. Joseph Hoet, still ill in bed, was delighted and immediately ordered some lilies. Several family members drove the Bests to the Brussels airport: "We were sorry to say goodbye to the Hoets. We always have a happy time with them."

Arriving in Montreal from Europe on the *Corinthia* the Bests were invited to dinner by Omond and Elizabeth Solandt. Omond had recently been appointed Vice President Research of the Canadian National Railways. Fellow guests awaiting the Bests' arrival made bets about how soon they would mention famous names. Omond described what happened. "Margaret initiated it by prompting, 'Oh, Charley, tell about the time we had lunch with Queen Mother Elisabeth of Belgium.' Nearly all of Charley's close friends were a little uneasy about this as it created a bad impression."[657] J.K.W. Ferguson, director of the Connaught Laboratories, who, like Solandt, had known Best since 1929, offered a kinder assessment: "Genial, quick-witted and handsome, Best greatly enjoyed his fame, and liked to reminisce about his encounters with royalty and the eminent of the world. Unfriendly critics called this name-dropping. To me it seemed just exuberant enjoyment of knowing so many interesting people. He was always good company."[658]

Three days later the Bests headed for Québec and Maine with Linda, staying at the home of Jean and Agathe Lacourcière Lacerte, where Henry spent two happy years in Quebec City. From Berthier, the Bests took the government boat *Grosse-Ile* the six miles to the island where Henry was administrative officer. When the island was a quarantine station in the mid-nineteenth century, between twenty and thirty thousand mostly Irish immigrants were buried there, victims of cholera and smallpox. During the Second World War and after, it was an experimental station for bacteriological warfare. Best had been involved with the Defence Research Board's plans for the island after the war, but he had never been there. On this occasion, Best visited the labs with director Dr. Peter McKercher. By 1956, it was used mainly by the federal Department of Agriculture as an experimental laboratory, and later, as a quarantine station for imported animals.

At Schooner Cove Farm, the sweetpeas and the petunias were in full bloom. Charley had fun writing verses about "the tide yesterday when it seemed to be making up its mind whether to come or go. He said, 'Robert Coffin would have written a poem about this.'" Best's poem was titled "We Watched the Tide Make up Its Mind."

> Our Schooner Cove was full to the brim
> Salt water lapped the pine and spruce rim
> Even "The nubble" and Mariner's hay
> Were well covered with great Fundy's spray.
>
> We donned our gear and hurried to find
> If the old beach road was buried in brine
> Down the lane under a mackerel sky
> Went Margaret, Linda, Henry and I.
>
> The new inflow did not keep its pace
> The true outflow was soon a mill-race.
> The cause of these changes is hard to find
> But we watched the tide make up its mind.[659]

Margaret wrote, "I have been driving a little up the road each day but I am not capable yet of driving a real journey." Charley's back had been causing him pain but it eased up enough for him to drive them back to Toronto.

On 5 February, 1957, the Bests left Toronto for New York and Boston. Best was to appear briefly in a TV re-enactment of the discovery of insulin for The Kraft Hour, in colour. Max Rosenfeld was involved and Jim Salter went from the institute as an adviser; Jim Salter was a young scientist for whom Best had great hopes, but unfortunately these were never realized and Salter disappeared completely from the scene. The Canadian actor William Shatner played the young Best. "Charley appeared at the beginning sitting at a desk opening mail. Then at the very end he was shown again and he spoke, seated behind the desk. There was a photograph of Fred Banting on the desk. The show was far better than the Canadian one — Max wrote both of the scripts but this last one was greatly improved and on the whole done much better. I found it very moving and others felt the same way about it. Charley told 'Fred Banting' and 'Charley Best' that they were so good that he would be in danger of thinking of them in the future as 'Banting and Best.'"

Sandy was becoming more and more involved in politics and had been a delegate to the 1956 convention that chose John Diefenbaker as Conservative leader. Sybil Bennett, MP for Halton, died, and the loss hit Sandy hard. "Sandy really loved that woman," Best wrote, "and he finds it — I guess the first grief he has ever had. He didn't know his grandparents really. He wasn't old enough."[660]

Henry arrived from Québec, and the whole family went out to Milton for the Conservative nomination of a candidate for the anticipated federal election. George Elliot, a Milton lawyer, nominated Sandy. His mother noted that he was wearing a Macdonald tie in honour of Sir John A. and of his great-great-grandmother, Mary MacDonald Macleod. The other candidates were the Presbyterian minister from Norval, the Rev. G. Lockhart Royal, and Mac Sproule, a farmer from near Acton. Sandy won on the first ballot.

Henry came home to help Sandy in his election. His father had bought a 1950 Dodge for Henry to use in campaigning. At a rally in Toronto's Massey Hall Premier Leslie Frost spoke, followed by John Diefenbaker. George Hees, the perennial Tory MP and cabinet minister, introduced "Mr. Charles Alexander 'Sandy' Best, just twenty-five years old and unmarried — here's a package for you girls."

With the election approaching, Margaret and Charley, who before had never shown any interest in politics, spent more time in Halton County. On 6 June there was a rally in the Legion Hall in Georgetown, with speeches. Charley said a few words, and Sandy told a story that was risqué for the 1950s. He had knocked at a door and, when a little girl answered, asked to see her father or her mother. She said "No." "Are they both out?" "No, they are both in the bathtub."

Margaret and Charley went in to Toronto to vote in their own riding and then back to the farm. On the evening of 10 June, 1957, Sandy Best took an early lead over the Liberal, Ken Dick, and held it, winning by nine thousand votes. The Conservatives were in power, but not with a majority. Among the phone calls and letters was a message of congratulations from his godmother, Liberal Senator Cairine Wilson. Margaret and Charley were proud of Sandy's electoral victory and were caught up in the excitement, riding in a convertible behind the triumphant candidate.

In Toronto, the long-awaited gold collar of the Pontifical Academy of Sciences had arrived. Cardinal McGuigan had speeded up the process. With a reporter there, Charley stated that it looked very nice around Margaret's neck, but she thought "that the Pope might take a dim view" if he saw a picture of her wearing it.

Best's brief appearance in February 1957 in the Kraft Hour TV re-enactment of the discovery of insulin had certainly revived his memories of that period. Also, three years earlier, following Sir Henry Dale's request to "know fully and exactly what happened" during the purification and development phase of insulin, Best had written him a detailed account of the period. Shortly after the Kraft Hour TV show, Dr. W.R. Feasby, who, in 1956, had started writing a biography of Best, asked him about the discovery and early development of insulin and the controversy over the Nobel Prize.[661]

In reply to Feasby's question Best talked of the roles played by Macleod and Collip in 1921 and 1922. Best wrote about Macleod, who was not in Canada when Banting and Best made their discovery:

> [Macleod] saw an opportunity, by taking charge of the development of insulin, to recoup his losses and, of course, Collip played a very important part there. As soon as Collip failed to tell Banting and me what was happening and made his reports directly to Macleod, you had a split in the personnel ... You had Banting and Best who felt that they had made a discovery and invested their time and effort, alone, before anything promising had come out of the work — you have these two on one side and you have Macleod, supported by Collip, on the other.

> It seemed to me that these two full professors saw their opportunity to steal a fair share of the credit for the discovery. That may be too strong a statement, but I have thought about it over the years and that certainly was Fred Banting's reaction. ... [Banting reacted] by losing his temper and raging about, and getting support from people like Sir William Mulock and Billy Ross and others; he probably did it pret-

ty effectively. I don't think I took it quite as seriously at that time. I don't know that I realized exactly what was happening, but it seemed to me that I had more faith in good work being its own reward, and that I would eventually get credit for the things that I had actually done.[662]

In a letter to Feasby dated 6 May 1957, Best commented on Macleod's letter of September 1922 to Colonel Gooderham:

> There are a number of extremely useful statements in it and many which are not accurate. I have been wondering ever since I first read it, how Professor Macleod selected the successful procedures which Fred Banting and I used, and claimed them as his own suggestions.

Best went on to say that Macleod had never claimed publicly or in print that he had made these contributions and suggestions regarding the procedures used.

> I really think what happened is that Professor Macleod confused what he taught me as a student with the advice that he thought he gave to Banting and me. I was particularly puzzled by his statement that he had helped in solving the difficulty in making insulin on a larger scale ... He was never in the laboratory except perhaps for a few minutes' visit ... It was certainly not Professor Macleod who introduced open evaporation of alcoholic extracts in a warm air current into the insulin process. I had done it long before he knew anything about our success with alcoholic extracts of foetal and adult beef pancreas.

> He would not have dared to do it. Banting and I would have challenged them instantly. Macleod certainly read statements in the literature which Banting and I published about the procedures we used. He never stated in print, as he has done in this unpublished document, that he claimed credit for the use of these procedures. He distributed this document to several of his friends and may

have made the same claims in speaking or writing to Professor Krogh who is said to have reported to the Nobel Committee. I must say that in 1922 I was blissfully ignorant of what was going on behind the scenes ... Only Professor Macleod appreciated the possible significance of Krogh's visit.[663]

Best acknowledged that as a student he had admired and respected Macleod whose "text was a bible to me." Best remembered him "with gratitude as my finest and most friendly teacher during my undergraduate course." Nonetheless, Macleod's actions around the time of the discovery of insulin were truly those of a rival, not an advisor and friend.

A very different view of Professor Macleod's role and the motivations for his actions is given in a book by Dr. Michael J. Williams, a consulting physician at the Aberdeen Royal Infirmary's Diabetic Clinic.[664] He wrote a sympathetic and thoughtful account of Macleod's career, attributing to him the major role in the discovery of insulin.

On 18 June 1957, Margaret and Charley left Montréal on the *Empress of Britain* for the UK. They returned for a few days to Ulster where, rather ironically, they were royally received, in contrast to Margaret's non-conformist Mahon ancestors who had left Londonderry in 1761. CHB attended a dinner given by Viscount Brookeborough, the premier, for Viscount Montgomery. Lord Wakehurst gave a reception for them at Government House. Genealogy seemed to have taken a back seat.

In London on 12 July 1957, Best gave the Osler Oration to the Osler Club, meeting at the Rembrandt Hotel with Dr. William Copeman, president of the club and of the historical section of the Royal Society of Medicine. The title was "The Discovery of Insulin," the topic uppermost in his mind due to Feasby's recent interviews and the Kraft Hour TV dramatization in February. Margaret wrote, "It was a consideration of the documents submitted by Fred, Charley, and Dr. Macleod in response to a letter from Colonel Albert Gooderham, chairman of the Insulin Committee at the University of Toronto. Colonel Gooderham wrote that Dr. Dale was coming from England in September 1922, and that 'in the interests of the University of Toronto, it would be advantageous to remove all points of discord.'"

Best took this opportunity to clarify the roles of various participants, as he saw it, in front of this distinguished audience. Among the guests in

1957 were Dr. Harry Platt of Manchester, president of the Royal College of Physicians, Lord and Lady Evans, physician to the Queen, and Sydney Pierce, Canadian deputy high commissioner. Margaret noted that "Charley knew that it would not be published. He wanted to be certain that the record was straight from his point of view but he did not want to stir the hornets' nest of the protagonists of Dr. Macleod and Dr. Collip."

Sir Henry Dale was there and was asked to speak. "Sir Henry said, 'When I arrived in Toronto in 1922 there was only one person who had his feet solidly on the ground and who knew exactly what had to be done and that was Charley Best.'"[665] In fact, the lecture was the first public recounting of many details of the events in Toronto of 1921 to 1923. Best finished his speech, "It would have been easy to omit all these personal details. Historians who are not directly involved will be able to appreciate better than we can, the magnitude of the advance. Many of them will ignore both the valleys of dissension and the peaks of personal loyalties and friendships. The seven months of harmonious, intensive work which Fred Banting and I carried on together in 1921, was the period which we both considered to be that of the 'discovery of insulin.' The picture of those days, which I have tried to paint for you, is the one that I hope you will carry away in your minds."[666]

The Bests went to see *The Prince and the Showgirl* with Sir Laurence Olivier and Marilyn Monroe — "a strange combination, the two playing together. It was quite fun." Lady May Mellanby had lunch with the Bests and talked of André Maurois writing the life of Sir Alexander Fleming. "Lady Fleming lives in Chelsea — very sad, May says, and keeping everything, even Sir Alexander's clothes just as they were."

People may make deprecating remarks about Royal Garden Parties, but most who are invited are delighted to attend. On 18 July, 1957, Charley, in rented finery from Moss Bros on Regent Street, and Margaret, in a linen dress and long white gloves, walked from the Stafford Hotel to Buckingham Palace. "The Queen was lovely in a powder blue coat dress and a little feather hat. They had been briefed and Prince Philip began at once to talk about diabetes and insulin. He said, 'What about these new pills?' They were obviously tremendously interested in medical affairs. Sir Winston and Lady Churchill went by. He is really tottering now. She looked wonderful."

Three months later the Queen and Prince Philip were in Ottawa on 14 October 1957 for the opening of Parliament. Margaret, Charley, and

Henry were there, proud to see Sandy Best, member for Halton, take his seat with the new government. Walking along Elgin Street in Ottawa the day after the opening of Parliament, Margaret fell and broke her arm, two ribs, and had a big lump on her head. Charley gave her a sedative, and she went back to Toronto lying in the back seat of the family car, supported by pillows. In Toronto Bob Janes took more x-rays and confirmed that she had broken the radius and the tip of her elbow. Almost three weeks later the cast came off. "It took some time to get it off. I have been warned that my arm would look like something that had been under a log but I was agreeably surprised to see it come out quite brown. Then Dr. William Spence asked me to move it which I did and the next thing I knew I was lying on the floor. I fainted two or three times."

The new MP for Halton gave his maiden speech in the Commons on 9 December 1957, responding to a motion by Stanley Knowles to set up a committee to deal with various celebrations, including Canada's centennial. He later spoke in favour of a resolution to create a committee "to promote and accelerate scientific research in Canada" — a subject that he had discussed with his father. Ian Macdonald later wrote to Margaret and Charley, "Sandy's speech in the Commons on April 6th was first rate, and I am sure that it must have had a good effect on his colleagues, not only in giving them some understanding of the problems of research, but also in stimulating them to make some bold decisions for the future."[667] As a member of the committee on agriculture, Sandy spoke on motions to require humane slaughter of farm animals and to establish a productivity council. He became vice-chair of a committee on conditions among the Inuit and on encouragement of their art. His contributions were well received; he was well prepared and could think on his feet.

The Bests were not in the habit of ordering food to be sent in but they developed a liking for Chinese food from Toronto's Lichee Gardens, where George, the manager, took very good care of them. On Margaret's fifty-seventh birthday, on the 30 November 1957, George sent up a nice meal. Sandy telephoned from New York, where he was part of the Canadian delegation to the United Nations, and Henry called from Québec.

At an open house at the Best Institute, Dr. Bernard S. Leibel had introduced himself to Margaret. Charley later explained to her that Leibel was attached to Mount Sinai Hospital in Toronto and that he had a very large diabetic practice. Bernie and Queenie Leibel were very thoughtful and helpful to the Bests for many years. They were the Bests' hosts at the Primrose

Club in early December at a dinner for the Empire Chapter of B'Nai Brith. Best spoke and was presented with a cheque for $3,000 for diabetes research.

English sculptor Dorothy Russell started working on a bust of Best in the garden room of the basement floor of the Bests's house. Margaret did not seem to know much about it except that the CDA was involved and that Russell had done a bust of Prime Minister Diefenbaker. On the second or third day, Russell appeared in the doorway of the living room, "Oh, Mrs. Best, it has collapsed." Apparently the clay was too wet. "I got her some pieces of wood and some implements. I think that all goes well now." Later Margaret wrote, "It is excellent, very like him. She spoke on TV twice and said that Charley was the most intelligent sitter she has ever had." A few days later, "Mrs. Russell has finished her head of Charley — an excellent likeness. I hope it won't get smashed before she has it cast in bronze." No one, at the CDA or elsewhere, knows what became of it.

Henry and Lydia Mahon arrived from Duxbury for Christmas, but Margaret was down with bronchitis. The Vin Prices came for dinner on Christmas Day when Margaret got dressed and Charley showed some old sixteen-millimetre movies. In Ottawa, Sandy had been introduced to Eileen Thompson by his godmother, Senator Cairine Wilson. Eileen, as assistant editor of *The Presbyterian Record*, had gone to interview Senator Wilson for an article. Margaret remarked, "We have met Eileen Thompson, the Irish girl from Belfast twice now and she is very attractive." A first-class church organist, Eileen had come to Canada with her parents when she was twelve.

The New York Academy of Medicine on 25 February introduced three guests who had done the most to facilitate use of anticoagulants in clinical medicine: Charles Best, Dr. Armand J. Quick of Marquette University Medical College, and Dr. Karl Link of the University of Wisconsin. Irving S. Wright, the chairman, was the greatest clinical expert on anticoagulants. Best had initiated and directed work that led to purification of heparin and proved that it could prevent various types of thrombosis; Quick had developed tests to control use of anticoagulants; and Link had isolated and made dicumarol, the oral form of heparin. David Schulte, a tobacconist turned investor, financed the meeting; many years earlier Best and Gordon Murray, who had undertaken the first clinical experiments, had gone to New York and given Schulte heparin when he was very ill. In New York, Margaret went to see *The Entertainer*, a new play by John Osborne, who wrote *Look Back in Anger*. "They refer to John

Osborne as 'the angry young man.' It didn't seem to me to be much of a play. It is about a vaudeville entertainer played by Laurence Olivier who is entirely no good. Laurence Olivier is always a splendid actor but it seemed to me that he was wasting his talents on *The Entertainer.*"

On 26 February 1958, Margaret and Charley flew to Caracas, Venezuela, for a week of meetings, despite recent political disruption. Richard Bower, the Canadian ambassador, and his wife, Barbara, were present at the convocation of the University of Caracas when Best received an honorary degree. CHB was particularly impressed by the work at the brain institute, under Dr. Marcel Roche.

Back in Toronto, "We had Sandy and Eileen for dinner — and Sandy told us that he and Eileen are planning to be married at the end of May or first of June 1958. We were all very thrilled. She is a dear, beautiful girl. It was an exciting day for the Best family. Henry opened a bottle of sparkling cider from St-Benoît-du-Lac last night at dinner time and we drank to Eileen and Sandy's health."

The Conservative nomination meeting took place in Milton on 14 February 1958 for the federal election called for 31 March. Sandy's parents were there, and Henry flew back from Québec. Eileen Thompson was sitting beside Margaret, and when there was a request for someone to play "God Save the Queen," she went forward. The meeting chose Sandy, standing unopposed, as candidate. Sandy and Henry flew to Sudbury and to the riding of Algoma East to speak — one in English, the other in French — for Basil Scully, the Tory candidate in Lester Pearson's riding. In February, Sidney Smith, ex-president of the University of Toronto, now secretary of state for external affairs, offered Henry the post of executive assistant; Henry was to go to Ottawa after working for Sandy's re-election. On 31 March 1958, Margaret and Charley once again proudly joined Sandy's victory cavalcade through Georgetown, Glen Williams, Acton, Milton, and Oakville. The Conservatives had won a massive majority, taking many seats in Québec for the first time in thirty years.

Since Sandy was living at the Stewarttown farm — first called Strawberry Hill, but renamed Greenock Farm — Margaret and Charley had been looking for a place for themselves nearby. Nassagaweya Township, in northwest Halton County, provided undulating land, old stone houses, and fairly reasonable prices. "I believe that we own another farm — the Moffat one in Nassagaweya — the one with a big square Georgian stone house. I have only seen it once. It is a very nice house and something could be made of it. I think it is in my name." said Margaret.

Eileen's parents, Mr. and Mrs. Arthur Thompson, came to Greenock Farm for dinner. Margaret wrote, "Her parents are very Irish and I could scarcely understand them." The parents, unfortunately, had very little in common, and Margaret Best never developed a rapport with Margaret Thompson. Eileen was soon busy with Sandy's business. He had bought her a Jaguar, several years old, and it was fine when the brakes worked. He decided to join the Presbyterian church formally before their wedding.

Sandy and Eileen's upcoming wedding day brought many showers and other parties. Margaret helped Eileen pick Sandy's *speciosum rubrum* lilies for her bouquet. Margaret and Henry went to Jensen's and bought cuff-links as gifts for the ushers: Dal Browne, a friend from Montréal; Wally Nesbitt, MP for Oxford; John Pallett, MP for Peel; Ted Pengelly, a biologist; and Billy Thompson, Eileen's brother. Gisela Wenke, Eileen's maid of honour, was very busy, as was Henry Best, as Sandy's best man. The service took place on 6 June 1958 in Knox College Chapel at the University of Toronto with the reception in the college's library. Dr. John McNab, editor of the *Presbyterian Record* and newly elected moderator of the Presbyterian Church of Canada, performed the ceremony. "Dr. McNab made the service very simple and dignified. Eileen was wearing a pearl necklace and pearl earrings that Sandy had given her. At the reception Dr. McNab proposed the toast to the bride. Sandy responded, talking of Eileen's ability to ride horseback, drive a car, and fly a plane. He said that it was not hard for her to like lilies, but pigs might prove more of a problem." In addition to raising lilies Sandy had just embarked on a new venture buying an additional farm to raise Landrace pigs.

On 11 June, Margaret and Charley sailed from New York for Southhampton and ten days in England. CHB lectured several times and chaired a day-long session on ageing at the Ciba Foundation. He and Margaret saw the Dales, Lawrences, and Cousin Mary Scott as well as Marguerite Hoet, Pierre, and Anne Marie, who visited from Belgium. They spent a weekend at Clopton, Northants, on the farm of Ian Winterbottom — a stock-breeder friend of Sandy's.

On their return, during the Bests' annual stay in Maine, Eleanor Mahar Hurst, whom Charley had known all his life, sold them some land on the shore near Haycock Harbour for $500. "Margaret's Cove" was two to three acres and had four hundred feet of ocean frontage. Eleanor said that she was very appreciative of all that Dr. and Mrs. Herbert Best had done for her family. Margaret gave her a kiss. "I kissed Charley once," Eleanor said playfully, "playing post office at a party of Styles Bridges." Charley took a copy of his *Selected Papers* to Dr. Hurst, Eleanor's husband. Margaret noted in her diary, "Everytime I write in this book I think, 'Well, surely there won't be anything more to write about this trip,' but there always is — something fascinating seems to happen every day."

At the end of September 1958, Henry Best and his parents were all in New York. Henry, Tom Delworth (Sidney Smith's departmental executive assistant) and Lois McIntosh (the minister's private secretary), all at the United Nations, joined the Bests at a reception and dinner given by Charles Pfizer and Company at the Hotel Pierre. In an interview at a TV studio, Charley had to sum up a whole series of meetings. "He has had to work awfully hard. I don't like it. It has been a conference on a new oral drug for diabetics. It was under the auspices of the New York Academy of Sciences and all arranged by the Pfizer Company."

When they returned to Toronto, Sandy announced very happy news, that Eileen was to have a baby. Margaret and Charley went to see the film made by Leslie McFarlane of the National Film Board on the discovery of insulin: *The Quest,* starring Dennis Stanway as Charley and Leo Ciceri as Fred Banting. McFarlane had been in correspondence with CHB for several years about the content of this film.[668]

At the installation lunch for Claude Bissell as president of the University of Toronto, the Bests were hosts at one table. Brough Macpherson, the outspoken professor of political science, who thought Margaret scintillating, said, "They put you at this table instead of giving us drinks." At the installation ceremony, Mgr. Irenée Lussier, recteur of the Université de Montréal, received one of three honorary degrees conferred that day. "Dr. Lussier said that when he went to Paris to the Sorbonne and heard them talking about Dr. Banting and Dr. Best, he was proud to be a Canadian. From that moment he forgot that he was from Montréal."

Margaret finished diary number fifty-one with a quotation from Malcolm Lowry's *Under the Volcano* from Sophocles' *Antigone:* "'Only against Death shall he call for aid in vain, but from baffling maladies he hath devised escapes.' It might be a good quotation for Charley to use."

Within a few months, there was evidence of trouble in Sandy and Eileen's marriage. Sandy was in Ottawa much of the time and when he was at home the newlyweds were rarely alone. Before the Nassagaweya farmhouse was ready, every weekend, Margaret, Charley, and Linda arrived to stay at Greenock Farm. In Toronto on New Year's eve, Eileen asked Sandy to go to church with her. When he refused, she went alone to Yorkminster Baptist Church, much to the consternation of Margaret and Linda. Eileen felt that her marriage was off to a miserable start and that she was lost in the shuffle. CHB later said to her, "You have your faith. I think maybe we should have gone to church more instead of always going to the farm. Sandy had no faith. He was not comfortable with religion or church."[669]

On 20 February 1959, Charles Stewart Best, Margaret and Charley's first grandchild, was born. Don van Wyck, Eileen's obstetrician and son of Margaret's obstetrician, H.B. van Wyck, came to inform them, singing "Bonnie Prince Charley." Sandy was in Ottawa on a very crucial day for the Diefenbaker government: cancellation of the Avro Arrow jet project. The baby might well have been called Charles "Arrow" Best. Henry pulled a few strings and got Sandy on a plane for Toronto that evening so he arrived at the Toronto General Hospital in the middle of the night.

Margaret and Charley were elated by little Charley's arrival. They were overjoyed by the birth of their first grandchild. On his sixtieth birthday a week later, Charley, speaking after a dinner in Indianapolis given by Lilly's, said that his birthday had been rather overshadowed by another — that of his grandson. Knowing full well the answer, one of his friends called out "What's his name?"

To Eileen's relief, after months of having them come to Greenock Farm every weekend, the Bests slept for the first time on 14 March at their new Londonderry Farm, "the big square Georgian stone house." It was in Nassagawega Township, Halton County, nine miles west of Greenock Farm. They named the hundred acres for the city in Ireland, whence the Mahon family had sailed in 1761, and the settlement in the district of Nova Scotia where they were pioneers.

The house was solid stone, a full two stories high, with a rubble-stone coach house attached, with double doors in front and back so that a team of horses could be driven through. There was a large fireplace in the coach house for boiling maple syrup or making soap. There had been a bell on the roof for summoning the men in case of emergency or for meals, but it had disappeared, and Charley later found one to replace it. The interior of the house consisted of a large kitchen with a fireplace, a parlour with finer woodwork, and a series of three small rooms at the back, including a "tramp's room" for itinerants. Off the parlour was a grandmother's bedroom, rather like the one in the house in Maine. Upstairs were four bedrooms, one of which they converted into a bathroom. There was no running water, septic system, or heat. The large bank barn, typical of Ontario farms, was quite a distance away, near where the original log house had been built.

By early spring, Margaret was able to find many wildflowers at Londonderry Farm: wake robins, red trilliums, yellow, white, and dog-toothed violets, Dutchmen's breeches, bloodroot, hepaticas, and Jack-in-the-pulpits. Every weekend friends arrived for a meal, and Linda was always busy in the kitchen. Sandy had bought another farm for the pigs, but he also did a lot of work on his parents' new place, planting perennials and getting the fields in shape.

On 17 March 1959, Sandy called his parents to say that Sidney Smith had just died. Smith had returned to Ottawa from a short trip, gone to his apartment for a rest, and had died peacefully there. A short time later Mrs. Smith found him. The state funeral was in Ottawa two days later, and the minister was buried in Windsor, Nova Scotia. The Best family knew that Henry, aside from losing the man for whom he worked, had also lost an important mentor and friend, someone for whom he had great affection. Henry was also very fond of Mrs. Smith, and he helped her move to Toronto. She gave Henry an upholstered chesterfield and chair, and said, "Those were the first pieces of furniture Sid and I bought."

Hoechst and Upjohns pharmaceutical companies were sponsoring in Atlantic City a meeting on oral treatments of diabetes. Drs. Otto and Anka Sirek, Gerry Wrenshall, and Bernie Leibel from the lab were there as well as the Bests. When Margaret called home, Linda told her that Dochet, her poodle, had been in a fashion show at the Royal York Hotel and had lifted his leg and wet on a bush on stage — the audience laughed for five minutes.

On 12 June 1959, Margaret and Charley Best left Toronto for Montréal and the Cunard liner R.M.S. *Sylvania* for Britain. In London, Dr. James Liston, the permanent secretary to the minister of health, took the Bests to lunch at Lord's cricket ground to talk about a television show about diabetes with CHB and Robin Lawrence.

On 23 June, Charles Best received the first Dale Medal of the British Society for Endocrinology and spoke on "A Canadian Trail of Medical Research."[670] Frank Young moved the vote of thanks after Charley's talk. Sir Henry and Lady Dale were both there; the Hoets had come from Belgium, bearing news of three engagements in their family. The *conversazione* of the Royal Society was always a gala and formal occasion — white tie, long dresses, and decorations — Best had his CBE around his neck and his row of miniatures. For the Bests, it was a reunion of old friends: the Dales, Drurys, Haringtons, Hills, Himsworths, Lady Mellanby, the Peters, and the Todds. Another occasion in London was the celebration of the tenth anniversary of the Ciba Foundation for the Promotion of International Cooperation in Medical and Chemical Research. To the Ciba dinner, Best wore his Pontifical Academy chain.

One evening the Bests went to the Mermaid Theatre to see *Lock Up Your Daughters,* a new and very successful musical adapted from Henry Fielding's *Rape Upon Rape.* Seated nearby were Garfield Weston, his wife, Reta, and two of their daughters. "Charley used to ride with Garfield years ago at Woodbridge. They invited us to have lunch at Fortnum and Mason's.[671] It was great fun. We went up to the top of the store and were shown into a most beautiful boardroom where we all four had drinks. Then we went into another room for lunch — a wonderful dining room with a round table for four." Weston said to Best, "If you ever want a different sort of holiday, Charley, I will loan you my Chinese junk which is in the Mediterranean. I brought it from Hong Kong. It is equipped with a motor as well as sails."

The next day, Margaret and Charley went to the Dominion Day reception at Lancaster House to be presented to the Queen Mother. "We stood beside Lord Beaverbrook ... We talked about New Brunswick. When he heard that my father was a Presbyterian minister, he said, 'We have a lot in common.' He knows Nellie Mowat, Lucy Jarvis. He takes a real interest in New Brunswick." The Queen Mother "knew all about us and she murmured about the great work that Charley had done."

One evening, George and Alison Ignatieff took the Bests to a party. He was the deputy high commissioner at Canada House, and Alison's grandfather, later Principal Grant of Queen's University, had married Margaret's Macleod grandparents in Prince Edward Island. Later at Canada House, George and Fiorenza Drew and the Ignatieffs told the astonished Bests that the London *Evening Standard* had an article about Sandy flying over with spikes of his own blooms to the Royal Horticultural Society's Lily Show, and winning the Lindley Medal. He wanted to keep some for a few days to show at a dinner of neurosurgeons and neurologists at Claridge's, where he was to speak at the invitation of Dr. Allan Walters of Toronto.

On 17 July, the Bests left London for Edinburgh to attend the joint meeting of the British and the Canadian Medical Associations. On 22 July

1959 Margaret and Charley went to McEwan Hall of the University of Edinburgh for the conferring of honorary doctorates of law on Best, Adrian, and Penfield, among others. "Then Adrian spoke — I always love to hear Adrian speak — he was wearing, as always, his little half glasses with the steel rims. Then Wilder Penfield spoke and told about the story of McGill University. Hester Adrian said to me later, 'How wonderful that three such great friends, Charley, Wilder and Adrian should have been on the same platform together and received degrees in one ceremony.'"

Most of the speeches that Charles Best gave, or articles that he wrote, were strictly scientific, or about the history of insulin, heparin, or choline, but occasionally he spoke in a more philosophical way. At Northwestern University, near Chicago, he received an honorary degree in September 1959, and spoke on "Unfinished Researches." He talked of areas of experimentation in which he had worked where there was more work to do. He concluded, "The measure of success which was granted me at the beginning of my career may account in part for the fact that I have always been, and continue to be, most optimistic in attacking research problems. We physiologists and biochemists feel that substances found in tissues must serve some interesting purpose. We feel that 'man's inability to comprehend' is our limiting factor, and not 'Nature's unwillingness to reveal.'"[672]

At home, Garnet Lunny of the National Film Board visited the Best Institute to take pictures of Best. He came to Londonderry Farm and took one of the most frequently reproduced pictures ever taken of him, sitting in an old rocking chair with young Charles Stewart standing on his lap.

In November, Sandy had taken some of his Landrace pigs to the Royal Winter Fair in Toronto. He won a prize for the grand champion boar and the highest number of points for any Landrace breeder in the show. The next day one hundred people went to the farm for an auction of pigs. In a short time Sandy had risen to the top of this field. He became the president of the Canadian Landrace Association. However, as in other ventures before and after, he soon lost interest. Nothing ever would succeed fast enough for him. If he had had considerable capital behind him, perhaps it might have been different. Certainly, Eileen gave him all the support that a wife possibly could and the rest of the family helped in many ways.

Yousuf Karsh's *Portraits of Greatness*[673] included several Canadians. Karsh had taken photographs of Best several years before but had refused to send him the proofs, saying later that he knew his subject was unwell. Shortly afterwards Best had had a heart attack. For the photos that he used in the book, the photographer followed his subject around for a day in the lab; Professor Gerald Wrenshall spent part of the day photographing Karsh taking pictures of Best. The eminent photographer had sent ahead a list of questions to his subject. One was: "As director of a research department, what role do you play in the work? Do you make assignments and suggestions or just supervise the work in progress?" Best's reply was: "Chance often plays a role in research but usually alert and well-trained people recognize the opportunity. As a director I sometimes just advise when asked. In other cases I suggest problems, supervise work and when possible participate. Up to the time of the war I was a very active participant." Another query was: "What would you say is the most important contribution that has been made to medical knowledge in the last ten years?" The reply was: "The chemical basis of heredity."[674] Marsh Jeanneret, the head of the University of Toronto Press, made a tape of Karsh, Leonard Brockington, Floyd Chalmers, Chancellor Jeanneret, and Best talking about the book.

Best had promised to do a broadcast for young people for Shell Oil with Leonard Bernstein, conductor of the New York Philharmonic, and Margaret bought a copy of his new book, *The Joy of Music*. Charley read the volume so that he could mention it in his talk. The Shell show, on 26 March 1960, was broadcast from Carnegie Hall, New York City, with first Leonard Bernstein and the New York Philharmonic, and then "Best speaking on the problems of feeding the world. It was a splendid hour. Bernstein had young people performing — two young conductors, a very young violinist and a boy cellist."

A social visit turned into one of the most important occasions in Margaret and Charley's lives. On 1 April 1960, Garfield and Reta Weston, whom the Bests had seen recently in London, came for tea with their daughter, Barbara Mitchell, and her small son called after his grandfather.

Margaret described the occasion: "Garfield and Charley sat on one side of the room and talked while we (the ladies) sat on the other side but near to them and talked. Garfield had intimated to Charley that he wanted to do something to help his research. Pretty soon Garfield got up and came across and said 'Margaret, I have just given Charley a million dollars.' He said, 'No one has anything to say about this but Reta and I. We are the sole trustees.'" Their lawyer would prepare the documents. "He wanted everything done just as Charley wants it. Charley had contemplated for some little time setting up something to endow the Banting and Best Department and then along came this generous and thrilling gift."

Many people as they age become concerned that what they have built will not carry on after they are gone. This was certainly true of Charles Best, and the Weston Fund would go a long way to achieving his aims. "There was quite a lot of hugging and kissing in the end. Reta said to me 'Charley deserves it. He is a wonderful man. He has done so much for Canada.' I said, 'They are both wonderful men — each in his own field.' Reta said, 'Yes they are, Margaret' and her eyes were filled with tears."

Also in early April 1960, Anka Sirek passed her PhD orals in physiology. Otakar, or Otto, and Anka, or Anna, Sirek had both graduated in medicine from the University of Komenius in Bratislavia, Czechoslovakia. Best had read a paper by Otto on choline, written while working in Sweden, and invited them to Toronto. Otto received his PhD in physiology in 1954. Anka was working at the Hospital for Sick Children with the cardiovascular team of Drs. Bill Mustard and Laurie Chute and wanted to practise medicine. Because she had a child she had great difficulty gaining accreditation with the medical authorities, who told her to go home and look after her family. Best suggested that she work at the Best Institute. The Sireks worked in the same lab and published over eighty scientific papers. In a profile written for *Prime Mentors of Canada* in 1990, Anka recalled, "Dr. Best offered me the support and encouragement I needed to dare to combine a scientific career with raising a family … Dr. Best's approach was to allow great freedom. The atmosphere was exciting and stimulating and I was always given fair credit for my contributions to the work that went on in his lab."[675]

A rare occasion requiring formal attire arose at the state dinner in Toronto on 21 April for President and Mme Charles de Gaulle. The Bests had been invited to go early to be presented. When Best shook hands with the general, he said, "I am very honoured, sir." General de Gaulle responded in English, "I know your work, Dr. Best, and I am very honoured to meet you."

As spring approached, Sandy and Eileen had a great deal to do on the farm. Lily orders for the United States were taken to Buffalo to be forwarded. Twenty- five Landrace pigs were shipped to Roumania. Her father-in-law did not approve of the fact that Eileen did so much work with the pigs. Some of them were very large and heavy, and he was concerned that she might be injured. While Sandy was in Ottawa, Eileen's hands were more than full, not only with the practical sides of the lily and pig businesses and all the secretarial and book-keeping duties associated with them, but also the time-consuming requests from the constituency, to say nothing of an active one year old.[676]

On 17 June 1960, Margaret and Charley flew from Toronto to London economy fare and thought it worth the $200 saved on each ticket. Ciba House had become a second home to them. At Burlington House, Charley presented the official congratulatory message from the University of Toronto on the tercentenary of the Royal Society.

That evening the Bests took Joseph and Marguerite Hoet, who were in London for other meetings, to dinner at the Athenaeum Club. The next day, they went to the Parliament Buildings for tea with members of the Parliamentary Scientific Committee. They did not know who their host was. "Our host said to Charley, 'Don't leave us alone. There is no telling what we would be up to.'" Margaret noted, "He and I were becoming very good friends. I said, 'But, you don't wear your name and I don't know what it is.' Then we learned that he was Herbert Morrison," recently elevated to the House of Lords after many years as a Labour minister in the Commons. He was the president of the Parliamentary Scientific Committee. At a University of Toronto dinner at Hammersmith Postgraduate Hospital, Lord Coleraine proposed the toast to the University of Toronto, and Best replied. One speaker said that Best would be immortal, and Cousin Mary Scott "applauded madly." One has to allow for a certain degree of family bias.

The Dales joined the Bests for dinner at Bentley's. "Lady Dale is truly remarkable. She sees very little and carries a white cane. It is very hard for her to walk. Sir Henry is quite bent but both of them were in gay, happy spirits and we had a wonderful time — sherry, then smoked salmon, then sole Bentley (which is delectable) and a bottle of Liebfraumilch. I have a beautiful letter from Lady Dale, written in her own hand, since we dined together. After dinner we all four went on to the Royal Society conversazione at Burlington House. Lady Dale was wearing a long red dress and her necklace of rubies. Sir Henry said that during the war he turned in all his gold medals and bought that necklace for Lady Dale."

On their only Sunday in England, Margaret and Charley went to see Robin and Anne Lawrence. Robin was much better than the previous year and was regularly seeing patients. That afternoon a special train took the delegates to Glyndebourne to see Mozart's *Don Giovanni*. "It was superb. An Australian girl had one of the main parts — Joan Sutherland. She is very big — long face but a grand voice."

367

After a short visit to Cambridge, Garfield and Reta Weston invited the Bests again to lunch at Fortnum and Mason's. Scotch salmon and lobster were on the menu. That evening, the Tercentenary Banquet of the Royal Society took place in Grosvenor House — 1,300 guests — another full-dress affair. Prime Minister Harold Macmillan, Lord Adrian, Principal Cyril James of McGill University, and Professor Hugo Theorell, director of the Nobel Medical Institute's department of biochemistry, were the speakers.

The next day, Charley went to hear Bernardo Houssay give the second Dale Lecture of the British Endocrine Society, "An Argentinian Trail of Hypophysical Research." Best had given the inaugural lecture the previous year. "Sir Charles Dodds introduced Dr. Houssay and said very nice things about him. He also said that everyone in the audience must be stimulated to have two such giants in endocrinology present as Dr. Houssay and Dr. Best."

It had been difficult for Charley not to speak publicly about the Westons' generous gift, but on 28 October President Claude Bissell announced the formation of the Charles H. Best Foundation and the presentation of the Weston cheque for one million dollars. All three Toronto papers provided detailed reports. One said, "Dr. Best's foundation is in charge of all medical research at the university." Margaret commented, "That would not be happily received by everybody." Some people even thought that the money went to Best personally.

After a month in Maine, the Bests and Linda left on 2 November 1960 for six weeks in Europe and Israel. Linda wrote regularly in her lively and amusing style to Jessie Ridout at the Best Institute. Dr. Ridout carefully kept these missives under the heading "Dear Jessie."

The first stop was Lisbon where the Bests found a large welcoming committee from the medical school, including the president of the Society for the Protection of Poor Diabetics (the oldest diabetic society in the world), Dr. Pedro (Peter) Lisboa, who was to act as the "liaison officer," and several photographers. Linda was impressed by the reception. "I can see that travelling with the Bests is going to be quite different from slipping in and out of countries under my own steam."[677]

The Canadian ambassador, Dr. Philippe Panneton, author of *Trente arpents* under the pseudonym "Ringuet," was an interesting host. On their first evening in Lisbon Margaret tripped on a rug in the hotel and broke her right wrist. A senior surgeon set it the next morning. The next stop was Madrid where Ambassador Jean Bruchési, the author and ex-senior Québec government official, entertained the visitors. It was their first time in Spain and the Prado with its works by Goya and Velázquez was just as impressive as they had expected.

Margaret's arm had to be re-broken and set. The surgeon at the San Francisco hospital found that an operating room was available only when the sister in charge was informed that Charles Best was a member of the Pontifical Academy of Sciences. Margaret is reported as saying that the operating room was full of people to "see the fun."

The next stop was Rome. The time there was very short but Margaret and Charley wanted Linda to see as much as possible. The Pontifical Academy sent a car and driver to take them to Vatican City — the beautiful Academy building and the Sistine Chapel. Linda was amused that everyone bowed to Best saying, "Excellency, whatever you wish." She signed that letter, "Celestially yours."

Then came Athens. Margaret and Linda, being minister's daughters, were delighted to see the Market Place in old Corinth where St. Paul spoke to the Corinthians. Those who made the visit to Greece so happy were referred to as "friends of John's," meaning relatives or friends of Dr. Logothetopoulos who had been a professor in the Banting and Best Department of Medical Research since 1956, and, with his wife, Ismene, had done so much to arrange matters in advance.

The flight from Athens to Tel Aviv was delayed overnight due to mechanical problems. On their arrival in Israel on 17 November, the Bests were met by a car and driver to take them to Jerusalem. Max Rosenfeld, previously in Toronto, was very much in attendance. Itzhak Ben-Zvi, the elderly president of Israel, received the Canadian visitors, and he and Charley had an animated discussion about Israel.

Aside from many medical people, the Canadians met other people of interest. Abba Eban, the minister of education and culture, formerly Israel's first ambassador to the United States and to the United Nations, entertained the visitors to lunch. He and Charley talked about many things, including golf. Best's major lecture to the Hadassah Medical School was a great success. Charley, Margaret, and Linda had a four-day tour of the country. All Christians have a picture in their minds of Nazareth and many are disturbed by what they find. Linda was disconcerted, "The cave where Mary lived and where, according to tradition, the angel appeared to tell her that she would give birth to Jesus, is a simple cave on the outside but, as one goes down underground, one finds not one but three altars, most elaborate, made of marble brought from Italy. You

369

can hardly see the little cave. Somehow it spoiled it for me and it did not seem real. I think it's better to have one's own idea of where Mary lived and how she lived — more satisfying somehow."

They spent the night at the Galei Kinnereth Hotel in Tiberias, waking with delight the following morning to the sound of waves of the Sea of Galilee breaking below their window. In Haifa, Margaret got in touch with Mary Maxwell Rabbani, the widow of the leader of the Baha'i faith. She was a cousin of the Maxwell brothers, architects in Montréal and St. Andrews. Her husband was the grandson of the founder the Baha'is. The visitors went to see the shrine and to Mrs. Rabbani's home. "She has quite a regal manner as if she is used to being the 'top one,' and she used very exotic perfume. She has been in Haifa for twenty-four years now and has only been back in Canada twice."

The last evening in Israel, Margaret Meagher, the Canadian ambassador, gave a dinner for the Bests. Our first woman ambassador, Linda described her as, "quiet, poised, and has an extremely pleasant, thoughtful face."

The Bests were certainly pro-Israeli. This is not surprising since their hosts were Jews and the Bests had many Jewish friends in Toronto, in the ADA, and elsewhere.

They then had a short visit to Vienna to see the famous Spanish Riding School and attend a concert of the Vienna Boys Choir and the opera *Fidelio* before flying to Denmark. In Copenhagen they were met by Dr. Hagedorn. "He has Parkinson's disease now, and has lost a great deal of weight, but really looks rosy and well, aside from the trembling. His white sideburns are still magnificent, and he looked as natty and impressive as ever." It was quite a short visit in Copenhagen, but a full schedule. Dr. Hagedorn sent a car to take the Bests to his home at Gentofte. After tea, Best lectured at the hospital. Professor Cai Holten, Head of Medicine at the University of Aarhus, thanked the guest speaker, saying that "he had done more for the cause of peace by going to so many countries than any other kind of ambassador."

Best was one of five scientists invited to give a lecture as part of the Karolinska Institutet's 150th anniversary celebrations in Stockholm in 1960. On 30 November, the Bests were met there by Canadian Ambassador Kingsley Graham and his wife, Eileen. They were old friends of Margaret's from their school days in Toronto. He had been named to Stockholm by Prime Minister John Diefenbaker. Tom Delworth, the first secretary at the embassy, had worked in Sidney Smith's office in Ottawa with Henry.

Margaret and Charley had first met Professor Yngve Zotterman of the Wenner-Gren Centre and his wife Britta in 1926 when he was working in London with Sir Thomas Lewis on "Vascular Reactions of the Skin to Injury."[678] They gave a dinner for their old friends with a wonderful menu: fish soup, rack of reindeer, and a soufflé with cloudberry sauce. There were many toasts and reminiscences of previous meetings.

The Nobel officials and staff of the Karolinska Institutet went to great lengths to welcome the Bests. Dr. Ulf von Euler accompanied them to the Nobel House for a party, given by the staff of the Karolinska Institutet, held in the apartment of the rector, Professor Sten Friberg and his wife, Gudrun. "He is a really handsome smoothie — tall, lean, bald, and quite young." Dr. Axel Wenner-Gren[679] was there with his wife, Marguerite, whom Linda described as, "just as wild as ever, but certainly keeps him eating out of her hand. He seems to think that anything Marguerite says or does is the last word. She has to be seen to be believed. She sort of weaves around in sweeping satin, with a few little old white minks as a cape, and the diamonds one simply couldn't count — bracelets from wrist to elbow, and earrings and rings to match."

On 3 December 1960, the Karolinska Institutet marked its 150th anniversary in Stockholm's city hall. The guests wore evening wear; Best had difficulty tying his white tie — Margaret usually did it, but of course could not because of her broken wrist. A valet was called but no success, and two maids had no better luck. Finally the head waiter succeeded, and Charles Best entered with the procession to the famous Blue Room where the lectures were held. Margaret was seated between Lady Brain of London and Dr. Walter Bauer of Harvard; Sir Russell Brain was also a special lecturer for the event, as was Dr. Bauer. Best's lecture was entitled "Insulin and Some of its Scientific Offspring."[680] Professor Gøran Liljestrand, Secretary of the Nobel Committee on Physiology and Medicine, gave the history of the Karolinska, and Professor Hugo Theorell, also from the Karolinska and a Nobel laureate in 1955, spoke on "Medicine and Chemistry." The guests mounted the stairs to the Gold Room for the banquet. Linda found it "a dazzling sight." The Bests were given seats of honour at the head table, Margaret next to Liljestrand. It was a long evening, lasting seven hours, but very interesting. Margaret and Charley Best were presented to seventy-nine-year-old King Gustav VI Adolf; the Bests had been at the meeting of the Royal Society in London the previous year when he was made a foreign member.

There had been little reference in Linda Mahon's letters to Margaret's arm. She had been having a lot of pain and Charley was determined to have the cast removed. A Swedish surgeon, Dr. Tor Hiertonn,[681] took the cast off and found a large ulcer above her wrist. He replaced the cast, and at least now she did not have the great pain she had been suffering for so long.

Linda described some of the people attending the Nobel Prize ceremony on 10 December. It was a gala occasion at the Concert Hall, with the women in colourful dresses, the men with their decorations, the flags, and bowls of flowers. The Nobel laureates and the members of the committee and foundation took their places on the platform. A blare of trumpets heralded the King and three princesses.

After presentation of the Nobel prizes for physics and chemistry, Sir Frank Macfarlane Burnet of Melbourne and Sir Peter Medawar of London received the prize for physiology or medicine, for their work in immunology. The final presentation was for literature to the great poet Saint-John Perse, (Alexis Léger), a French diplomat resident in the United States. Linda described him as "a slight, grey-haired man with pouches under his eyes."

The banquet was held in the Gold Room of City Hall where once again the Bests were at the long head table. Dr. Axel Wenner-Gren sat next to Margaret Best; a young man from the ministry of education was on her other side and cut up her meat for her. Saint-John Perse's speech seemed to make the greatest impression. "He spoke in French, and while he is difficult to follow even in English, it did not seem to matter as he is a born mesmeriser — his liquid tones almost make the subject matter immaterial." For Best it had been an honour to be one of five scientists invited to speak at the 150th anniversary celebration of the Karolinska Institutet and they all were impressed by the Nobel Prize ceremony. Why did the Nobel officials include Best in these celebrations: was this a consolation prize?

In London, the Ciba Foundation was, as always, comfortable and welcoming. There were no official events and there was time to see old friends and visit old haunts. Liberty's was a favourite stop for scarves and ties, and sometimes for other things, as Linda explained to Jessie: "As we were leaving, whom should we spy, but Charley. He had quite a sheepish look about him, and upon probing, we discovered that he had purchased, of all things, a leather elephant! This is much bigger than the pig and made of lighter leather. Margaret was quite incensed and went off up the street and bought herself a white satin hat she had been hankering after. Quite right too! An elephant — I ask you. He must think he is a Democrat or a

Republican — I can't remember which party is linked with 'eleflunks,' as the boys used to say." The pig he had bought some years before at Liberty's was a great success with Little Charley, so why not an elephant?

Linda concluded, "Before bringing these memoirs to a close, however, I think it is only fitting to show that some of culture's bloom has been rubbed off on this earthly soul and shall quote a few well chosen lines from our Nobel laureate friend, Saint-John Perse."[682] And, so she did!

It had been a long trip — 2 November to 15 December, with many different flights and hotel rooms. Margaret Best did not give up despite her bad arm and the complications therefrom. Once again, the insistence of senior medical people in dealing with situations that they no longer managed regularly led to unnecessary problems.

When they returned to Canada they learned of other health problems in the family. Henry Mahon in Duxbury, Massachusetts had a recurrence of tuberculosis and needed to rest most of the time and take a great deal of medicine. Henry had suffered from "weak lungs" as a boy and had spent a winter in Edmonton with his Uncle Bruce in the hope that the Prairie air would improve his health. At the end of the Second World War he had been in hospital in Washington, DC because of chest problems. Yet, he had won his "letter" for prowess on the track while at Harvard and had played a good game of golf all his life. On a previous visit to Florida a doctor in Delray Beach took x-rays of Margaret Mahon Best and found old TB scars.

Margaret could not use her broken wrist until late February 1961 when she was able to start writing in her diary again. One of her first entries was to record that "Alexander Macdonald Best was born on Jan. 31 at 7.15 in the morning — a Tuesday. I don't think he looks at all like little Charley (who was very blond when we saw him first.) Alexander has brown hair. He is a little beauty — a doll. Eileen has two wonderful babies."[683] There was competition to see which child resembled which side of the family. Margaret decided that Charles Stewart was a "Best in looks" which was quite true. "We haven't quite decided who Alexander is like, but possibly like Eileen — blue eyes and dark hair."

Following the announcement in October 1960 of the Charles H. Best Foundation and the presentation of one million dollars from the Westons, Best referred to an attack early in 1961 on the Banting and Best Department of Medical Research:

My first knowledge of the "attack" came when I received advance notice of certain reactions of Mr. Arthur Kelly, then Chairman of The Insulin Committee. I called on Mr. Kelly at his office and was given a warm reception. I found, however, that he had been briefed, quite incorrectly, by some unknown antagonist of the Banting and Best Department. Mr. Kelly was pleased to learn my interpretation of the history and present position of the department. … When President Sidney Smith was told of this episode, he remarked: "Methinks I see herein the fine Italian hand of Mr. MacFarlane." My old and trusted friend "Mac" first appeared as an open antagonist when I informed him by telephone (I have never discussed this whole matter directly with him) of the Garfield Weston gift.

Mr. Weston wished to set up a foundation outside the University and to have the money used specifically and solely by the Banting and Best Department. Furthermore he, quite independently, arranged that if anything interfered with the activities of the department as described in the University Calendar the money would be transferred to the support of activities outside the University of Toronto. "Mac" was against all this. I was for it. President Bissell gave it his blessing, and this is the way it is. "Mac" had apparently approached the heads of a number of departments in the Medical Faculty. There may have been those who agreed with him. Several heads of departments came to tell me that they did not agree with the Dean. More than one stressed his opinion that the Banting and Best Department would be prized by any university in the world. "Mac" told one of these professors that there was already too much medical research. Just what he meant I do not know. There may be too little first rate teaching. There is certainly not too much first rate research. … Professor Ray Farquharson recently asked Professor Duncan Graham his ideas about the future of the Banting and Best Department of Medical Research. Professor Graham, who knows the whole story of the department as few do, replied in terms which Fred Banting would have approved whole-heartedly, and I certainly do: "The University of Toronto is morally obligated to support the Banting and Best Department of Medical Research in perpetuity." I believe that the department will always, also, be a credit and a help to other sections of our university. My files and the "archives" contain many tributes from world famous investigators to the researches of past and present members of this department.[684]

Following this attack, at meetings of the American Association of Physicians in May 1961, Best was in a room with about fifteen or twenty heads of medicine from different American universities and he told them that he was being pushed around. "I think almost every one of them said, 'Well, Charley, all you have to do is pick the university in this country, and a Banting and Best Department of Medical Research will be created.'"[685]

Dr. Peter Lisboa and his wife, Mary Adelaide, who had been so helpful and hospitable to the Bests and Linda in November when they arrived in Lisbon, were in Toronto at the lab for a month before going to Boston. They named their youngest child "Charley" after Best. Dr. Jack Davidson and his family from Atlanta had been in Toronto for five years. On 6 June he did his PhD oral examination, and Best said that he did as brilliantly as any student he ever heard. This called for drinks at the house and dinner at Lichee Gardens.

Margaret and Charley and Linda were in New York for three days at the end of June for ADA meetings. At the banquet Best spoke on "Forty Years since the Discovery of Insulin." Dr. Rachmiel Levine received the Banting Medal. At one gathering, Linda told how when she was fifteen, she broke her leg, and Fred Banting, using the Mahon kitchen table, put a cast on it. She said, "I can't remember now which leg it was but it is quite a famous leg." Dr. Frank Allan added, "a historic leg."

On 3 July 1961, Margaret and Charley flew to London. They attended meetings of the British Diabetic Association, the Parliamentary Scientific Committee, the Ciba Foundation, and the Imperial Cancer Institute. They saw the Dales and went to performances of the Sadler's Wells and the Leningrad State Ballet, and an all-Liszt concert by Sviatislav Richter at the Albert Hall. Margaret made a brief visit to the National Gallery. "There was no time to make new friends among the pictures, so I went about and saw some of my old friends."

The University of Toronto Press was to publish some of Best's papers from over the years, and that summer of 1961 in Maine, Charley worked in his room in the barn, looking out to Cobscook Falls, writing "bridges" to join the papers chosen for publication. Margaret recorded that one day Charley did all of his "favourite pastimes." "He played golf, painted, drove to the point in his jeep, then went over to Eastport and bought some tinker mackerel and stopped to have fish chowder and blueberry pie."

Best had bought a small Mercury outboard motor to put on the *Sandpiper* — it made short picnic trips much easier. The distance from Toronto and relative isolation made it hard for the younger Bests to get to Maine. Sandy and Eileen were very busy, with children, politics, pigs, lilies, and Sandy's PhD thesis. Henry was writing his PhD thesis, but he and his dog, Luke, arrived on 3 September, his parents' thirty-seventh wedding anniversary, bringing a bas-relief wood sculpture of a boat and a man. Lea Reiber sent an old Bennington bowl as a present, and others, antique china.

The Bests had thought for many years about buying the peninsula between Schooner Cove and Long Cove. Charley had painted it repeatedly, at all times of day and in all weather. He asked his old friend Harold Blackwood to make the arrangements with Earl Ashby, the current owner. He had a weir in Schooner Cove and thus owned the weir rights. Finally, Best agreed to pay $1,400 for the twenty acres, without the weir rights.

They had calls from two of Charley's old teachers. First came Mrs. Alina Bridges, mother of Styles and Ronald, and her daughter Doris. "Charley thinks she was his first teacher." Ronald had died, and they reported that Styles, dean of the American Senate, was quite ill. Doris, also a teacher, talked of her first school at Young's Cove. She had "boarded down" with Frank Mahar. Carrol Fisher, another teacher and his wife, dropped by, and Mrs. Fisher and Margaret compared photos of their "grandbabies."

Back in Toronto, life was full. The long-delayed extension to the Best Institute was now under construction, helped by a grant of $200,000 from the Wellcome Trust; it included a conference room, new labs, and the bridge for a small museum connecting the Best Institute to the Banting. Robert Thom, from Detroit, was in Toronto on behalf of the Parke Davis Company to do a painting of Banting and Best as they were in 1921 for a series on the history of medicine.

When the director of the Ciba Foundation, Dr. Gordon Wolstenholme, and his wife, Dushanka, arrived in Toronto, the Bests entertained them and introduced them to the university's medical people. They had never been to

Ottawa, so the Bests decided to drive them there and then on to Montréal, taking the Québec side of the Ottawa River. "It was one of the most beautiful drives — the colours were magnificent — glorious tapestries of colour on the hillsides. Gordon and Dushanka were ecstatic about it." They enjoyed lunch at the Seigneurie Club. In Montréal the assistant manager of the Ritz showed them to a lovely room with a sitting room, courtesy of the general manager, M. Contit, who was a diabetic. Margaret described him as "very nice, a hand-kissing gentleman."

In mid-October, Charley had two sets of meetings in Ottawa — as an adviser to the Medical Research Council and as chair of the DRB's Advisory Medical Committee. Margaret went to the Parliamentary Library to see Henry, who was searching old newspapers, particularly *La Minerve* of Montréal, for information about Sir George-Etienne Cartier, his PhD thesis subject.

Each year the presentation of the Gairdner Foundation Awards was a special occasion. In 1961, one recipient was Ulf von Euler, the Bests' friend from the University of Stockholm, who stayed with them in Toronto. Margaret Best and Margaret Haist went to the Gairdners' home in Oakville on Lake Ontario to a lunch for wives of the recipients, and Charley attended the awards dinner at the Royal York Hotel. The next morning Best chaired the meeting where the recipients each spoke. The Bests then took von Euler to the Royal Winter Fair, where they saw Sandy escorting an enormous Landrace pig to its pen.

On 20 November 1961, the Toronto Diabetes Association held a meeting at the Best Institute to celebrate the fortieth anniversary of the discovery of insulin. "Charley spoke first — a splendid talk — then Walter Campbell and Almon Fletcher spoke — the first two clinicians to use insulin. It was quite an historic meeting. I was glad to be there." For Christmas 1961 the Canadian Diabetes Association made a card of Best's *Wind in the Pines*, painted at Greenock Farm (the old Strawberry Hill); the family later gave the original to the Best Institute to hang in the entrance hall alongside one of Banting's paintings.[686]

Fortieth-anniversary celebrations for insulin also took place in New York. The Bests asked Eileen to go with them to give her a break from the lilies and pigs and political meetings. She was not sure if she could go until the last minute, but she was able to arrange for little Charley and Alexander to stay with her parents. Eileen was then able to join Margaret and Charley on the overnight train to New York where they stayed at the

Hotel Pierre. The first night, 30 November 1961, there was a party for Margaret's sixty-first birthday. Then they went to *The Sound of Music*, starring the von Trapp family, and enjoyed it immensely. Margaret and Eileen went to hear Charley lecture first thing the next morning. At the celebration that evening, all the ADA stalwarts were there, and a number of special guests, such as Billy Talbot, a severe diabetic, and member of the American Davis Cup team. Best received a bronze bust of himself — an excellent likeness by Ruth Lowe Bookman. "Charley made a very nice speech. You could have heard a pin drop and when he finished they all stood up in his honour. Altogether we all had a thrilling time."

The next day, "Eileen, Charley and I went to the Museum of Modern Art to see the Marc Chagall stained-glass windows which will be placed in the Medical School at Jerusalem. They are fascinating, twelve of them, very strong colour — the twelve tribes." On Saturday afternoon they went with Gretchen Graef to the Metropolitan Museum to see the famous new acquisition, Rembrandt's *Aristotle Looking at the Bust of Homer*. "It was wonderful."

Early in 1962, Margaret and Charley went to meetings in several American centres. In Chicago, they were met by reporters, photographers, and officials of the local diabetes association. At their dinner, Ham Richardson, another diabetic Davis Cup tennis player spoke. "He told about learning that he had diabetes when he was fifteen years old and about finding a doctor who said that he could go on playing tennis. He was in the hospital at first and he said it gave a fifteen-year-old boy almost his first chance to think about life. He had his mother bring his tennis racquet to the hospital and he practised backhand in front of a mirror. He said he wanted to thank Charley for his life. It was a most encouraging talk for other diabetics." In his own speech, as on many other occasions, Best managed to work in James DeMille's poem "Fair Maiden of Passamaquoddy." He never said so, but he probably took the title as referring to Margaret, who was born on the shores of Passamaquoddy Bay.

Next came Pasadena, a lovely place for golf, but Best also gave a talk to a group of doctors and another to nine hundred lay diabetics. His topic was "Past, Present and Future of Diabetes and Insulin." When they were in California, Linda called to tell them that Dr. Joslin had died on 28 January 1962. It was the loss of a mentor and great friend going back to 1922.[687]

In March 1962, Margaret made reference to Sandy having financial problems, with "a consultation" at the office of Vincent Price. This was followed by a note about Charley and Morley Sparling meeting regarding

"Sandy's problems." There was also question of selling some of the Emily Carr paintings. The Taylor Farm, which Sandy had bought for the pigs, now belonged to his mother as payment for debts that his parents paid for him.

After a long period Sandy had finished his PhD thesis, and he had his oral examination on 9 April. The oral went very well, but the thesis was sent back to be more compressed. It was exceedingly difficult, despite Eileen's tremendous help in handling his duties as an MP, his farms, and his academic work. Henry had taken a job as a trouble-shooter with Conservative national headquarters for the federal election of 1962 and travelled the country putting out "brush fires." The Diefenbaker train was losing steam.

On 27 April 1962, Sandy Best was nominated by acclamation in Halton County. Margaret and Charley were in the back of the hall. David Walker, minister of public works, was the guest speaker. He told of being at a garden party at Buckingham Palace the previous year and had followed the Bests in the line to be presented. Prince Philip asked, "Who is the greatest Canadian?" Walker replied, "John Diefenbaker." Walker added, however, that he thought that Prince Philip had had Charles Herbert Best in mind.

A photograph from this period, taken for election purposes, showed the grandparents and parents on each side of little Charley. It was later published in a biography of Sandy's godmother, Senator Cairine Wilson. The Bests were frequent visitors to her home in Ottawa, the Manor House in Rockcliffe Park, and to "Clibrig, her home in St. Andrews, New Brunswick, where in 1937 they had celebrated their thirteenth wedding anniversary. She took an active interest in the senior Best's work, attending a luncheon arranged by him to spearhead the establishment of the Canadian Diabetic Association and contributing substantial funds to the Charles H. Best Institute of the University of Toronto."[688]

While in France in June, Margaret and Charley received letters from Linda and Henry about the federal election on 18 June — the election had been close, but after the ballots cast by armed forces members overseas, Sandy lost by ninety-eight votes to the Liberal candidate, Dr. Harry Harley. On their return to Canada, they learned that there had been threatening calls about the children during the campaign. Sandy and Eileen did not tell the police until later, but little Charley had stayed in Toronto with his Great-Aunt Linda, and Alexander with his Grandmother Thompson. Little Charley did not realize that the election was over and happily told people to "vote for Diefenbaker and Sandy Best."[689]

In March 1962, CHB was delighted when four young scientists at the Best Institute sailed through their PhD orals, fulfilling his belief in the value of a combined medical and research training. Jan Blumenstein was a medical graduate from Toronto in 1958 and a research fellow in the Banting and Best from 1954 to 1962. Kenneth Gorman, a diabetic, received his MD from Queen's University, Belfast, in 1956 and did post-graduate work at the Joslin Clinic. John Logothetopoulos, a medical graduate of the University of Athens, became a highly respected and productive scientist. Pierre Potvin, a medical graduate of Laval University, where he later became dean, was an old friend of Henry's. While in Toronto, he lived in the small apartment at 105 Woodlawn.

That summer, following the tradition established at Strawberry Hill, the Bests had a picnic at Londonderry Farm for people from the lab. Hamburgers and fruit pies were the staples. Charley loved having his colleagues and friends relax in the beautiful rolling countryside and admire the 1860 stone house, which Margaret had furnished with old Ontario pine. There were no horses to ride or drive at that point, but visitors walked over the farm and looked at Lou Hanover and the cattle. Jamie Campbell, aged seven, son of Professor James and Mary Campbell, asked Margaret how long they had owned the house. "Then, 'How much did it cost?' When I said it cost quite a lot, he said, 'It must have cost millions.'" Jamie often called Margaret on the phone just to have a little conversation.

On 30 July 1962 the Bests left Toronto for Maine, taking little Charley with them — Alexander was at the Thompsons. Little Charley was happy travelling with his grandparents and Great-Aunt Linda. He made comments like, "I love the rivers, I love the mountains," and would say about a hideous house, "What a nice house," and then would laugh. The wee fellow asked, "What is your name, Grampy?" "Charley Best." "Then I am a Grampy too." When they arrived at Schooner Cove Farm, Winnie Leighton had the house open and the window boxes full of petunias. Little Charley quickly found the barn again and the toys that had belonged to his father and uncle. Grampy had bought a swing and a slide.

Henry, with Luke, arrived from Montréal. An enormous porcupine had been eating the apples under the trees, but something had to be done because of the dog. "Operation Porcupine" went into action, and "my friend Porky," as little Charley called him, was put into a box and taken up to the empty old schoolhouse to "attend classes." The youngster was sorry to see him go but satisfied with the explanation. Predictably, little Charley was the centre of attention wherever he was taken, and understandably resisted any form of discipline when he returned home to his mother. Eileen reminisced: "It was hell to pay when he came back because he'd been spoiled rotten. So, it took a month to get him straightened out, that he wasn't just king of the whole walk, and the sun did not rise and set on Charles Stewart Best!"[690]

On 24 September, Eileen Best had her third child, a girl, Margaret Cairine, named after her two grandmothers, Margaret Best and Margaret Thompson, and her father's godmother, Senator Cairine Wilson. The grandparents went immediately to see the new arrival. "She is a pet — brown hair. Her eyes were closed. They are nicely spaced and I saw one precious little ear." On 1 October there was a family party in honour of the new baby, who was on a couch in the dining room. Grammy Best used dishes belonging to the baby's great-grandmothers Best and Mahon. Little Charley sat, as usual, in his highchair beside big Charley.

Weekends at Londonderry Farm resumed. Sandy and Eileen's boys were often there as well. The two Charleys planted spring bulbs, and Alexander later went around and pulled up all the markers. Another campaign was in progress to complete Sandy's revised PhD thesis.

John Diefenbaker called a federal election, and on 26 October 1962, the Conservative nomination meeting took place in Milton. There was opposition to Sandy in several areas of the county. While he had made good contributions to debates on the importance of medical research, agricultural reforms, and other areas that interested him in the five years he spent as an MP, Sandy had not paid sufficient attention to the day-to-day concerns of his constituents and this was catching up with him. He was always short of money and his financial and family situations were not good, in spite of all Eileen's devotion and hard work. John Pallett from Peel and Hal Jackman from Toronto-Rosedale both supported him by speaking at his nomination. Two others ran against Sandy, but he carried the vote. At the same time lily bulbs were being forwarded to his customers. On 29 October, he received his PhD in botany.

The Bests went to the bar mitzvah of John Alan Rothschild, son of their friends Bud and Sybil, at Holy Blossom Temple. Rabbi Gunther Plaut officiated. "Some of the service was in English and part in Hebrew. At one point the Rabbi said in English, 'The Lord bless you and keep you,' exactly the grace our father always said before a meal," Margaret wrote. Someone said to her, "'You must have found the service very different and unusual,' but I said, 'There were many familiar things.'"

On 6 November 1962, a meeting of Toronto's Academy of Medicine commemorated the fortieth anniversary of the publication of the first clinical paper of insulin. Charley went to a dinner at the University Club as part of the celebrations. Two of Almon Fletcher's daughters entertained the wives at their father's home in Wychwood Park — Mrs. Charles Best, Mrs. Walter Campbell, Mrs. Bert Collip, and Mrs. Wallace Graham. At the Academy, with Dr. Graham as president, "Charley spoke first. He quoted entirely from the first three papers which he and Fred Banting had written alone. It was truly splendid. He showed a few slides" and mentioned all the participants. "Everything was 'taped' that evening so we will be able to hear it again." Bert Collip spoke next. "He has lost many pounds of weight and looks quite different." Margaret did not refer to Collip's speech but he mentioned "the two senior members of the team, Fred Banting and J.J.R. Macleod," but not Best.[691]

"Then came Walter Campbell. He was both erudite and amusing. Then, Almon Fletcher spoke and, of course, we are all very fond of him. Almon and Walter were the first two clinicians to use insulin. A cast had been made of the Frances Loring bust of Fred Banting and also one of the Ruth Lowe Bookman bust of Charley. The Eli Lilly Company had done this." They were presented that evening to Lady Banting and to Charley, respectively, who in turn presented them to the Academy. A few days later the Bests went to Boston for Best to deliver the first Joslin Memorial Lecture.

Like many people in their early sixties, Charles Best did not look forward to retirement. Confident as he was in the abilities of those he had brought along in his two departments, he was only too aware of the difficulties that he had himself experienced, including Dean MacFarlane's attempted takeover early in 1961 of the Banting and Best Department of Medical Research. How would they manage? Would the emphasis on diabetes research remain? He had been head of the Department of Physiology for thirty-five years and of the Banting and Best Department of Medical Research for twenty-one.

He had a meeting with President Claude Bissell who reassured him. In Margaret's words, "He told Charley that while the retiring age is sixty-eight, rules were made to be broken and also that his university could never express its gratitude sufficiently to Charley for remaining in Toronto and keeping productive research activities at a consistently high level." An example of continued activity was Best's appointment as a member of the Advisory Committee on Medical Research to the World Health Organization. This meant an annual meeting in Geneva for four years.

In the midst of Best's own activities came a happy family occasion. Sandy received his PhD at a ceremony in Convocation Hall, wearing the red hood that Linda gave him. His father was on the platform in his London DSc gown. Margaret and Charley were still searching for ways to raise money to deal with Sandy's debts. Ayala Zacks[692] had suggested that if they wanted to sell any of their paintings by Emily Carr they should consult gallery owner Gerald Morris.

On 9 February 1963 while in California, Margaret and Charley received a letter saying that Douglas Harkness and George Hees had resigned from cabinet and that an election had been called for 8 April. There was turmoil in the Conservative Party and much bitterness between the pro- and anti-Diefenbaker forces. Both Sandy and Henry supported a change in leadership.

Vincent Price, the family's trusted friend and adviser, called from Toronto to discuss a number of problems concerning Sandy's affairs. It was quite obvious that his election campaign was not going well. Against the very strong advice of Price and others, Henry had become his brother's campaign manager. He set two conditions: first, no expenditures would be honoured unless he had authorized them in writing; second, all debts from the 1962 election would be settled before any new accounts were paid. There would be enough money to mount a reasonable campaign, but in the event of defeat neither the Halton Riding Association nor Sandy Best personally would be saddled with political debts.

Sandy was in deep trouble and threw all caution to the wind in his personal behaviour. Eileen coped very well with it all — election, business, and family. New figures in Halton politics were very helpful. George and Meredith Kerr were lawyers in Burlington and both graduates of Dalhousie Law School; George was the new Conservative provincial candidate in Halton. Other couples, such as Louis and Lee Keene, provided support as well. The Best family turned out for political gatherings such as a church supper in Campbellville.

Margaret and Charley were aware that Sandy was having a difficult time in his campaign and was being cavalier about it. On 4 April John Diefenbaker was the special guest at a large rally in Hamilton. The Bests watched TV in Toronto as Sandy bounded to the platform to join "The Chief" against whom he had rebelled. On 8 April, the Tories lost many ridings around the country, giving the Liberals a minority government. Sandy lost by 9,742 votes to the Liberal candidate Dr. Harry Harley.

Charley blamed politics for causing all Sandy's personal and financial problems. Henry, however, knew that Sandy admired rich and powerful businessmen who seemed to be able to write their own rules. None of his own enterprises with lilies and pig breeding, modestly successful though they had been, achieved for him the kind of wealth and independence Sandy craved.

In late March, two officers of the Mounted Division of the Toronto Police went to Londonderry Farm to see the two black mares that Sandy had received in payment of a debt. In turn they now belonged to his father. When Henry had tried to buy a retired police horse for his father, he found out that the waiting list was very long, but when he mentioned that they had two black mares — untrained — things began to happen. Shortly after, two large pensioned black mares arrived at the farm, both beautifully trained. Henry and his father got a great deal of pleasure from Lady and Princess. On Easter morning they visited several of the neighbours on horseback.

Margaret and Charley left Toronto on 21 April 1963, for New York, London, and Athens. At the fiftieth-anniversary celebrations of the Rockefeller Foundation in New York, John D. Rockefeller III and U.S. Secretary of State Dean Rusk received the guests, including Det and Helen Bronk, the Glen Kings, Mgr. van Waeyenbergh from Louvain, and Dr. Sten Friberg, rector of the Karolinska Institute. The speakers were J. George Harrar, president of the foundation, Rockefeller, and Rusk.

In Greece on 27 April 1963, Charley received an honorary degree from the Aristotelian University of Thessaloníki. "The Professors all wore black gowns with a pattern of gold braid around the neck and down the front and a medallion picture of St. Demetrius on one side at the top. A gown was placed around Charley's shoulders — there were no hoods — and he was given a blue case holding two parchments. Then Charley was asked to speak and he lectured for about half an hour on 'The History of Insulin.' He had some slides. A woman did a small amount of translating." The next morning Professor Demetrius Valtis took the Bests to see the big military cemetery from the Great War — there had been three Canadian hospitals in the area. Visiting four Byzantine churches, they were especially impressed by the mosaics in the oldest — St. George's. "There is a ring of saints around the dome inside, set against a glittering golden background."

Back in Athens, Dr. and Mrs. Thomas Doxiadis gave a dinner for the Bests.[693] Dr. and Mrs. Dickinson Richards, old friends from New York, and the Canadian Ambassador and Mrs. Antonio Barrette were there. Dr. Richards had won the Nobel Prize in 1956 for his work in cardiology.

The next morning, Best went to the diabetic centre, directed by Dr. N.S. Papaspyros, a diabetic who had worked with Robin Lawrence in London. The centre had thirty thousand patients on its registry. Best lectured at Dr. Doxiadis' hospital. An elderly doctor came to see Charley — Dr. Cabhadias, who had lived in London during the Second World War and had asked Charley to help Greek children who were without insulin. Best had arranged for insulin to be sent from Canada and distributed by the Greek Red Cross.

On to Beirut, Best gave the opening lecture of the scientific program of the thirteenth Middle East Medical Assembly on "The History and Present Position of Insulin." Sir Wilfrid Sheldon, a distinguished paediatrician from London, spoke on "The Role of the Pediatrician." Charley lectured again the next day and attended other sessions.

On their return to Toronto, they found that Sandy was looking for a job, since he was no longer in politics, had lost interest in lilies, and the pig business was failing. He obtained a post with Trans-Canada Freezers as an agricultural consultant. He then set up his own firm, Alexander Best Associates, specializing in the import and export of beef cattle and semen, especially the "exotic breeds" from Europe.

At the beginning of June, Margaret and Charley went to Mount Pleasant Cemetery and chose a plot. "There is an oak tree beside it. I found it rather trying but I am relieved that it is done. Then Charley took me to the Ports of Call and we had a delicious lunch in the Polynesian Restaurant."

In June in Geneva, Best attended meetings at the Palais des Nations, his first as one of the nineteen members of the World Health Organization's Research Advisory Committee. He and Margaret enjoyed lunch on the balcony of the eighth-floor restaurant of the United Nations building. Mme Albert Renold, wife of the professor of medical research in Geneva and a specialist in diabetes research, took Margaret to her mother's house on Lake Léman, which had a magnificent view of Mont Blanc. Marcel Choffat, manufacturer of Auriole watches at Le-Chaux-de-Fond, took the Bests to dinner; both he and a brother were severe diabetics. A new acquaintance told Margaret that when her boys were young they were given two white mice, which they named "Banting" and "Best."

Other committee members in Geneva were Bernardo Houssay; Sir Harold Himsworth; Chief the Hon. Sir Samuel Manuwa, a graduate of the University of Edinburgh and inspector general of medical services in Nigeria; and Dr. Saul Adler from Israel. Margaret wrote very warmly of Adler, who was "absolutely devoted to Charley."

Margaret had earlier mentioned Sam Lunenfeld, a native of Galt, Ontario, who was very successful in business and now a resident of Switzerland. Dr. Bernard Leibel and Leonard Brockington, CMG, rector of Queen's University and first chairman of the Canadian Broadcasting Corporation, introduced the Lunenfelds to the Bests. In Geneva Sam Lunenfeld came with his Rolls Royce and chauffeur to take them to Montreux and the Palace Hotel. They saw his daughter, Sybil Lunenfeld Kunin, and her family at their chalet high above Montreux. Sam bottled his own wine with authentic-looking labels saying *Château Faute-de-Mieux*, which greatly amused the Bests. Over the next few years in Canada, Europe, and Israel they spent many evenings together. Lunenfeld was very helpful in raising money for research and also with the family's financial problems.

At the beginning of August 1963, the Bests with little Charley went for their annual visit to Schooner Cove. On 8 September, Margaret wrote in her diary that she was very worried about big Charley — the first indication of a major problem: "Charley was not at all well yesterday afternoon and night. He seems better this morning. He had a frightful depression — most unusual for him. We miss Henry."

Little Charley, at four, sensed the situation. "Last evening he sat down at the dining room table and said wisely, 'Sometimes Grammy worries about me and sometimes I worry about Grammy.' He climbed up on Grampy's bed last evening and said, 'I want to have a talk with you Grampy.' Grampy said, 'What do you want to talk about Little Charley?' He replied, 'About tractors, Grampy.'" The next day the little boy helped his grandfather pick up golf balls from the mud flats. Eileen then arrived with Alexander for a short visit. The children were a joy to the grandparents.

At the beginning of October the Bests flew to London for a symposium on diabetes at Ciba's and for meetings of the BDA. They saw many old friends, the Dales, Lawrences, Youngs, and enjoyed receptions, delicious dinners, and of course, the theatre. On October 13 1963 they sailed to New York on the *France*. "After five times crossing the ocean by plane since the end of April, here we are making our sixth crossing by ship — a pleasant and restful change."

The Bests travelled to Washington, DC for the centennial of the National Academy of Sciences, the senior American scientific group of which Best was a foreign member. Many old friends, including Alex Todd and an impressive number of other Nobel laureates, were there. On 22 October, the Academy held a convocation in Constitution Hall. Det

Bronk, the retiring president, and his successor, Dr. Frederick Seitz, professor of physics at the University of Illinois, both spoke, followed by President John F. Kennedy. "He is a very attractive person."

The whole family was stunned a month later when President Kennedy was assassinated on 22 November 1963. Then came the shooting of the assassin. "Those days were violent and dreadful." On 29 November Margaret wrote in her diary, "Tomorrow Winston Churchill will be eighty-nine and I will be sixty-three. Gordon Ross will be sixty four." Gordon Ross, a doctor in California, was a friend from their student days at the University of Toronto who always sent Margaret flowers on her birthday.

In November, Eileen, six months pregnant and now separated from Sandy, had rented a house on Balmoral Avenue close to Woodlawn. Greenock Farm was to be sold. Margaret wrote, "All week we have been helping Eileen to settle in at 40 Balmoral. It is a cozy little house."

Charley went alone late one evening to Eileen's. He was desperately worried about the relationship between Sandy and Eileen and the welfare of the children. Charley told Eileen that she should not take Sandy back as he believed that Sandy had no intention of making their marriage work. He knew how much Eileen had contributed to Sandy's political and farming ventures and admired her loyalty and devotion to the children. He told her that he had advised Sandy to find a job elsewhere, possibly in the cattle business in South America, and he would look after her and the children.[694]

At Londonderry Farm the well had gone dry, as had many others in the area. Henry hauled water in milk cans. He had adopted several of Sandy's dogs, giving one or two away, but keeping three St. Bernards. Whenever possible Henry rode with his father at the farm. He had never ridden as a child as did Sandy, but he really enjoyed it. Looking out the window, little Charley, now aged four, was heard to say, "Those damned guys are very slow." Margaret said, "That sounded a little rude, Charley. Whom did you hear saying that?" He replied, "Uncle Henry."

One day in December, Professor G.S. Morgan of the School of Social Work came to the house. "He brought to Charley a small parachute, the one which pulls out the bigger one. It was the parachute which Fred Banting was wearing when he was killed. It was given to Professor Morgan by Mr. J.P. Hefferman of St. John's West, Newfoundland, who had in some way secured it at the time of the accident. Professor Morgan met this man on a plane. (The man had the parachute with him and when he heard that the professor came from Toronto, he gave him the parachute and asked him to give it to Charley.)" No one seems to know what happened to it.

An organizing committee chaired by Best had been set up for the first meeting of the International Diabetes Federation (IDF) to be held in North America to take place in Toronto in July 1964. Dr. W.R. Feasby, who had started researching and writing a biography of Best in 1957, had been appointed the Executive Secretary. Feasby became ill so Charley telephoned Henry, who was researching his PhD in Ottawa, and asked him to take over at short notice.

On 27 December, Margaret wrote guardedly about Henry's Christmas guest. "Little Janna Ramsay who came for Christmas dinner brought a cyclamen plant." Janna Mairi de Grasse Ramsay, from the island of Islay in Scotland, and a graduate of St. Andrews University, had been working with an international medical congress in Montreal before coming to Toronto in November to work with the fifth IDF Congress.

On New Year's Eve, Margaret and Charley went down Woodlawn Avenue to the Guy Saunders's house — the original "Woodlawn," built by Chancellor William Hume Blake of the university in 1830. On New Year's Day, the Bests gave a party for people at the lab who were away from home — from China, Czechoslovakia, India, Japan, and Yugoslavia, as well as a few Canadians.

Margaret and Charley were writing reminiscences. Margaret recorded, "I have been working on our book. The chapter on my childhood is more or less done and I am working on chapter one, 'The Beginnings.'" Chapter one was about the first of the Best family to come to Nova Scotia. Chapter two was about the Mahons, and chapter three was for the Macleods. "Part of chapter four contains Charley's thoughts."

On February 5, 1964 the Bests flew to San Antonio, Texas. On arrival they were met by Colonel Robert Stonehill, USAF Medical Corps, with a message from Linda that Eileen had had a baby girl, Melinda Jane. Charley gave the Malcolm Grow Memorial Lecture next day to the Medical Corps. They then flew to California where Charley had many meetings and lectures. Margaret received from Linda a "very good picture of Sandy with little Charley, Alexander and Margaret in our living room at 105." Charley, though exhausted, was distracted by his busy schedule; but the pictures reminded him of Sandy and Eileen's problems awaiting them in Toronto.

They both relaxed at Smoke Tree Ranch in Palm springs, with Charley riding, bowling and doing a pastel of the mountains and the desert. When their old friend Gordon Ross from Pasadena suggested more meetings, Margaret insisted that Charley must rest and not take on any more commitments. Charley had a cheerful sixty-fifth birthday party hosted by Leon Koerner of Vancouver, one of many good friends at Smoke Tree.

However, the trip home from Los Angeles was a nightmare. After an early start they flew to Chicago, arriving late due to bad weather, and missing their plane connection to Toronto. It took hours to retrieve their baggage. At the ticket office in Chicago there was again a long wait to get train accommodation. Charley, exhausted and unwell, didn't want to disturb Margaret by discussing his worries about Sandy's problems. But Margaret was disturbed about him. She telephoned Henry at the farm to ask him to meet them the next morning at Union Station, explaining that his father was very depressed.

Naively, Henry thought that seeing his two grandsons would cheer his father up, so he called Eileen and asked her to have little Charley and Alexander ready to go with him to the station. "Grampy" walked right out to Front Street, paying no attention to the boys. "Grammy" was wearing dark glasses, as she usually did when she was very upset, and the boys asked her to take them off. At home, Charley went right to bed. Dr. Farquharson was called. Bill Greenwood came to the house to compare heart records. It was just ten years since Charley had had a series of heart attacks, but he had been monitored regularly since. He was driven to the Medical Arts Building at Bloor and St. George to have chest x-rays.

Two days later Henry took his mother to see Melinda Jane, her new granddaughter. "She was one month old yesterday. She is a splendid baby — nice head, well spaced eyes, ears close to the head, dark hair." Sandy was not living with Eileen, but was in and out. Eileen agreed to go with him to take the children to cheer their grandfather. Margaret hoped that pretending that everything was fine between Sandy and Eileen would make it so. She got out several coats that had belonged to Sandy and Henry to give to the next generation.

Hoping that rest and quiet attention would help Charley come around, Margaret took him on long walks — one to the Isaacs Gallery on Yonge Street and then to the Morris Gallery on Avenue Road, to see if the paintings by Emily Carr that they had put up for sale had attracted any worthwhile interest. They returned home by the bus up the Avenue Road hill. Vin

Price came for a talk, and Ray Farquharson was in several times. Margaret hoped fervently, "My darling Charley. He must get rested and well again." But on 13 March 1964, Charles Best entered St. Michael's Hospital. A few days earlier, he had taken a box of pharmaceutical samples sent to doctors and lined up some that were potentially harmful beside his bed.

After he entered hospital, a letter arrived at the lab from the USAF Medical Corps thanking him for the Grow Memorial Lecture that he had given in San Antonio — contrary to custom, the sponsors would like to invite him back. Linda Mahon showed the letter to Henry, who decided to take it to the hospital, hoping to make his father feel better. Charley had told them that the talk in San Antonio was no good and that he was out of date and unable to keep up with younger scientists, particularly in mathematics and statistics. He read the letter but commented only, "You asked him to write this, didn't you?"

Dr. Aldwyn Stokes, the Oxford-trained professor of psychiatry, was in charge of Charley's treatment. He was an able and careful man, but the family especially relied on Ray Farquharson's wise counsel and comforting support. Farquharson reassured Henry that his father would probably make a complete recovery within two years. Best was administered a series of electric shock treatments. Henry was concerned that shock treatments must be destructive, but no viable alternative was proposed, and gradually the patient seemed to improve.

After three weeks Margaret was encouraged, "It is wonderful to have Charley home again and well. He is not going back to the lab for some time. He does some work at home. Don Clarke came up and went over estimates with Charley. It is the time for the income tax too. Darling Charley, he worked far too hard on that Cincinnati, San Antonio, Los Angeles trip — lectures, lectures. He must never work so hard again. He is sixty-five years old now and must take life more easily. Then he got a virus infection in California and he was really sick when we arrived home. I am not going to write about that. It makes me too unhappy."

Charley may also have had a virus infection, but he was certainly suffering from severe depression. Margaret did not understand his depression any more than she had Dr. Herbert Best's illness. There was a predisposition to depression in the Best family, what Charley called the "Woodworth strain." His two Woodworth grandmothers (first cousins) and both his parents were depressive. Charley was certainly exceedingly distressed by Sandy and Eileen's marital problems, which he felt helpless to do anything

390

about. He was really concerned about the children. Sandy's financial problems were a constant worry. Especially since Margaret and Charley had always been prudent and responsible in managing money themselves, bankruptcy seemed shameful, and Charley refused to consider such a step for his son. The strenuous lecture tour in itself would not have made him ill. But in trying to spare Margaret he bottled up his anxieties.

Linda was acting as "guardian at the gate" at the lab. Some long-time colleagues were permitted to visit Charley but could not raise any issue that might be disturbing. It cannot have been easy for them either, not knowing what the future held for them and for the Institute.

On 18 April, Margaret, Charley, and Linda drove to Londonderry Farm and sat in the sun there. The crocuses were in bloom, and the daffodils in bud. On 23 April, Margaret and Charley went to the lab for an hour. Dick Connelly, executive director of the ADA, and Edwin Gates, a board member, had arrived to meet with Henry Best, Don Clarke, Reg Haist, and Gerry Wrenshall about the Fifth Congress of the International Diabetes Federation that July in Toronto, and went to 105 Woodlawn for a visit.

Margaret recorded, "In the afternoon Charley and I went to see one of his doctors." Another time she spoke of "Doctor D," Dr. Arthur Doyle, chief psychiatrist at St. Michael's Hospital, who administered the electric shock treatments. By early May, Charley was going to the lab for a short while each day. Margaret wrote in her diary, worked on a chapter of their memoirs, and cleaned books, glass, and china. "We go for walks. We have been to the dentist. We are coming along slowly."

At the farm, Charley was able to do a little more each week. One day Henry Best found his father sitting in a chair, holding a book upside down. He went down to the barn, saddled Lady, and led her back and forth on the lawn. After a few minutes, Charley jumped up and said, "What are you doing with my horse?" Henry replied, "If you are not going to exercise her, someone has to." Whereupon his father mounted Lady and rode away up the lane. Margaret was beside herself. Henry ran back to the barn, put a bridle on his mare, Princess, and rode bareback down the gravel side road. About a mile away, he caught up with his father, who was riding along unconcernedly, with one hand in his pocket. When a neighbouring farmer came out to say "Hello," Henry asked him quietly to call his mother and say that everything was fine. Charley's early experience with horses held him in good stead.

Another of Sandy's properties in Nassagaweya Township was sold, which was a relief. Henry's mare, Princess, had a foal; the colt was chestnut, like his Arab sire, and Henry named him Kyrat after Uncle Bruce's horse that went to the First World War. On 23 May, Margaret wrote, "Charley is still not very well but perhaps a little better. His three doctors are most attentive. I can't write about that." She could write that Henry had been at McMaster University to debate with George Grant, the author of *Lament for a Nation*. Henry lost the debate.

Margaret tried to be positive and to encourage Charley to be happy. The Prices were celebrating their fortieth wedding anniversary on 28 May. "That same year on 3 September, Charley and I were married. I wore Ruth's train. I am seriously considering burning my wedding dress veil. I have dusted off boxes for forty years and I feel sure that no one is ever going to wear them again."

Plaintive phrases keep appearing: "We always seem to have problems." As well, Charley complained about the house being either too hot or too cold. Invitations continued to arrive at the lab. On 27 May, a letter came from Cordoba in Argentina wanting the Bests to attend a meeting. They could not accept, but Margaret got out her diary for 1951 and read the section about their visit there.

After having him at home for almost nine weeks, Margaret and Henry took Charley back to St. Michael's Hospital on 2 June. "Perhaps they will be able to conquer the troubles." He had a second series of electric shock treatments. Margaret tired herself out going to the hospital three times a day; the Mahons offered to come, but Margaret suggested that they carry on with their summer plans to go to Schooner Cove Farm and fish for salmon on the Dennys River and come to Toronto when Charley was out of the hospital. The patient was "somewhat better. I hope he may come home soon. He longs to come home and I long to have him."

Encouragement came constantly. Dr. Don Baker, a radiation specialist, and his wife were leaving the lab to go to the Brookhaven National Laboratory in New York City, and he told Margaret how much Charley had meant to him. Many flowers and messages kept arriving. Leon Koerner of Vancouver and Palm Springs sent several dozen red roses.

On 27 June, Sandy took his father home for a few hours. Then Charley went home every day but returned to the hospital each evening. He was able to go out for lunch or dinner. At York Downs, he was amused when a waiter from Swift Current, Saskatchewan, told him that his school was divided into four houses: "Best" House for Charley, "Carman" for poet Bliss Carman, "King" for W.L. Mackenzie King, and "Scott" for skater Barbara Ann Scott.

After five and a half weeks based in hospital, Charley went home again on 10 July. People were beginning to arrive for the IDF Congress, and naturally they expected Charles Best to be there. The Bests, therefore, moved out to Londonderry Farm so that they would *not* be available. Old friends said, "But I am sure that they will want to see us." Terribly distressed special friends such as the Hoets, Robin Lawrence, and Fritz Gerritzen talked to the Bests on the phone. Henry and Lydia Mahon arrived and were a great support to Margaret.

At the congress's opening session, Reg Haist, who had taken over in Best's absence read a message from Charles Best. Toronto Mayor Philip Givens announced that two streets near the university would be renamed for Banting and for Best, but this never happened. At a special university convocation, Joseph Hoet, Robin Lawrence, and Randall Sprague received honorary degrees. Sprague, from the Mayo Clinic and a diabetic for forty-three years, spoke on behalf of the graduands. The university gave a party at the Faculty Club for about seventy-five people. Henry, who had taken over as executive secretary of the congress when Bill Feasby took ill, reported to his parents each evening by phone on the events of the day. Janna Ramsay ran the secretariat and kept the congress on budget. When the congress adjourned, the Mahons returned to Boston, and the Bests prepared for Maine.

On 5 August, Henry drove Margaret, Charley, and Linda to the east coast. The views of Schooner Cove and Cobscook Bay, the flowers and the birds, and the old house gave them great pleasure. Henry and Lydia Mahon paid a visit; again, their kind but practical manner was always very helpful. On the 14 August, Janna, two friends, Sonja Lobe and Yeiko Izumi, and Luke, Henry's yellow Labrador, arrived with Henry's car. He showed his guests the local sights before all four left for Québec and Toronto.

Margaret was very careful about not tiring Charley and accepted few invitations for meals. It was a lovely time of year — cool, clear days and nippy nights. The several small restaurants in the area served excellent food, and almost every day the Bests went to one or another for a meal and usually saw friends or acquaintances. Dr. Herbert Everett was always on call; twice he took Charley to St. Stephen to the Chipman, Dr. Herbert Best's favourite hospital.

Pembroke and Schooner Cove were in Washington County, which was not a prosperous area, and burglaries and vandalism were becoming more common. Empty houses were prime targets, and their contents would end up in antique stores in Massachusetts, impossible to trace. Margaret put all the brown and white china that she had been collecting for years, added to by many gifts, on the dining room table, listed it and photographed it. She did the same with her varied collection of pressed glass. Margaret said that she had packed up the Coalport tea set — her mother-in-law's unusual Canton pattern — to take back to Ontario, adding, "I suspect that I may want to give it for a gift to a relative!"

"The Birthplace" in West Pembroke was now in pretty good shape, and Margaret and Charley went to see the house. Both Charley and his sister Hilda loaned items such as their father's roll-top desk and several pictures, as well as Herbert Best's diplomas: "One is for Doctor of Medicine, University of City of New York, 1896," Margaret wrote, "one is for Operative Surgery and one is a picture of a class, New York Post-Graduate course, 1904."

In late September, the weather was very foggy and dreary, but most important, Charley's health deteriorated. Margaret wrote to Henry: "I wonder how we will get through another week — however, I suppose we will. I am very disappointed that he is not a great deal better now — it is a terrible struggle. … I think he has been more troubled and depressed as the days go on. I phoned H. [Dr. Herbert Everett in St. Stephen] this morning and suggested that … he should go into the hospital again. Henry, it is all heart-breaking after all these weeks. I have tried so desperately hard. You have only to ask Uncle Henry and Aunt Lydia. My darling Charley is very far from well. … You had better phone Dr. Farquharson and tell him Daddy is bound to need help when we get home."[695] Although Margaret never ever mentioned in her diary that Charley was suffering from depression, she knew that was what it was. It was an illness very difficult for her to comprehend.

Sandy, Eileen, and little Charley arrived at Schooner Cove and they all returned together to Toronto — Sandy drove one car, and Eileen, the other. The night they got home, Ray Farquharson came to see Charley, and he soon saw his other doctors as well. Margaret said simply, "He has had three calls since he came home. On the whole they feel that he is better."

Margaret continued to act as if Sandy, Eileen, and the children were still one happy family. Eileen's one-year lease of the Balmoral house was almost up and she had to move. She was having great difficulty in finding another house for herself and her "gang of four," as she referred to them.[696] Eventually she moved to 108 Helena Avenue, which was in very bad shape — Margaret called it "a modest house." Little Charley stayed with his grandparents for a while, and Margaret walked him to and from Brown School on Avenue Road. As often as possible, Eileen and the children spent the weekend with Henry at Londonderry Farm. He stayed there to look after the animals, commuting during the week to Toronto where he had started a job as the assistant to Murray Ross, president of York University. This was a positive event to celebrate on Thanksgiving weekend. Charley, Margaret, Linda, Henry, Janna Ramsay, and Jessie Ridout were at Londonderry. On 9 October 1964, Henry's thirtieth birthday, Margaret and Charley gave him his grandmother's Coalport china, which they had brought back from Maine. Charley started to ride again at the farm as if he had never been ill.

To most people who wanted to see them, Margaret explained that Charley had been very ill, and visitors were tiring for him. She tried to organize easy outings. Charley was playing some golf in Toronto and evidently enjoying it; Margaret thought long walks very beneficial, and they walked all the way to the Art Gallery of Toronto to see the Canaletto exhibition. They had dinner at the new airport at Malton, where the paintings in the restaurant were by Harold Town.

Well-trusted friends were allowed to visit or take Charley out. Sam and Elizabeth Lunenfeld were in Toronto and invited the Bests for dinner with Leonard Brockington and Bernard and Queenie Leibel — Charley did not feel up to going, so Henry went in his place. When the Lunenfelds were back in Toronto later, they came to the house for a drink. A few days later they sent their Rolls Royce and chauffeur, both brought over from Switzerland, and the Bests went for a two-hour drive. MacCharley [Dr. Clarence MacCharles from the DRB] took Charley to lunch at the Military Institute.

In mid-November 1964, Ray Farquharson won the Gold Medal of the Canadian Pharmaceutical Manufacturers' Association on the occasion of its fiftieth anniversary. Physically Charley was well enough to attend the ceremony, but was not able to take part in conversation. Omond and Elizabeth Solandt came for a visit. Omond Solandt recalled, "Reg [Haist] and I noticed that after he became ill, Margaret a little too obviously managed Charley's affairs."[697] Charley liked and respected his former student, and Henry consulted Solandt, Reg Haist, and Laurie Chute about his father's condition.

On 3 November 1964, Professor Aldwyn Stokes, head of psychiatry at the University of Toronto, wrote a letter marked "very private and confidential" to Dr. John Hamilton, dean of medicine, about Best's condition. "His despondency has been profound, associated with a deal of self-blaming, self-doubting and indecisive immobility. There have been times when it has been necessary to appraise suicidal risk. Hospital admission and control have been required. The illness, although prolonged, has been running a usual course and over the last month there has been considerable betterment." The cause of his illness was close to home. "The mistakes and failures unfortunately came from within his own family. He was confronted with a situation in which his good name seemed in jeopardy and his financial resources in danger. With the weight of these events pressing hard upon him, he found himself less able to live up to his professional role and in fact the depression started when on an important lecture tour he found himself unable to match the standards he had set for himself and the standards which other people expected of him. This was not a case of burned out effort but of a threat to himself which he had never previously experienced." Stokes urged that the university provide a very good pension — "generous in the eyes of international observers rather than in relation to the University pension plan" — and an appropriately sizeable role "in the eyes of the many groups interested in Best and what he stands for," in the Banting and Best Department — two matters of importance to Best and to the university.[698]

Sandy's problems and CHB's worries over the well-being of Eileen and the children may have triggered the depression; but those were not the only worries. The future of his departments and his approaching retirement also contributed.

It is interesting to note the differences in interpretation and tone from Dr. Stokes' letter of 1964 with what Dr. Allan Walters said 1981. Walters was a neurologist on the staff of the Faculty of Medicine at Toronto. He was in the first class that Best taught in physiology; his own interest was in neurophysiology, a field that he believed Best underestimated. In London in 1959 Walters had invited Sandy to show and talk about his prize lilies at a meeting of neurologists. He did not know either Best, father or son, well. Walters claimed that Charles Best was "very brilliant, very conceited — knew he was good, wanted to be told he was good, wanted to have his talents used productively at the international level — bright, good-looking, pink-cheeked, with those blue eyes — a happy combination of ambition, ability, brains and applied science." Walters compared Sandy with his father: "They were not manic depressives. With the Bests you got a kind of expansiveness, and then a withdrawing in cycle — 'I'm-not-comfortable-until-I'm- first syndrome.'"[699]

Walters' comments smack of the common Canadian compulsion to cut down the tall poppy. Ken Ferguson, director of the Connaught Laboratories from 1955 to 1972 had known Best since 1929. Ferguson pointed out that Best, with positions of authority, "had access to facilities and finances which were most advantageous ... it was inevitable that Best should be the object of envy and jealousy." Ferguson always enjoyed Best's company and his "genuine sense of humour which was never malicious. ... Selfish ambition was not in my opinion a notable feature of Charley Best's character. With his great authority and ability he clearly felt a responsibility to create what would now be called a 'centre of excellence.' In doing so, he unselfishly advanced the careers of many younger scientists. Many of them, I know, remember him with affection, a tribute seldom accorded to a chief of great egocentricity. My memory of Charley is of a man of great generosity, great interest in other people, and a great sense of responsibility."[700]

Henry called from Montréal on 8 November to announce that he and Janna Ramsay were engaged and would marry between Christmas and New Year. Margaret wrote, "She is a very bright little girl and we are lucky that we will have another lovely daughter-in-law." Janna did not like being called "little"; however, at five foot one, she did look "little" beside Henry's six foot three. Charley was genuinely happy at the news. Margaret, despite her optimistic comments, was unsure. Linda was furious, saying that Henry had no right to do anything of importance when his father was ill. Henry had left the amethysts that he bought in Brazil in 1959 in the family's safe. Margaret wrote, "I handed over to Henry the lovely amethysts which he got in Rio. He will have an engagement ring made for Janna first."

Chapter Eight

Golden Anniversaries, 1964–1978

Freda Ramsay had placed the announcement of Janna and Henry's upcoming wedding in two British papers — the *Scotsman* and the *Times*. Margaret was curious about the wording of the wedding invitations — "'Mrs. Iain Ramsay Yr.' will puzzle some of our friends. Grandmama in London is still alive and she is Mrs. Iain Ramsay. 'Yr.' stands for younger — something new to me."[701] Margaret was planning what to wear to the wedding but was concerned about cost. She bought a hat for half-price at Morgan's. "It is quite lovely but I am afraid I will never wear it again after the wedding. My thrifty half-Scottish nature is troubled by that thought." Henry and Janna bought the marriage licence. "They went to the City Hall and Henry teased the serious woman behind the desk by asking, 'Who pays the five dollars, the bride or the groom?' She looked uncertain. Then Henry said, 'I suppose they usually go Dutch.' Janna joined in the fun — she opened her purse and put down $2.50."

Charley's health was slowly improving. Margaret Best's sixty-fourth birthday took place on 30 November 1964. The previous day, Charley had driven the car for the first time in many weeks, when he, Margaret, and Linda went to Sunday service at Melrose Presbyterian Church, where Eileen was organist. The following week Charley went to the university to talk to Dr. John Hamilton, dean of medicine, about future plans. Dr. David Scott took Charley to the funeral of Dr. Almon Fletcher, one of the first clinicians to use insulin.

There was a Scottish flavour to Janna and Henry's wedding on 28 December 1964, a bright, clear day with no snow but cold enough that the ground was hard and there was no mud. Rev. Wilfred Butcher, previously of St. Andrew's Church in Québec and secretary of the Canadian Council of Churches, officiated. Both Henry and Janna admired his ecumenical views, and his knowledge and understanding of the rapid changes taking place in Québec society. Janna's attendants, dressed in rich red velvet, were Sonja Lobe, with whom she shared an apartment, and Anne Sutherland, a colleague at the IDF Congress. Sandy was best man; his wee boys Charley and Alexander were kilted pages; the ushers were Henry's oldest friend Tony Rolph, Dal Browne from Montréal, Bruce Stewart and Dave Price, classmates from Henry's short career in medicine, and Bill Morrison, also wearing a kilt, a political friend with whom Henry had lived in Ottawa. Eileen played the very difficult little organ. Bill Bitcheno, head of Marconi Canada Limited, who had flown with Janna's father to test radio for planes in the 1930s, escorted the bride.

An informal reception followed at Londonderry Farm. Freda Ramsay had made the wedding cake — a real fruit cake with marzipan and icing; the ushers poured champagne, and Reg Haist, with whom Janna had worked on the IDF congress, gave the toast to the bride. Fortunately, the women of the church had prepared large quantities of robust sandwiches, as, although 150 people had accepted invitations, some brought visiting friends and relatives, thus boosting the numbers to 200. Lieutenant-Governor Keiller MacKay wore his kilt, as did his sons. Margaret wrote, "I have never been to a wedding that went off more smoothly and beautifully. No-one will ever forget it. Charley was wonderful and I know he enjoyed it all." Even Linda seemed happy, despite her displeasure at the timing of the wedding.

After their honeymoon in Québec, where Dr. and Madame Lacerte held a special wedding reception for them, Henry and Janna returned to their Toronto apartment on the top floor of John and Connie Eltons' house on Highland Avenue in Rosedale. Henry was research assistant to Dr. Murray Ross, president of Toronto's new York University; Janna was teaching French and Spanish at Bishop Strachan School. Eileen and the children were staying at Londonderry Farm because the furnace at their new home in Toronto did not function. The farm was a busy place, with all the people, two St. Bernards, a litter of Great Pyrenees puppies, and with Henry, Janna, and dog Luke added on weekends.

Charley continued to worry about the amount of land that the family owned and was relieved when he sold the remaining fifty-eight acres of the Georgetown property. Margaret listed what was left. "This house is our joint property. Londonderry and the Taylor Farm are mine, Schooner Cove is Charley's, and the Best Point Property in Maine is owned jointly by Henry and me. Then Margaret's Cove in Maine belongs to us too!" The last two were small, undeveloped parcels with no buildings.

On 4 February 1965, three weeks before his sixty-sixth birthday, Charles Best received a letter from D.S. Claringbold, secretary of the board of governors, advising him that he had been reappointed professor of physiology and director of the Banting and Best Department of Medical Research. The next day Dean Hamilton wrote to Best that even if he relinquished the chair of physiology his salary would remain the same. On 15 February, Best informed the dean that he would like to retire from physiology as of 1 May.[702]

By the time Charles Best retired as chair of the Department of Physiology, he had held the position since 1929, thirty-six years. Reg Haist succeeded him, which pleased Best. Inevitably, the department's focus changed somewhat, especially towards neurophysiology. Best continued as director of the Banting and Best Department of Medical Research, where Don Clarke was temporarily in charge.

Gradually the Bests life became more normal. Two events drew favourable comment in Margaret's diary. The first was the arrival of the insignia as a knight of the Order of St. Lazarus of Jerusalem. Secondly, in the first week of April 1965, Janna and Henry told his parents that they were expecting a baby. "We were very thrilled. And they both looked so happy."

Both Margaret and Charley continued to be interested in reading and painting. Charley read Hal Borland's *Beyond My Door Step* and Donald Culross Peattie's *Almanac for Moderns*. Margaret was proud of her membership in the Champlain Society, and she, Charley, Henry, and Janna went to a reception for Dr. Kaye Lamb, dominion archivist and retiring president of the society. Margaret had belonged for twenty-one years. She and Charley went to see the Ontario Society of Artists' Show at the Art Gallery of Toronto — "on the whole exceedingly modern. It makes me feel old not to understand what they are trying to do. For instance — a canvas in one colour with three rectangles in different colours on it. Another canvas was white with splashes of different colours down each side — all the rest white. I saw a pretty blonde girl looking at them — perhaps eighteen or twenty years old. I said to her, 'You are young. What do these picture mean to you?' She replied, 'A stomach ache.'"

As Charley's health improved Margaret was more positive about his medical team. "What wonderful doctors he has had!" Dr. Heinz Lehmann, professor of psychiatry at McGill, renowned for his contribution to the field of psychopharmacology, was in Toronto, and the Bests met him in Professor Stokes's office; he spoke first to Charley alone and then to them both together. Margaret found him "very kind, very nice. He told me it had been a great honour and a great privilege to meet my husband. I liked him very much."

On a visit to Montreal, Henry had an appointment with Dr. Wilder Penfield to discuss his father's treatment. At the last minute Sandy wanted to go too. Surprisingly he admitted to Penfield that he had contributed to his father's illness by burdening him with all his problems. Penfield reassured them that their father was getting appropriate treatment and confirmed Dr. Farquharson's view that CHB would recover from the depression.

Margaret and Charley were able to resume some activities. Charley went regularly to the lab for short visits. Dr. Wilhelm Meier of Hoechst Pharmaceuticals in Frankfurt, West Germany, and film producers Dr. and Mrs. Georg Munck were in Toronto in connection with a film — *The History of Diabetes.* Charley said that he would speak briefly at home rather than in a studio. The crew was, as Margaret feared, at the house for five hours. Bill Feasby, as his own health improved, was able to work on his biography of Best again, and Margaret and Charley spent a few days with the Feasbys at their farm in Caledon.

As Charley's health gradually improved, they turned their attention to more normal matters. Margaret was busy looking for various papers that Bill Feasby wanted. Sir Henry Dale sent a much-appreciated letter, and Margaret and Charley replied with congratulations on his ninetieth birthday. Best resigned from all connection with the Defence Research Board in 1965. A letter from Morley Whillans at that time said, "I shall never forget your wise and foreseeing role in setting up our Committees and Panels. We couldn't have done it without you."[703] The DRB had occupied an important place in Charles Best's life for twenty years.

Just as life seemed to be getting better they had a dreadful shock. Ray Farquharson died in Ottawa on 1 June at the young age of sixty-seven. As well as being a professor of medicine and chief of the Toronto General Hospital, he was the first chair of the Medical Research Council of Canada. He was a wonderful friend and counsellor to the Bests and to many others. Margaret Best wrote, "Poor Ena, how dreadful for her. How can we get along without him? Our kind and wonderful friend and physician!" Margaret, who hardly ever went to funerals went with Charley and Henry to the service at St. James the Less Chapel on Parliament Street.

Then Dr. Ed Hall, president of the University of Western Ontario, sent Charley a telegram to say that Bert Collip had died at age seventy-two, on 19 June 1965, and to ask him to attend the funeral. Charley did not feel up to going, but he sat down and wrote Mrs. Collip a letter. He had never forgiven Collip for some of his actions in 1922, and was uncomfortable talking in public about the discovery of insulin when Collip was present, but they had worked harmoniously at the NRC and elsewhere for many years. The relations between Best and Collip were cordial, but they were never friends.

Leonard Brockington was now a part of the Bests' life. He was the first chairman of the Canadian Broadcasting Corporation from 1936 to 1939, special wartime assistant to Prime Minister King in 1940–1, and later rector of Queen's University, and he remained very active, though he was bent over with arthritis. He had a quick wit and wry sense of humour. On one of his infrequent stays in hospital he asked a visitor if he knew what an "ADC-in-Waiting" was? Chuckling he continued, "An Arthritic Diabetic Cardiac, Waiting to get the hell out of here!" His office was Room 200 in Toronto's Lord Simcoe Hotel, where he periodically started a fire when his cigar ash fell into the waste basket. He looked after some of the arrangements for Sam Lunenfeld's contributions to the Charles H. Best Foundation. He often summoned Henry in the evening to drive him home, always entertaining for the chauffeur.

Sandy's lily business was long gone and most of Sandy's remaining lilies were moved to Londonderry Farm where Margaret enjoyed them thoroughly. Many were new hybrids, often the only stock available anywhere. Now with his own agricultural consulting company Sandy was one of the first to introduce "exotic" European breeds of cattle to North America. He imported them to Canada where they were quarantined on the island of Grosse-Ile in the St. Lawrence, with which both his father and his brother had had different connections earlier.

Charley resumed golfing with David Scott and others at York Downs and not far from Londonderry at the new Halton Country Club — "a delightful place, high on the escarpment." Janna and Henry were at the farm every weekend; Janna's baby was due soon, and Margaret thought that she should stay close to Toronto.

Janna Ramsay Best had agreed to officiate at the opening of the Ramsay Wright Building, the new home of the Department of Biology at the University of Toronto. Professor Wright had no direct descendants. His first cousin was Janna's grandfather and she was his closest relative in Canada. Ramsay Wright had come from Scotland in 1874 as the first professor of Natural History. Before he left home, John Ramsay, his uncle, and Janna's great-grandfather, had given him a microscope and financed the purchase of books, travel, and living expenses since he would not be paid until the end of his first year. Ramsay Wright became the first vice-president of the university in 1901.

On the morning of the opening of the building, 17 September 1965, Mairi Mahon Ramsay Best was born three weeks early. When Henry called Dr. H.J.C. Ireton, in charge of ceremonials, to tell him that Janna had had her baby that morning and would not be present at the opening, his dismayed response was, "But I've got the programs printed!" Henry did the honours, and he, Margaret, Charley, and Linda went to the ceremony and on to the dinner at Hart House.

Two days later the Bests went to the Toronto General Hospital to see their new granddaughter. "She did not open her eyes. They are well spaced. She had neat little ears and a darling mouth — dark hair. She is a lovely little pet. Then we went along to Janna's room but did not go near to her. Of course, it would be dreadful if she got an infection. I wrote to Freda Ramsay in Islay yesterday to tell her about her dear little grand-daughter." Margaret found the penguin doll that Henry used to love and sent it to the baby.

On 2 October, Janna, Henry, and their baby went to 105 Woodlawn for dinner. Charley was genuinely delighted by little Mairi. Margaret was unsure about her gaelic name, but Janna played a record of the song "Mairi's Wedding," which reassured her that it was a "real" name.

Just as Farquharson and Penfield had predicted, Charley's health improved dramatically over the next weeks. Omond Solandt remarked, "Charley made a pretty good recovery, but he never regained the sparkle."[104] Henry took his parents to the new campus of York University at Keele and Steeles where the new buildings impressed Margaret and Charley. They were joined at lunch by Professor John Conway, master of Founder's College, who had moved from Harvard with his wife, Jill Ker Conway, who was teaching history at the University of Toronto, and by Professor Tom O'Connell, also from Harvard and head librarian at York.

Early in October 1965, Joseph P. Hoet lectured at the institute, and Best moved the vote of thanks — the first time that he had spoken in public since he took ill in March 1964. The Mahons and the Bests attended the official opening, which Henry co-ordinated, of the main campus of York University; Maureen Forester was the guest soloist. Another university occasion that Margaret and Charley were very proud to attend was Omond Solandt's installation as chancellor of the University of Toronto.

Gerry Wrenshall and Bernie Leibel had edited the proceedings of the Fifth IDF Congress, which Charley had missed the previous year. On 11 November 1965, they presented the first copy to him.[705] Best's lab continued to attract scientists from many parts of the world. Gerald and Consie Wrenshall entertained for Dr. Y. Tahooka, professor of medicine at Nagasaki University, and for two couples from Japan who were working in Toronto, the Tashakas and the Rikuo Ninomiyas. In the absence of "The Chief," other senior people looked after the social duties of the Best Institute.

Despite appearances, all was not well for the future of the independence of the Banting and Best Department. First Banting and then Best as head of the department always had reported directly to the president of the university. In addition, when Best became head of the Banting and Best Department of Medical Research in 1941, he was already head of physiology. Since then the two departments had worked well together. There was now a plan to separate the two departments and have each report to a dean instead of directly to the president. On 30 October 1965, Dr. Gerald Wrenshall, a brilliant physiologist and a severe diabetic, wrote a three-page memo:

> The Banting and Best Department of Medical Research represents the combined fulfillment of the lifelong ambition of the two great scientists who founded and directed it. Their purpose was to establish the same unfettered complex of teamwork which was evident in the discovery of insulin where each partner exploited his own special talents and skills for the advantage of the total program. Such a system is superior to that in special departments where the energies of the creative researcher are often dissipated by routine teaching responsibilities, where the range of interest is narrowed by the limited sphere of the respective department, and where new ideas remain unborn because of the lack of intimate communication with other departments which is a major feature amongst the numerous sections of the Banting and Best Department.[706]

The Department of Physiology was to become completely independent once more after twenty-four years of combined research, planning, and administration with the Banting and Best Department. Some of the many advantages that had resulted from that connection were eventually lost. After listing some of the accomplishments of the latter department, Wrenshall outlined the possible results of its demise, and prescribed preventive action:

> In order to prevent this sad fate of a department which perhaps more than any other has brought fame to its university, in order to preserve its leadership in medical science which has been established, and in order to maintain a tradition of loyalty to the Discoverers, it is necessary to proceed with the following solution. A careful analysis of the individual sections should be carried out to determine their requirements for seasoned senior creative personnel and young productive workers. A search for the ablest men to fill these posts ... For them, laboratory space will be necessary, and it would be well to decide upon a projected plan for the next ten years which would include the research aims of the department as well as the necessary physical accommodation for the various sections. Finally it is essential to provide an expanded income of money because profound scientific research is expensive.[707]

Best, "assisted by a Council of his colleagues," could direct this process.

Early in 1961 Dean MacFarlane had led an attack on the Banting and Best Department of Medical Research. He was furious that Garfield Weston had given Best one million dollars to set up a foundation specifically and solely for medical research at the BBDMR. Mac MacFarlane died in mid-April. He and Charley were friends but they did not always agree, and Mac had a fiendish temper. Unfortunately after his death, his wife, Marguerite, burned his notes on people and events — or perhaps they self-combusted!

Uncertainty over the future of the Banting and Best Department of Medical Research abated. Best hoped that after his eventual retirement the focus of the department on *medical research* would not change. A later memo stated that the department would probably "form the nucleus of an expanded medical research program. Dr. Solandt and others will, I feel sure, guard against a negative approach to the department and he has given assurances that Dr. Best's interests will be protected. I think that the

405

morale within the Department has improved, due in large part to the increased activity of Dr. Best."[708]

Margaret Best's sixty-fifth birthday was celebrated with much singing of "Happy Birthday" over the phone, cards, and gifts. She received the new biography of newspaper publisher Roy Thomson as a present. A few days later, at the wedding reception for Sigrid Solandt, daughter of Omond and Elizabeth, Margaret fainted. Three doctors — Harris McPhedran, a cousin of Elizabeth Solandt's, Bill Feasby, and Irwin Hilliard, chief of the Toronto Western Hospital, all attended to her. Hilliard ordered an ambulance to go to the Western. There he took an electrocardiogram and other tests, and Margaret spent the night. In the morning, the woman in the other bed was talkative: "You needn't think you are going home this morning. They will tell you, just as they told me — twelve hours, then twenty-four hours, then five days, then a week, and so on." Margaret found her a distressing companion.

In the morning, Reg Haist drove Charley to the hospital. Dr. Hilliard was there. "It must be very unusual for the physician-in-chief to wheel the patient to the door." There was, of course, fear of a heart attack, but Margaret had long had low blood pressure, and if she stood for too long she became faint. When she got home Linda and Jessie were both there. Within a few days Margaret was back for a series of appointments at the dentist's — surely unwise under the circumstances. During the next several weeks she was thirteen times in the dentist's chair.

Henry, Janna, Mairi, and Luke, the now old yellow Lab, were the first to arrive on Christmas Day. Sandy, Eileen, and the four children kept appearances by attending such events *en famille*. Despite the grandparents' concern that Luke might not take kindly to new baby Mairi, he lay across the doorway to her room to prevent strangers from entering. If she crawled on top of him and fell asleep, he would not budge.

On 2 January 1966, towards midnight, Margaret Best suffered a heart attack. She recalled saying to Charley, "I think I am very ill." Three days later she wrote, "I will be in the house for six weeks. I can't write much about it. It is too troubling. There are so many things waiting to be done — in the house particularly and of course, my main worry is that I won't be able to help Charley — to go on long walks with him and so on." Moray Jansen, who succeeded Ray Farquharson as the family's faithful and careful physician, had been on the spot within minutes, and Bill Greenwood, the chief of cardiology at the Toronto General, had taken an electrocardiogram. Only family members were permitted to visit Margaret for a time, but many people sent messages of concern and affection.

One day, the technician who came to the house to take blood samples from Margaret blew on the spot before he applied a bandage. She and Charley did not want the young man to lose his job, so Charley merely told him that he thought such a practice unwise. He answered, "I know that scientists are very particular but you must realize the importance of speed and perfection," — all they could do was laugh. K.J.R. Wightman, the new professor of medicine, paid a visit, and Margaret found him "kind and gentle." The grandchildren wanted to see Grammy, but Margaret found them too rambunctious at first. She did not answer the phone lest she might have an overly talkative caller.

In mid-January 1966, the biggest snowfall since 1945 blocked all the roads. From her bed, Margaret could see through the large windows of their solarium bedroom the sixteen inches of snow that fell and listen to reports of calls from the family in the country. The next day was lovely and sunny, typical after a winter storm. Happily marooned after a weekend in the country, Henry rode Princess from Londonderry Farm to the village of Moffat to get provisions.

On 9 February 1966, Margaret and Charley took a very short walk outside. Progress remained slow, but there was improvement. By mid-February, she was ready for a short drive. Margaret busied herself sorting Charley's many coloured slides. In the evening, he would set up the projector, and they would look at them. Later they went through their sixteen-millimetre moving pictures from the 1920s on. Margaret also wrote a few letters each day. Dr. Bill Greenwood continued to monitor her condition. "He is awfully nice and it is wonderful to have a heart man whom I know. He is quite frank. He doesn't tiptoe around the subject of my coronary. He tells me what to do. That is the way I like a doctor to be."

The grandchildren usually knew instinctively how to say the right thing. Margaret told little Charley, "You are my first little grandchild and I will love you all your life and you will love me." He replied, "Yes, Grammy, and I think you will have a long life." This number one grandchild, being congratulated on getting all As at school, said that Albert Schweitzer had all As as a child. "If you don't believe me, ask God."

Margaret had kept various items of clothing and books from her own childhood or that had belonged to Sandy and Henry. When Mairi was six months old, her grandmother sent her a copy of Robert Louis Stevenson's

A Child's Garden of Verses, which had been given to Margaret in 1908. In the spring, Charley asked Henry to help him look after the farm, so Henry and his family moved out there for the summer.

Margaret and Charley had hoped to go to Rome in April for the meetings of the Pontifical Academy of Sciences, but she had not recovered sufficiently. Sam and Elizabeth Lunenfeld wanted the Bests to join them in Gibraltar for part of the winter as well, but that was too soon. However, when Best received an invitation from the Free University in West Berlin to receive an honorary degree in June they hoped she would be well enough to go. Dr. Hans Giese, Hoechst's representative in Montréal, promised that the trip would be carefully organized and all expenses covered. Margaret made a good recovery. The first-class flight to London en route to Berlin on 24 May 1966 was very comfortable, and Linda was along to help her sister. Mr. Cuthbert of Hoechst met the plane and drove the travellers to the Stafford Hotel.

At Leonard Brockington's suggestion, Dame Laura Knight, eighty-eight years old, invited them for drinks and dinner. In 1928, when she had seen some of Dame Laura's portraits of the royal family at a show at the Royal Academy, Margaret had written, "I call them really repulsive — all very bad." After thirty-eight years Margaret had forgotten her earlier reaction. "We climbed stairs to her studio at the top of her house, a very large room. She greeted us warmly … She moves rapidly and has a fine memory. Her hair is white and she wore a black bandeau. There were many of her own pictures — ballet dancers and horses." They admired a long panel of ballet dancers. "She gave Charley her book of reminiscences, *The Magic of a Line,* which came out recently. She pretended that she had been quite nervous all day about meeting us because Leonard Brockington had taken half an hour on the telephone from Toronto to tell her about us and then she said, 'And of course you take pages in *Who's Who.*' We could not have had a more entertaining and delightful evening. We love her and I hope we will meet again."

Robin Lawrence had had another stroke. "They told us that Robin is in a wheelchair now but he came walking into the room — very thin and wasted but with some of his old charm still evident. Dear Robin, he has been our good friend for many years. We love him. Adam poured drinks for us all. His father had an orange drink and when Adam asked him if he would like more he said, 'No more of this drink — a Scotch and soda.'" They also saw Lady Dale, who was ninety-three and completely blind but otherwise little changed, her memory excellent; Sir Henry, at ninety-one, used a walker. Several months later the Dales moved to the Evelyn Mirking Home in Cambridge to be near the Todds. "They were not happy about being in two rooms without their own things around them."

The Bests visited Carnaby Street in Soho, "where there are boutiques which cater to the boys and girls who wear the mod clothes. The boys have long hair, tight trousers. You can scarcely tell the boys and girls apart, but now the girls are wearing skirts several inches above the knees and long hair hanging down their backs."

A car and driver took the travellers to the British European Airways flight for Templehoff Airport, Berlin, where Dr. Wilhelm Meier of Hoechst met them and drove them to the Schloss Hotel in the Gerhaus district. There, Hans and Gisela Giese danced attendance on them. Charley was very pleased with the meals — venison, fresh asparagus, and strawberries. "Twice we climbed up steps and onto a lookout place in order to see over the Berlin Wall better. The first place looked into a cemetery. The second was 'Checkpoint Charlie.' We looked across at big buildings. It is a very depressing sight." Dr. Fritz Lindner, head scientist at Hoechst, and his wife gave a theatre party for the Bests and the Meiers. The performance was of *Salome*, music by Richard Strauss — "terrific, cruel story, good voices, wonderful setting and costuming. Salome a beautiful red-headed girl (possibly a wig). The orchestra was splendid."

In the evening of the next day, the three Canadians were driven to the Old Clinic of the Free University. Canadian, West German, and West Berlin flags decorated the lecture hall. Dean Wilhelm Masshoff of the Faculty of Medicine conferred the honorary degree of doctor of medicine on Charles Best, who had been presented by Heinz Goerke, professor of the History of Medicine at Heidelberg. Best gave a short speech, finishing in German. (At lunch that day, he had lost a front tooth, so he tried not to smile too much.) In the evening Dr. Lindner and Hoechst hosted a banquet for two hundred people.

The next day there was a showing of the film made by Hoechst and produced by Dr. and Mrs. Munck on the discovery of insulin. The Bests thought it well done. There was a postgraduate conference on diabetes going on, presided over by Professor Gotthard Schettler, and he and his wife hosted a luncheon in the city's tall radio tower. In its large assembly hall, Charley received a miniature replica in china of the Berlin Liberty Bell and a beautiful book about the city.

The next morning, Hans and Gisela Giese took their guests to see the new Kaiser Wilhem Memorial Church built next to the ruins of the old church. The walls and the bell tower were fashioned of small squares of coloured glass made in Chartres and set in concrete. At a meeting of the Lay Diabetic Association of West Berlin, at the City Hall, Drs. Meier and Best both spoke — the former translating the latter's words into German. Charley made several short speeches in West Berlin, but the schedule was much more relaxed than usual.

From Berlin, Margaret, Charley, and Linda flew to Frankfurt. Dr. and Mrs. Rolland Muller of Hoescht met them and drove them to the Schloss Hotel Kronberg on the slopes of the Taunus Mountains, where they had the royal suite. "We see that our rooms cost two hundred twenty marks a day, which since the mark is now twenty-seven cents, that would be $59.40 a day. Hoechst are being very good to us … The ceilings here are enormously high and are of wood in fancy pattern — oak, I think. There is an enormous stone fireplace in the sitting rooms and another in the bedroom. There are old carved chests — oak and walnut — ancient portraits on the walls, big old mirrors. Our beds are large and made of brass — old but just the sort of thing that has come back into vogue." Charley was driven to the Hoechst plant in the town of the same name. Hoechst had 25,000 employees in its plants. Margaret and Linda joined him there later, and they all had a tour with Dr. Lindner and several of the scientists.

One evening, Joseph and Marguerite Hoet paid a surprise visit with their son Jean and his wife, Christian. "They thought that Charley looked much better, also that Charley was wonderful. He is quite tanned now from our various times in the sun and he was the perfect host — bringing Jean and Christian into the conversation. It was Charley — well again."

On 10 June, Margaret, Charley, and Linda flew direct from Frankfurt to Toronto, and Henry drove them home, where Janna had supper ready. Margaret was exhausted, but Moray Jansen encouraged her by saying that her heart was fine. Both Margaret and Charley had been able to undertake the schedule, and that was very reassuring. Charley soon went to the lab and had several meetings with his colleagues and with visitors.

On 7 July 1966, Janna and Mairi left for London and Scotland. Janna cabled from London, signing "Angelic Peanut" — Henry's pet name for Mairi. Sir Henry and Lady Dale were very anxious to see "dear Henry's baby," so Janna took Mairi to their flat for tea. Lady Dale, who was blind, took Mairi on her knee and felt her little features with her fingers. While his family was away, Henry spent every possible hour on his PhD thesis, in addition to his work at York University, and haying at the farm. When his father was there, they both rode their mares. Margaret, Charley, and Linda enjoyed weekends at Londonderry Farm, going on antiquing expeditions with Henry in the nearby country villages where they found an old dry sink to use as a changing table for the baby. Charley also loved to spend time with Harry Dunkie, a retired farmer, discussing the cattle that Harry looked after in the summer months on the pasture.

Margaret had bought Boris Pasternak's novel *Dr. Zhivago* when it came out in English, and she and Charley had both read it and were anxious to see the film. "It is a wonderful picture. The photography is splendid. It was very long, three and a half hours, and I was very tired that evening and the next day." It was the first time in several years that they had been to a movie theatre.

In the sixties Canada saw great expansion in universities and the University of Toronto was developing its satellite campuses at Scarborough and at Erindale in Mississauga. Margaret and Charley drove out to Scarborough, and Margaret was disappointed. "It looks like a fortress — cement, I suppose — very heavy and I did not like the architecture. I went expecting to be thrilled by it." Professor G. Ron Williams worked on choline deficiency at the BBDMR for several years before becoming head of biochemistry and then principal of Scarborough College. Later he revealed that there was always an air of expectancy on Best's part of new and spectacular work from his colleagues, and that he was sad if this did not occur.[709]

Two old friends of the Bests died in September 1966. Leonard Brockington was seventy-eight when he succumbed to his many bravely borne afflictions. He had been a very helpful friend. Within a few days, a letter came from Colombo to say that Dr. W.A.E. Karunaratne, the Bests' very kind host in 1952, had died.

On 4 October, the Toronto Academy of Medicine made Charley Best an honorary fellow. Reg Haist presented CHB for the honour. Margaret enjoyed her two interesting dinner companions at the Granite Club: on her left was Dr. Irwin Hilliard, the president of the Academy; on her right was the Rev. Dr. Ernest House of Bloor Street United Church, recently elected moderator of the United Church of Canada, and, Margaret discovered to her delight, a graduate of Dalhousie and Pine Hill, like her father.

Margaret continued to have several ailments. Eileen said that she was like Job who had so many worries and boils. "I opened my Bible and read about

411

Job at that point and poor Job really had a miserable time. Eileen made me laugh anyway. I am ashamed to mention any more ills to the family. They will begin to think I am one of these characters who always has something wrong." The family did come to understand that the term "heart attack" was used too broadly. Dr. Moray Jansen later confirmed that some of the "heart attacks" were actually bouts of angina — worrying just the same.

On 7 January 1967, Bruce Macleod Ramsay Best was born to Janna and Henry. "He is a darling — chubby cheeks, neat ears, dimples in his elbows." A week later the grandparents went to visit the new baby in the house that Henry and Janna had rented in north Toronto. Margaret remarked that "Mairi seemed mildly intrigued by him."

The Bests flew to Dallas on 17 January for an ADA meeting, where Charley was made an honorary citizen of Dallas. "Charley was many years ago made an admiral of the Texas Navy. He was once given the golden key to the city of Dallas — once we were both given large Texan hats. I think Charley has twice been made an honorary deputy sheriff of Texas County. There can't be any honours left to give him." Five days later they flew to New York where they went to the new ADA offices on 48th Street, near Madison, and talked to the staff. They both went to the Whitney Museum on Madison Avenue, an exciting new building. "We found many of the exhibits too modern for us — a long plank painted red was one. It just leaned against the wall. Another was a short flight of stairs with a beige carpet." They went on a tour of the new Lincoln Center and admired "the enormous Chagall paintings — figures floating about and blowing horns."

Charley Best had been in good health for some time, but he suddenly developed a sharp pain, and on 15 February, Henry drove his parents to the emergency department at the Toronto General Hospital. Dr. Jansen asked Dr. Bob Mustard for a consultation. Margaret wrote on 26 February, "I don't write these days in my diary. I go every morning to the hospital and stay for 12 hours. At noon I go over to the institute and have a sandwich with Linda, lie down for half an hour and go back to my darling Charley. Dr. K.J.R. Wightman, Dr. Farquharson's successor, comes every day as well as Moray Jansen and Dr. Stone, the young resident surgeon, and others. It has been puzzling because there have been complications. It began with gall bladder and then involved other parts. There was talk of a rub (pleurisy), of an abscess in the liver, etc. but there has been no operation. I don't know whether they are going to operate. They don't tell me." The news that Charley was in the hospital always spread quickly, and many doctors would drop by to chat. After almost a month, Charley was sent home. "He has no pain, no temperature now but I feel that it has not been resolved."

On 17 March, Dr. Mustard removed Best's gall bladder, which had been causing all the trouble. Margaret summarized what had happened. "When Charley went to the hospital first, February 15th, the gall bladder had perforated. That made it difficult to get x-rays. Also, that caused the rub (in the chest) pleurisy and other complications. When he went in on March 15th, that had subsided and Dr. Mustard was able to operate. At least that is the way I understand it."

A dinner for 240 guests at Hart House on 15 June 1967 marked Charles Best's retirement as director of the Banting and Best Department of Medical Research. He had retired as head of Physiology two years earlier. Reg Haist, who had succeeded Best as head of physiology, was the chairman. Margaret sat between President Bissell and Dean Chute, who gave speeches, as did John Hamilton, vice-president of medical sciences, and Best. Chancellor Omond Solandt presented the honoured guest with a cheque for one thousand dollars. Most members of the family were at the event, including little Charley, now eight; Alexander, just fifteen months younger, was very insulted that he could not be present as well. Days later little Charley said, "Grampy is much more merry since he got that money." His grandmother asked, "What money?" "Oh, the money he got at the big dinner."

More events marked Charley's retirement. The technicians at the Best Institute held a lunch at Pepio's with 150 people present and gave their departing chief luggage and silver Centennial spoons. Keith Bowler, the comptroller, had organized the event. Christine Bissell asked Margaret to give her a guest list of people for a dinner at the university president's home on Highland Avenue. It was a lovely evening, and the sixty guests were able to have their drinks outside. The Bests were very happy, surrounded by old friends, and sat at a table with the Bissells, the Chutes, the Solandts, and the Keiller MacKays.

Months later the university gave a dinner at its Faculty Club for members who were retiring. The Bests sat at a table with two couples whom they knew well, the Alex MacDonalds and the Eric Arthurs. Eric Arthur was professor of architecture and had published several interesting books on Toronto.

Margaret really wanted to go to Expo '67, and she and Charley took the Rapido train to Montréal, where Dal and Elizabeth Browne looked after them at their apartment on Simpson Street, on the south face of

Mont-Royal. Dr. Carleton B. Peirce, a radiologist and naval colleague of Charley's, with whom Janna had worked in Montréal, and Ben Hofley, assistant to Expo's general manager and a friend of Henry's in Ottawa, welcomed them to the world's fair. They were driven in an electric car to the art gallery, where Gordon Shepherd of the National Gallery of Canada showed them around. The Wilder Penfields and the Duncan Grahams were there the same day. Mr. and Mrs. Yousuf Karsh were also present at the lunch of arctic char — "better than smoked salmon" — and buffalo steaks.

Margaret, Charley, and Linda spent almost every weekend in the country. Henry and his family had moved again to Londonderry Farm for the summer, keeping an eye on the cattle and getting the hay in. They organized a celebration there on 1 July 1967 for Canada's Centennial. Margaret, Charley, and Linda decided that the party with many people might be too much for them, so the coach house was kept decorated with flags and mementos until the grandparents arrived the next day. Charley and Henry rode and Charley enjoyed keeping tabs on the farm work. Alexander asked Margaret, "Do you think that some people have sad faces, Grammy?" "Yes, some do. Who were you thinking of, Alexander?" "The dogs — the St. Bernards."

Margaret and Charley's memoir proceeded very slowly. "This morning Charley and I looked into the zippered bag where I keep the chapters for our book that I had already written and also notes as well as my very early diaries. We have real fun looking at them. How we will enjoy getting on with our book in the autumn. Charley had once made an outline of chapter headings. This morning he said, 'It is too medical.' We must get a good title for our book — <u>most important</u>." Margaret was determined, but Charley was less keen as he had spent a lifetime looking forward, not back. The prospect was daunting, and he simply did not have the interest or energy to relive his life.

The trip to Berlin had gone so well that when an all-expenses-paid invitation came for the Sixth IDF Congress in Stockholm in 1967, Charley accepted. The organizers had received a good start with the considerable surplus from the 1964 meeting in Toronto, which had been donated to them. Charley complained about discomfort in his chest, and Dr. John Morrow came to take electrocardiograms of them both — neither showed any fresh lesions. Moray Jansen diagnosed a hiatus hernia, but advised them to go to Stockholm. Because he was ill Charley had missed the 1964 IDF Congress in Toronto, and he was, therefore, especially determined to attend this one. But Margaret was anxious: "the important thing is to be careful not to run risk of trouble while we are away. In the meantime we are about completely packed."

On 28 July 1967, the Bests flew to Kennedy Airport in New York, and from there to Oslo and Stockholm. It was an uneasy flight, with two youngsters, aged two years and fifteen months, who "cried and screamed most of the night." Dr. Rolf Luft, professor of medicine at the Karolinska Institute, and Dr. Bo Andersson, the secretary general of the congress, met the plane, looked after the luggage, and drove their guests to the Carlton Hotel. Reporters were busy, and pictures of the Bests and of Bernardo Houssay appeared in the newspapers the next morning. Houssay, at eighty, was overheard saying that "Margaret Best is the most lovely lady in the world."

Rolf Luft hosted a cocktail party at his book-and painting-filled apartment overlooking the harbour. The next day, there was a lunch at the home of Ulf and Dagmar von Euler, and Ingve and Britta Zotterman were there. "Ingve has changed not at all — he was full of reminiscences about our many meetings. We have known them for a long time — first of all in London in 1925 or '26. Ulf von Euler we met first in 1926 in Lund where he was a student — twenty-one years old."

Bo Andersson's car came to take the Bests to the Konserhuet for the opening ceremonies of the congress, attended by two thousand delegates. Charles Best, Joseph Hoet, Bernardo Houssay, and Robin Lawrence, all past presidents of the IDF, were on the platform. At the back of the stage a small orchestra played Scandinavian music. Elisabeth Söderström, singer to the court and international opera star, sang Swedish folk songs. Prime Minister Tage Erlander welcomed everyone. Like Best in 1964, the president of the IDF Congress, Dr. Howard Root of Boston, was ill and unable to attend so Joseph Hoet read his speech.

In the evening, the delegates went by boat to the Drottningholm Court Theatre to hear Pergolesi's *Il Maestro di Musica* — "all in Italian of which I understand not one word. However, it was not a complicated plot and they had lovely voices. There were two acts and at the end, Charley slipped out and appeared on the stage and presented the bouquets and shook hands with each of the four … Dan Lawrence and I teased him afterwards by saying that he should have sung a note or two while he was up there."

Charley enjoyed the meetings and went to a number of sessions. Dr. Leonard L. Madison of Dallas gave the Iacobaeus (Jacobean) Lecture. Charley had once given this address, and the Insulin Foundation entertained him, Madison, and other previous lecturers at the Stallmästargården (Stable Master's Garden). Best was proud of the contributions to the congress from people at the Banting and Best Department; John Logothetopoulos, for example, presented a paper at a session chaired by Reg Haist. The congress banquet for 1,200 people took place in City Hall — in the Blue Room, which was not blue, but red brick, where the Bests had attended a dinner in 1926. "We had a delicious dinner beautifully served — smoked salmon, filet of beef, ice cream and tiny cakes, and all sorts of little side delicacies and wines. The speeches were all short and were spaced throughout the dinner." Albert Renold toasted the women and started off by proposing, "Dr. Nancy Erickson and Mrs. Best." "Dr. Nancy Erickson is president of the Swedish Diabetic Association and a member of parliament. There was a high platform set up in the hall and two young men, brothers, played marvelous table tennis, a most unusual entertainment for a big dinner party. One of the boys is a diabetic."

Both Margaret and Charley went to hear Rolf Luft give the closing speech of the congress and to congratulate him on the excellent arrangements. That evening the Bests had dinner with the Hoet family, Joseph and Marguerite, Jean and Christian, and Marie-Noëlle, and they discussed where they could next meet.

The Bests flew to Copenhagen, where Dr. and Mrs. Jacob Poulsen of Novo Nordisk met them and drove them to the Palace Hotel, and later to see Hans and María Hagedorn at their home near Staverly, south of Copenhagen. "Dr. Hagedorn, of course, has been very ill with Parkinson's disease and he is a great deal thinner than he used to be, but still an unusual and arresting figure. He can speak very little and in a low voice. Mrs. Hagedorn has been ill too but now she is better and really very little changed — quick as a flash on her feet. They are both seventy-nine years old." Margaret thought she might never see them again. It was hard for Charley to see the powerful man whom he had long known and admired reduced to a shell. On 9 August, the Poulsens took the Bests to the airport for their flight to Canada.

Having not been to Schooner Cove for three years due to Charley's illness, the Bests returned to the east coast in August 1967. They took the trip east more easily, spreading it over four days. Erich and Dorothy Baer from the lab stopped at the farm by the sea for a meal. "Dorothy was intrigued by our funny old furnishings. I am rather intrigued myself. It is like meeting old friends again — after three years absence." Colin and

Mary Lucas, also from the institute, spent a night and went on to Nova Scotia without ever seeing the cove because of the fog. Margaret was reading the second volume of Harold Nicolson's *Diaries and Letters, 1939–1945* — "wonderfully interesting."

The widow of James D. Havens, the first American to receive insulin, had asked Carl Hersey to take three of his coloured woodcuts to Charley — "very delicate and beautiful. One is called 'Shy Veery' — we often see this particular thrush in our garden at 105 Woodlawn Avenue West. Another is called 'Corn Husking Bee' — a squirrel in a tree working on a cob of corn. The third is a portrait of himself called 'Done With Mirrors.' Charley has written to Mrs. Havens this morning to tell her how pleased he is to have these pictures done by her gifted husband."

News came from Toronto about the national Conservative leadership convention, where John Diefenbaker wanted to succeed himself. Henry and Sandy both supported the winner, Robert Stanfield — a great prime minister that Canada never had. For the federal election on 17 October, Radio Canada television hired Henry as pundit for its election desk in Toronto, but a producers' strike in Montréal prevented French TV coverage, so he switched to the radio.

After just a month in Maine, the Bests returned to Toronto in two and a half days. Charley and Margaret asked Henry if he and his family would like to stay on at Londonderry Farm and a formal rental agreement was worked out. Mairi's birthday was on 17 September 1967, and the whole family joined in the celebration. Mairi was a "terrible two" and on a visit to Toronto had found a handy key to turn on the outside of the cloakroom door at 105 Woodlawn thereby locking her mother in. Margaret commented, "Pretty smart little girl."

The Bests resumed their fall routine with a typical stream of visitors coming and going. Sir Douglas Menzies of Melbourne stopped on his way home from London especially to see the Bests. Henry and Lydia Mahon arrived for a few days before going to Florida for the winter. Joe and Pep Hoet came from Belgium to visit various labs in North America.

On 23 October, CBC Radio in Toronto put on an hour-long radio broadcast — "Charles Herbert Best and the Islets of Langerhans" with many old friends and colleagues taking part. Omond Solandt said that Best tried to make a story out of each scientific investigation — what came to be called "systematic thinking." Laurie Chute described Best as "not grandiose" and "not content to be a pure scientist, he wanted to see the results — a true physician." Clarence MacCharles emphasized Best's "intense capacity to concentrate." Colin Lucas compared Banting and Best, saying that the former liked young people, and the latter liked bright young people; Best's early discovery created "great expectations and great strain." Gerry Wrenshall described how, as one of three diabetics working in the Best Institute, he was "in awe of The Chief." Sandy Best reported that he was brought up to believe that he had a duty to contribute to society, and Henry described his father as "dominant but not domineering." Finally, Charles Best himself said that the discovery of insulin in 1921 was certainly the "high moment" of his career. He added that he later regretted not having training in mathematics and statistics.

At Reg Haist's suggestion, Best had started meeting with second-year medical students, one at a time, in his office three days a week to discuss their future plans. Charley derived great pleasure from their youth, energy, and enthusiasm. Everyone seemed to enjoy the informal sessions. There were so many students, however, that he had to see them two at a time. "Charley says it will not be so satisfactory. When one comes alone he confides in Charley — they will be more inhibited when two are together." He attended events on campus such as the laying of the cornerstone of the new Medical Sciences Building, where one occupant would be his old department, Physiology. The separation of Physiology from the Banting and Best Department of Medical Research, which he had opposed, was taking place.

In 2002, all of the documents concerning the future of Best's two departments in the mid-sixties were sent to Dean David Naylor of the Faculty of Medicine for help in understanding the possible rationale of having the Banting and Best Department no longer reporting to the president and the separation of the department of physiology. In a careful and thoughtful reply, he said in part:

> The rationale for special status for BBDMR was doubtless stronger when it was led by one of the individuals to whom the department was, as Charles Best put it, "a living memorial." However, I can see no particular administrative rationale for having a department within a faculty bypass the Dean and the Provost, and report direct to the President. I would surmise instead as the Faculty and University were growing in size and complexity, there was

a desire to create a more conventional set of administrative accountabilities. In other words, the change had nothing to do with sinister motives, malice, or rivalry, and everything to do with common sense and management. … In a University that now has a budget in the hundreds of millions of dollars, it is not conceivable that the President would give the BBDMR the close attention that it deserves. There are a number of research institutes and units across the University that function within and across departments without full departmental status. They report variously to department Chairs or Deans, and have the same special focus on research that characterizes BBDMR. I would also note that the growth of research activities within the Faculty of Medicine suggests that one does not need BBDMR-type structures for excellence to be achieved … Last, on the matter of the separate status of Physiology and BBDMR, science has moved on dramatically and this association would today make little sense. Physiology is at what I might call the "downstream" end of the basic medical sciences with a focus on organs and organisms as well as molecular and cellular functions. If anything, the work of the BBDMR is closer conceptually to more "upstream" science being done in the Departments of Biochemistry and Medical Genetics.[710]

At Christmas, Margaret was rather sad. "We hope to see all our children over the holiday but we are no longer equal to having the big family party. I wish we could." Sandy went to see his parents on Christmas Eve. On Christmas afternoon Margaret, Charley, and Linda drove to Londonderry Farm and had dinner there with Henry and his family, including Freda Ramsay and a student from Hong Kong. The next day Henry and his father had a good ride, and later Eileen arrived with the four children.

Two dear friends died within a few months of each other. Lady Dale, ninety-three, died in Cambridge on 23 November 1967. A few days earlier she and Sir Henry had celebrated their sixty-third wedding anniversary. "She was a dear and lovely person and for all these years since Charley and I went to London in 1925, she had been our wonderful friend." On 13 February 1968, a cable announced the sudden death of Joseph Hoet. "Dear Joseph.

419

We have known him and loved him for so long. I have just finished writing the chapter in our book about Charley and Joseph working together at the National Institute for Medical Research in 1925–1926. That Christmas of 1925, we visited Joseph's mother in Antwerp. Joseph and Marguerite and the baby Joseph were there. We have had so many happy times together and the most recent was in Stockholm last summer at the International Diabetes Congress."

It was mid-April before the Bests went to the farm again, when Charley enjoyed riding his mare, Lady. All the grandchildren gathered there to see Margaret and Charley before they went to Rome on 17 April 1968 for their first meeting of the Pontifical Academy of Sciences. They flew tourist class on Canadian Pacific and enjoyed the flight. Dr. Helmut Sadee and Dr. Corrado Mochi of Hoechst met them and drove them to the Hotel Reale, via XX Settembre 30. Hoechst provided a car and driver for the duration of the visit.

Drs. Sadee and Mochi took their guests to the Casena Valadier Restaurant. "In 1932 Charley and I had dinner there on the balcony, looking down over Rome. It is a very old and famous restaurant. First we stopped on a terrace on the *pincio* (near the Borghese Gardens) and looked down on the Piazza del Popolo — a great obelisk in the centre, a large church at either end of the piazza, and away in the distance, St. Peter's. We had dinner in a small room — a most delicious dinner — Campari to drink at first and then a fine white wine — Frascati. I had smoked salmon and then a rather complicated veal dish."

The next day they were at the Piazza di Spagna and the Spanish Steps. In the evening the chauffeur took them to the Canadian Embassy Residence to a cocktail party given by Ambassador Gordon Crean and his wife. There was a conference on foreign aid meeting in Rome; Maurice Strong, president of Power Corporation and a United Nations official, was at the party.

The Bests went to Sunday service at the Scottish Presbyterian Church and afterwards talked to the Rev. Dr. Colin MacLean. They made good use of the car and driver to see the sights. On one occasion, they took Dr. and Mrs. Gerhard Herzberg to Castel Gondolfo, the pope's summer residence. At the Sistine Chapel the lift was out because of a power strike, and Margaret could not climb the one hundred steps. They were glad to see the paintings in the Villa Borgese that they had seen in 1932, particularly the works of Bernini. Margaret threw three coins in the Trevi Fountain so that they would return to Rome.

One evening, Dr. Mochi invited the Bests to dinner at the rooftop restaurant of the Hilton Hotel. The big Fiat had stalled on the steep street above the Piazza di Spagna, where a student celebration of some kind was going on, and twenty or thirty young people pushed the car to the top of the hill. Then the Bests had a welcome cup of tea at Miss Babington's English Tea Room in the Piazza di Spagna. Passing through a tunnel their car stalled again. "It was an alarming place to be stalled because the traffic was tearing past us all the time. They set up a triangle on the road behind us to warn cars not to run into us but I must say I was quite alarmed." The next day they changed both car and driver.

Margaret and Charley met Father Daniel O'Connell, president of the Pontifical Academy, and Dr. Pietro Salviucci, the chancellor. On 28 April, the members of the academy and their wives gathered in the garden of the Vatican before a papal audience. Most of the men wore tails with a black waistcoat, their academy gold medal around their necks, and miniature medals. Margaret had balked at wearing a long black dress, but before she left Toronto, she had had one made with a high neck and long sleeves. "I will look awful in it. I almost never wear black — neither Charley nor I like it. When we come back home I can have it cheered up at the neck, etc."

Cardinals, academicians, and diplomats gathered for the audience with Paul VI. "Then the Pope entered and sat on a throne at the end of the room. He read an address in French. He was in white with red velvet cape and long embroidered stole and tiny white skull cap. He came down and first shook hands with all the cardinals (two of whom, very old, had fallen asleep during the Pope's address). Then he walked up and down the two rows of Academicians, and shook hands with them. He had been told about Charley's work and he asked about Toronto and said that he had been there. He then shook hands with the front row of ladies and he shook my hand and I bowed. A few men fell on their knees."

On the official visit to Castel Gondolfo, Mgr. L.G. Ligutti, official permanent observer of the Holy See to the United Nations Food and Agricultural Organization (FAO), took the Bests to see the herd of Aberdeen Angus cattle. Charley went into one of the barns to see the Holsteins, including a bull donated by Stephen Roman of Toronto.

On their last evening in Rome, the Bests visited more of the places that they had first seen in 1932. Then, as they left the Victoria Hotel, to Margaret's delight they saw the new crescent moon over the city's walls promising "another month of happiness." Dr. Mochi came to see them to the airport. William J. Cameron, manager for Canadian Pacific Airlines in Rome, took the Bests to the plane and installed them in first class. They had a good flight home. "We had a wonderful two weeks. We feel that we know Rome much better now. The Pontifical Academy will meet again in two years time."

As so often happened after a trip, Margaret was sick in bed for a week. Her eyes were causing a lot of trouble. She missed several events, such as the farewell party for the Jack Davidsons, who were returning to Atlanta after a very successful stay in Toronto. Some years later, the Davidsons established the Charles H. Best Memorial Lectureship in the Department of Physiology. And, Dr. Jessie Ridout, seventy-one, who had worked with Charley since 1922, retired from the university.

Margaret and Charley really wanted to go to the ADA meetings in San Francisco. "Charley could not go without me but I know they would be devastated if he is not there. I must be well." She was, and the Bests were able to go to San Francisco. At a meeting of the ADA council in Atlanta ten years earlier Drs. Edwin Gates, Bill Omsted, and John Reed, and the ADA's attorney discussed creation of a foundation to purchase Charles Best's birthplace in West Pembroke, Maine. The attorney and Gates had already been there to talk to Harold Blackwood, who told them the history of the house. Dr. Edwin Gates of Niagara Falls, New York, and Dr. George Cahill of Boston then founded a group of trustees who bought the house and restored Dr. Herbert Best's office "as it was in the early 1900s when it was in very active use. From Dr. Charles Best we were able to obtain his father's portable operating table and roll-top desk." Charley and Margaret had co-operated fully with the restoration as they had long wanted Dr. Herbert Best's office to remain as a memorial to him. Also on loan were his surgical instruments and medical diplomas. Charley's sister, Hilda Best Salter, also loaned furniture and other items and took an active part in restoring their father's office.[711]

At San Francisco in 1968 the trustees turned over the deed of the "Birthplace" to the ADA. Gates said that the ADA "is proud to announce its acceptance from the trustees of the Charles H. Best Birthplace Trust. … The residence and site will be maintained as a symbol of gratitude from all those who owe their lives and their well-being to the historic discovery of insulin in which he shared, and to the subsequent research performed by him and those under his direction."[712]

It had been six weeks since Margaret, Charley, and Linda had been at Londonderry Farm when they went out on the 1 July holiday weekend.

There were no longer any cattle in the fields; Henry and Janna were now boarding standardbred horses from the Mohawk Raceway, including several mares and foals. At one point they had forty horses on the property.

Margaret allowed herself a few lines in her diary about Sandy's marital problems. "These are very troubling days for us. We have so much on our minds and in our hearts. I keep saying to myself, 'Let not your heart be troubled.'" Eileen and the children moved to a good house at 19 McMaster Avenue, just down Avenue Road from 105 Woodlawn.

On 16 July, both Sandy and Henry saw their parents off to Maine. The three-day trip was one of the hottest they could remember, and they were happy to feel the sea breezes. Canada had a postal strike, so news reached Maine by phone. Henry called to say that Sir Henry Dale had died, just eight months after his wife. "The dear old gentleman — we loved him very much. For so many years, he had been our good friend. How we will miss his letters." Since he first met him in 1922, Charley Best had relied on Dale's judgment more than that of any other person, except Margaret. On 11 October 1968, there was a memorial service in Westminster Abbey. Margaret and Charley would very much have liked to have been there.

A *festschrift* or special collection of papers honouring Best had recently been published. Because of the postal strike no letters could reach him from Toronto, but a few people, such as Rachmiel Levine, the new president of the IDF, called to express pleasure at receiving a copy. Two dear friends wrote short messages at the beginning of the book. Omond Solandt observed:

> Literally millions of diabetics all over the world feel personally indebted to Banting and Best. As with Dr. Banting, wherever Dr. Best has gone, he has been engulfed by an intense personal recognition of himself and his work. He has received quite exceptional public as well as professional acclaim for his achievements. … Historians of the future will recognize the discovery of insulin as the greatest contribution to science in Canada's first hundred years. They will also see the tremendous personal influence that Dr. Best has had on the development of science in general and physiology in particular in the University of Toronto, in Canada, and throughout the world.[713]

Laurie Chute wrote:

> Like all true physicians, however, he has always sought for the application of his scientific discoveries to the relief of human suffering. He encouraged his surgical confreres to adapt heparin to the control of thrombosis. He persuaded voluntary organizations to set up camps for diabetic children and encouraged the development of Day Care Centers for adult diabetics. He is Honorary President of the International Diabetes Federation. The Best Institute has attracted keen young investigators from all corners of the globe. His active interest and concern for their personal as well as their scientific welfare has thus provided him with scores of friends in all lands.[714]

From Buenos Aires, Bernardo Houssay wrote expressing thanks for having received a copy of the *festschrift* and remarked in his expressive English:

> Your life has been like a fairy tale. Being still a young student you made with Banting one of the greatest discoveries of this century and of all times in medicine. It was due to genial insight and persistent and able work by precocious utilization of your ability, sound judgment and laboriosity … Your kind, stimulating, lovable personality has won the affection of all who had the privilege of knowing you, like your work of scientist has arisen the admiration of all scientists, you are also one of the greatest benefactors of humanity.[715]

Upon their return to Toronto there was more sad news from England — Robin Lawrence had passed away in his sleep. "Sir Henry died while we were in Maine. Both A.V. Hill and Adrian have written to us about his death. Alison and Alex Todd had gone to Australia. To think that Joseph, Sir Henry, and Robin should all go in one year. They were dear and wonderful friends." There was soon word that Dr. Heymans of Ghent, whom they had seen in Rome, had died, and a few days later, Ena Farquharson, Ray Farquharson's widow, whom they had known well since the 1920s. Charley, Margaret, Linda, Jessie, Janna, and Henry all went to her funeral at St. James the Less.

Margaret and Charley Best no longer had to travel. Charley no longer needed to make and maintain the important network of contacts with scientists around the world, which, for over forty years, had been so vital for the work with his colleagues and students in Toronto and Canada. Receiving and accepting invitations to lecture, however, reassured CHB that he still had something to say that people wanted to hear. Also, they enjoyed seeing new places and people. On 12 September 1968, they flew to Chicago and on, with stops for CHB to speak at Louisville, Kentucky and Knoxville and Chattanooga, Tennessee. There were several receptions and dinners — at one they were served "the biggest, thickest steaks I have ever seen." They were interested to learn that it was Charolais beef, as Sandy had been the first person to import this breed into North America.

Having vacated the director's quarters, Charley and Linda were installed in their new offices at the Best Institute, and Margaret went several times to help go through papers. Some items were taken home for safekeeping since Charley recalled that, after Fred Banting's death, some papers disappeared from the files. They went to the Ontario Science Centre to see "The Discovery of Insulin Lab" — "a replica of Fred and Charley's lab in the Medical School where they discovered insulin. It was very fascinating and Charley was able to give some suggestions."

For Thanksgiving 1968, Margaret, Charley, and Linda went out to Londonderry Farm. Henry went in to Toronto to pick up Gilles Vigneault, *doyen* of Québec *chansonniers,* and his partner, Alison Foy. Gilles and his musicians were to perform at York University. While at the farm, Gilles was fascinated by a muscovy duck called Peter and followed him around. Later, he included recollections from his travels in a poem "Je t'ai rapporté"[716] of "Peter, le canard, chez les Best en Ontario." Having looked after Londonderry Farm for some years for his parents, Henry and Janna had been looking for a place of their own closer to Henry's work at York University. They had made an offer on a lovely old farm near Bradford. Charley, when he realized that they were serious, wondered who would keep Londonderry Farm going. Vin Price advised Margaret and Charley to sell the property to Henry, which they did; he and Janna now had their own place. The older generation could still come regularly to visit, and Charley could ride whenever he wanted.

Early in 1967, Charley had received Canada's Centennial Medal. On 21 December 1967, a letter arrived from the governor general's secretary announcing that he was to become a companion of the new Order of

Canada (CC). This honour was to take precedence over the CBE or any other decoration that he had received. On 11 November 1968, Remembrance Day, Margaret, Charley, and Linda went to Ottawa for the Order of Canada investiture at Rideau Hall. Charley was not very well; he had had the first angina since his heart attack in 1954, and Moray Jansen had advised an electrocardiogram. "We were packed but not at all sure that we were going until less than an hour before leaving the house."

At the Skyline Hotel, Ottawa, Charley dressed in his tails and medals, and Margaret in a blue and gold brocade dress and gold shoes. "We all met at the Albert Street entrance at five o'clock and went by bus to Government House. It had been a very stormy day, snow, wind. We stepped gingerly through the slush and up the steps of our bus." At Rideau Hall Governor General Roland Michener, an old friend of the Bests, made the presentations to the twelve people receiving the Order of Canada.[717]

Margaret regarded Janna's mother as unwelcome competition. She wrote, "Mrs. Ramsay is expected to arrive from Scotland on Saturday, to visit them again!" Freda Ramsay expected to be treated as an equal by Margaret and Charley. But Margaret saw her as competition for *her* grandchildren, and she resented that Henry got along so well with his mother-in-law. Margaret could not understand Freda's life on the isolated island of Islay in the Inner Hebrides, while at the same time moving in distinguished academic circles. Later Freda published two books on Scottish history, including a history of eighteenth-century Islay, and both volumes were well received. She made many interesting friends during her research travels in Canada and the United States.

Wider family gatherings were not easy either, as Margaret had decided some time after Dr. Herbert Best died in 1942 that, for reasons that are not entirely clear, she no longer wanted any contact with Charley's sister, Hilda Best Salter, or her husband, Ralph. From the late forties on they stopped seeing each other. Again, Margaret saw Hilda as a rival, in this case because of her close relationship to Charley. At the end of December 1968, Debbie Whitley, a daughter of Hilda and Charley's first cousin, Isabelle Hallam Whitley, married John Rodaway in Christ Church, Deer Park, five minutes from 105 Woodlawn. Isabelle and her husband, Harold Whitley, had always remained friends. Margaret, Charley, Henry, and Janna went to the wedding. Hilda's daughter, Dr. Joan Salter Bain, and her husband, Dr. Stan Bain, were there. Encouraged by Vin and Ruth Price, who had always continued to be friends with Hilda, Joan and Henry decided to forget the family rift and they and their families became great friends.

Margaret, however, always welcomed contact with Mahon and Macleod relatives. The following May an invitation to the CDA's annual meeting in Winnipeg provided an opportunity to see Margaret's Scott cousins, the children of her mother's younger sister, Aunt Linda Macleod, and her husband, Uncle Walter Scott. The Bests had last been in Winnipeg eleven years earlier for Uncle Walter's ninetieth birthday on 29 October 1958. He was the son of a Presbyterian minister who, like A.W. Mahon, had served at St. Columba's parish in Prince Edward Island. Margaret had always been close to her cousin Kirk Scott Wright who was only three weeks her senior. Also the Bests had spent much time with Kirk's older sister, Mary, when they were in London, and the youngest sister, Margaret Scott Henderson, and brother, Bruce Scott, often saw them in Toronto.

Over the Christmas holidays, Sandy and Eileen's children had lunch at 105 Woodlawn and were introduced to oysters. Little Charley was the only one to swallow one. "The two little girls retreated under the table."

On Easter Sunday 1969, Margaret, Charley, and Linda had their noon meal with Janna, Henry, their children, and Freda Ramsay at the farm. Freda was in Canada for the launch of her book on nineteenth-century Islay emigrants to Ontario.[718] Margaret noted the positive changes to the house, especially the library, made by Henry and Janna since they bought the property.

Margaret had finished another chapter of their memoirs, up to Sandy's first birthday at Maine in July 1932. Charley would make the occasional suggestion but was not doing any writing himself. He was not interested in writing his memoirs. He had always been forward looking and interested in what lay ahead. At this point, he really did not want to relive his life. In the one period in the 1950s when he had relived the events surrounding the discovery of insulin he had hated experience.

Charley did, however, enjoy hearing about advances in research. Margaret and Charley flew to Indianapolis on 4 May 1969 for a conference on pro-insulin, a precursor of the insulin molecule, chaired by Dr. Donald Steiner, professor of biochemistry at the University of Chicago. Albert Fisher, John Logothetopoulos, and Cecil Yip were other delegates from Toronto. Dr. Dorothy Hodgkin of Oxford was one of the speakers, and CHB was very impressed with her presentation; she had won the Nobel Prize for chemistry in 1964 for her analysis of the structure of penicillin, insulin, and vitamin B12.

Dr. Bill Kirtley, director of medical research at Eli Lilly and Company, and others on his staff were as always very welcoming. Margaret and Charley had dinner with Eli and Ruth Lilly at their home on Sunset Lane. "Eli and Ruth don't play bridge. Eli told us that the first time he played he made a grand slam and the second time he trumped his partner's ace, and then he gave up bridge. 'As for golf,' he said, 'I would rather lean over a fence and look at a fine hog.' His interests were history, farming and growing orchids." They also saw the new Lilly Center, which would house, among other things, Eli's orchids.

They also went to Boston for the centennial of the birth of Dr. Elliott P. Joslin, and Charley spoke at the ceremony. They spent the weekend in Duxbury with the Mahons. In Boston the Joslin Foundation provided them with a suite at the Ritz that had a lovely view of the gardens, the swan boats, and beyond. Mary Joslin Otto took them to a meeting of the foundation and then to a general meeting, where Dr. Alex Marble, director of the Joslin Clinic, Dr. Frank Allan, Dr. Allen Joslin, Dr. Leo Krall, and Dr. Priscilla White spoke. Mary Holt, retired librarian of the Harvard Medical School, and the Edwin Gates from Niagara Falls, New York, were among the guests. Marian Minot, widow of Nobel laureate Dr. George Minot and a diabetic, was at the dinner that followed. The next morning, at the clinic, Charley spoke to a group of patients.

In Toronto, Bill McNeill of the CBC took the Bests for lunch with Robert and Signe McMichael, the generous donors of the McMichael Canadian Art Collection at Kleinburg, Ontario. A.Y. Jackson, aged eighty-seven, a distinguished founding member of the famous Group of Seven artists, greeted them. "Mr. Jackson went on a little tour with us. He took us around the Jackson Gallery. He told us little stories about the different places — Québec, north shore of Lake Superior, the far north, etc. Sometimes Fred Banting painted with him." As they were parting, "a class of school children were leaving. Mr. Jackson stood in the middle of them and talked with them a little. They were introduced to Charley. One little girl who shook hands with A.Y. said, 'Now I will never wash that hand.' Later she shook hands with Charley — her left hand that time, and she said, 'I will never wash that hand either.'"

Stan Hartroft, chief of research at the Hospital for Sick Children, included "The Chief" in a new special advisory body. The other members were Americans, including Dr. Charles Huggins of Chicago, Dr. Charles Janeway of Harvard, and Dr. Fred Robbins of Cleveland. Both Huggins and Robbins were Nobel laureates. The CDA's annual meeting took place at Emmanuel College and attracted an overflow crowd. The next day a picture, often reproduced, appeared in the *Toronto Telegram* of Charley with a little boy named Brian sitting on his knee. He had brought a pen engraved with "Gratitude Dr. Best" as a gift.

In July 1969, it was reassuring to return to the old haunts in Maine and to visit with friends — both local and from away. On walks to the point, they saw wild pink roses in bloom, and warblers, white throated sparrows, chickadees, pine grosbeaks, and gold finches. Eileen and the four children arrived for a few days. Despite fog and rain they went on walks, and Grampy taught them how to drive golf balls into the cove. Charley continued to be interested in anything affecting health in the area. He spoke about his various researches at a meeting of a group organized by the local medics, Drs. Jim Bates and Rowland French, who were attempting to preserve the Eastport Hospital.

In the autumn of 1969, the BBC was making a film on the discovery of insulin, *Comets among the Stars,* for the fiftieth anniversary in 1971. A Mr. Wilson, the representative in Ottawa, arranged for Dr. Stephen Black and Philip Daly to spend several hours with Charley; then they went to see the exhibit of the lab at the Ontario Science Centre. The BBC wanted to hire a horse for Charley and also to take pictures at York Downs Golf Club, but he was too tired for either. "They were very interested to find that Charley showed no bitterness about the Nobel Prize. They talked about the animosity between Fred Banting and Bert Collip, and they appeared surprised when Charley told them that Fred and Collip were quite friendly in later years." Best had shown bitterness about the Nobel Prize in the fifties after his heart attack, but after his depression he no longer dwelt on that. He was looking forward to the celebrations of the fiftieth anniversary of the discovery of insulin. Best enjoyed being interviewed by Dr. Jan Blumenstein, a classmate of Henry's when the latter was a medical student, who made a film of himself talking to CHB on endocrinology. He had completed his PhD in 1962, working on choline and methionine.

Margaret wrote, "Then, on October 15th, Sandy and Eileen appeared in the divorce court. After an hour or two with their lawyers they appeared before the judge and now they have what they call a *decree nisi.* I think the divorce becomes final in two or three months. It is heartbreaking but we have known that it was coming for a long time. Relations had been tense for some time." Eileen was not anxious for a divorce, nor was she bitter, but Sandy was obviously not going to return to her and had developed other romantic interests. Margaret looked every morning at the *Globe and Mail's* Osgoode Hall reports, and the following February, she saw Sandy and Eileen's names on the list of "Divorces Absolute." It was sad, but also probably a relief.

In December 1969 Henry, Janna, and the children went to Québec City where Henry defended his PhD at Laval, a biography of Sir George Etienne Cartier, Sir John A. Macdonald's partner in the Confederation of Canada in 1867. Henry's Québec "parents," Docteur Jean Lacerte and Madame Agathe Lacourcière Lacerte, gave a wonderful reception for Henry, his family and friends to celebrate his passing *cum laude*. Margaret, Charley, and Linda celebrated the occasion when they went to Londonderry Farm for Christmas.

Margaret and Charley were looking forward very much to their return to Rome on 8 April 1970 for the meeting of the Pontifical Academy. At a reception at the Argentinian Embassy, the Bests admired the fifteenth-century Palazzo Patrizi, and enjoyed meeting other guests, including a Chinese cardinal. There was the customary audience with the Pope. Afterwards, the Bests talked to the British ambassador to the Vatican, Sir Michael and Lady Williams.

On Sunday morning, Charley read the lesson at St. Andrew's Church — The Epistle of Paul the Apostle to the Romans, chapter one. "... To all that be in Rome, beloved of God, called to be saints; Give to you peace from God our Father, and the Lord Jesus Christ!" After the service someone said, "No bishop could have done better!" That afternoon Dr. Don McRae, the medical officer at the Canadian embassy, drove the Bests to Casino. "We went down by the big through road and came back by the sea. Gardens were being cultivated and fruit trees were in bloom. The great Benedictine Monastery stands high on the mountain. We drove up the winding road. Casino was destroyed in the fighting between the Germans and the Allies in 1944." The Bests were very impressed with the rebuilt monastery and the statues of St. Benedict and of his sister, St. Scholastica and were moved by role of the Polish and Canadian troops. "We stood at the balustrade and looked down over the hillside and toward the Polish cemetery."

On their last day in Rome, Margaret and Charley once again took a taxi to the Trevi Fountain, talked to a young couple from Paris who were on their honeymoon, and threw a coin in the fountain to ensure that they would return. That evening, Dr. Luigi Travia, professor of medicine at the University of Rome and a diabetic specialist, had a dinner for the Bests at his apartment, via Spallanzani 22. "His apartment is beautifully furnished — rugs, furniture, pictures. In the dining room I was delighted to see several very fine George Morlands[719] on the walls. In the living room one of the paintings was a Canaletto."

On their return to Toronto, Margaret and Charley were pleased to find that Sandy's life had taken a happy turn. "On Sunday morning, we had coffee at Sandy's house on Tranby Avenue, in the Annex. The improvements to the house are going ahead down there." Laurie MacTavish, Sandy's American fiancée, was in town for two or three days from the west. Later in the summer Margaret and Charley drove from Schooner Cove to Prince Edward Island where they visited Sandy and Laurie and Sandy's four children at Dundas Farms. Sandy was building up an important cattle breeding centre there for the owner, Howard Webster. Sandy was travelling a lot on business and Margaret said, "He works very hard, and I think he looks tired." Very quietly, Sandy Best and Laurie MacTavish married on 30 September 1970 in Hart House Chapel at the University of Toronto. "They came to see us last evening on their way to the airport. They were flying to New York. We are very happy. Laurie is a dear girl."

Researchers who worked at the Best Institute regularly moved on to posts elsewhere. Stan Hartroft, who had gone from Toronto to St. Louis and back to the Hospital for Sick Children in Toronto, was now off to Honolulu to help launch a new medical school. Geza Hetenyi was going to the University of Ottawa to chair the Department of Physiology. Dr. Sailen Mookerjea joined the Banting and Best Department first in 1957, returned to India, and came back to the University of Toronto in 1966. He conducted studies on the role of lipotropic factors in cholesterol synthesis and discovered "the occurrence of four different glycosyltransfereases in human amniotic fluid." He later became head of biochemistry at Memorial University of Newfoundland. Mookerjea recalled: "Dr. Colin Lucas and Dr. Best were champions for precise writing in scientific literature ... Dr. Best was a great man who made a tremendous contribution to scientific and medical research, while maintaining a caring and respectful relationship with all fellows and students fortunate enough to have worked with him."[720]

At a special convocation in connection with the opening of the new Medical Sciences Building at the University of Toronto on 7 October 1970 — "a glorious warm day" — Best received an honorary LLD.

[Omond Solandt] made an eloquent and quite touching speech about Charley at the luncheon. Charley is very proud that Omond, the chancellor, Laurie Chute, dean of medicine, and Reg Haist, professor of physiology, were all his pupils … Charley was the one speaker at the luncheon. He did it beautifully. He worked in Professor James DeMille's poem on the place names of New Brunswick and there was much laughter. John Hamilton (the vice-president, health sciences) read the citation for Charley and Omond placed the gorgeous scarlet hood over his head. Then was the ceremony of the official opening of the great new building — Premier Robarts used the golden key.

After the ceremony, the Bests saw John Alfson's portrait of the late "Mac" MacFarlane, which shocked them. "It must have been painted when he was a sick man." Others agreed.

Charles Best's connection with the Connaught Laboratories went back to January 1922, and for years he and his colleague and friend Neil McKinnon had ridden horseback at the Connaught Farm on Steeles Avenue, as had Sandy Best and Jane McKinnon. The Robert Defries Building opened on that site on 20 November 1970. The audience included Bob Defries and Ken Ferguson, past directors of the lab; Albert Fisher, past secretary of the university's Insulin Committee; Milton Brown, Mort Orr, and David Scott, all active in research and production at the lab. "It was a nice day — pouring rain but the weather did not dampen our spirits. That new building is the Insulin Production Laboratory not much like the little old Y.M.C.A. building where it was made almost fifty years ago. Of course, at the very first, Charley and David Scott made it in the basement of the old Medical Building, in the winter and spring of 1922."

The following week researching and writing Best's biography came to an end with Dr. Feasby's sudden death at his farm in Caledon. Bill Feasby, loyal friend and courageous man, was sycophantic in his biography-in-progress on Charles Best, but his research is useful — a number of his interviews are the only ones with many subjects.

The Bests flew to Bermuda for the first time on 2 December 1970. "The airport is perhaps ten miles from Hamilton, winding, narrow roads all the way, some parts like Devonshire lanes. We came through the main street of Hamilton, Front Street, and on to Waterloo House, Pembroke. It

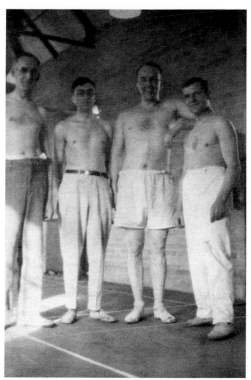

Drs. J.G. FitzGerald, E.W. McHenry, Charles Best, and Neil McKinnon on the track at Hart House, University of Toronto, c. 1929.

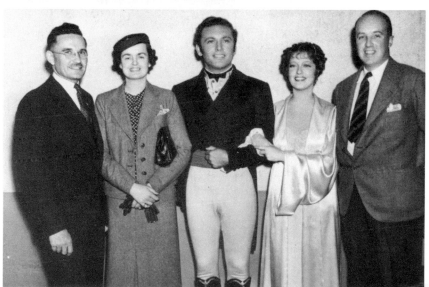

Dr. Elmer Belt, Margaret Best, Alan Jones, Jeanette MacDonald, and Charley Best on the set of *Firefly*, MGM Studios, Hollywood, California, May 1937.

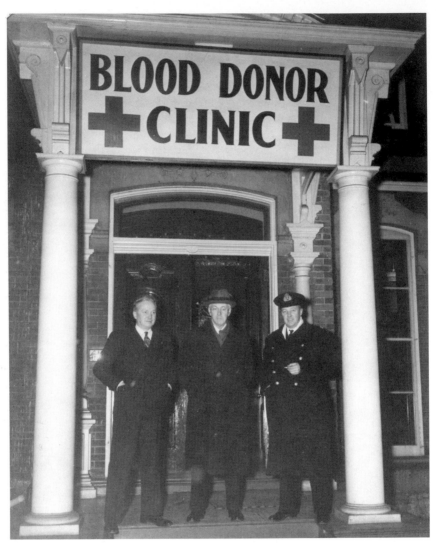

G. Roy Sproat, Sir Henry Dale, and Surgeon Lieutenant-Commander
Charles H. Best, Red Cross Blood Donor Clinic, 410 Sherbourne Street,
Toronto, January 1942.

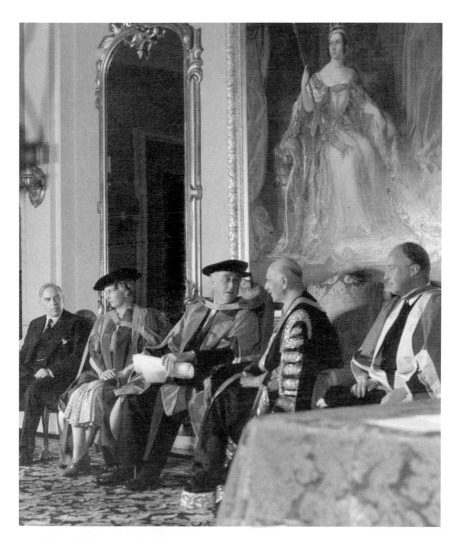

Prime Minister W.L. Mackenzie King, Princess Alice, President F.D. Roosevelt, Lord Athlone, and Charles H. Best, on the occasion of Best's presentation of President Roosevelt to Lord Athlone for an honorary degree from the University of London, England. Rideau Hall, Ottawa, 25 August 1943.

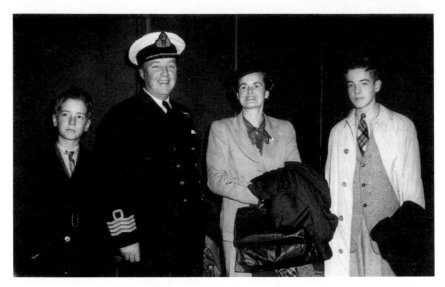

The Best family arriving in Vancouver: 27 June 1944.

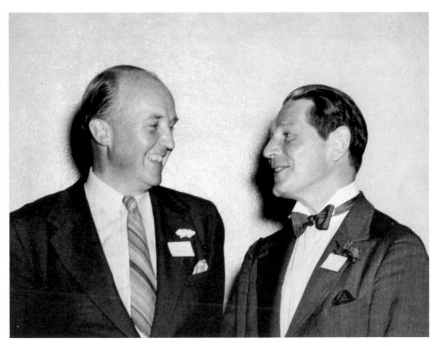

Charles H. Best and R.D. Lawrence, London, 1946.

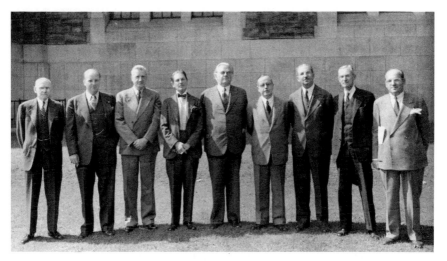

An unusual gathering in one photograph of experts on diabetes and insulin at the 25th anniversary of the discovery of insulin in conjunction with the sixth annual meeting of the American Diabetes Association, Toronto, September 1946.

Elliott P. Joslin of Boston, C.H. Best, Russell Wilder of the Mayo Clinic, R.D. Lawrence of London, H.C. Hagedorn of Copenhagen, B.A. Houssay of Buenos Aires, Joseph Barach of Pittsburgh, Eugene Opie of the Rockefeller Institute, and Cecil Striker of Cincinnati.

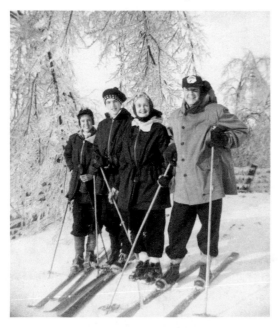

The Best family at Strawberry Hill Farm, Stewarttown, near Georgetown, Ontario, Christmas 1946.

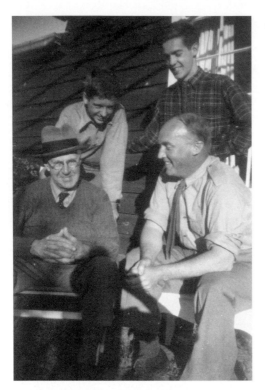

Sir Henry Dale, Charley Best, Henry and Sandy Best at Strawberry Hill Farm, Stewarttown, near Georgetown, Ontario, 1947.

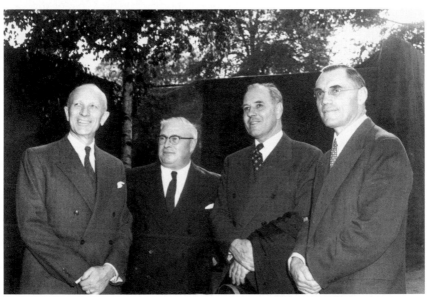

Four distinguished Canadian medical men: Wilder Penfield, J.B. Collip, R.F. Farquharson, and O.M. Solandt, c. 1947.

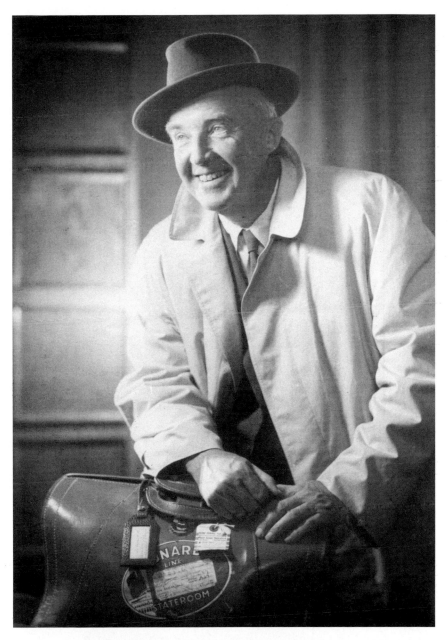

Henry Best's favourite photograph of Charley Best, c. 1950.

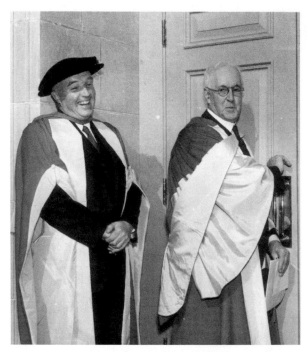

Charles H. Best and Sir Henry Dale at the official opening of the Charles H. Best Institute, University of Toronto,15 September 1953.

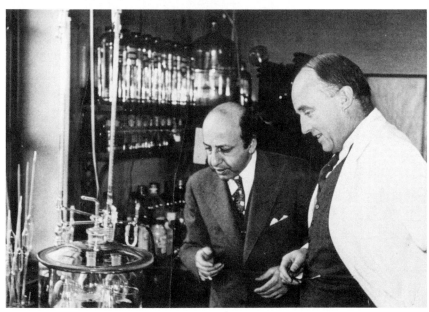

Yousuf Karsh and Charles H. Best: Karsh came to the Best Institute to photograph CHB.
Photo by Dr. Gerald Wrenshall, June 1958.

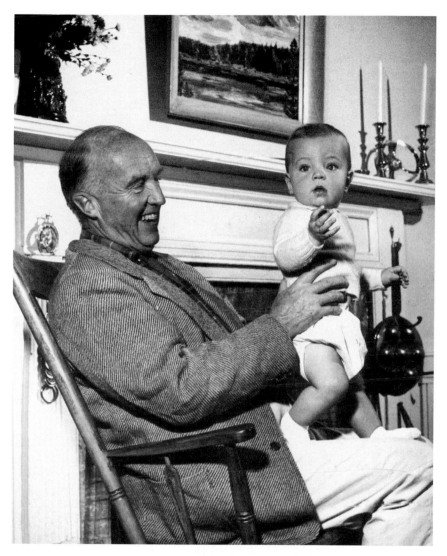

Charles Herbert Best with Charles Stewart Best, his first grandchild, son of Sandy and Eileen Best, in 1959 (photo Garnet Lunny, NFB).

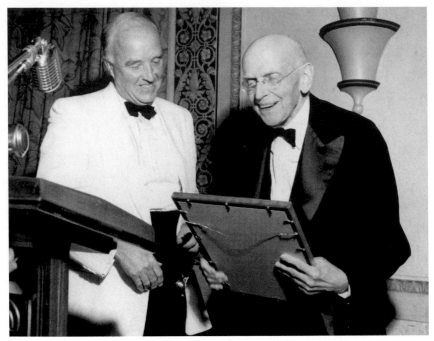

Charles H. Best and Elliott P. Joslin, aged 90,
at ADA meetings, Atlantic City, 1959.

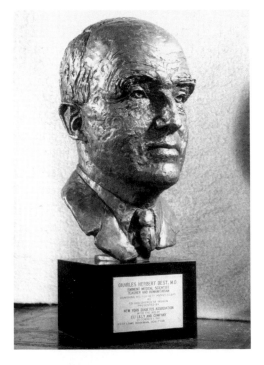

Bust of Charles H. Best by
Ruth Lowe Bookman.
Presented by the New York
Diabetes Association with
the aid of the Eli Lilly
Company, 1 December
1961, in commemoration of
the 40th anniversary of the
discovery of insulin.

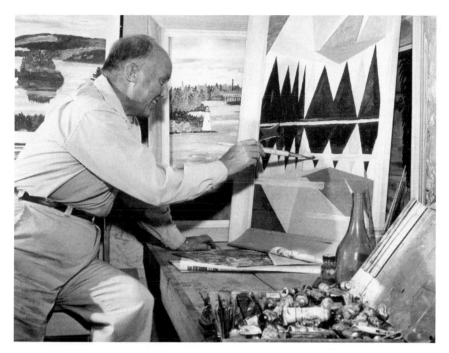

Charley Best, painting in the furnace room of 105 Woodlawn Avenue West, Toronto, c. 1962. His only attempt at non-objective art, though the scene is Schooner Cove like the majority of his canvasses.

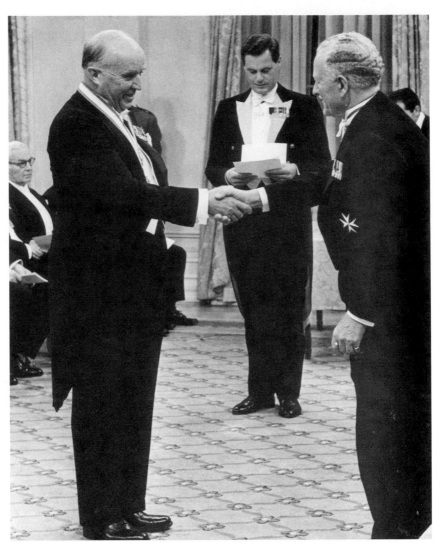

Governor General Roland Michener presents the Commander of the Order of Canada to Charles H. Best (Esmond Butler, secretary to the governor general, is in the background), 12 November 1967.

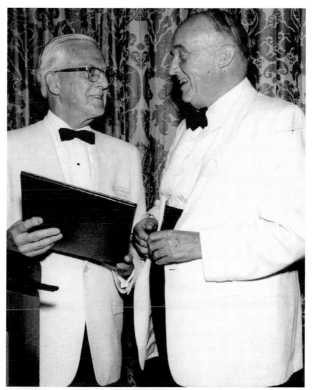

Dr. Edwin Gates, president of the American Diabetes Association, presenting a document recording the acquisition of the birthplace of Charles H. Best in West Pembroke, Maine, signed on 15 June 1968.

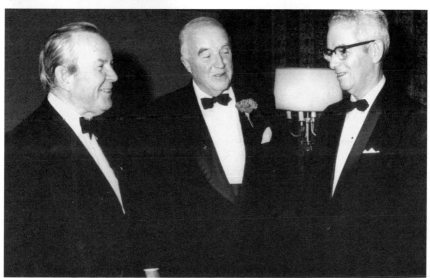

Lester B. Pearson, Charles Best, and Dr. Randall Sprague of the Mayo Clinic, at the Canadian Diabetes Association dinner celebrating the 50th anniversary of the discovery of insulin, Toronto, 8 November 1971.

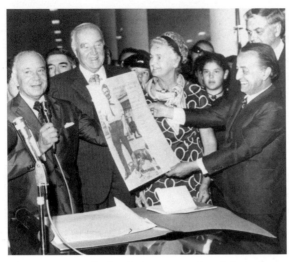

Presentation of
Biennial Science Prize
to Charles H. Best,
Sao Paulo, Brazil,
4 September 1971.

l to r: Dr. Edmundo Vasconcelos (chairman of the Biennial Science
Committee), Charles H. Best, Margaret Best, Dr. Zeferino Vaz
(president of the University of Campinas), and Barry Steers
(Canadian Ambassador to Brazil).

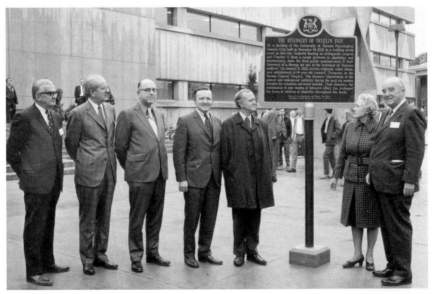

Unveiling of the plaque at the site of the old Medical Building, University
of Toronto, commemorating the discovery of insulin, 25 October 1971.

Drs. R.E. Haist, Albert Fisher, A.L. Chute, Harold Alexander, president
of the CDA, Professor J.M.S. Careless, representing the Historic Sites
Board of Ontario, Lady Henrietta Banting, and Charles Best.

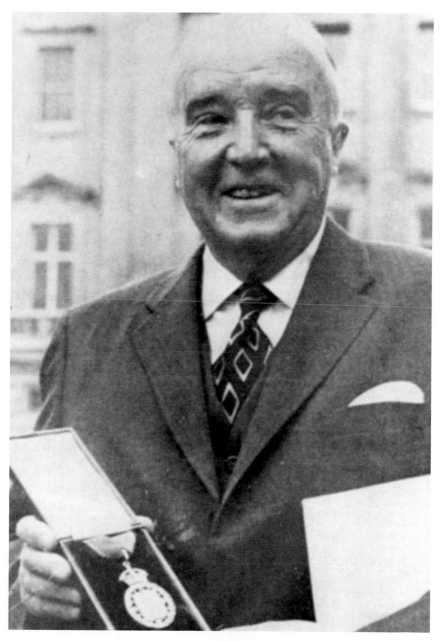

Charles H. Best as he left Buckingham Palace, London, just after having been presented with the medal of the Companion of Honour by Queen Elizabeth II, 16 December 1971.

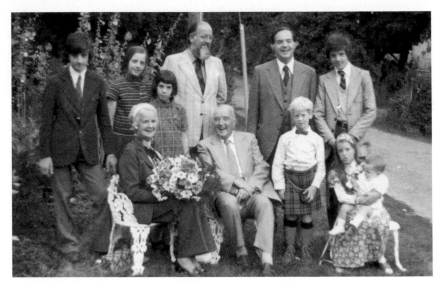

The 50th wedding anniversary of Margaret and Charley Best at
Londonderry Farm, Moffat, Ontario, 3 September 1974.

Front row: Margaret, Charley, and Bruce and Mairi — children of Henry
and Janna Best. Mairi is holding Susan MacTavish Best, daughter of Sandy
and Laurie MacTavish Best. Back row: Alexander, Margaret Cairine,
Melinda, and Charles Stewart — children of Sandy and Eileen Best —
with Henry and Sandy in the centre.

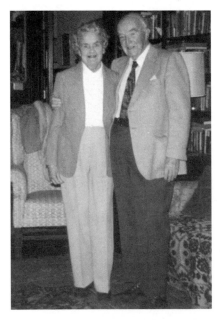

Margaret and Charley Best at their
home, 105 Woodlawn Avenue West,
Toronto, taken by Linda Mahon
before they left for New York,
22 January 1978.

is a pink stucco place, charming, with steps up and down, tropical plants, little courtyards. Our room looks directly on the Harbour, and there are boats of all descriptions coming and going constantly — sailboats, fishing boats, tugs, ferries, destroyers and freighters."

On the Sunday morning, the Bests attended St. Andrew's Presbyterian — "the only pink church I have ever seen. We saw a plaque on the wall in memory of a minister who had been here from 1891 to 1908 (Rev. Andrew Burrows, MA, DD). That was evidently the time when my father was asked to come to Hamilton as their minister. I would be seven years old then. I remember very well the decision being made to stay in St. Andrews, New Brunswick. The trip to Bermuda was one of the happiest we have ever had — my seventieth birthday present."

Sue and "Mac" MacTavish, Laurie's parents, arrived in Toronto for a visit in early February 1971. "On Wednesday evening they came here for dinner — our first meeting and we like them very much. They are both tall and we think Laurie looks like her mother. Mac's father was born in Scotland, Inverness district, I think. Mac is a graduate of McGill University. He has retired now from the Chase Manhattan Bank, New York." They had a tour of the Best Institute, and Sandy took both families to the Albany Club.

There was a rare reference in Margaret's diary to events outside science and the family. "The great excitement last week was the unexpected marriage of Pierre Trudeau, our prime minister. He married a beautiful twenty-two year old girl, Margaret Sinclair, of Vancouver. I think most people are delighted."

Fiftieth Anniversary of the Discovery of Insulin

Nineteen seventy-one marked the fiftieth anniversary of the discovery of insulin, and the Bests received far more requests than they could handle. "Every day invitations came to go here and there. Everyone wants Charley in this wonderful golden year of insulin." Mairi and Bruce helped put together a small album of photographs of the six grandchildren for Grammy to take with her on her travels.

Margaret and Charley Best flew to New York on 5 April and checked in at the Waldorf-Astoria. Mac and Sue MacTavish were waiting for them in the lobby. Dick and Wilva Connelly of the ADA took the Bests to the Barbetta Restaurant on 46th Street and then to the musical *Applause*, starring Lauren Bacall. "Lauren Bacall is an amazing woman — a most strenuous part and she was splendid. We really enjoyed every minute. Charley and I had not been at a theatre for ages."

The next morning, Charley gave interviews at the studios in the Roosevelt Hotel for World Health Day. Margaret wrote, "I firmly refused to be interviewed. However, a photographer took several pictures which I fear will not be flattering as I was tired and not in a cooperating mood. However, Charley looked rosy and happy." After lunch with the MacTavishes, Laurie went with her father-in-law back to the NBC studio, as she had considerable experience in the media. That evening, the MacTavishes were hosts for drinks at the Canadian Club on top of one of the Waldorf towers. From there they all went to Club 21 for dinner. "Two of the owners came to talk to Mac — one had a diabetic mother. I ate Nova Scotia smoked salmon, roast duckling with orange, etc. and banana ice cream — appropriate drinks! It was a gay and successful evening."

At six the next morning, Dick Connelly took Charley and Laurie to 50 West 55th Street, the NBC studios. There Charley was made up to be interviewed by Ed Newman and Barbara Walters for TV's "Today Show." "I watched the show at the Waldorf in our bedroom. It went off splendidly. It was in colour. It lasted about fifteen minutes — perhaps a little longer. It was seen all over the U.S. and, of course, in Toronto. Laurie knows so much about television shows."

On 14 April 1971, Margaret and Charley flew first class, free, courtesy of Air Canada, to London and then on to Holland and Denmark for a series of events to mark the fiftieth anniversary of the discovery of insulin. A deputation from the British Diabetic Association (BDA) — Peter Allard, Dr. John Butterfield, James Jackson, and Alan Nabarro — met them at the airport, along with several photographers. "All interesting but rather exhausting." Butterfield, vice-chancellor at the University of Nottingham, drove them to the Stafford Hotel that they knew so well.

"We had a short rest yesterday and then things began to hum — thirty-five or possibly more reporters and photographers assembled at the hotel. As Charley and I entered the Breakfast Room on the ground floor there they were standing — a formidable crowd. They fired questions at Charley for more than an hour. Then he had a private interview with the *Times* correspondent. They took literally hundreds of pictures — a few out of doors. Charley did three taped interviews for radio broadcasts."

There was a stop at Moss Bros on Regent Street to arrange for a morning coat for the service at St. Paul's Cathedral. For the first time, the Bests saw the new quarters of the Royal Society at 6 Carlton Terrace. In the evening they enjoyed the farce *The Philanthropist*, by Christopher Hampton, aged twenty-four, at the Mayfair Theatre.

On Monday, Charley unveiled a plaque in memory of Robin Lawrence at the BDA offices. Both Adam and Dan Lawrence and their wives were there. It was a fitting ceremony, "but we are very sad that Robin is gone." Lunch at the Royal Society preceded Best's lecture there, and guests included Dr. Alan Hodgkin, the president, Sir Frank and Lady Young, and Lady Todd. In the audience for the lecture were Marguerite Hoet, Philippe, and his bride, Roselyne. CHB spoke on "Fifty Years of Insulin." Afterwards, the new agent general for Ontario, Allan Rowan-Legg, and his wife held a reception.

The next day the Bests moved to the Ciba Foundation. The BBC interviewed Charley, and then they went to a reception held by the Royal College of Medicine at Chandos House. Margaret did not go: "I don't feel very well — tired out, I think. It is a very strenuous trip. I went to bed at two o'clock and did not move about again until the following morning — a rather severe intestinal attack." Charley took Margaret to Chandos House the next day to see the rooms. That evening, they had dinner at Verrey's on Regent Street and then on to the Globe Theatre to see *Kean* with Alan Badel in the title role. "It was splendid — a translation of the Jean-Paul Sartre play about Edmund Kean," the early-nineteenth-century London actor.

Then the Canadians went to the Tate Gallery. "I particularly wanted to see the Turners again — especially the late Turners. They were very beautiful. Again, I was not feeling very well — dizzy — so I went to bed and did not get up again until yesterday morning. I was very much afraid that I would miss the service of thanksgiving for the discovery of insulin in St. Paul's Cathedral."

On Sunday, the Bests had lunch at Ciba with Gordon and Dushanka Wolstenholme and Frank and Ruth Young. It was pouring rain as they walked up the steps to St. Paul's — "a crowd of people gathered on the steps and many photographers — within the cathedral, one thousand people. We were escorted to the front row of pews and there we sat with Mr. and Mrs. Charles Ritchie (the Canadian high commissioner) and Lord and Lady Fiske." Lord Fiske, president of the British Diabetic Association, had come to see the Bests a few days before. He was in charge of introducing the new decimal monetary system in Britain which Charley found interesting. Margaret continued, "It was very impressive as we looked up into the chancel — great bunches of flowers — red and yellow — carnations, tulips, snapdragons, gladiolas, daffodils, etc. The full length of the chancel was lighted by red-shaded lights. A procession was led into the chancel — the Lord Mayor of London and his wife and other city dignitaries wearing beautiful chains of office. Then the Duchess of Kent and her lady-in-waiting were escorted to two chairs immediately in front of us."

"Charley read the first lesson, 2 Kings 4: 18-37, '... and when Elisha was come into the house, behold, the child was dead, and laid upon his bed. He went in therefore, and shut the door upon them twain, and prayed unto the Lord. And he went up and lay upon the child, and put his mouth upon his mouth, and his eyes upon his eyes, and his hands upon his hands and he stretched himself upon the child and the flesh of the child waxed warm ...' The dean of St. Paul's, the Very Rev. Martin Sullivan, gave an appropriate and dynamic sermon for the occasion — he talked of the discovery and of the wonderful fact that one of the discoverers was with us. He said that a few days ago, he was presenting prizes at a nurses' graduation and that a man nurse and a woman had won them. He took a close look at the books he was presenting and saw that they were *The Living Body* by Charles H. Best and Norman B. Taylor."

After the service, the Bests went with the Ritchies and Dr. Black, the official scientific adviser, in the high commission's limousine, with the Canadian flag flying, to the official residence on Upper Brook Street. There was a tea there for about two hundred people. The Bests had made sure that Cousin Mary Scott was invited. Dinner took place at the Apothecaries' Hall, the first building burned in the Great Fire of 1666, rebuilt two years later; a bomb in the Second World War created the gaping hole in the front of the hall. Margaret found John Butterfield and Dr. D.M.F. Bishop — past master of the Apothecaries — amiable dinner companions. "Eventually we arrived at speeches — Lord Fiske spoke about the debt of diabetics to the Toronto discovery. John Butterfield proposed a toast to Charley and to me. Charley replied and proposed a toast to the BDA. When Charley stood up the whole dinner party rose and gave us an ovation. It was very moving. Alan Nabarro, the honorary secretary of the BDA, replied to Charley's toast to the BDA. He had a written speech telling of his struggle as a boy diabetic before the discovery of insulin — very moving." He had been taking insulin for fifty years. "Afterwards, both

Charley and I signed dozens of menu cards — mothers came to tell me of their young children who lead happy lives because of insulin."

The BDA branches met the next day at the Bloomsbury Central Hotel. Frank Young chaired the gathering. Best spoke on "Insulin in Retrospect and Prospect." Later, BBC television interviewed John Butterfield and Charley. That evening, the London branches of the BDA held a dinner at the House of Commons, hosted by Nigel Spearing, Labour MP for Acton. Charley spoke to the four hundred people present, "Then scores of people crowded around to get not only Charley's signature, but mine also!" On all these occasions, speakers invariably mentioned not only Charley, but also Margaret. "I have been very proud." After over fifty years of devotion, particularly through severe illness, Charley wanted Margaret to share in the recognition.

The next stop was The Hague, where Fritz and Ruth Gerritzen met the plane. Organon, the Dutch manufacturer of insulin, supported the visit. Young Fritz Gerritzen and his wife were there; he had developed a large diabetic practice since he had worked at the lab in Toronto. Next day, at the University of Leiden, Charles lectured on "Fifty Years of Insulin" to a medical audience. The following day, the Bests visited a Diabetic Children's House near Utrecht, where they met many diabetic children and their parents. The children sang "My Bonnie" in English and performed folk dances. Using pink hyacinth blooms, they formed the name "Best" on the grass. "Finally we had to say good-bye and drove out to the road through an avenue of waving children. It was a thrilling experience."

The visitors went the next day to the Mauritshuis Museum in The Hague to see the Rembrandts and Vermeer's *Head of a Girl* and *View of Delft*. In late afternoon of the next day, a car arrived from Belgium with Marguerite Hoet, Pep, her son Matthew, and Marie-Noëlle. Jo arrived later with several more of his children. By the next day, when they sat down to dinner, there were twenty-two Hoets from three generations to see the Bests.

Jacob and Kirsten Poulsen met the Bests' plane in Copenhagen and drove them to the Palace Hotel. Mrs. Hagedorn seemed very well, but her husband was no longer able to communicate. CHB lectured at the Nordisk Laboratories in Gentofte. Margaret thought this perhaps his best speech of the trip — "at least I thought so, his choice of words was always so perfect."

Back in London on 9 May, they enjoyed Robert Morley in Alan Ayckbourn's *How the Other Half Loves* — "He is a most hilarious stout fellow." Another evening, there was a performance of Enid Bagnold's *The Chalk Garden*.

"Gladys Cooper played the leading part! She is in her eighties and still beautiful." Miss Cooper died only a few months later.

In spite of the demanding schedule, the Bests found this special month-long visit to Britain and Europe particularly thrilling, "a wonderful trip." It was a time of many honours for Charles Best. At the end of May 1971, he received an honorary degree from Laurentian University in Sudbury, Ontario. Dr. R.J.A. Cloutier was acting president, and William B. Plaunt was chairman of the board of governors. The heads of the federated universities of Laurentian were at the ceremony. At the dinner that evening, "I got to know Mr. and Mrs. Plaunt. They were great friends of Jack and Ethel Robertson," Margaret's cousins. "Charley had his beautiful hood — blue with a touch of yellow." "Dr. Lee (of the School of Nursing) took us to Laurentian University, splendid — on a hill beyond Ramsey Lake. It was very fine — the buildings are new, and modern and striking. We climbed up a story or two in one and saw the fine views of Ramsey Lake and another lake," and the cottage that had been built by the Robertson cousins, which now belonged to the university.

The CDA held a meeting in Toronto in connection with the anniversary of the discovery of insulin and presented CHB with a colourful scroll. A few days later Margaret and Charley went to Alliston; Gordon Wright, principal of the Banting High School, had organized the visit. His father-in-law, Professor John Baker of Guelph University, had been a colleague of Charley's in the navy and was over eighty. Margaret judged him "just about the best storyteller I have ever met." Edward Banting, a son of Thompson's and a nephew of Fred's, was at the dinner with his wife. Charley had a big day — speeches to two groups of nine hundred students, a lunch courtesy of the mayor, a meeting with local doctors and those from Camp Borden, dinner, and then his lecture. Ken MacTaggart, whom the Bests had known when he worked for the *Toronto Telegram*, was master of ceremonies. "It was a long day and a heavy one for Charley."

On 11 June 1971, it was announced that the Queen was awarding Charles Best the Companion of Honour. A few days earlier, Lord Dunrossil, counsellor at the United Kingdom's high commission, had called from Ottawa with the news. There were many calls, pictures in the newspapers, and cables from Britain. The Bests would be off to London in December for the investiture. There had also been much communication about an award from Brazil, the first Brazil Science Biennial Prize. The presentation was to take place at Sao Paulo in August.

The family decided to sell the last of Sandy's farms. The Taylor place on the Second Line of Nassagaweya was a lovely property, with an old log house and a good barn, but the Bests could not afford to keep it. Margaret noted that it was listed at $69,000 and brought $45,000. "Henry Best came to see us on Friday. Laurie was there when he came and they met for the first time."

It was the time for the annual trip to Maine. Margaret, Charley, and Linda set out on 30 June. At Schooner Cove Farm, "the rabbits are as tame or more so than last year — sitting on the lawn nibbling. The white-throated sparrows are singing. It is all glorious."

But even in Maine they continued to receive invitations. Dr. Rachmiel Levine called to invite Charley to open his new Metabolism Building near Los Angeles in February. Best was not sure that he would be up for this, and did not give a definite answer to the invitation. Sam Lunenfeld phoned from Toronto wanting the Bests to go to Israel for Christmas, where Charley would receive an honorary degree from the Hebrew University of Jerusalem and give a lecture. Linda would go to be of help, and the Israeli government would foot the bill.

By early August there had been several letters from the Queen's secretary about the Companion of Honour. The idea was to go to Israel by way of London in December. After more correspondence, 16 December was decided for the royal ceremony. The mail on 6 August brought invitations to Uruguay and to Vancouver, but the Bests did not think that they could fit those in.

In Maine, the old friends who came for the summer and those who were permanent residents kept the social schedule busy. Hilda's son, Charley Ralph Salter, and his family stayed for a few days at his mother's cottage at the point. They had the Bests down for supper and the next day had a tour of the house in Pembroke where Hilda and her brother had lived.

Margaret Mahon Best's sixty-ninth diary covers the period from August 1971 to April 1972. In those months the Bests made eleven trips of some distance, three within Canada and eight to the United States or further — four outside North America — quite remarkable, given their age and their health history.

The Bests left Toronto on 28 August 1971 to catch a nine-hour flight from New York to Rio de Janeiro. On arrival in Rio, there was "much showing of passports, etc. and then a frantic scene when the luggage was claimed, there was no porter to help collect them, and it was terribly hot in the shed.

Customs inspection was very slow but no trouble otherwise." Dr. Carlos Chagas Filho, Brazil's scientific ambassador to UNESCO, was in charge of arrangements. Their room at the Copacabana Palace Hotel faced the ocean.

Charley lectured at the Institute of Biophysics for Dr. Chagas, who was also its director, on "History of Insulin and Recent Developments." Lord Adrian attended the lecture. That evening Professor and Sra Chagas entertained at their own home, and the other guests were Ulf and Dagmar von Euler of Stockholm, Dr. John Kendrew of Cambridge (a Nobel laureate in 1962 for his work on protein chemistry), Adrian, and several Brazilian doctors. Their host told of his father — the discoverer of Chagas' disease — going to Toronto in 1922 to obtain insulin for his wife, the first person in South America to receive it.

At São Paulo, Dr. Arnoldo Sandoval, secretary general of the diabetic association, met the plane. Dr. Edmundo Vasconcelos, head of a large private hospital and chairman of the Biennial Science Committee, joined them at the Othon Hotel. The Bests and Professor Kendrew went for a drive into the country the next day and saw the new University of Campinas. They met the rector, Zeferino Vaz, a small, dynamic man, and Kendrew spoke to a medical audience. The professor of physiology told Margaret that it was "as though Santa Claus had come, unbelievable."

Margaret and Charley were both very careful not to eat raw fruit and vegetables, but Margaret developed an "extreme form of an intestinal disturbance." Charley had sounded a bit hoarse on Thursday, looked flushed on Friday, and became really sick on Saturday. Mrs. Vasconcelos took her guests to the police headquarters to get their passports. "Charley was getting more and more weary. We came back to the hotel, missed a dinner party that had been planned, and went to bed. Charley developed a temperature and Dr. Sandoval came to see him and gave us medicine."

The next morning they both felt better, and they went to the Biennial celebrations. Senhor Ermelino Matarazzo, the donor, presented this first Biennial Science Prize, but not the U.S. $25,000 in prize money — "It will be sent to a bank in Toronto." Charley received two parchments — for the Biennial Science Prize and for membership in the Military Medical Academy — and a colourful medal from the academy.

Back at the hotel, Charley's fever rose to 103 degrees Fahrenheit and even with drugs refused for some time to go down. He had viral pneumonia and everyone wanted to help. There were reports on the functions that they were missing. At a dinner given by the diabetic association, Dr.

Sandoval read a poem that he had written for Charley and Margaret and the English translation. "He is a most unusual, fascinating man." The hotel room was full of flowers sent by Canadian diplomats and various others.

The next day, Charley had a fever of 104 degrees and Sandoval decided to admit him to the Gastroclinica — a private clinic owned by Dr. Vasconcelos, designed by Oscar Niemeyer, the architect responsible for Brasilia. X-Rays and blood counts followed. "We are installed in a suite of rooms on the top floor of this very modern, beautiful hospital. Mrs. Vasconcelos was here and has helped in telephoning to Henry at Londonderry Farm. Henry answered the phone at once and Charley explained to him what has happened and that we would not be in Toronto tomorrow. A bed for me has been made up in this large room. There is also a sitting room and two bathrooms." By the next day the patient had improved.

"Yesterday much coming and going in our room — doctors, nurses, and even newspaper reporters. Charley and I were lying in our beds and I was horrified when I realized that the photographer had taken pictures of both of us. This morning many visitors coming and going … From our windows here — top, sixth floor of the clinic, we see down below us the landing place for Dr. Vasconcelos' helicopter." Patients came with their relatives to meet the Bests. Margaret made a list of the thirty-nine people who came; beside some names she wrote, "Reasons for visit unknown." One reporter stayed for one and half hours.

Paul Théberge, the Canadian consul, drove the Bests to the airport. "The scene was beyond description — thousands of people milling about. Without Paul we would have had great difficulty. They took our passports and we did not get them back until ten minutes before we went out to the plane." Edmundo and Eliza Vasconcelos and Arnoldo and Catherine Sandoval came to wish them "Bon voyage."

Both Margaret and Charley were exhausted by the time they reached home on 11 September. From Argentina they received the very sad news that the Bests' old and valued friend Bernardo Houssay had died in Buenos Aires. Charley not only admired his colleague as a great scientist, but always was grateful for his unwavering loyalty.

By 30 September, however, the Bests were on the road again, this time for a short trip to New York for the nineteenth annual symposium of the Clinical Society of the New York Diabetes Association. They were well looked after — a room at the Waldorf and a limousine to ferry them around. Laurie once again spent some time helping them in New York. Mayor John Lindsay had been supposed to receive them, but he was off electioneering, and Vice-Mayor Ted Palmer presented Charley with a large gold key, "certainly *not* gold," said Margaret. Irving and Gretchen Graef of the ADA entertained the Bests at their apartment at 25 East 86th Street. Charley was honorary chairman of the symposium the next day at the Barbizon Plaza Hotel. That afternoon, Joseph Lubin, science editor of the *Voice of America*, interviewed Charley.

The next trip was to Mont Gabriel in the Laurentians, north of Montréal. Hans Giese of Hoechst had organized a workshop on insulin, and Ken Gorman, Reg Haist, Peter Moloney, and Otto Sirek from Toronto made presentations. Moloney received a citation — the first Charles H. Best Medal given by Hoechst of Canada — and a cheque for one thousand dollars.

The Bests flew on 17 October to Indianapolis where CHB gave the introductory lecture for Lilly's 50th Anniversary Insulin Symposium, entitled "Summer of 1921." Henrietta Banting and Albert Fisher were down from Toronto. Dorothy Hodgkin and Philip Randle of England and George Cahill, Leo Krall, Arnold Lazarow, Rachmiel Levine, and I. Arthur Mirsky of the United States were some of the participants. Charley and Randy Sprague made a TV program together. One day, Margaret and Charley arrived in their hotel room and were amused to find forty-eight bottles of beer and mountains of ice cubes in their basin and bathtub, apparently not for them but meant for an American Legion meeting.

Charles Best had a very high opinion of the scientific expertise and the integrity of the Lilly company and close friendships with some of its officers, particularly G.H.A. Clowes and Bruce Peck, as well as members of the Lilly family, especially Eli and Ruth. Mrs. Otto Behrens, wife of the associate director of research, took Margaret to the art gallery on the property of J.K. Lilly, Jr. "It is an amazing place with enormous grounds and the gallery is huge and very modern. We spent quite a long time there — paintings from many periods — English, Italian, Flemish, American — Mexican and Peruvian pottery — ancient Roman and Greek jars, etc." The Eli Lillys were at their home at Wawasee, but neither was well, so the Bests decided not to go to see them but instead talked with them on the phone.

On 24 October 1971, there was a service of thanksgiving for insulin at St. James' Cathedral in Toronto. Eileen, with her four children, and Henry and Janna, with their two, were there. Charley read the first lesson,

2 Kings 4: 18-37, the same as at St. Paul's Cathedral in London. The next day, Henrietta Banting and Charley unveiled a historic plaque marking the site of the lab in the old Medical Building where insulin was discovered. "The wording is very good but we were a little surprised that it was in English on both sides (not one in French and one in English)." Years later the wording was changed to expand the role of Macleod and Collip, and fit in with a revised version of the events of 1921–22. Then, in the lobby of the Medical Sciences Building, Margaret unveiled Ruth Lowe Bookman's bust of Best. There were copies of the same bronze in the living room at 105 Woodlawn Avenue, at the Academy of Medicine, and at the New York Diabetes Association.

A couple of days later a special convocation at the University of Toronto marked the installation of the new chancellor, Pauline McGibbon, and the fiftieth anniversary of insulin. Walter Campbell was presented for an honorary degree by Ian Macdonald; Robert Defries, by Bernard Bucove, the last director of the School of Hygiene; Knud Hallas-Møller, director of Novo in Copenhagen, by Reg Haist; Leo Krall of the Joslin Clinic, by Irving Fritz; Peter Moloney, by John Logothetopoulos; and David Scott, by Ken Ferguson. Hans Christian Hagedorn was to have received a degree, but he had died. Omond Solandt addressed the audience. "His references to Charley were very touching to me and he said words to this effect, 'that few couples are so beloved around the world as Charley and Margaret Best.'"

Charley gave the final lecture of the Symposium on Insulin Action, held from 25 to 27 October. He wrapped up his talk with: "For twenty years, my wife and I were among the youngest at these Insulin Conferences. We are now at the other extreme but we still enjoy them. The chief reason is that so many of you younger people are our good friends."[721] Other participants included Dorothy Hodgkin, Arthur Rubenstein, Donald Steiner, Cecil Yip, John Logothetopoulos, and Mladen Vranic.

The Gairdner Foundation gave a luncheon on 29 October for the recipients of its 1971 awards. Several family members were included: Linda, Sandy and Laurie, Charley's niece Joan Salter Bain and her husband Stan Bain, as well as Don and Sally Fraser. The Gairdner Foundation's sessions began with a lecture by CHB, followed by Dr. Frederick Sanger, a Nobel laureate from Cambridge, and then by Dr. Rosalyn Yalow of New York, who was to win a Nobel prize in 1977.

In the evening, Mr. and Mrs. James A. Gairdner, the Bests, and Dr. Ramsay Gunton, acting president of the foundation, and his wife greeted the guests at a dinner at the National Club. "It was a most beautifully arranged affair. Every detail had been carefully thought out." The recipients of the Gairdner Awards were Solomon Berson of New York, Charles Best, Rachmiel Levine, Frederick Sanger, and Donald Steiner. Lady Banting presented a scroll and a cheque for five thousand dollars to CHB, who gave out the other awards. On 1 November, Henry Best drove his father to the Canadian Club, where Charles Best spoke on "Medical Research in Canada."

The Bests' next stop was Minneapolis, where their hosts tried not to be too demanding. Margaret was taken to the Walker Art Center, "very modern outside and in — stark white walls which are splendid for background. They have a show of Joan Miró sculptures. He has been a name to me previously but now I have really seen him, some are weird — many called simply 'Woman,' others 'Personage' — some of metal, some of stone, many women with a bird sitting on the head." There were television and radio interviews. At the dinner the governor presented Charley with a plaque. "Now, therefore, I, Wendell R. Anderson, Governor of the State of Minnesota, do proclaim Thursday, November 11, 1971, as Dr. Charles H. Best day." Charley spoke on "Diabetes Research: Fifty Years Ago, Today, in the Future."

Back in Toronto, Margaret was much troubled by a hiatus hernia. She was afraid that she would miss the banquet at the Inn on the Park on 18 November given by the Toronto district, and by the national office of the Canadian Diabetes Association, but she was able to go. Margaret Gorman was organizer for the occasion. Linda, Sandy, Laurie, and Bill Banting were there, and Randy Sprague from the Mayo Clinic. Janna came from Londonderry Farm, picking up family friend Freda Herbert in Georgetown. Linda introduced them both to Laurie whom they had not met before. Henry was teaching at York University and arrived later. The first speaker was Lester B. Pearson, the former prime minister. Then, "Randy Sprague briefly reviewed the insulin story and his own history, followed by Laurie Chute, who said, 'I am not going to talk about the scientific achievements of Charles Best but of Charley Best the man,' and he told several stories about his oral examination with Charley, the histamine story (the overdose) and about helping Helen by providing heparin when their first baby was born. He said that Margaret and Charley were loved by everyone." At the time of his MA oral, Charley asked Laurie, "What is the water content of the human body?" A very unsure Laurie answered, "ninety-five percent," to which Charley calmly replied, "No, that's a cucumber."

In early December, the Bests attended a dinner sponsored by the Shaari Shoncoyhn Brotherhood, a synagogue on Glencairn Avenue in Toronto. Linda, Janna, and Henry were also invited. All the men, including Charley and Henry, wore yarmulkes. On a canoe trip in the summer re-enacting the Nor' Westers' fur-trading at Fort William, Henry had grown a patriarchal beard. "Henry, with his splendid beard, looked very fine." Dr. Norman Rasky, a dental surgeon, was chairman. "Bernie Leibel introduced Charley in a delightful way and Charley spoke for about half an hour, showing slides, 'The History of Insulin.' Rabbi Forman thanked Charley — a most eloquent and beautiful speech and presented Charley with the Jerusalem Medal, which came from the Shaari Zeeleh Hospital in Jerusalem, brought by hand by a member of the Toronto Synagogue — a very beautiful medal encased in glass on a small wooden stand."

Margaret and Charley would soon be in Jerusalem themselves. On 14 December 1971, the Bests and Linda Mahon left Toronto for London and the investiture of the Companion of Honour by the Queen. J.G.L. Jackson and Peter Allard of the BDA met them and took them to the Stafford Hotel, where they were greeted by Mr. Brown, the owner, and members of his staff. Charley was driven to the BBC to record a TV broadcast. The next morning there were photographers from *The Times*. At Margaret's request Charley wrote a detailed description of the audience at Buckingham Palace on 17 December 1971. He described his arrival at the palace and being escorted by two young officers to a large beautiful room where the Queen was standing.

> The Queen came forward as I walked toward her and we shook hands. She picked up the case containing the decoration, opened it and presented it to me. I said that I was very honoured to receive it, that it was very beautiful and thanked her. Her Majesty asked me to sit down and we talked about various matters for about forty minutes. She asked me about the early work on insulin, how Fred Banting and I knew where to search for insulin, and how long we worked before we were certain of success. She was very interested in diabetes and had a friend who had been taking insulin for over thirty years. The friend had kept very fit, but recently had some trouble with her feet.

445

> The Queen said, "Great Scot, Professor Best, she would have been dead many years ago without insulin."

The Queen mentioned her visits to Canada and Toronto. She was soon to leave for Africa and was receiving injections to prevent yellow fever. Charley told her that he and Margaret were going to Israel for which they had been vaccinated against cholera.

> Her Majesty asked if great progress had been made in the field of insulin in recent years. I said that many advances had been made in the laboratory studies and we hoped for more application to the treatment of patients. She asked how many people had received insulin and I told her that the statisticians estimated that nearly one hundred million had taken it — some for short periods, others for up to 49 years. I told her that we regretted that so many diabetics in underdeveloped countries could not obtain insulin.[722]

The Queen thanked Charley for telling her about recent work on insulin. They shook hands and he thanked her for the great honour, stepped backward, bowed, and left. Charley was disappointed that Margaret could not be present. The investiture of the Companion of Honour is made to the recipient alone in private audience with the Queen.

From London, security was very strict for the El Al flight to Tel Aviv — the Bests travelled first class, guests of the Israeli government. Sam Lunenfeld, Professor Eleazar Shafrir of the Department of Clinical Biochemistry at the Hebrew University of Jerusalem, and Avner Shavitsky, assistant to university president Avraham Harman, met the plane and drove their guests to the King David Hotel.

Professor Jacob Katz, rector of the university, and his wife gave a lunch for the Bests at the Belgian House (the faculty club). Dr. Hanna (Anna) Gelber was there, as were Canadian Ambassador Charles McGaughey and his wife, Jessie.

The next morning, Charley talked to faculty members and students at the Hadassah Medical Centre. Margaret and Linda went to the synagogue to look at the twelve Chagall windows that they had seen in New York in 1961. "They are very beautiful and fascinating — no human represented but birds, fish, animals. The colours are wonderful — yellow, blue, red and green."

Charley made a television broadcast, and then they all went to the Knesset. After passing through the strict security, Mrs. Harman, a member of the Knesset, gave them a personal tour. Eunice Kennedy Shriver was there with a group of American girls. The Bests met Mrs. Grossman, chair of the Knesset's Public Services Committee, who represented the non-Jewish people of Israel. The Bests found the enormous Chagall tapestries "magnificent. They were woven in France — the colours very beautiful. They depict biblical scenes — human figures as well as animals in these tapestries. On the floor here and there were mosaics, also Chagall's, and on one end wall close to the great windows was an enormous mosaic in rather bright colours — strong and delicate at once — the Wailing Wall, figures of people, a great Menorah — a star in the sky."

The Bests visited Old Jerusalem on foot. Charley bought Margaret a Christmas present of a gold brooch with tiny rubies. They enjoyed the sights, sounds, and smells of the Souk. That evening, at the convocation, Best received the degree of honorary doctor of philosophy from Dr. Harman. They did not wear caps and gowns, but Charley received an exquisite scroll in Hebrew and in English and he spoke on "The History of Insulin and the Present Position." Ambassador McGaughey, Sam Lunenfeld, and Anna Gelber were among the guests. Back at the hotel late in the evening the Bests found a six-foot Christmas tree in their room, decorated with tinsel, real candles, birds, and baby dolls. Anna Gelber, thinking they might miss Canadian Christmas decorations, had thoughtfully placed the tree there. Gifts arrived at their hotel — flowers, a jewellery box of mother-of-pearl from Anna Gelber, a gift basket with wine, chocolates, and candied fruit from the Harmans. Charley phoned Mrs. Harman to thank her and to ask about her husband's health. Anna Gelber said that "she had never known such reverence and affection to be displayed at any convocation, as was shown last evening."

The Canadians visited Israel's president, Zalman Shazar — "a bright-eyed, elderly man who has been president for ten years." He talked about diabetes and insulin. He was born in Russia and was educated in Freiburg, a city that Margaret and Charley knew well.

The King David Hotel provided a dinner of turkey and red cabbage on 24 December. Then, Mr. Weiss, an experienced driver from the university, drove the three Presbyterians to Bethlehem — "very heavy traffic, many checkpoints for the car. Presently, through the rain, we saw to our left the lights of Bethlehem on the hillside. We drove up the steep hill —

447

thousands of people climbing, hundreds of buses and cars — high stone walls and stone houses climbing the steep streets."

Leaving their car they climbed further. "The university authorities had gone to a great deal of trouble to make the arrangements for us to visit Bethlehem, and particularly for us to get into the church and be seated there." Margaret described the church as fortress-like. "We went through a last barrier where Mr. Weiss told one of the policemen that it was Professor Best of Toronto and his party. The policeman said, 'I know that he is in Israel. He saved my mother's life.'" They sat near the back for an hour and a half before the lights near the altar went on and the service began with the singing of *Adeste Fideles*. Then they walked to Manger Square in the light rain, and drove back to Jerusalem. "From far off we saw the lights of the Holy City."

On Christmas morning, Weiss drove them to the Scottish Church — St. Andrew's. The music was beautiful — two hymns with words by Christina Rossetti — "Love Came Down at Christmas" and "In the Bleak Mid-Winter" — and "Once in Royal David's City." Linda described St. Andrew's, "built after World War I and beautiful inside and out. Of course, the hymn speaks of 'Jerusalem the Golden' and this is really true because everything is built of stone which is a beautiful golden hue."[723] Then they returned to Bethlehem to see the Church of the Nativity, the mosaics, and the grotto. That evening, Dr. Alexander Keynan, professor of biology and a vice-president of the university, and his wife entertained for them. Dr. Anna Gelber received them at her home at 15 Ben Yarmon Avenue. The Bests had dined there with Edward and Anna ten years earlier. "We were able to sit most of the time. It was a very friendly, happy party."

On their previous visit, the Bests could not enter East Jerusalem, so this time they enjoyed seeing the historic sites and the university's Mount Scopus Campus. Several people, including Mr. Avner Shavitsky and Dr. Eleazar Shafrir, took the Bests on tours. They saw some of the archeological excavations, the Dome of the Rock. Linda described their walk "through narrow Via Dolorosa to the Ecce Homo Convent which stands on the top of the Roman Fortress where the judgment of Jesus took place. Here a little bird-like sister took us down to the excavations made in the 1930s which brought to light the original floor. There she gave us a lecture and if ever an actress was lost to the stage it was she. Her very voice changed, she stood on tip-toe, flung out her arms, hissed (when she was a Roman soldier), whispered at dramatic points, all the time fixing us with an eagle eye to be sure our attention had not strayed — as if it could!"[724]

On 10 January 1972, in Toronto, the provincial government gave a dinner at the Ontario Science Centre to celebrate the fiftieth anniversary of the discovery of insulin. Bert Lawrence, the minister of health, was the host. "In Charley's speech, he had commented on the fact that Bill Banting and our two sons were present and they were all three distinguished alumni of Windy Ridge Nursery School." The Brazilian ambassador came to Toronto to present the promised Biennial Science Prize money to Charles Best on 7 February 1972, and there was a reception at the consulate. Ambassador Frank Moscoso told the Bests that his mother started taking insulin in 1928 and lived for many years. After the presentation, Margaret and Charley went to the bank and deposited the very welcome cheque — US$25,000, less bank charges — $24,995.30.

The next trip was to Ottawa to make up for the earlier cancellation in September 1971 caused by Charley's illness in Brazil. Geza and Caroline Hetenyi were their hosts. The staff of the University of Ottawa's Department of Physiology included John Cowan, who had done his PhD in Toronto under Gerry Wrenshall. Charley did two television interviews, including one with Peter Jennings. Dr. Jean-Jacques Lussier, dean of medicine, was host for a dinner at the Cercle Universitaire. Margaret sat between Père Roger Guindon, the rector — "a delightful person" — and Roger Séguin, a lawyer and chair of the board of governors. Charley spent the next day at the physiology labs, and then came the convocation, where he was made an honorary doctor of medicine.

In Rome, in early April, the enjoyable pattern of previous visits repeated itself. The Hoechst Company again provided a car and driver for Margaret and Charley. The Hotel Reale was as comfortable as ever. Their room was full of flowers — orchids from the chancellor of the Pontifical Academy, daisies and roses from Hoechst, and purple lilacs that they bought from a street vendor at la Ponta Pia. They avoided the tours arranged by the Pontifical Academy as they were too long and too tiring. With their own car and driver, they could go where they wanted, not have to walk too far, and could return to the hotel when they were tired. One of their favourite destinations was the Museum of the Villa Giulia, the Etruscan Museum. "The gardens were lovely this week in the courtyards of the museum — purple stock, white stock, tulips with myriad of forget-me-nots among them, yellow iris, marigolds, lemon trees with large lemons hanging there — it was beautiful."

At the Pontifical Academy Best gave the opening address, "The History, Discovery and Present Position of Insulin" — in the Academy building in the garden of the Vatican. The printed forty-eight-page version, complete with charts and photographs, gave Best's views on the subject of insulin in his later years.[725]

At the academy banquet that evening, Margaret talked to Father Daniel O'Connell, the president, and Professor Alfred Ubbelohde, a brilliant physical chemist from the University of London. The next morning, the Bests went to St. Andrew's Church, where Charley read the New Testament lesson — John 10:1-16. "… I am the good shepherd and know my sheep, and am known of mine. As the Father knoweth me, even so know I the Father: and I lay down my life for the sheep. And other sheep I have, which are not of this fold: them also I must bring, and they shall hear my voice; and there shall be one fold, and one shepherd." Ambassador Ben Rogers and his wife were there.

Before the Bests' departure for Toronto the ambassador had asked the new Canadian Pacific Air representative in Rome, John Smidon, to look after the Bests at the airport. On their way they again drove to the Trevi Fountain: "We always go there before leaving Rome to throw in a coin to ensure our return."

In spite of well over a year's strenuous travel to celebrations of the fiftieth anniversary of the discovery of insulin, both Margaret and Charley had been remarkably well, apart from his bout of viral pneumonia in Brazil. On 10 May 1972, however, Margaret had severe pain that she at first thought was the hiatus hernia, but then that it was a coronary attack. "Moray Jansen came and gave me a shot in the arm. It is distressing to write about it — more than six years, since January, 1966, when I had the previous coronary. Charley kept me at home and he is nursing me. I wrote that the pain began lower down. It quickly rose from my abdomen to my throat. What blessed relief when that subsided. Moray comes every day — there have been several electrocardiograms taken. Six years ago, I was kept in bed for six weeks. The treatment for heart attacks has changed. The week after next, Moray thinks I will be able to go for a little drive." She and Charley cancelled trips to Atlanta and to Newfoundland. It was unlikely that Margaret had suffered a coronary. Moray Jansen later confirmed quietly to Henry that she was suffering from a hiatus hernia and angina, probably both exacerbated by fatigue. For the rest of 1972, however, Margaret kept writing in her diary that she had had "another heart attack."

Family members paid short visits. Melinda, aged eight, said, "It is lucky you did not die," a direct if surprising statement. Margaret wrote on 23 May,

"I am getting stronger but am very tired each evening. Moray remarked that I am doing better than he expected at first — I told him it is because I am at home, not in a hospital, that Charley is nursing me, and that he is taking care of me. Charley has had a great deal of experience in the hospital and with many nurses during his several illnesses beginning with the coronary in 1954. He said that the essence of good nursing is to do everything quietly, to be unobtrusive but efficient." Charley took Margaret out for a short drive in their new car — a grey Buick Skylark — on 26 May.

Margaret was improving but experienced angina, which she described as "the pressure" in her chest. She could not travel to Washington for the ADA meeting. "Charley is going alone and it is many years since he has gone on a trip without me. It will be the big celebration of the American Diabetes Association for the discovery of insulin. I will be very forlorn to see him go off." Bill Greenwood did an electrocardiogram at the Toronto General Hospital — "he thinks I am getting over this very well." Charley kept in constant touch from Washington, and all their friends expressed disappointment at Margaret's absence. "Tributes were paid to Fred Banting and to Charley. Charley also received a very beautiful framed scroll which is now hanging in our hall." Dr. Stefan Fajans, professor of internal medicine at the University of Michigan and president of the ADA, took CHB to the White House for a meeting with President Richard Nixon, but he was otherwise occupied. "At the time we did not realize that those were the beginning days of the Watergate scandal."[726]

Everything was going well, and on 5 July, Margaret, Charley, and Linda left Toronto for Maine, which they found very reassuring. From the Wharf Restaurant in Eastport, one could see the constant activity of fishing boats and small ferries. Several weeks after arriving, Margaret had what she referred to as another heart attack, though it was more likely another bout of angina. She remained inside to convalesce, and was able to enjoy Pierre Berton's two volumes about the Canadian Pacific Railway, *The National Dream* and *The Last Spike* while recovering.

The arrival of young Charley, aged thirteen, in West Pembroke, cheered Margaret up, and he was very helpful with firewood and other chores. His grandfather took him on several expeditions when someone could stay with Margaret. Eileen called to say that she was leaving for San Francisco and then Mexico. In 1970 Eileen became bursar of Knox College at the University of Toronto. Now that her children were bigger she was able to do some of the travelling that she had never been able to do before. Young Charley was to leave Schooner Cove to go to Prince Edward Island and Laurie flew a single-engine plane to the St. Croix airstrip, near Calais, Maine, and picked him up.

Best spoke, as he had done the previous year, at a meeting of those who were trying to save the Eastport Hospital. Dr. Nelson Stott from Eastport came to see how Margaret was recovering, and gave her a prescription for valium to ease the tension. He also brought Swiss chard, beans, and rhubarb from his garden. It was six weeks since they had left Toronto, and Margaret wanted very much to get outside.

On 20 August, Margaret wrote, "Red Letter Day. I got dressed this morning, the first time in four weeks, and then sat out in the sun with my darling Charley for half an hour. Six weeks ago today we arrived here and four weeks ago I had the heart attack." She was anxious to be able to do more. "I get quite breathless when I attempt too much. I have made my bed, bathed myself and washed my pajamas ever since I became ill and have gone out to our funny little toilet. I dare say that all of this activity has prevented me from becoming too weak."

Charley took Margaret out in the car on 23 August. Dr. Herbert Everett came and took her blood pressure and arranged for an electrocardiogram in St. Stephen, New Brunswick, and the same day, Dr. Nelson Stott was over again from Eastport. Every visitor brought flowers, vegetables, or magazines.

"This is our anniversary day — forty-eight years," Margaret wrote on 3 September. "It is a dreary, dull day but happy nevertheless because so many friends have remembered us. Yesterday a truck from Calais drove up with a tremendous basket of fruit and an arrangement of yellow and white chrysanthemums — all from Janna, Henry, Mairi and Bruce. Sandy and Laurie called from Prince Edward Island." Many local friends arrived with cards and gifts.

After their return home, on 28 September, Dr. John Evans was installed as president of the University of Toronto. Margaret could not go and Charley did not want to leave her, but they regretted not being present. They watched the thrilling, final hockey game between Russia and Canada. How could a university ceremony compete with that? The Canadians won 6 to 5.

The NFB film, *The Discoverers,* was shown again on CBC. The actors were all different from the 1959 production. "It had been changed somewhat … The one who played Charley's part looked most unlike Charley. The man who played Joe Gilchrist was really more like Joe than Charley or Fred were like themselves. However, everyone seemed to like it and of course other people were not around as I was when Charley and Fred made the discovery."[727] Henry called to say that Mairi and Bruce had stayed up for the occasion. Bruce was not interested and played with his cars; Mairi sat on her father's lap and when it was over asked, "Did Grampy really do all that?" "Yes, he did." "Good for Grampy. I'm hungry."

Margaret Best was ill again, having two attacks of angina on 24 October, and Moray Jansen was quickly on hand. Within two weeks, she seemed to be on the mend. Charley went to some events at the university, including a dinner at Massey College for Sir David Martyn, the Scottish executive secretary of the Royal Society of London since 1947. Jo and Pep Hoet from Belgium were in Toronto and visited the house, bearing flowers and a present from Marguerite.

On 9 November, Margaret Best had more severe pain. Jansen gave her nitroglycerine, then an injection, before the pain subsided. He and Bill Greenwood were very attentive. "I am getting stronger but as I told Moray I am perhaps losing confidence in myself. There have been so many heart attacks. I read and Charley reads to me — dear Charley, and so the time passes. I long to be up and around and doing things. This last week we would have spent in Denver, Colorado, if I had been well. This week we would have flown to Bermuda on the 22nd." There was another attack of angina, but by the end of November Margaret was able to work on her scrapbooks. "Charley set up a card table in our room and I finished pinning in the clippings about Brazil. Today I have been sorting and getting ready to put in the many references to our doings after Brazil — a year ago this autumn — there are many, we never stopped."

For her seventy-second birthday, 30 November, Margaret was touched to receive Laurie's needlework picture Schooner Cove Farm. "Laurie worked a lovely reproduction of Schooner Cove for us. She has never been there. I asked her to go with Charley to choose a frame." Every few days, Margaret recorded her progress with her scrapbooks. "Never before did I get behind with the scrapbooks, but 1971 was too much for me." She seemed to be a little unsure herself of the details of each episode of heart trouble. On 14 December, she wrote, "Today for the first time I got out. Charley took me for a drive and I saw some Christmas decorations. I had not been out since October 24th when I had certainly had a heart attack and then on November 9th, the very severe attack."

For the second time, one of Charley's paintings, *Low Tide, Schooner Cove*, was being used for Christmas cards — this time by the British

Diabetic Association and the Twin Cities Diabetic Association of Minneapolis and St. Paul. The CDA reissued cards with a reproduction of *Wind in the Pines*, done at Strawberry Hill Farm.

On Christmas Eve, Sandy and Laurie and his children dined at 105 Woodlawn. Charley had had the piano tuned, and the house was full of flowers and many other gifts. On Christmas Day, Henry and his family arrived for dinner; Janna had cooked the turkey and made asparagus soup. Eileen and her children and Henry and his family gave Margaret and Charley cable service for their TV and Linda a small TV set for her own bedroom. Sandy and Laurie and his four young people arrived in time for dessert. "The children played with their gifts and I was very happy to have Sandy and Laurie and Janna and Henry and all six of our grandchildren here together."

As the new year dawned, Margaret noted, "Many people have been saddened by the death of Lester B. Pearson — 'Mike.' Yesterday was the funeral in Ottawa. A little more than a year ago, he was at the big dinner party celebrating the discovery of insulin given by the Canadian Diabetes Association at the Inn on the Park (see my scrapbooks). I sat on his right hand (between Mike and Charley), and we had a very happy time. Years ago, when both of our boys were in politics in Ottawa, we were waiting to take a train from the old station opposite the Château Laurier — Mike was going through, saw Charley, came over to us and said, 'Charley, those are two wonderful boys of yours.' (Mike is a Liberal and our boys are Conservatives.)"

The children from St. Veronica's Separate School, who had been to the house to interview Charley, called to say that they had written fifty-two pages about Charles Best and the discovery of insulin. "They have decided to write to the Nobel Committee in Stockholm to tell them that Charles should get the Nobel Prize! This was rather startling to us — there was no point in discouraging them. The Nobel Committee will take care of that. One of them said to me yesterday on the telephone, 'Your husband is a great man. And you are wonderful too.'"

Margaret had recovered enough for them to fly to Florida on 11 April 1973 to stay for the third time at the University Inn at Coral Gables. In Miami, Margaret used a wheelchair in the airport for the first time. She had intestinal troubles and was dizzy. Charley had a swim every day in the pool. "This is a very relaxed, pleasant life and I would be very happy if I felt really well. For the first time today, I had to let Charley go off by himself to do any little bit of shopping."

In Toronto, Dr. Paul Lacy, professor of pathology at Washington University in St. Louis, gave the third Charles H. Best Lecture of the Toronto Diabetes Association. Lacy had worked in the Banting and Best Department. "He has devised a method of preparing isolated islands of Langerhans and has recently shown that when injected into the hepatic artery they flourish in the liver and provide sufficient insulin to maintain the host dog after complete pancreatectomy. This is a very exciting development."[728] This work has led recently to further developments at the University of Calgary.

The Bests drove on 23 May, to the new Charles H. Best School in Burlington, where they liked the colourful interior and the demeanour of the teachers and the students. "Charley said how proud we are that their splendid school carries our name. When he showed them a picture of Margaret in 1920, the principal asked if the children knew who it was. A chorus answered, 'It's Mrs. Best,' and then added, 'She's pretty.'"

The ADA meetings were to take place in Chicago in late June 1973, and a new group on the council wanted major changes. "We, as well as many others, were distressed by the decision of the Executive Committee to ask Dick Connelly to resign. Charley has had long talks with Edwin Gates and Cecil Striker on the telephone. Jack Davidson will present a protest against the decision at the meetings. Where could they find a more wonderful and dedicated person than Dick?" On 4 July, Margaret wrote, "Word has come today that Dick Connelly will no longer be the executive director of the American Diabetes Association. How terribly we will miss him if we ever get to meetings again. There could be no one like Dick. Edwin Gates and others feel as we do."

Charles Best continued to attract attention. A journalist and a photographer from an Italian magazine, *Famiglia Christiana,* came to the house. Margaret and Charley went to Toronto's City Hall Square to draw the winning numbers in a lottery that raised some eighty thousand dollars for the Huronda Children's Diabetic Camp. The Bests went to Kitchener in late July to open Charles Best Place, part of a development by Gerhard Matthaes, whose daughter Birgit was a diabetic. Charley received a porcelain eagle made by Karsen Porcelain in Germany.

After the heavy travelling for the "Golden Celebrations" of 1971 and 1972, and Margaret's heart problems, they were quieter in 1973. Their main interest was keeping track of the comings and goings of the next two generations. Sandy was preparing for his "Multi-Breed Production Sale" at

Howard Webster's Dundas Farms in Prince Edward Island, which Sandy had built up to a mammoth undertaking. Henry and Janna flew to the Maritimes after a busy summer at York University, the Ontario College of Art, and on the farm, arriving in Prince Edward Island just after the giant sale that had grossed over $1 million in one weekend. Henry enjoyed riding the quarter horses with his nieces and nephews, all good riders, but Melinda was the star circus performer. The sale was the pinnacle of Sandy's professional career and a remarkable recovery from the financial failures of a few years earlier. On their forty-ninth wedding anniversary Margaret wrote "Charley talked to Sandy and Laurie and Charley Stewart in P.E. Island. How lucky the four children are to be down there at the end of their lovely summer holidays. The Dundas cattle sale had been a big affair over the weekend and a big success."

Buyers came from all over North America and beyond. With Sandy's expertise in agriculture and cattle breeding Dundas Farms was an impressively successful enterprise. The *Globe and Mail* published an article on the sale, with several good colour pictures of Sandy and Laurie, and of the farms.[729] Laurie, who was expecting a baby in November, acted as a ferry pilot, flying people to and from Moncton in a rented single engine plane. Sandy bought a spacious house on the Cardigan River that needed a lot of work but would make a great family home. Laurie enjoyed looking for antiques on the island that would be appropriate for the house.

On 13 September, the Bests heard the sad news from Winnie and Kenneth Leighton that Schooner Cove Farm had been burgled. The farm was the last place on the road, so robbers could work without interruption. The Franklin stove and pipe, four antique chairs, the bed linen, old cooking pots, and the model Gaspé schooner were all gone, and there was no point in looking for them.

Margaret was reading Virginia Woolf's *To the Lighthouse* and *Mrs. Dalloway*. She had first read the former in 1937 and the latter in 1930. "There has been renewed interest lately, in both Virginia Woolf and Victoria Sackville-West because of recent books about them. I think that Nigel Nicolson may have been too revealing about his mother's life in *Portrait of a Marriage* (1973). We telephoned Lea Reiber the other day, before we left home. He asked Charley, 'Is Margaret shocked at the revelations about Vita's life?' Charley said, 'No, Margaret isn't easily shocked.'"

Laurie wanted her baby to be born in Prince Edward Island, as she expected that the family's future lay there. On 7 November 1973, Susan

MacTavish Best entered the world in Charlottetown; the baby's great-grand-mother, Flora Cameron Macleod Mahon, was born there in 1867. Laurie had pleurisy after the birth, which delayed the return to Toronto with her new baby by a month. Charley and Margaret were in Coral Gables, Florida, and did not see their seventh grandchild until after their return on 19 December. They went first to see Laurie, still suffering from pleurisy, in the Toronto General Hospital. Then they saw Susan for the first time at the house on Tranby Avenue. "She is adorable — dark blue eyes, auburn hair, chubby cheeks — a darling baby. Sandy held her and then I held her."

In February Charley and Margaret went to Londonderry Farm three days before his birthday for lunch. Jack and Janet Simpson were there. Jack was the son of old and dear friends, Roy and Elizabeth Simpson. Mairi and Bruce, Henry and Janet Simpson all skated on the frozen pond. "I was charmed to see the children skate so well," said Margaret. For the birthday lunch Henry and Janna had haddock, sole, and mackerel sent by their friend, Fred Green, of the Ferry Wharf Fish Market in Halifax, and Mairi had made the birthday cake "which we are to take to Florida."

Charley Best's seventy-fifth birthday was on 27 February 1974. Best had an appointment on the same day with President John Evans to discuss the disposition of his papers. Later in the day, two University of Toronto policemen arrived at the home with a large box. One of them said, "May I congratulate you sir, I believe this is your seventy-fifth birthday," and they shook hands. The box contained a lovely cake with "Happy 75th Birthday" as part of the decoration. There was a note: "Dr. Best, with best wishes and many happy returns on your 75th birthday from your University, John Evans, February 27th, 1974."

Two days later Laurie and Sandy gave a surprise birthday party at their home on Tranby Avenue. Sandy had arrived from Ireland with a whole fresh salmon and a whole smoked salmon. As well as their seven grand-children, there were six of Margaret's Macleod cousins and many old friends, including Jessie Ridout, Vin and Ruth Price, Laurie and Helen Chute, Omond and Vaire Soldandt, Reg and Margaret Haist, Mary Fraser and Donnie and Sally, George and Catherine Scroggie, Queenie and Bernie Leibel, Moray and Margaret Jansen and Morley Sparling. Susan, the new baby, was the centre of attention.

On 5 March the Bests were off again for Coral Gables, Florida. Margaret had said that she would never fly in a jumbo jet because it was too big, but she did, and enjoyed it. They were soon back into their

Florida routine — Charley swam every day, they made some meals in their own unit, and they walked to nearby stores for a change of scenery. They were distressed to hear of the death of Dr. Earl Sutherland, the fifty-eight-year-old professor of physiology at Vanderbilt University in Nashville who had worked on insulin and glycogen. "He discovered cyclic AMP, a very important substance which is involved in very many vital processes. Dr. Sutherland said, 'Everything from memory to the toes.' He won the Nobel Prize for his work on cyclic AMP. He moved here to the University of Miami, possibly last year. Charley knew him quite well and he is mentioned frequently in Charley's *Selected Papers*."

It was rare for Charles Best to go anywhere without Margaret, but on 14 June he flew to Atlanta to attend the ADA meetings, and was gone four days. Jack and Bebe Davidson looked after him. At the banquet, Charley presented Charles H. Best Medals to Senator Gale McGee of Wyoming, Senator Richard Schweiker of Pennsylvania, and Gail Patrick Jackson, past chair of the ADA's board. The speaker was Senator Howard Baker of Tennessee. Jack Davidson, professor of medicine at Emory University, took his former chief to the Diabetic Clinic.

Federal election day was 30 June, and Margaret Best showed her colours: "Trudeau won, I was very disappointed. I had hoped that we might have a change and that Stanfield would win. It is time we had a Conservative government." Margaret was not particularly interested in politics, but both her sons were strong supporters of Robert Stanfield.

In July 1974 Sandy and Laurie moved into 30 Rosedale Road. Margaret wrote, "It is a very large house. They have done a great deal to improve it already — painting, sanding floors, etc. It will demand a great deal of furniture. Laurie is away in Idaho with Alexander. The dates had been arranged long ago and unfortunately, the moving took place at the same time. I think they started off at Boise, Idaho, to take the Raft Trip on the Salmon River."

Golden Wedding Anniversary

Originally Sandy and Laurie were going to host the party for the Bests' fiftieth wedding anniversary in their new house. However, the alterations and painting had not been completed. Henry and Janna were about to leave for a sabbatical year in Nova Scotia, Québec, and the West and they had rented the farm to a young couple for the year. They borrowed back Londonderry Farm for the party on 3 September. The weather was cool, but it improved; fires were burning in the living room and in the coach house, making it more comfortable for the one hundred guests. Many friends and neighbours helped provide the meal by bringing casseroles prepared at home. All the grandchildren, except Susan who was too little, had a hand in making the three-tiered cake. Peggy Ritchie, a floral designer at Robinson's Flowers in Guelph, where Janna had been the bookkeeper for several years, beautifully recreated Margaret's original bridal bouquet from cosmos grown at the farm.

Members of both sides of the family — Salters, Whitleys, Scotts, Hendersons, and Robertsons — were there. Allen and Barbara Joslin came from Boston, Geza and Caroline Hetenyi from Ottawa, and Hans and Gisela Giese from Montréal. Vin Price was toastmaster. Lauric Chute spoke, as did Solicitor General George Kerr, MPP for Halton County and also a personal friend. Helen Lawson with her daughter, Ruth Kindersley, arrived to say that her husband, the former lieutenant governor of Ontario, Ray Lawson, was unwell; but a half-hour later he arrived by limousine, saying right away that he wanted to make a speech, which he did. Everyone was very happy. "Over and over again our friends say, 'It was the best party I was ever at.'" As Vin Price said, it was truly a golden day.

After the very happy celebration life settled down again, and Charley gave an occasional lecture to medical students. He spoke to an audience at the South Waterloo Hospital in Galt on the discovery of insulin. The next day he and Margaret drove through Mennonite country to see the farms and the cities of Galt, Hespeler, and Preston, all recently combined into Cambridge. Sandy and Laurie were both in Europe. Susan's nurse brought her to visit her grandparents, who saw her take her first steps. "Charley says that each time she took a step I clapped my hand on my knee, just exactly as my Father used to do when pleased, and also laughed with joy."

Charles Best was increasingly concerned that he had received so many honours and Margaret none. He tried to make up for this omission by giving her things and nominating her for honours in her own right. Charley attempted to have Margaret awarded an honorary degree from the University of New Brunswick, in the province where she was born, and a medal from the City of Toronto, but with no success. She never asked for anything herself, but a blonde mink coat from Charley for Christmas 1974 delighted her.

Charley prepared a fifteen-page c.v. of Margaret — really a short biography. He wrote, "Her interest in people, and her thorough knowledge of the history of insulin and of the thousands of people who have contributed to the development of our knowledge of it, have made her a wonderful help to me." His next comment underlies one of the problems of the biographer — "It is not feasible for me to make a list of our friends around the world. It would be a fascinating record of research personalities over the past fifty-two years in sixty different countries. It would take a good bit of work but many of these names are in Margaret's diaries."[730]

Henry, Janna, Mairi, and Bruce had spent the first part of their marvellous sabbatical year from York University in Nova Scotia at the old family home of Mim (Meredith Spicer) Kerr, wife of George Kerr, before moving on to Québec in December 1974. For New Year's, Linda, with Eileen and three of her children, joined Henry, Janna, Mairi, and Bruce in their spacious flat in the Château St-Louis. The cousins enjoyed skiing at Mont Ste-Anne and skating on the open-air rink on the Plains of Abraham.

Early in the new year Freda Ramsay arrived from Scotland to stay at the flat, and Margaret and Charley Best flew to Québec to visit them. Peter Price, general manager of CP Hotels, a friend of Henry and Janna's, provided the senior Bests with a small suite at the Château Frontenac on the fourteenth floor looking over the St. Lawrence. The grandparents had dinner at Janna and Henry's flat in the Château St-Louis each evening and heard about the children's schools, Mairi at the Couvent des Ursulines, and Bruce at St-Louis de Gonzague. Unexpectedly, Sandy and Laurie arrived from Toronto, taking a suite in the Château Frontenac on the same floor as Sandy's parents. It was Laurie's first time in Québec.

One evening, Dr. and Mme Marcel Carbotte, who lived in the apartment across the hall, came to visit. "Mme Carbotte is the very well-known Canadian writer Gabrielle Roy, who wrote *Where Nests the Water Hen* and *The Tin Flute*. Her descriptions of her father (when she was very young and a boyfriend came to call and sat beside her) were most amusing. She got up from her chair and, playing the role of her father, paced up and down the room, casting stern glances in the direction of the sofa where his daughter and the boy sat. We were all in gales of laughter, including her husband."

When the Bests had moved in, Henry's dear friends Jean and Agathe Lacerte had warned Mairi and Bruce to be very quiet because Mme Carbotte wanted peace to write — the previous occupant of the Bests' flat was a quiet person; she had died at 102 after thirty years in residence. In

April, when Janna and Henry left Québec, he deposited a box of chocolates at the Carbottes' door with a note saying that he hoped the children had not disturbed her. Gabrielle Roy wrote a note of thanks saying that she had never heard the children, but that she had often heard their father. Henry Best has a laugh that can be heard above the din in a large, crowded room.

Charley was busy at his office going through papers with Linda. Another senior researcher was retiring from the Banting and Best: Gerald Wrenshall had dedicated thirty years to his lab; he had a double PhD, in physics and in physiology, and was a severe diabetic. Wrenshall worked on the assay of insulin, used computers in analyzing data regarding the incidence of diabetes, and studied the islets of Langerhans.

When Henry and his family arrived home from Québec in early April 1975 before heading west, both his parents were unwell. They both had had a series of debilitating dental appointments, his mother had an attack of acute angina and his father had fallen at least twice. Bill Greenwood gave Charley a thorough examination and discovered high blood pressure. He soon improved, and Moray Jansen told Henry that he did not expect any great problems, so he, Janna, and the children left for the West. Henry called his parents from Colorado and was not happy with their response as everyone seemed to be ill, so he called Jansen late that evening and kept in touch regularly. Sandy was in Tunisia but was not well. Laurie was in the Toronto General Hospital as she had recurring back problems that had to be treated periodically with traction. Charley was much better, but Margaret had an infected kidney, and, much to their regret, they were unable to attend the Pontifical Academy sessions in Rome. By mid-summer 1975, Henry and his family returned from their once-in-a-lifetime trans-continental trip, which had taken them from Nova Scotia and Québec to the southwest of the United States, up the west coast and back through Canada.

On 3 September 1975, Henry took his parents to Londonderry Farm for five days. It was their fifty-first wedding anniversary, and there was a dinner party that evening. Charley hadn't been riding in the year Henry had been away on sabbatical, and now he took pleasure in getting back in the saddle. "It did my heart good to see Charley, Henry, and Mairi all riding together."

On 11 September, Margaret made the first mention in her diary of Sandy's heart trouble. "He had a great deal of angina." Moray Jansen had been looking after him, but they had had a disagreement as Sandy refused to take Moray's advice. Margaret was discouraged: "What dreary things I report just now." In October worsening relations between Sandy and

Laurie certainly troubled Margaret and Charley Best deeply. "Laurie and Sandy have reached the parting of the ways. Laurie has rented a house somewhere near Guelph. Sandy has put 30 Rosedale Road up for sale. It is a <u>very</u> large house and is in much better shape than when he bought it, I think a year ago last April. They moved in a year ago July. We see Sandy almost every day. Of course we are unhappy."

Margaret wrote on a happier note on 13 October: "Yesterday Charley and I returned from a wonderful visit to Londonderry Farm." Janna drove them out and Henry arrived later from York University. "It was his birthday and he opened his presents. We gave him an unusual one — the big silver loving cup with deer-horn handles that had been given to Uncle Bruce in January of 1904 by his friends in Woodstock, New Brunswick, when he left as manager of the Bank of Nova Scotia to go to Edmonton. I had found the letter from his friends and a list of their names. Henry has them now. Uncle Bruce had left these in my care." Grampy rode twice with Henry and Mairi, and he and Margaret had several short walks. Janna showed movies of their trip west. Margaret enjoyed hearing the children practising on their great-grandmother's piano and Henry playing while everyone sang the hymns and old songs that his father so liked. Charley drove the fifty miles back to the city — his first long drive for a considerable time.

Henry and Janna were off to Massachusetts. They visited the Mahons in Duxbury, but they did not report that Uncle Henry was very confused, and that Aunt Lydia was in tears to see him in such a state when he had had such a good mind. It was the last time they saw him. They went on to Smith College in Northampton to see their friend, Jill Ker Conway, previously a professor of history and vice-president of the University of Toronto, installed as president. Professor Conway was the first woman to head this outstanding women's college, and alumnae gathered from all over the globe for this historic happy occasion.

Another old colleague of Charley's, Bob Defries, died, J.G. FitzGerald's successor as director of the Connaught Labs and of the School of Hygiene. Best was an honorary pallbearer, along with Ken Ferguson, Albert Fisher, and Peter Moloney. Margaret accompanied Charley, "just to be helpful. He was less confident about going to such occasions alone." Many old friends had gathered whom the Bests did not see very often, including Don Cameron, Mary Fraser, Chancellor Eva Mader Macdonald, and Neil McKinnon. Rev. Robert McClure, the missionary surgeon and moderator of the United Church from 1968 to 1971, Margaret noted, "is amazing. He looks young — is going to new work in Peru, high in the mountains northeast of Lima. The minute he saw me, and I had not seen him for years, he said, 'Harbord Collegiate, 4A, I was in 4C, I did not take Greek.'"

Charley enjoyed the 1975 Gairdner Awards ceremonies at the Royal York Hotel, with Lieutenant Governor Pauline McGibbon making the presentations. John Keith and Bill Mustard, both well-known heart specialists in Toronto, were winners, along with Dr. Ernest Beutler of Duarte, California, Dr. Baruch Blumberg of Philadelphia, Dr. Henri Hers of Brussels, and Dr. Hugh Huxley of Cambridge.

On 12 November, Margaret and Charley were very pleased to return to Bermuda. They had their favourite room, No. 10, at Waterloo House. They were delighted to see Bishop Henry Marsh, a university and army friend of Charley. On their graduation in arts in 1921, Henry Marsh, Clark Noble, and Charles Best had their picture taken together to save money. The Bests also met Jon Vickers, the Canadian opera singer, now a resident of Bermuda. Greetings came for Margaret's seventy-fifth birthday on 30 November.

Margaret and Charley had trimmed their Christmas card lists and refused some invitations, but still bought a twenty-one-pound turkey. Many relatives and friends came to visit; Henry, Janna, Mairi, and Bruce were there for Christmas dinner. Several days later, Laurie came to see them, and the next day Sandy brought Susan to 105 Woodlawn. "Sandy has a visit from Susan every Sunday. She was as usual in fine spirits. She loves her Daddy and also 'Margit.'"[731] On New Year's Day, Margaret returned to her older son's health. "Sandy has not been at all well and the doctor had seen him — bronchitis and the possibility that he had a slight heart attack. We worry about him."

The whole family was interested in a visit that Charles Stewart Best, now sixteen, had had in Ottawa with John Diefenbaker through the good offices of Duncan Edmunds. The eighty-one-year-old former prime minister invited him to his home, and they talked about his book of memoirs. Margaret noted that Mr. Diefenbaker had recently received the Companion of Honour from the Queen, the same award that Charley had received in 1971.

Henry Mahon died suddenly in Winter Haven, Florida, on 28 January 1976. Linda had arrived there a few days earlier. When Margaret wrote of him as "a wonderful brother," she meant it, and she put a notice in the *Globe and Mail.* Family ties were very important to all the Bests and

463

the Mahons, and Henry was a favourite with everyone. Janna, Henry, and their children drove in April to meet Lydia Mahon as she arrived near Washington, DC on the car-train from Florida. She was happily surprised to have Mairi and Bruce rush down the platform to greet her. Henry and Janna drove her home to Duxbury and in the short time available helped her go through a lot of Uncle Harry's papers. Henry made arrangements to have his uncle's ashes buried beneath a military grave marker in the cemetery of the Anglican church in South Duxbury.

By May 1976, Sandy was living at 105 Woodlawn. Margaret wrote, "The Rosedale Road house had been cleared out of furnishings but has not been sold yet. His belongings are here, at McMaster (Eileen's house), at George Yost's, and in storage. Sandy does not look well. His heart condition worries us." In June, "Little Margaret" won a general proficiency prize at Bishop Strachan School. "She is a clever and a beautiful girl" and looked very like her grandmother. "Well, all of our grandchildren are exceptional."

A few weeks later, the Bests lost their most trusted adviser and very great friend. Vincent Price had always provided his legal services free of charge, including for many of Sandy's complicated business affairs. Margaret never had many words for the things that really mattered. She wrote, "Our dear Vin. We all loved him, what a wonderful friend he has been." Charley did not feel well enough to drive to the funeral in Guelph.

Margaret was not always approving of Charley's taste in books. He read very little outside of scientific periodicals, but he loved action stories such as the Captain Horatio Hornblower series by C.S. Forester in the *Saturday Evening Post* and stories about horses. It was a pity that he never discovered the Dick Francis mysteries. Janna had compared notes with her father-in-law about Zane Gray and his tales of the American desert, and she and Henry found a twenty-one-volume set for Charley's seventy-seventh birthday in February 1976. He immediately emptied the small bookcase beside his bed and installed Zane Gray.

The Hannah Institute for the History of Medical and Related Sciences showed on 29 June 1976 the ninety-minute British film *Comets among the Stars* (1973), with Sir Ralph Richardson playing J.J.R. Macleod, Alan Howard as Banting, Nigel Havers as Charley, and Susie Blake as Margaret Mahon. "We liked it only fairly well. Professor Macleod was too vehement and ranting. Charles was a thin-faced, dark-haired boy, not at all like Charley, and so on." Bill Banting was at the event, but Lady Banting was very ill with a brain tumour. Dinner followed at the York Club hosted by

Dr. Jason Hannah, founder of Associated Medical Services (AMS), and his wife, Ruth, and several officers of AMS and of the Hannah Institute.

Margaret remarked that she was writing less frequently in her diary. Both she and Charley were operating in low gear and they did not go to Maine in the summer. There had been another break-in at the farmhouse there, followed by a further intrusion a month later, which brought Margaret and Charley to a sad conclusion: "We think we must try to sell Schooner Cove Farm. It is heart-breaking because we love it." By September they had made arrangements to sell the farm, along with the other parcels of land they owned in the area — Best's Point, Margaret's Cove, and Morrison Mountain. The farm itself comprised about eighty acres lying between Schooner Cove and Cobscook Bay, and included the 175-year-old house and the barn. To pack their possessions, Margaret and Charley left shortly after their fifty-second wedding anniversary, flying to Fredericton where they were met by Henry and Mairi who had driven down east to help them.

In Maine, caretakers Thursa and Clayton Sawyer of Charlotte were most understanding and helpful. Styles and Beatrice Carter, who owned an antique store in the village, bought everything that was not being shipped back to Ontario. Mairi cooked, dug clams, persuaded her father to go for a swim off the big beach, wrapped china and glass, and generally cheered everyone up.

Margaret remembered where each item came from. "I found it very hard to know that my beloved old chairs and tables were leaving us — the dining room table, the corner cupboard, the beautiful red lamp in the living room ceiling, the old rocking settee for mother and baby, old lamps, etc. We sold them all directly rather than waiting and having them on consignment. The piano we did not sell." The corner cupboard was one of a pair made by Captain W.E. Leighton; the piano was Lulu Best's. It was a sad and poignant time for Margaret and Charley.

Several years earlier Charley wrote a twenty-two-page memoir about Schooner Cove, expressing why it meant so much to him. "To distill the essence of Schooner Cove Farm would be a difficult task for a much better chemist than I. We have spent many vacations with our children there and two of our grandchildren have already chased the huge flocks of sandpipers, watching them wheel in perfect flight formation and land like leaves falling on a still autumn day. My wife, who has none of my childhood memories of the immediate area to influence her judgement, says that it is the loveliest place in the world. It is a country where, as T.S. Eliot wrote, 'The salt is on the briar rose, the fog is in the fir trees.'"[732]

Maine was the place where Best did most of his paintings — Schooner Cove from every angle, in every weather and time of day. "I paint seascapes there every summer. My efforts are usually received by the family with commendation or silence … The Canadian Physicians Art Association never noticed my work. A little later I shipped the same picture to the American Physicians Art Association where it won an Award of Merit. Not only that, but I was elected the first honorary president of the Association!"

Best reminisced about meeting President Roosevelt in 1936. It was on Campobello that the president had contracted polio, diagnosed by Dr. Eban Bennet, of Lubec, Maine: "The president told me that he got the infection while swimming in the cold waters of Herring Cove. I said, 'I used to swim as a boy for hours in that same cold water.' 'Oh,' he said, 'I know what you're thinking, Dr. Best — I don't mean that I got the virus from the water, I mean that my resistance was lowered so that the virus got hold of me. Isn't that a good theory?' 'Yes, sir,' I said meekly."[733]

After five sad days packing and arranging for the sale of other items, Margaret and Charley left Schooner Cove Farm, with Henry and Mairi accompanying them. "The question of selling four pieces of property and the selling of our possessions I found troubling. I have often said, 'I love Schooner Cove more than any place in the world.' Charley and I stood and looked, perhaps a last look, at the cove before we climbed into the car to drive away."

Henry had persuaded his parents to take a longer but much-loved route. They went to Eastport, where, a few days earlier, they had closed out their bank account of long standing, and from there took the ferry to Deer Island. "We drove across Deer Island, going right down to the end of the wharf at Chocolate Cove. The Deer Island villages looked prosperous with the houses freshly painted. At the far end we took the Letete ferry to St. George. The little trips on the water were lovely."

In St. Andrews, they visited all the well-known places of Margaret's childhood, had lunch at the Shiretown Inn (Kennedy's Hotel in her day), and shopped at the Charlotte County Cottage Craft. Charley was looking at a yellow tweed jacket (goldenrod colour); he said that he had all the clothes he needed, but Henry convinced him to change his mind, and it was the last item of clothing that he ever bought. St. Andrews looked lovely, with the kirk, the manse, and the homes that had, and in some cases still did, belong to families that Margaret had known. The Bests stayed in

Fredericton for two days, visiting the cathedral and the Beaverbrook Gallery, and then they flew home.

Henry and Mairi drove back to Schooner Cove, where Clayton and Thursa Sawyer helped them pack the car very, very full. At the Calais–St. Stephen border, the customs officer asked, "Where are you coming from?" "West Pembroke." "And your name?" "Best." For twenty minutes there were reminiscences about Dr. Herbert Best who had brought this man into the world, while traffic built up down the main street of Calais. With a "Drive safely now," Henry and Mairi were dispatched on their way.

Arriving home they learned of the death of Dr. Alexander E. MacDonald — "Uncle Alex" to Sandy and Henry. He was an expert ophthalmologist and an internationally known collector of old maps, but he could be very difficult with people whom he did not particularly like. With the Bests — in his office, on the golf course, or elsewhere — he was thoughtfulness itself. At the same time there was a letter from Dr. Jacob Poulsen of Copenhagen saying that Maria Hagedorn, aged eighty-eight, had died. The Bests recalled their many fine visits with her and her husband.

In spite of the sad reason for their trip to Schooner Cove, it had gone well, and so Margaret and Charley accepted an invitation to the dedication of the Howard Root wing of the Joslin Clinic in Boston. The Leo Kralls met their plane, and members of the Joslin family were attentive. Many members of the original staff of the Joslin Clinic, including Drs. Alex Marble and Priscilla White, were at the celebration. The banquet for four hundred people was at the Harvard Club, with newspaper publisher William Randolph Hearst as guest speaker. Charley Best spoke, describing his many meetings with Drs. Joslin and Root. At a scientific session the next day, Dr. David Pyke, Robin Lawrence's successor at King's College Hospital in London, spoke on the possible situation of diabetics in the year 2000. Barbara Seavey Bradford took Margaret and Charley to see Lydia Mahon at the Jordan Hospital, where she was recovering from a hip operation.

Despite a restorative month in Bermuda, Margaret Best was not at all well in the last half of December 1976. She fainted and was confined to her bed for two weeks. Family and friends brought flowers and food over Christmas. On 2 January 1977, a rare family party at 105 Woodlawn brought together Eileen and Sandy, and Janna and Henry, and six of the seven grandchildren. Margaret recorded that they had a large roast of beef delivered from Duguid's on Yonge Street; Linda, as usual, was on hand to prepare the meal. Margaret remarked, "It has been wonderful to have Sandy living here with us." She also noted, "It has not been announced yet but we understand that Henry is to be the new president of Laurentian University in Sudbury!" A few days later, Henry brought Dr. Ed Monahan, the retiring president, to meet his parents.

There was a gathering in early February 1977 at the replica of the 1921 insulin lab at the Ontario Science Centre in connection with fundraising for diabetes research. Margaret was pleased with the write-up in the *Toronto Star* the next day and with the photo of herself and Charley. It was good to feel that they were not entirely out of the swim of events. A bit later, Albert Fisher took CHB to see Premier Bill Davis about funds for research.

Despite plans to go to Boston to take part in a film about Dr. Joslin, neither Best felt up to the trip. Margaret was working on a chapter for their book — the part on her Macleod ancestors in Canada. A current family event was the governor general's awarding of the Star of Courage to Cousin John Albert Mahon of Halifax; he had rescued a two-year-old child from a burning house. The Bests called his parents, Albert and Jean, to express their admiration.

For Charley's seventy-eighth birthday on 27 February 1977, Sandy was in Calgary, and Janna and Henry were in Québec with a group of students. Eileen and her four provided a much-appreciated musical evening, playing the piano, the flute, the guitar, and the trombone, and all singing. Charley "really had a good time. The musical evening pleased him greatly. He is talking of buying a piano so the children can play when they come here. I think he would really like to take piano lessons himself." Eileen did give him several lessons, starting with one of his favourite songs, "There's a Long, Long Trail a Winding, Into the Land of My Dreams," a First World War marching song.

On 19 March 1977, Charley and Margaret went to the wedding of Maria and Joe Diogenes in St. Sebastyao Church at Pauline and Bloor streets. Maria, from the Azores Islands, who had worked briefly for Sandy and Laurie at 30 Rosedale Road, was now helping at 105 Woodlawn. Over the next ten years, she was to become a much loved and important member of the household.

There were several happy occasions in connection with the meetings of the American Gastroenterological Society in Toronto in late May. Best received its Beaumont Medal; he had delivered the Beaumont Lecture of the Wayne County Medical Society in 1948. The Walter Palmers of Chicago gave a dinner for some of the delegates. He was a distinguished internist and retired professor of medicine, and Elizabeth Palmer talked to Margaret about her father, Dr. Howard Ricketts, a famous researcher on typhus and other infectious diseases, and about her brother, the Bests' old friend Dr. Henry Ricketts. The next evening society president Dr. Marrin Sleisenger of the University of California gave a large dinner at Casa Loma. In the midst of happy events came news that A.V. Hill had died in Cambridge at the age of ninety; shortly afterwards they learned that Dick Connelly, long-time executive director of the ADA, had died in New York.

Eileen was now administrative director of the Ontario Craft Council. She took her former parents-in-law to see the quarters on Dundas Street, and they enjoyed seeing the beautiful articles on exhibit. Eileen took Alexander, Margaret, and Melinda to Europe. They rented a Renault and saw a great deal in five weeks.

Best was speaker on 19 August at the president's luncheon of the Canadian National Exhibition. "Charley's talk was a great success and there was much laughter at times. He ended by telling about the meeting in Ottawa when Roosevelt was given an honorary degree from the University of London, presented by Charley. He mentioned Lord Athlone, Princess Alice, and then he added, 'Mackenzie King, I could not stand him.' There was a great applause at that point, apparently there were many present who did not care for Mackenzie King. Julian Porter, in thanking him said that Mackenzie King had heard him, and his dog too."

Don Harron, the well-known broadcaster, came to the house on 30 August to do an interview with Charley. "He is extremely nice and I think the interview went well." Barry Penhale conducted another interview in several sessions in June and August 1977 for the Ontario Medical Association's Oral History Project. The transcript records Best's answers to questions about his career. At the end, Penhale recorded his general impression: "Dr. and Mrs. Best are very gracious people ... he is at his most relaxed and most personable when he talks about horses. He spoke of his wife and his regret that she had not had the kind of recognition of her talents and her accomplishments that he believes she should have had."[734]

Sandy had a great interest in various art forms. He was involved in an exhibition at the Mira Godard Gallery on Hazelton Avenue called "Art of the Americas — Pre-Columbian sculpture, gold, jade, terra cotta, and stone — north-west Indian art — prehistoric Eskimo Art." He curated an exhibition of the works of Alex Janvier at the Royal Ontario Museum. Later he organized an exhibition of Indian quill work, also at the ROM, including many pieces from his own collection. He was also interested in many other art forms. His mother was pleased to examine some early Ontario weaving that he showed her.

For their fifty-third wedding anniversary on 3 September 1977, Charley bought Margaret Donald Blake Webster's *The Book of Canadian Antiques*; Linda gave them Margaret Atwood's *Dancing Girls and Other Stories*. Despite the family's reservations, Margaret and Charley wanted to go back to the Maritimes. They flew to Fredericton on 12 September. From there, they drove to St. Stephen and Calais. "We plan to go down to Schooner Cove tomorrow. It will make us sad to see the dear old empty house but we want to know how it is looking and also to have a glimpse of Schooner Cove." They drove down Leighton's Point Road. "I found it very sad, the grass is tall, the windows are all boarded up and Charley could not make the front door key work, we did not have even a glimpse of the interior. We looked across at Best's Point which we have sold this year." They visited the Kenneth Leightons, the Harold Blackwoods, and the Carl Herseys, with reminiscences at each stop.

Dense fog made the trip across the Bay of Fundy on the *Acadian Princess* calm. Scallops were Margaret's favourite seafood, and she enjoyed them in Digby, the great scallop-fishing centre. George and Phyllis Best of Cornwallis drove their cousins around King's County. They found the house outside Waterville built by Ken Fisher, a brother of Charley's mother, and the house where Lulu Fisher herself was born. George Best also pointed out the site of the original Burbidge house and the first Best house on Starr's Point. They returned to St. John's Church and saw the first church (moved from Fox Hill to serve as a garage and workshops) built by John Burbidge and William Best.

Visiting cemeteries may seem morbid to some people, but the Best family enjoyed ancestor-hunting in this way. Early on, the boys had become accustomed to having picnics in graveyards and being sent running up and down the rows of markers looking for particular names.

George and Phyllis offered to help with the driving to Prince Edward Island. They went to see the house that Sandy had bought in 1973 in Cardigan, King's County. "It is large and most comfortable, many rooms, open fireplaces, lots of windows and the most glorious trees around it, linden (lime)." Sandy furnished the house with antiques from the island and from Nova Scotia. He had a dinner to introduce his parents to some of his friends — Thomas McMillan, later MP for Hillsborough, and his wife;

Kelso Gordon, a neighbouring farmer, and his wife; and Marjorie Webster, divorced from Howard, Sandy's former business colleague on the island.

In Toronto on 12 October, Dr. George Cahill, an old friend from the Joslin Clinic, gave the Banting Memorial Lecture; he and his wife had gone to West Pembroke recently to look into repairs for "The Birthplace."[735] Charley went to the lecture, and they both went to the dinner at the Faculty Club. They were pleased to be among some of the active researchers, such as Dr. Charles Hollenburg and Dr. K.J.R. Wightman.

The senior Bests were in Sudbury at the end of October, before Henry's installation as president of Laurentian University. Margaret described the president's house at 179 John Street, how Henry and Janna's own furniture fitted in, and what more pieces they had bought. There were two dinner parties for cousins John and Teen Robertson, and for their new university friends. Margaret and Charley talked with Dr. Paddy Bruce-Lockhart, the Scottish vice-chairman of the board and his Ukrainian wife, Eve, and Dr. Jean-Noël Desmarais, chairman, and his wife, Colette. After the dinner, Charley enjoyed standing beside the piano while Paddy played and everyone sang. Unfortunately, Henry's parents were not going to be at his official installation — possibly they thought that there would be too many people or that their presence would somehow detract attention from him. However, while they were in Sudbury, his new robes arrived, blue and gold with a Henry VIII hat, and, to everyone's delight at one of the dinners, he tried them on over his kilt.

Margaret and Charley flew to Bermuda on 9 November. On the plane were Mr. and Mrs. Scotty Bruce. He was chair of the Old Boy's Association of Upper Canada College and was delighted that three graduates had recently been appointed presidents of universities: George Connell at Western Ontario, John Godfrey at King's in Halifax, and Henry Best at Laurentian. On the nineteenth, Margaret and Charley sent a cable to the family in Sudbury; Linda Mahon and Jessie Ridout flew from Toronto for Henry's installation. Eileen and her four children drove up. Sandy flew up in the morning and left partway through the ceremony to catch a plane back south.

In describing Christmas dinner for 1977, Margaret said that the eighteen-pound turkey cost twenty-two dollars. When she was young, the Mahons had to be very careful about money. "I find that we are most interested in my old diaries to learn what we paid for various things years ago, and so I record the price! Then dinner of turkey, peas and carrots together, potatoes, tomato scallop, cranberry sauce, the usual Christmas fare for the Best family." Sandy's baby grand piano was now at 105 Woodlawn, so every family gathering had plenty of music.

Linda took a picture of the Bests before they flew to New York on 22 January 1978 for a meeting of the ADA council. They enjoyed their suite at the Waldorf-Astoria. Rosalyn Yalow, who had recently won the Nobel Prize for her part in explaining the role of hormones in body chemistry, was there, along with Jack and Bebe Davidson from Atlanta. New friends included Dr. John A. Galloway from Lilly's; John L. Dugan, new executive secretary; and Wendell Mayes, new president of the ADA. The trip went well, and Margaret and Charley appeared in relatively good health. Linda sent a copy of the picture she had taken to Henry and Janna in Sudbury. On the back Linda had written, "Don't they look great?"

Sandy was in New London, Connecticut, on 12 February 1978 to see Susan. She spoke to her grandparents in Toronto on the phone, and Margaret happily recorded the conversation. "I asked her if she was going to school. 'Not today,' she said, 'This is Lincoln's birthday. But he is in the cemetery. Perhaps he will come out since this is his birthday.'"

Chapter Nine
MMB Solo,
1978–1988

In February 1978, Charles Best reminisced about his life in medical research. It was mainly autobiographical, starting from his youth: "Environment, opportunity and heredity played an important role in influencing my future." Of the summer of 1921, he wrote, "Things did not go well at first but being young and enthusiastic, we were able to withstand our initial disappointments and to begin again. It seemed a long time before we achieved success but, in actual fact, we were convinced by the end of July that we had solved a problem which had baffled previous investigators for generations." Of his most influential mentor, he said, "All of us who had the privilege of working under the benign and vigorous guidance of Dale found his sustained and meticulous approach to research contagious. He left his mark on all of us." Of Margaret, he wrote, "She has always helped and encouraged me in every venture and has become a continual source of inspiration. By her charm, intelligence, and understanding, she has created goodwill in all our travels and won the admiration and affection of people in countries the world over."[736]

CHB recalled some of the high points. He mentioned the fiftieth anniversary of the discovery of insulin and particularly "the happy and memorable events which took place in London, the award of the Companion of Honour by Her Majesty the Queen, reading the lesson in St. Paul's Cathedral at the Thanksgiving service attended by twelve hundred diabetics and their families, lectures at the Royal Society and before the British Diabetic Association, as well as the many pleasant social activities."

On 27 February, Eileen organized a seventy-ninth birthday party for "Dr. Charley." Her four children and Sandy were there. "What a lovely birthday he has had. Our grandchildren are very accomplished musicians and both Eileen and Sandy are full of music."[737]

In early March, Sandy travelled to Sudbury to advise a group of people who wanted to buy the Burwash Prison Farm on Highway 69 to raise cattle. Surprisingly, since he had never ever done this before, he called and asked if he could stay with Janna and Henry. They had a good evening together, with no arguments. The entry in the guest book was, "March 9th, 1978, Sandy Best, 32 Front Street, Toronto" — his business address, not 105 Woodlawn where he was living with his parents.

Early on Saturday, 25 March 1978, Henry and Janna were awoken by the telephone. It was Henry's father, who told him the shocking news that Sandy had died suddenly of a massive heart attack at the age of forty-six. Henry, Janna, and their children flew to Toronto as soon as they heard the news. The next evening, Sunday 26 March, Charles Best collapsed. Henry and Janna, young Charley, and Dr. Moray Jansen were at the house within minutes. CHB reached out to Janna and said quietly, "Don't let them take me to the hospital!" He suspected the worst. Moray Jansen called the ambulance, and as the attendants wheeled the stretcher out of the bedroom Charley said softly, "I'm sorry, Margaret." He had been deeply shocked by Sandy's death.

The next day was found on his desk a tribute to his elder son's life, which he was writing when he collapsed. Margaret put this into a scrapbook, later giving it to Eileen. Charley wrote: "Charles Alexander Best, born in Toronto, July 7, 1931, accomplished more in his short span of 46 years than most men do in four score years and ten. He was interesting and intelligent from a very early age … Sandy's passing, March 25, 1978, leaves a gap which never can be filled in the hearts and minds of all of us who loved and admired him, but we must carry on perhaps with heavier loads because he would have wanted it that way."

Eileen, young Charley, and Henry went to the funeral home to make arrangements for Sandy's funeral. They requested not one of the fancy coffins on display, but a simple, pine coffin with wrought-iron handles, beautifully made in Lindsay, Ontario. Meantime, Charles Best was in hospital acutely ill. Dr. Douglas Stewart of St. Andrew's Church planned a graveside service for Sandy at Mount Pleasant Cemetery on Monday 27 March.

A memorial service was planned for Friday 31 March in St. Andrew's Church. Dr. Stewart had talked to all the family members before the memorial service and had taken special note of the thoughts of Sandy and Eileen's children. He spoke sympathetically, but honestly: "Sandy made mistakes and that is why you related to him. Who finds it easy to companion with men who never miscalculate? The distinctive thing about Sandy seems to be that like his accomplishments, his miscalculations were always man-sized. He was resolute, determined and tenacious even in the midst of reversals. He was a man born under a great man, who was in search of his own greatness. Endowed as he was with such a breadth of skills and insights, it seems he had to try them all."[738]

Early on the morning of Sandy's memorial service, Charley died. For Margaret the sudden deaths of Sandy and Charley were an incredible double-blow. It was 27 June before she could write in her diary.

> Henry took me down each day to the hospital in the morning, in the afternoon, and again at night, and we were able to stay until midnight. We sat in a little lounge but often I went into the room where Charley was lying — a room by himself — and for the first day or two he knew me and put his hand up to caress my cheek and once on my forehead. He knew me then. You could tell from his eyes. There was so much apparatus, wires and complicated things. His colour was always good, I thought, and I really thought that he might get well. They told me it was an aneurysm of the aorta. Dr. Bernard Goldman operated twice. There were several doctors about, Dr. Bob Mustard, Dr. Bill Mustard, Dr. Bill Clark, Bernie Leibel, etc. I am not sure but perhaps an aneurysm of the aorta means that there was internal bleeding.
>
> On Friday, March 31st, early in the morning I was told that he was gone. That same day, the memorial service for Sandy was held in St. Andrew's Church. I was too ill to go either to the cemetery when Sandy was buried or to the memorial service for him. On the following day, Saturday, 1 April, the funeral service for Charley was held at the grave. I was able to go to that. Charley and I had chosen some years ago a plot in Mount Pleasant Cemetery, and there Sandy and Charley were both buried a few days apart. The pallbearers for Charley were Jamie Bain [Joan Salter Bain's son], Jimmy Campbell, Donald Fraser, Omond Solandt, and Bruce Scott [her first cousin, son of Aunt Linda and Uncle Walter of Winnipeg]. The pallbearers for Sandy's funeral were Henry Best, Charles Stewart Best, Alexander Best, and

three of Sandy's colleagues, George Yost, Alex Havilant, and Warren Gear.

On Monday, April 3rd, a memorial service was held for Charley in Convocation Hall and I was there. Dr. Stewart took the service. He was wonderful through all of those sad days. Mr. Douglas Bodle, who is the organist at St. Andrew's Church, played the organ. The hymns were "Abide With Me" and "Unto the Hills Around." Laurie Chute gave a beautiful eulogy. I had heard Charley say, years ago, very casually, that he liked those hymns very much and would like them sung at his funeral. I made a note of that at the time.

I also heard him say to Laurie Chute (I think it was in the Quadrangle of Hart House before the dinner on Charley's retirement) that he hoped Laurie would be the person to talk about him when he passed on. There was nothing morbid about Charley, these were just remarks that he had happened to make.

The kindness of people has been overwhelming. I have not mentioned the flowers. They were everywhere, at our home here, at Convocation Hall, everywhere, plus telegrams, phone calls and letters. Some of our friends baked cakes, roasts, turkey — whole dinners were sent in, and that was most helpful since there were always many people here. The telegrams and cables were listed as they came in as well as the letters. I have now answered more than 425 letters. Everyone loved Charley and our dear Sandy had many friends. This is, I know, a most inadequate telling of what happened during that terrible week.

Before the memorial service for Charley, she had asked Henry to ask Eileen and Janna to buy her a black dress as she thought that it would be expected. Henry wondered out loud what his father would say since he detested black and so did she; she wore blue. One of the most touching moments was when the doorbell rang and Henry asked Cousin Bruce Scott to come in. He refused, but took a roll of bills out of his pocket and said to take it. He knew that, particularly with the suddenness of events, there could well be problems with frozen bank accounts.

Many people travelled from out of town for the memorial service for CHB, and in the weeks that followed many more visited the house. Margaret Best showed her strength of character and stood up very well. Friends thought that Margaret should not try to answer all the letters that she received, but she wanted to do it and wrote ten each day, which proved to be therapeutic. Dr. Fred Whitehouse, who attended the service on behalf of the ADA, recalled: "It was clear to me … that Margaret Best was a remarkable human being who greatly enhanced the aura about your distinguished father."[739]

After Best's death in 1978, Dr. Norbert Freinkel, president of the American Diabetes Association said, "Some of the greatness of the 20th century has gone out of our world with the passing of Charles H. Best. Dr. Best translated science into terms that the whole world could understand, and into service that enabled our efforts. He was a beacon of civilization, typifying the true goals of science and medicine … improving and saving human lives."[740]

A somewhat tangled story that involves the ADA concerned what was known as "The Birthplace," the house in West Pembroke, Maine, where Charles Best was born in 1899. He and Margaret had long envisaged something being done with the small office wing at one end of the house, primarily to perpetuate the memory of Dr. Herbert Best and also to mark the place where his son was born. As was related earlier, the group of trustees, who bought the property, turned over the deed to the ADA in 1968.

There followed a period of upheaval in the administration of the ADA during which the structure of the house deteriorated and a decision was made in 1978 after Charles Best's death to give the property to the U.S. National Trust. Unfortunately, some items were lost, including Dr. Herbert Best's framed medical diplomas and graduation photographs; other items of furniture loaned by family members, including Dr. Herbert Best's roll-top desk and chair, portable operating table and surgical instruments were sold with the house. A plaque outside the office door read: "Charles Herbert Best, CBE, MD, FRS, co-discoverer of insulin was born in this house February 27, 1899. With the discovery of insulin, control of diabetes became possible and the lives of millions of diabetics have been saved. The American Diabetes Association donated this historic property to the National Trust for historic preservation in the United States for sale subject to protective covenants to help assure the future preservation of the property as a memorial to Dr. Best." In fact the National Trust contributed nothing to the preservation of the house and it was sold, with the contents loaned by the Best family, to a private buyer.

By July, Margaret and Linda began accepting invitations to lunch — at the Faculty Club, the Yacht Club, and elsewhere. On 9 August: "I write very seldom in my diary now. I will be very glad when all the problems are settled, perhaps they never will be. I try very hard to keep in mind all of the various things I am supposed to know." Many people wondered how Margaret would cope after so many years when all decisions of importance were made with Charley. Actually she managed very well; she concentrated on what she had to do, and people were willing to help her.

Charley had made a reservation to go to Bermuda in November 1978, but Margaret did not want to go alone. She left Toronto only once during the next ten years, to go to Sudbury, but she maintained her interest in what was going on in the world. The funeral of Pope Paul VI brought back memories of Rome and the Pontifical Academy of Sciences. She added, "Who will be the next Pope?"

Her health was quite good, but occasionally she fainted and hurt herself in falling. Linda slept on the second floor of the house, and although she tried to do everything in her power to help her sister, she did not always hear her calls. She often stayed home from the office where she still went part-time.

Young Charley had been a great help to his grandparents for some years, but now he enrolled at Queen's University. "How I will miss him! He has some of the thoughtful, kindly qualities of his grandfather." Eileen and the three remaining children who were in Toronto were of immense help to Margaret. Eileen was changing jobs to become general manager of the Young People's Theatre Centre, continuing to make a very good reputation for herself in arts administration. The Sudbury family came to visit as often as possible. Moray Jansen agreed that a daily Scotch and water was good for Margaret, and Henry kept her supplied.

The third of September 1978 was a difficult day for Margaret, but family and friends remembered Margaret and Charley's anniversary with calls and flowers. The unsold properties in Maine were on Margaret's mind. Katherine Raser from the next property to Schooner Cove Farm called to say that there were six places for sale on Leighton's Point Road. Henry had meetings on Canadian studies at the University of Maine in Orono, and he and John Conway drove to Pembroke. He reported that Schooner Cove Farm looked lovely, but that "The Birthplace" was neglected and in bad shape.

The tenth of October was Charles H. Best Day in the Faculty of Medicine, and Ed Sellers, Sr., was the chief organizer. Henry and Janna came from Sudbury to accompany Margaret on the occasion. The National Film Board film *The Quest* was screened, and also the Hannah Institute's film on CHB, which formed part of *Making Canadian Medical History*. Classes were cancelled, and the auditorium was packed. Dr. Brian Holmes, dean of medicine, chaired the gathering, and Dr. James Ham, the university's new president, spoke. Dennis Timbrell, Ontario's minister of health, announced a grant of one million dollars to endow a research chair in Charley's name. Rachmiel Levine talked about the history and discovery of insulin, and Robin Harris, the university historian, gave a paper.

In the afternoon, Geza Hetenyi, a student and colleague of Charley's, received the Charles H. Best Prize of the Hoechst Company. Dr. Oscar B. Crofford, director of the Diabetes Endocrinology Centre of Vanderbilt University in Nashville, Tennessee, spoke on "Diabetes as a Current and Future Problem." Laurie Chute gave a talk on "Charles H. Best — Teacher, Physiologist." That evening Linda, Eileen and young Charley, Henry and Janna accompanied Margaret to a dinner at Hart House. "It had been a very exciting, wonderful day."

Alexander and his grandmother were taken by limousine on 21 November 1978 to the new Charles Best Elementary School, near Bathurst Street and Finch Avenue in North York (now Toronto). Dr. David MacLennan, acting head of the Banting and Best Department of Medical Research, and his wife were there, as were others from the institute, the staff of the school, and the trustees. A large photograph of Charley was unveiled, and three students who had suggested the name received books. Mr. Mullin, the principal, pleased Margaret by saying, "I thought you were going to be a little old lady." Despite illness and sorrow, she did not look her almost seventy-eight years.

An x-ray of Margaret's knee at the end of November showed that a bone had been broken in a fall in August and had not mended. Moray Jansen set out the options: replace the knee, put metal pieces on either side, or do nothing. "I didn't have the presence of mind to ask him whether it would get progressively worse if nothing were done. I would choose to do nothing. After all, I have been putting up with the pain since August 18th when it happened. After so many heart attacks, I think an operation would be dangerous." She discussed the matter several times with Henry, and he talked to her doctors. "This is really too much to bear at Christmas time. It will be difficult enough anyway. Well, I still have pain but I praised myself to Linda last night when I got the bad news and I said, 'Well, I have spunk. My mother had spunk and I have not complained very much although I have had a good deal of pain.'"

The next morning she took a taxi to the bank, "got some cash and so if they should pop me into the hospital, I will be more or less prepared. But I would die in the hospital. Charley never let me be away from home when I had the heart attacks. He knew it would be wrong for me." When the matter was sorted out, it was the cartilage that was broken, and there was no longer any question of an operation. Stairs remained difficult for Margaret and Linda helped her in and out of the bath.

Nineteen seventy-nine did not start off very well for Margaret. She was housebound for five weeks with flu and angina, while Linda stayed at home to look after her. Margaret kept in touch with the family, read the paper, and followed the news on television. The departure of the Shah of Iran from his country reminded her of the gift from the Iranian Diabetic Association on their fiftieth wedding anniversary — a portrait in carved wood of Avicenna, the great eleventh-century Persian scientist. "Charley had written a short biography and put it on the back of the lovely frame, wood inlaid with gold." In 1971–2, there had been correspondence about possibly going to Iran.

Margaret was concerned about the Best Family Papers:

> Then there will be another problem, what to retain in the family. There are the diaries, more than seventy of them, the scrapbooks, forty-three of them: Series I, more about medical affairs, Series II, more personal, and Series III, our friends. Then, the chapters of the book I was writing about our lives, then letters and papers, snapshot albums, mainly of family interest but also some of important medical people.[741] There are also many photographs, principally of family interest, Charley's paintings, etc, several pieces of silver inscribed to Charley, Charley's portrait by Charles Comfort, Charley's books, his own medical writings which he gave to me as well as his many medals. It is a real problem for me to know how best to leave these very precious and interesting things.

Increasingly, Margaret would make lists of "problems" to discuss with Henry by phone or when he was in Toronto, which he usually was several times each month. Bills seemed overwhelming. "The tax bill for this house has come. I have paid Wylie Ivany's enormous bill (my lawyer) and the oil bills came thick and fast. I find it all quite alarming." She insisted on preparing the draft income tax return, but worried about it.

CHB's eightieth birthday was duly celebrated. Flowers came from several people, and Margaret remembered the previous year, when they had both gone to Yorkdale for lunch and enjoyed Nova Scotia scallops. "We were very happy!"

On 2 March, Margaret was out for the first time in more than a month. She went to the branch of the Bank of Nova Scotia in Forest Hill Village, where she had had an account for many years. She was very careful about money, investing every dollar that she could in Canada Savings Bonds.

Young Margaret was in a play at Bishop Strachan School, and her grandmother and Linda went to see it. "*The Women* by Clare Boothe Luce — a poor choice for the girls but they did very well. Margaret had one of the principal parts. She played Mary (Mrs. Stephen Harnes). She was splendid, looked lovely and acted beautifully."

A parcel arrived from Dr. Yoshitake Nishizume of Japan on 23 March. In a red velvet case was a thin golden chain with a round black enamel locket. Dr. Boniface Lin at the Best Institute translated the card, "An offering on the first anniversary of Dr. C.H. Best's death, 1979." Margaret Best wrote, "In two days, Sunday, March 25th, one year since our dear Sandy died. And then on Saturday, March 31st, six days later, my beloved Charley. Those who say it gets easier as time goes by don't know what they are talking about. It will never get easier." On 31 March, she added, "One year ago today my dear, dear Charley died. I can not write about it. It hurts too much."

Eileen, Alexander, Margaret, and Melinda went to 105 Woodlawn for dinner on Easter Sunday, and the Sudbury family called. Several people brought flowers and food. Reg and Margaret Haist were the most faithful of friends, often taking Margaret and Linda to the Faculty Club or to the Yacht Club for lunch.

There were fewer visitors "from away" now that Margaret was on her own. In mid-April, Mladen Vranic brought Rolf Luft, visiting from Stockholm. He was president of the IDF and had chaired the committee for the Nobel Prize in physiology and medicine. Don Fraser of the Hospital for Sick Children brought Margaret the scroll of honorary membership in the Canadian Society of Endocrinology and Metabolism to which Charley had been elected just before he died. Charles Stewart worked at the Hospital for Sick Children for the summer, which pleased his grandmother. Other documents appeared. Reg Haist brought a copy of the obituary that he had written for the Royal Society of Canada.

When she felt well, Margaret enjoyed going out. At the end of April, Henry appeared between meetings and took her to the York Club for lunch with Dean Boyd Neel of the Faculty of Music, always a lively and witty companion; Henry had recently participated in a CBC program about the doctor-musician. On other occasions, Henry and Margaret went to the University Club. While having lunch at Murray's at Yonge Street and St. Clair Avenue one day with Linda, Margaret fainted away for several minutes. She persuaded the ambulance crew to take her home rather than to the hospital. Moray Jansen came at once and talked of inserting a pacemaker. There had been no angina or other symptoms. Margaret finishes this paragraph in her diary, "Enough about that."

The activities of the family were, as for many her age, the centre of interest. Eileen took her to the Young People's Theatre to see *The Curse of the Werewolf.* "The play was done excellently but I was surprised that some of the very young children were not terrified in spots. I think I might have been at six or eight years of age but then I had not watched television as they have."

On 22 May 1979, Margaret Best, with the help of Heather Phillips from the small apartment in 105 Woodlawn, went down the street to vote. "It was quite an effort for me to walk down and back. I took my cane and we went very slowly." Early in the day she had written, "I want to try to get out for Joe Clark, the Conservative." Margaret followed closely news about the strike at INCO in Sudbury, which lasted nine months. She knew that it created tension in the community and made Henry and Janna's tasks more difficult.

Margaret was still concerned about what to do about the family archives. She, Henry, "jovial and with his big cane," and Ed Sellers met at the Thomas Fisher Library in early June with the custodian, Richard Landon, and the university's president, Dr. Jim Ham. Things did not go well and Margaret left in tears. "I still am quite uncertain about what is the best to do."

The Canadian Diabetes Association did not forget Margaret Best. At its 1979 meeting, Ken Gorman came to take her to the dinner at the Plaza II Hotel. "When Ken introduced the head table he left me until the last and said words to the effect that I was the guest of honour. They all clapped, hundreds of people and then suddenly they all stood up and really I was very moved and happy about the wonderful welcome they gave me. It was honouring my dear Charley." When the International Biochemical Association met in Toronto that year, it presented Margaret with a copy of the IBA's journal, a "Special Issue dedicated to the memory of Charles Herbert Best on the occasion of the first anniversary of his death." Dr. David MacLennan of the Best Institute wrote: "It has been said that the discovery of insulin changed research in Canadian Universities from a sideline to an essential activity. Dr. Best not only led the way for this change but set an example as a Scientist-Teacher that will be difficult to match again."[742] In November, Mladen Vranic brought Margaret a special copy of the proceedings of the International Conference on Exercise and Diabetes, published as a supplement to *Diabetes*, the ADA's magazine, and dedicated to Charles Best.

On 13 June, Margaret had an appointment with Dr. John Morrow, "the heart doctor," who did an electrocardiogram. "He did not appear to find my heart in any worse shape. He surprised me by talking about strokes. He found something on the right side of my head, something that runs up to the brain, a cord, a thread, what is it? ... he told me to take two Aspirin every day, one at breakfast time, one at dinner."

Sad news came from Duxbury, Massachusetts — Lydia Mahon was very ill. Henry flew down to see her in the hospital in Plymouth, and she was stoic as usual. A month later she died, and Henry and Janna travelled to the funeral. Henry went through some of the contents of the house with Lydia's nieces, and Mairi flew down from Sudbury to help.

Despite help from Linda, Henry, and Eileen and her children, Margaret found it difficult to cope with her home, but not so difficult that she wanted to move. "If only I could stay well now I think I could manage." Something always needed fixing: pipes, garage doors, appliances; some of the tradesmen were most helpful, others the opposite. Margaret talked of having to buy a new washing machine. "Very dull news for my diary but what can I expect when I am ill so often. I am not getting sorry for myself, only disgusted."

MMB had been concerned for some time about getting a stone for Charley and Sandy's graves. With help from Henry and young Charley, she picked what she thought appropriate at McIntosh Granite on Yonge Street. Margaret at first wanted only MD after Charley's name but later agreed to have several of his most significant honours included: CC, CH, CBE, MD, DSc, FRS. On their fifty-fifth wedding anniversary, 3 September 1979,

Margaret read some of her earliest diaries. "What a wonderful life Charley and I had."

On 28 May 1980, historian Michael Bliss paid his third visit to 105 Woodlawn concerning his book on the discovery of insulin, and Margaret showed him various items. "He is interviewing many people. In the autumn, he plans to go to England." On 28 November, he visited Margaret again. A number of people had advised Margaret not to co-operate with him, unsure of what he would write, but Henry had advised his mother to be as helpful as possible. Margaret wrote to Randall Sprague, "I did a great deal of reading of letters and documents of Charley's in order to give information to Dr. Bliss. He always wants a little more, but the eye specialist and my doctor say I must not work at it at present. I am so glad that you have helped Dr. Bliss. I only hope that it has not been too much work for you."[743] Margaret also made a list of names of people whom she wanted to talk to Bliss: "George and Peggy Clowes; Elliott Joslin's daughter, Mary Otto; Dr. Hagedorn's successor, Jacob Poulsen; Dr. Houssay's successor, Dr. Rodriguez; Robin Lawrence's son, Dan; Joseph Hoet's wife, Marguerite; Frank and Ruth Young in England; Sir Joseph Barcroft's son, Henry, and his wife, Biddy; Randall and Anne Sprague; Eduardo Braun Menéndez's wife, Maté, in Buenos Aires; Edwin and Agnes Gates; the Solandts; the Sellers; the Haists; and, the Sireks."

The Best Family Papers contain two letters from Bliss to Margaret, dated 2 and 29 June 1980. He asked for more letters and other documents about events in 1921–2, and stated his intention to write to all the people whom she had suggested. A later item concerning Bliss is a note that Margaret wrote to herself asking, "Why such a detailed description of the scientific work? Many people will skip all of that detail and concentrate on the personalities. <u>And</u>, how did he write so fully about the scientific aspects — details of laboratory work — he would have needed a very concentrated course to understand it. Who did that for him — was it the Sireks? He mentions much help from Otto."[744] Another note to herself showed concern about Bliss's intention of writing a biography of Fred Banting because, "He did not admire him and criticized him over and over again." After the publication of *The Discovery of Insulin*, Margaret saw Bliss at the opening of the Diabetic Clinic at the Toronto General Hospital. She said to him, "I understand you are now writing a biography of Fred Banting. Don't be too hard on Fred."

Later Margaret was interested to watch a television drama, *Glory Enough For All*, a joint production made by the Canadian Broadcasting

Corporation and Thames Television, based on *The Discovery of Insulin* by Michael Bliss. She thought R.H. Thomson excellent as Banting, but was disappointed in the portrayal of Charley. Unfortunately, the director of the film refused to tell Leah Pinsent, who played Margaret, that she was still alive and would have been delighted to talk to her. Much later Miss Pinsent was unhappy when she realized that she lost the opportunity to interpret her part in more depth.

At the request of the editors of *The Biographical Encyclopaedia of the World,* Linda Mahon had written a fifty-four-page *Account of Charles H. Best: His Background, Scientific Work, and other Pertinent Information,* which contained much valuable material. The last paragraph summed up his career. "To Charles Best, medical research was the most fascinating occupation in the world. He was always optimistic in attacking new problems and felt that one should be willing to invest one's efforts in the study of any interesting phenomena, exploring and eliminating unnecessary material until the main problem became more well defined and simple. To him, this was a real challenge and he often said, 'Our work is, of course, never finished.'"[745]

In June 1980, Henry suggested that his mother and Linda go to Prize Day at St. Andrews College in Aurora where Bruce was now a student. They were very eager to go but unsure. "Henry said he would have a car come to take us. I have never been outside Toronto since Charley and I went to New York in January 1978. I have not been well enough for long drives or flights." Headmaster Tom and Mary Hockin were very hospitable. Premier Bill Davis was the speaker, Bruce received a scholarship, and Margaret and Linda thoroughly enjoyed the outing.

Margaret's vision troubled her. "My eyes were behaving strangely. I could not see very well from the left eye. I would only see part of the room. It gave me a very strange feeling. I have had all these days the strange floating figures which go from me to the left side. I look up and these strange things are going by. It is quite weird." Specialist Dr. Keith MacDonald concluded "that the outside of each eye has lost the vision. He talked of the arteries behind my eyes being at fault, temporary lack of enough blood to that section of the brain, a slight stroke." Writing about all this in her diary was difficult, but she was determined to keep a record.

Margaret flew to Sudbury to visit Henry and his family in late August 1980, and enjoyed the guest suite in the president's house. Cousin John Robertson came for dinner and reminisced about 1921, when he was ten years old and Margaret stayed at their house in

Coniston. Various people came for meals, and there was a visit to see the family camp, or cottage, at Page Lake.

"Toronto, Friday, September 3rd, 1980. This was our beautiful wedding day, fifty-six years ago. The sun was shining, just as it is today." Eileen brought a large bunch of cosmos, remembering her mother-in-law's wedding bouquet. Albert and Mary Fisher entertained Margaret and Linda, along with Arthur and Aileen Kelly. Judge Kelly had chaired the Insulin Committee of the Board of the University of Toronto, and Albert Fisher had been its secretary. "What nice people Mary and Albert are! I am very fond of them both."

Henry had plans for his mother's eightieth birthday, but she did not feel confident enough. Then she developed shingles. "Why do I have to have so many miserable afflictions? My 80th birthday will not be the jolly day we once looked forward to. Now, concerning shingles. It is a horrible, outrageous disease."

In spite of the shingles, the family tried to make Margaret's birthday as festive as possible. "The great surprise in the morning was the front door opening and in came Henry. He had flown down from Sudbury. It became a big and happy day for me, although many of my children [MMB referred to all of her descendants as her "children"] could only look through the front door or stand in the vestibule and not come close to me because of the shingles. Henry, Alexander, Bruce and Linda stayed for lunch. There was champagne. There were flowers and phone calls."

Eileen was able to buy her own house in 1978 and she and her family moved to 179 Lyndhurst Boulevard in time for Christmas that year. Eileen made the spacious house comfortable and welcoming and Margaret and Linda enjoyed many happy occasions there, as did Janna and Henry and their family. In early March 1981, Eileen took Margaret to the Art Gallery of Ontario to see the show "Vincent van Gogh, and the Birth of Cloisonnism at the End of the Nineteenth Century." She had seen some of the canvases in Holland and enjoyed being wheeled through the gallery. Both Margaret and Eileen derived great pleasure from many such outings to the Art Gallery of Ontario.

A parcel arrived with several copies of the *Harvard Medical Alumni Bulletin* for December 1980, with a very good article by Mary Sunday; the cover had a portrait of a handsome young man supposed to be Charley, except that it was not. Young Charley visited his grandmother in May 1981 and introduced a friend, Amy (Anne-Marie) Yamamoto, whom he later married. Margaret would have liked to go to their graduation at Queen's, but it was not possible.

Ed Sellers was the right person to advise Margaret on many subjects, especially concerning the University of Toronto. He took her to meet Dean Frederick Lowy at his office in the new Medical Sciences Building, to discuss what items might complement the busts of Banting and Best in the foyer. "It should be a very good place for a selection of interesting things because medical students must come and go there constantly." For the display cases in the entrance to the Best Institute, Margaret had gathered together Charley's gold and scarlet DSc gown from London, books, degree parchments, medals, and several of his paintings. Amongst photographs could be included the three schools bearing his name, that in North York already mentioned, the Doctor Charles Best Junior High School opened in Coquitlam, B.C. in 1971, and the Doctor Charles Best Public School opened in Burlington, Ontario in 1973.

Several attempts to organize displays in the Medical Sciences Building and in the Best Institute are only now becoming a reality. Ted Wood and Dr. David MacLennan from the Best Institute spent two hours talking to Margaret about the disposition of many medals and scrolls. President Ham wrote to her about the documents going to the Thomas Fisher Rare Book Library. Since that time, Mladen Vranic, John Challis, and John MacDonald, successively chairs of the department of physiology, Dean David Naylor of the faculty of medicine, and Dr. John Friesen, the director of the Banting and Best Department of Medical Research, have all taken an interest and some items that are included in the list of documents to be deposited in the Fisher Library are already on semi-permanent loan to the appropriate departments. In late 2001, the department of physiology refurbished several secure display cabinets to hold manuscripts and medals.

Henry had been concerned that if Linda retired and was home all the time, she and her older sister might well get on each other's nerves. Fortunately, there were still many useful things for her to do at the lab on a part-time basis. On 29 June 1981, Margaret wrote in her diary, "Linda is taking a holiday now for July and August. It is very pleasant to have her at home. I am sometimes a little lost and lonely here by myself. But I manage very well and I love this old house."

On 17 August, Henry and his mother went to another meeting about the archives. Margaret now seemed happy to think of their papers deposited at the University of Toronto. Ten days later, Richard Landon and Katharine

Martyn of the Thomas Fisher Library came to the house to look at some papers and the first series of the scrapbooks. Margaret had set aside items that she did not think should go to the university. Volume 75, the last of Margaret Mahon Best's diaries, was started in October 1981 and contained sporadic entries up to 1985. Charley had written his name on the first page, intending to use the book himself. She also noted, "I almost gave up writing diary notes but here I am again."

Margaret would have liked to attend a dinner in the Great Hall of Hart House on 30 October 1981 to mark the sixtieth anniversary of insulin, but did not feel up to "being with so many people, old friends some of them." Henry and Mairi, however, came from Sudbury and joined Linda, Eileen, Charley, Alexander, and Melinda at the dinner; Peter Moloney called Margaret to give details of the evening and described Henry's speech. Margaret's eighty-first birthday was quiet, but many people remembered her with flowers, books, and cards. The same was true at Christmas. "Everyone is good to us."

Linda's health was not good either, and she talked of taking final retirement from the university. She was working with Katharine Martyn of the Fisher Library on papers at the institute. Some went directly to the library, others were taken home. She wanted Margaret to decide what to do with them. Margaret recorded that Henry had had breakfast with Michael Bliss at the Park Plaza and that the latter's book on the discovery of insulin was progressing well.

Margaret loved her big house and certainly did not want to move. But occasionally, especially when she had a call from an old friend who was in Belmont House or another retirement home, Margaret would ask Henry if she should not move there. His answer was always, "Do you want to?" and she would always reply, "No." As well, early 1982 was unusually cold. The two furnaces gobbled up oil, and there always seemed to be trouble with a pipe or an appliance. Henry reassured her that she had enough money to keep the house going. As long as she was living there, she felt an obligation to her tenants, Dorothy Thompson and Mary Davies on the top floor and Heather Phillips in the small apartment.

On 29 April 1982, a party marked Linda Mahon's record fifty-four years on staff of the University of Toronto. President Ham, Dr. David MacLennan, and Dr. Jessie Ridout all spoke. With a touch of condescension, Margaret said that her younger sister "made a very short pleasant speech." Many old friends were there, including Jim Campbell, Don Fraser, Reg Haist, and John

Logothetopoulos. Linda, an accomplished shopper, now took to going out regularly to shop or see friends. Margaret kept track of the travels of family and friends. "I can not travel any more. I do not feel up to it. But I have done a great deal of travelling in years gone by. I have counted for fun: twenty-six trips across the Atlantic which means I have crossed it fifty-two times. Some of these trips by sea, some by plane — all the early ones by ship, of course. (The first time I ever flew was the flying boat trip from Southampton to South Africa.) Enough reminiscing!"

Linda became ill in the winter of 1983 and was in bed with pneumonia for over a month. A VON nurse attended for a week and Margaret was up and down the stairs with meals. Soon after this Linda decided to sleep downstairs. Various members of the family did what they could, but the sisters had no regular help and would not have any except for the weekly visit of Maria Diogenes.

Old friends from near and far came to visit Margaret and Linda. Laurie and Helen Chute had been in Edmonton for an exhibition of paintings by Helen's mother, Laura Evans Reid, and brought them a copy of the catalogue. Jack Dugan, former executive director of the ADA, and his wife stopped by. Barbara Joslin, former wife of Dr. Allen Joslin, was involved with an art gallery in Toronto, and she brought news of the Joslin family. Dan Lawrence called from London, England, for a chat. Omond Solandt arrived for tea, and Margaret enjoyed the talk of mutual friends and of the trip from London Bridge to Leningrad with both Omond and his older brother Don in 1935.

Margaret was delighted when young Charley received his MBA from York University. Henry was never sure how his brother's offspring and his own felt when he took part in an academic procession wearing his presidential robes of bright blue and gold and his Henry VIII hat, but he was proud to participate in the graduation of Sandy's eldest child.

In 1983 Eileen sold her house in Toronto and moved to Prince Edward Island to make the large house that Sandy had bought on the estuary of the Cardigan River the centre for their children and friends. Margaret was sad to see her leave; but she had happy memories of "Sandy's house." George and Phyllis Best had driven Charley and Margaret to P.E.I. in September 1977 when they had visited and been entertained by Sandy in that house surrounded by "beautiful big linden trees."

Henry and Janna were completing their seven years in the president's house at Laurentian University and were preparing for a year-long sabbatical, 1984–5. Margaret was not able to attend the fine occasions organized in their honour in Sudbury. Young Charley and Amy went up for the last convocation. Margaret was sorry not to see Alexander graduating from the University of Toronto in June, "but everyone else was there and described it to me. I am so proud he has his B.A." Henry and Janna and Freda Ramsay joined Eileen and her family and a large group of friends at a dinner at the Faculty Club to celebrate Alexander's graduation. Eileen was staying with Margaret and Linda at 105 Woodlawn. "We are very happy to have her here with us. She is back off to the Cardigan house this morning — I call it Sandy's House."

Once on sabbatical, Henry called every week from wherever he was lecturing — in Scotland, Ireland, Belgium, England, Italy, or Israel. Margaret was always interested to know where they were and what they were doing in places that she herself had visited. She gave no indication that things were not going well in Toronto.

When Henry and Janna arrived back in Toronto in September 1985, they were shocked. Margaret was mentally sharp, but physically in poor shape; Linda had fallen several times, her hair and dress caked with blood, and had deteriorated mentally. They would not ask for help and were living on ice cream and ginger ale which they ordered from Duguids. Henry and Janna had great trouble getting them to accept any help, but gradually they assembled a team of caregivers who came during the day. Maria, who for years had been coming to help one day a week, now agreed to be their housekeeper. She arrived every evening as the other carers left, attended to all household affairs, prepared their meals, and helped them get to bed. Her loving, cheerful, and practical way of dealing with the housekeeping was a source of great comfort to Margaret and Linda, and of enormous relief to Henry.

The ten years after his father and brother died were the best that Henry had ever experienced with his mother. She and Linda were always pleased to see him. They had long talks about all sorts of subjects. After 1985 Henry gradually took over matters concerning the house and finances, and Margaret and Linda were both very appreciative.

Dr. Ken Gorman, newly appointed head of the Scarborough Grace Hospital, was no longer available to look after their health. Henry asked Dr. Barbara Hazlett, from the Diabetic Clinic at the Toronto General Hospital, who had known Margaret and Linda since she was a child, to keep an eye on them. This she did very faithfully, and it was she who called Henry on 26 January 1988 to say that Margaret had passed away. She died as she had hoped she would in her own bed at home.

The house was sold, and Linda, who never fully realized that her sister was gone, moved to Sudbury, where she spent the rest of her life in Janna and Henry's home overlooking Lake Ramsey. She died on 1 December 1989.

Thus ends this account of the remarkable times of Margaret and Charley Best. Their story lives on in the Best Family Papers ... and there is so much more to tell. Few people in the world can count as many friends as Margaret and Charley had, and fewer can appreciate what it could have been like to live as they did — on the cutting edge of medicine for decades, travelling in that special circle that would help make the scientific world a smaller place, with fascinating encounters far and near — and love for each other every day.

Glossary of Abbreviations

CHB	Charles Herbert Best, usually referred to as Charley but occasionally Charlie	
MMB	Margaret Hooper Mahon Best	

Margaret's Family:

AW	Alexander Wylie Mahon	Father
	Flora Macleod Mahon	Mother
ELM	Emma Linda Mahon	Younger sister
	Henry MacLeod Mahon	Brother
	Bruce Morpeth Macleod	Uncle, maternal side

Charley's Family:

HHB	Herbert Huestis Best	Father
LFB	Luella "Lulu" Fisher Newcomb	Mother
	Anna (Annie) Best Jenkins	Aunt, father's sister
	Dr O. Fletcher Best	Uncle, father's brother
LBH	Lillian (Lillie) Best Hallam	Aunt, father's sister
	Hilda Best Salter	Sister
	Iomene Newcomb	Cousin

Margaret & Charley's Children:

CAB	Charles Alexander "Sandy" Best
HBMB	Henry Bruce Macleod Best

Principal Names:

AG	Colonel Albert Gooderham	
ASW	Arthur S. Wall	Lab Technician
EPJ	Elliott Proctor Joslin	Joslin Clinic, Boston
FDR	Franklin Delano Roosevelt	
FGB	Frederick Grant Banting	
GMS	George M. Strode	Rockefeller Foundation

HHD	Henry Hallett Dale	London, England
JBC	James Bertram Collip	
JGF	J.G. FitzGerald Laboratories	Founder, Connaught
JHR	Jessie Hamilton Ridout	
JJRM	John James Rickard Macleod	
WRF	William R. Feasby	Military & Medical Historian

Principal Institutions:

ADA	American Diabetes Association
AOA	Alpha Omega Alpha Honour Medical Fraternity
BBDMR	Banting and Best Department of Medical Research, University of Toronto
BDA	British Diabetic Association (Diabetes UK)
BDH	British Drug Houses
CBE	Companion of the Order of the British Empire
CBMH	Canadian Bulletin of Medical History
CC	Companion of the Order of Canada
CDA	Canadian Diabetes Association
CH	Companion of Honour
CMA	Canadian Medical Association
CMG	Commander of the Order of St. Michael and St. George
CNR	Canadian National Railway
CPR	Canadian Pacific Railway
DMRAC	Defence Medical Research Advisory Committee
DRB	Defence Research Board of Canada
DSO	Distinguished Service Order
Fisher Book Room	Thomas Fisher Rare Book Room of the University of Toronto Library
FRCP	Fellow of the Royal College of Physicians
FRCS	Fellow of the Royal College of Surgeons
FRS	Fellow of the Royal Society
FRSC	Fellow of the Royal Society of Canada
IBM	International Business Machines
IDF	International Diabetes Federation
IHD	International Health Board, later Division, of the Rockefeller Foundation
IUPS	International Union of Physiological Sciences
JAMA	Journal of the American Medical Association
MBE	Member of the Order of the British Empire

MGM	Metro Goldwyn Mayer Film Studios, Hollywood
MRC	Medical Research Council (of UK, of Canada)
NAC	National Archives of Canada
NAS	National Academy of Sciences (U.S.A.)
NIMR	National Institute for Medical Research, Hampstead, London, England
NRC	National Research Council of Canada
OBE	Office of the Order of the British Empire
RAC	Rockefeller Archive Centre
RCAF	Royal Canadian Air Force
RCI	Royal Canadian Institute
RCN	Royal Canadian Navy
RCNVR	Royal Canadian Naval Volunteer Reserve
TGH	Toronto General Hospital
UC	University College, University of Toronto
UCC	Upper Canada College
U of T	University of Toronto
YMCA	Young Men's Christian Association

Charles Herbert Best: C.V.

EARNED DEGREES
1921   B.A., University of Toronto
1922   M.A., University of Toronto
1925   M.B., University of Toronto
1928   D.Sc., University of London

UNIVERSITY OF TORONTO APPOINTMENTS
Department of Physiology
    1920-22   Fellow
    1929-65   Professor and Head of the Department
    1965-78   Director Emeritus and Professor
Banting and Best Department of Medical Research
    1923-41   Research Associate
    1941-67   Professor and Head of the Department
    1967-78   Director Emeritus
Department of Physiological Hygiene
    1926-28   Assistant Professor
    1928-41   Head of the Department
Connaught Laboratories
    1922-25   Director of the Insulin Division
    1925-31   Assistant Director
    1931-41   Associate Director
    1941-78   Honorary Consultant

HONORARY DEGREES
1941   D.Sc. University of Chicago
1945   Docteur, Honoris Causa, Université de Paris
1946   Sc.D. University of Cambridge
1947   Doctor of Medicine, Honoris Causa, University of Amsterdam

1947	Doctor of Medicine, Honoris Causa, University of Louvain
1947	Doctor of Medicine, Honoris Causa, University of Liege
1947	D.Sc. University of Oxford
1949	LL.D. Dalhousie University
1950	LL.D. Queen's University
1951	Honorary Degrees from: University of Chile
	University of Uruguay
	University of San Marcos (Peru)
1952	LL.D. University of Melbourne
1952	D.Sc. Laval University
1955	D.Sc. University of Maine
1958	Honorary Doctorate, Central University of Venezuela
1959	LL.D. University of Edinburgh
1959	D.Sc. Northwestern University
1963	Doctor of Medicine, Honoris Causa, Aristotelian University of Thessalonika
1966	Doctor of Medicine, Honoris Causa, Freie University of Berlin
1970	LL.D. Honoris Causa, University of Toronto
1971	D.Sc. Laurentian University
1971	Ph.D. Hebrew University of Jerusalem
1972	Doctor of Medicine, University of Ottawa
1976	Doctorate Honoris Causa, Zagreb

HONOURS

1943	Award of Merit, The Navy League of Canada
1943	Award of Merit, The Canadian Red Cross Society
1944	Commander of the Civil Division of the Order of the British Empire
1947	King Haakon VII Liberty Cross Norway
1947	Legion of Merit, U.S.A.
1948	Commander of the Order of the Crown, Belgium
1953	Coronation Medal
1956	H.M. Queen Elisabeth of the Belgians Gold Medal
1958	Civic Award of Merit, Toronto
1958	Freedom of the City of Caracas, Venezuela
1962	La Grande Medaille d'Argent, Paris
1963	Humanitarian Award of the Canadian B'nai B'rith
1964	Knight of the Military and Hospitaller Order of St. Lazarus of Jerusalem

1966   Berlin Bell of Freedom
1967   The Centennial Medal
1967   Companion of the Order of Canada (C.C.)
1971   Companion of Honour (C.H.), Presented by H.M. Queen
        Elizabeth II
1971   The first Science Biennial Award of the Sao Paulo Biennial
        Foundation, Brazil - (Primero Primio de Ciencia Bienal de Sao Paulo)

SCIENTIFIC AWARDS
University of Toronto
1923   The Reeve Prize (Awarded to Banting and Best for the Discovery
        of Insulin)
1925   The J.J. MacKenzie Fellowship (Awarded to student obtaining
        highest grade in Pathology)
1925   The Ellen Mickle Fellowship (Awarded by the Council of the
        Faculty of Medicine to graduate with highest marks in the
        Medical Course)
1939   The Charles Mickle Fellowship (Awarded by the Council of the
        Faculty of Medicine to a member of the medical profession
        anywhere in the world considered to have done the most during
        the preceding 10 years to advance medical science)
(Dr. Best was the first to win both the Ellen and the Charles Mickle
Fellowships.)

OTHER SCIENTIFIC MEDALS AND AWARDS
1936   The F.N.G. Starr Gold Medal of the Canadian Medical Association
        (For achievement by a member of the CMA who has added
        distinction to the profession by his attainment in Science, Art, or
        Literature thus contributing to the humanitarian and cultural life of
        Canada. Also awarded to F.G. Banting and J.B. Collip.)
1939   The Baly Medal (Awarded by the Royal College of Physicians,
        England, for distinguished service in Physiology)
1949   The Banting Medal of The American Diabetes Association
1950   The Flavelle Medal of the Royal Society of Canada (Awarded by
        the Society for original research of special and conspicuous merit
        in biological sciences)
1953   The John Phillips Memorial Medal of The American College of
        Physicians (For achievement in internal medicine)

1955   The J. Howard Reber Medal of The Philadelphia Metabolic Association (For contributions toward the solution of social and economic problems which face the diabetic)

1958   Medal of the Royal Netherlands Academy of Sciences and Letters. (On the occasion of the 150th anniversary of the founding of the Academy)

1959   The Dale Medal of the Society for Endocrinology (Dr. Best was the first recipient)

1962   The Banting and Best Commemorative Medal of the Czechoslovak Society of Physical Medicine. (Coined in honour of the Discoverers of Insulin — bearing their profiles — on the occasion of the 40th Anniversary of the use of insulin in the treatment of diabetes mellitus)

1965   Awarded The First Joslin Medal of the New England Diabetes Association

1977   Awarded the Friedenwald Medal of the American Gastroenterological Association

FELLOW OR MEMBER OF FOLLOWING SCIENTIFIC SOCIETIES
Canada

1923   Alpha Omega Alpha (Hon. Medical Fraternity)

1927   Academy of Medicine, Toronto (Elected Honorary Fellow in 1966)

1931   Fellow of The Royal Society of Canada

1931   Fellow of The Royal College of Physicians and Surgeons (Canada)

1934   President Canadian Physiological Society

1948   President Toronto Diabetes Association

1952   Canadian Diabetic Association (First Hon. President)

1958   Membre Correspondent, La Societe Medicale des Hopitaux Universitaires de Quebec

1959   Hon. Member The Canadian Medical Association

Great Britain

1934   British Diabetic Association (Vice-President since founding in 1934)

1938   Elected Fellow of The Royal Society of London (Croonian Lecturer 1955)

1942   Royal Society of Medicine (Hon. Member, Section of Therapeutics and Pharmacology)

1952   The Royal Society of Medicine (Hon. Member, Section of Medicine)

1953   Hon. Fellow, The Royal College of Physicians (Edinburgh)
1957   Oslerian Oration, The Osler Society of London
1961   Fellow of The Royal College of Physicians (London)
1972   Elected Hon. Fellow, The Royal Society of Edinburgh

United States
1940   American Diabetes Association. Hon. Member since founding in
        1940; President 1948–49
1945   Life Member Dr. William Beaumont Memorial Foundation
1948   Hon. Member The American Academy of Arts and Sciences
1949   Fellow of The American Association for Advancement of Science
1950   National Academy of Sciences (Foreign Associates)
1950   American Philosophical Society
1950   New York Academy of Sciences (Hon. Life Member)
1954   Association of American Physicians
1963   Trustee of The Nutrition Foundation
1964   Elected Hon. Member, Society of Air Force Internists and Allied
        Specialists, United States Air Force

Pan American
Advisory Vice President Pan American Medical Association

SOUTH AMERICA
Argentina:
1951   Corresponding Fellow of the Scientific Society of the Argentine
Chile:
1951   Hon. Member of the Medical Society of Santiago
Uruguay:
1951   Hon. Fellow of the Biological Society of Montevideo
Venezuela:
1958   First Life Member of the Venezuelan Soc. of Endocrinology &
        Metabolism

EUROPE
Italy
1924   La Societa Medica-Chirurgion, Bologna
Germany
1932   Royal German Academy of Biological Investigation

Hungary
1938   Royal Medical Society of Budapest
France
1945   Foreign Associate of the Academy of Medicine (Paris)
Belgium
1946   Academie Royal de Medicine de Belgique
Netherlands
1946   Royal Academy of Sciences, Amsterdam
Sweden
1947   Foreign Member of The Royal Swedish Academy of Science
Czechoslovakia
1949   Czech Endocrinological Society
Denmark
1956   Royal Danish Academy of Sciences and Letters

INTERNATIONAL
1949   Hon. President of The International Diabetes Federation since
        founding of the Society in 1949
1953   First President of the International Union of Physiological
        Sciences (IUPS)
1955   Pontifical Academy of Sciences. Dr. Best was the first Canadian
        elected to this academy, limited to sixty members.
1962   Member of The International Foundation of Cos (Greece)
1963   Appointed to The World Health Organization Expert Advisory
        Panel on the International Pharmacopoeia and Pharmaceutical
        Preparations

ADDITIONAL APPOINTMENTS AND HONOURS
(Academic and Scientific)
1941-43 Dr. Best was a Scientific Director of The International Health
         Division of The Rockefeller Foundation. In 1943 he was elected
         Chairman of the Board of Scientific Directors for that year.
1946-48 Reappointed a Scientific Director of The Rockefeller
         Foundation for a further three-year term
1944   Appointed Member of the Advisory Medical Board, The
         Ontario Cancer Treatment and Research Foundation
1946   Appointed Member of the Metabolic Disease Study Section,
         National Institutes of Health and of the U.S. Public Health Service

1946	Appointed Medical Advisor of The Navy League of Canada
1949	Member of the Scientific Advisory Panel of The CIBA Foundation
1947-53	Chairman, The Josiah Macy, Jr. Foundation Conference on Liver Injury
1950	Member of the Scientific Advisory Committee of The Nutrition Foundation
1953	President of the XIX International Physiological Congress (Montreal)
1955	Elected to Board of Scientific Directors of the Roscoe B. Jackson Memorial Laboratory (for Cancer Research), Bar Harbor, Maine
1956	Appointed to the Active Consulting Staff of The Hospital for Sick Children
1957	Unanimously elected First Honorary President of The American Physicians Art Association
1960	Appointed Member of The Advisory Committee on Medical Research of The Medical Research Council of Canada
1968	Appointed member of the First Scientific Advisory Committee of The Research Institute, Hospital for Sick Children, and acted as Chairman
1968	Festschrift for Charles Herbert Best. *Canadian Journal of Physiology and Pharmacology*, vol. 46, no. 3, May 1968. This issue, containing articles on current work by colleagues and students of Dr. Best, was dedicated to him on the occasion of his retirement and "in recognition of his outstanding contribution to Medical Science in Canada."
1970	The Annual Charles H. Best Lecture of The Toronto Diabetes Association was established.
1971	Gairdner Foundation of Canada Award
1971	The Charles H. Best Postdoctoral Fellowship was established in the Banting and Best Department of Medical Research.
1971	Hoechst Pharmaceuticals established The Charles H. Best Prize to give recognition to an investigator in the basic or clinical sciences for outstanding original work in the field of diabetes conducted in Canada.
1995	The Charles H. Best Memorial Lectureship of the Department of Physiology of the University of Toronto established by Dr. John K. and Mary-Evelyn Davidson of Atlanta, Georgia.

Acknowledgments

The important financial contribution of the Sellers Foundation at the beginning of this project cannot be overestimated. It was instigated by the late Jean Sellers, widow of Edward Sellers, longtime fellow naval officer and scientific colleague of Charles Best. Both close friends of Margaret and Charley, they encouraged me to undertake this biography.

Without the sustained support of the Freda Ramsay Memorial Fund this volume could not have been completed. Ron Chrysler, Gerry Labelle, Gabrielle Miller, my colleagues in the History Department, and especially Rose-May Démoré, all of Laurentian University, made it possible to administer the funds for this project.

The major documentary source for this volume has been the Best Family Papers. All unidentified quotes are, as indicated in each chapter, from the eighty-four volumes of diaries kept by Margaret Mahon Best. Unless otherwise specified, all other sources are from the Best Family Papers held by Margaret Mahon Best at the time of her death in 1988, now in the possession of the author, along with all documents added from various sources. Dr. Joan Salter Bain kindly transferred to the author the important collection of papers which her mother, Hilda Best Salter, had inherited in 1942 from Dr. Herbert Huestis Best.

There have been so many people who have contributed to this biography. Janna Ramsay Best, Mairi Best, and Bruce Best all provided expert and thoughtful advice in the editing process, pointing out passages that might have seemed crystal clear to me, but which would have been less understandable to many readers. Bruce was also of invaluable assistance in solving numerous computer problems.

I am most indebted and grateful to my sister-in-law, Eileen Jane Thompson Best for her co-operation and insight. Her daughter, Margaret Cairine Best, kindly allowed me to reproduce the portrait of her grandmother.

I should especially like to mention Professor Mladen Vranic, the last post-doctoral fellow that Charles Best had and later chairman of the Department of Physiology; Prof. David MacLennan, past chairman of the Banting and Best Department of Medical Research; Dr. Donald Fraser; and Dr. Wilfred Bigelow for their repeated advice and support.

Claire Lecoupe, MA, my research assistant for three years, became a partner in this work. Her job description expanded very greatly as her thorough knowledge of the material and her dedication to the project grew. Claire's duties also included responding to the constant need for attention of Penny and Lucinda, the four-legged members of the family.

John Parry took on the onerous task of reducing my manuscript to a workable length. Cheryl Rondeau expertly photographed all the illustrations in digital format and prepared them for publication. Dr. Leena Patel worked with me when she was a student at Laurentian University and returned at a crucial moment to help after she had finished he PhD in Edinburgh.

Denis Dénommé, Sylvie Lafortune, and Frank Stradiotto of the Laurentian University Library Reference Service have been both helpful and patient. Always Rick Hauta has cheerfully assisted me.

Katharine Martin, Edna Hajnal, Richard Landon, and, more recently, Anne Dondertman and Jennifer Toews, all of the Thomas Fisher Rare Book Library at the University of Toronto, repeatedly provided exceptional advice and assistance over several years. Harold Averill of the University of Toronto Archives has also been of great help. The Canadian Diabetes Association, through James O'Brien and Bonnie Delany, was very co-operative.

Michael Eamon and Martin Lanthier of the National Archives of Canada repeatedly answered my queries about items in the papers of the National Research Council, the Defence Research Board, and the Medical Research Council — all bodies with which Charles Best was closely associated, as well as the army records for the First World War, and the navy records for the Second World War.

In the United States, Anita Martin and Lisa Bayne of the Eli Lilly Company Archives in Indianapolis; John Graham IV and Barbara Akin of the American Diabetes Association in Alexandria, Virginia; and Monica Blank and Thomas Rosenbaum of the Rockefeller Archive Center, just north of Manhattan, have all been very helpful.

In London, Keith Moore and Elizabeth Graham of the Royal Society answered many queries during and after the time I spent there myself. Dr. Tilli Tansey of the Wellcome Trust Archives has repeatedly showed her great knowledge of the relationship between Charles Best and Sir Henry Dale.

In Belgium, the papers of the late Joseph P. Hoet, Professor of Medicine at the Université Catholique de Louvain, and his wife, Marguerite, the Bests' closest friends in Europe, were generously made available to me by members of their family, who have continued to be of great assistance. These include the late Dr. Joseph Hoet and his wife, Pep, Dr. Pierre Hoet and Elisabeth, Anne-Marie Hoet and her husband, Xavier van der Borght, Dr. Philippe Hoet and his wife, Roselyne, and Mlle Marie-Noël Hoet.

Others who provided special assistance include: the late Dr. Omond Solandt and his wife, Vaire, and the late Dr. Laurie Chute and his wife, Dr. Helen Chute; the late Professor J.K.W. Ferguson and the late Dr. Albert M. Fisher of the University of Toronto, with their extensive experience and familiarity with many aspects of the story, gave me invaluable assistance and encouragement during the early stages of my research and writing; Dr. Jack Davidson and his wife, Bebe; Dean David Naylor, Dean Cecil Yip, Dr. Jim Friesen, Dr. John MacDonald, Dr. John Challis, and Jamie Katsoulakos of the University of Toronto Faculty of Medicine have been very supportive; Dr. Donald Barnett of the Joslin Clinic in Boston has answered many queries and provided valuable information; and Gail Menzel of the Pembroke Historical Society repeatedly answered questions about Pembroke, Maine.

In addition to the above, many other people were generous in providing interviews: Dr. Douglas Bilbey; Dr. James and Mary Campbell; Prof. Donald W. Clarke; Prof. Geza and Dr. Caroline Hetenyi; Sir Harold Himsworth; Jean Harris Horne; Eleanor Hurst; J.G.L. Jackson; Dr. Margaret Jansen; Dr. Louis Jaques; Dr. Oriana Kalandt; Dr. Adam Lawrence; Dr. Bernard and Queenie Leibel; L'Hon. Robert et Mme Andrée Lesage; Dr. John and Ismene Logothetopoulos; Dean Robert Lucas; Dr. Hugh MacMillan; Dr. Barbara McKinnon Hazlett; Dr. Sailen Mookerjea; Dr. Nina Morley; Dr. David Pyke; Dr. Henny Rappaport; Norman Rappaport; Prof. Arthur Rubenstein; Prof. John W. Scott; Margaret Scott Henderson; Catherine MacLeod Scroggie; Dr. Hans Selyé; Dr. Nelles Silverthorne; Professors Otakar and Anka Sirek; Barbara Solandt Griffin; Prof. Donald Steiner; Katherine MacKay Stewart; Dr. Ronald Tasker; Lord and Lady Todd; Prof. and Mrs. Beecher Weld; Helen Weld; Prof. G.R. Williams; Prof. Michael J. Williams; Sir Gordon and Lady Wolstenholme; and Sir Frank and Lady Young.

The International Diabetes Federation Congress held in Washington in June of 1991 provided the occasion for a number of invaluable interviews and contacts, greatly facilitated by the President of the Congress, Professor Joseph J. Hoet of Belgium. Interviews took place with Professors Rolf Luft; Virgilio Foglia; George Cahill; Rachmiel Levine; Pierre J. Lefebvre; Elezear Shafrir; Drs. John Galloway, James Anderson, Ernst J. Pfeiffer, John A. Colwell, Harold Rifkin, Pedro Lisboa, Jak Jervell, Rosalyn Yalow, Fritz Gerritzen Jr., J.S. Bajaj, Leo Krall, Juan J. Anderson, Raul Houssay; and Messrs. John L. Dugan Jr., Robert S. Bolan, Wendell Mayes, Jody G. Belmonte, and Noel B. Zabala.

Others who deserve thanks are: Joan Burns Addison; Lord Adrian; Sir George Alberti; Mary-Anne Alton; Dr. Ronald T. Baird; Ann Janes Banen; Robert D. Banting; Prof. Henry Barcroft; Isabel Bassett; Dr. James C. Bates; Dr. Colin Bayliss; Alexander Best; Marion Beyea; Barbara Billings; Frances Blackwood; Dr. Barbara McCallum Blake; Prof. Michael Bliss; Margaret Matheson Botterell; Senora Maria Teresa Cantilo de Braun Menendez; Prof. Vernon and Nancy Brooks; A.J.D. and Elizabeth Browne; Dr. Alan Bruce-Robertson; Prof. Dieter Buse; Lord Butterfield of Steckford; Miss Linda Cann; Prof. J.M.S. Careless; Dr. Juanita Casselman; Roberto Cipriani; Allen W. Clowes; Mrs. G.H.A. Clowes, Jr.; Prof. Oscar Crofford; Dr. George E. Connell; Michael Cooper; Stefan Coulombe; Prof. John Scott Cowan; Prof. Werner Creutzfeldt; Roger Dawe; Erica Deichmann Gregg; D. Haentjens Dekker; Sir Richard Doll; Prof. Israel Dostrovsky; Prof. Jonathan Dostrovsky; Dr. Jacalyn Duffin; Duncan Edmunds; Dr. David Evered; Kim Fahner; Dr. Stefan S. Fajans; Dr. H.A.M. Farquharson; Dr. Gordon Faulkner; Dr. W.R. Feasby; Dr. John Firstbrook; James FitzGerald; Dr. John Fowler; Dr. Clifford Gastineau; Jaap J.M Gerritzen; Dr. Bernard S. Goldman; Dr. David Gordon; Philip Gordon; Dr. C. Ken Gorman; John Gould; Gordon S. Green; Dr. Roberto Grosso; Mrs. Reginald Haist; Prof. C.N. Hales; Dr. Michael Hall; Beverley Hallam; Dr. John D. Hamilton; Dr. Rosemary Hawkins; Elizabeth Heffern; Prof. and Mrs. Carl Hersey; Dr. David Hill; Jean Harris Horne; Dr. Constantin Ionescu-Tirgoviste; Prof. Hubert A. Lechevalier; Dr. Alison Li; Donna Little; Sara Finnegan Lyett; Dean Andrew MacFarlane; Alaistair MacKay; Hon. Senator Heath Macquarrie; Dr. D. Maingay; Grant Maltman; Mrs. Henry Marsh; Prof. D.C. Masters; Prof. Shelley McKellar; Patricia McMichael; Hugh McNaught; Dr. Robert Metz; Prof. Frank C. Monkhouse; Alan Nabarro; Sir John Nabarro; Prof. Gunnar Nicolaysen; Krogh Nobel Museum; Dr. and

Mrs. Edward J.G. Noble; Nancy Nolin-Ethier; Rudy and Patricia MacIntyre North; Mina Ogiwara; Dr. Nancy Sparling Oke; Dr. Daniel H. Osmond; Dr. Abigail O'Sullivan; Prof. Paul Perron; Pat Piotto; Rabbi Gunther Plaut; Dean Pierre Potvin; Joan Lovatt Evans Prince; Norma P. Reynolds; Dr. Peggy Russell; Dr. Christopher Rutty; Ms. E.C. Shute; Jack Simpson; Dr. John Speakman; Mrs. Randall Sprague; Dr. Bruce and Lena Stewart; Elizabeth Sunding; Martin Taylor; Dr. Abigail O'Sullivan Tierney; Laurie Anne Price Wall; Miss Patti Walsh; Susan Watt; Brooke Webber; His Honour W. Scott and Sonya Wright; Dr. James R. Wright, Jr.; Norma and Don Young; and Dr. Bernard Zinman.

To any whose names I have missed, my sincere apologies.

A superb medical team succeeded in dealing with my recurring bouts of illness that repeatedly interrupted my writing of the text: Dr. John Jones, Dr. Tim Zmijowskyj, Dr. Eric Robinson, Dr. Roger Sandre, Dr. Jean-Guy Gagnon, Michael de Angelis, Diane Mastranardi and the Victorian Order of Nurses.

I am particularly grateful to my publisher, Dundurn Press, to Tony Hawke for his patience and understanding, and especially to Kirk Howard, whose faith in this project helped me persevere.

Notes

1   CHB's c.v. of MMB, p. 6.
2   CHB, "A Physiologist's Summer in Europe," Speech to the Physiological Society, University of Toronto, Autumn, 1950, p. 1.
3   Public Archives of Nova Scotia, MG3, No. 141, Account Book of William Best, Halifax, 1752–1759, p.105.
4   Joan Salter Bain Papers, Binder L61. HHB file.
5   The Medical Record Visiting List or Physician's Diary for 1898, Joan Salter Bain Papers, Binder L62. There is no information about Dr. Byron.
6   General Benjamin Murray was a lawyer and a Civil War veteran.
7   The Medical Record Visiting List or Physician's Diary for 1899, Joan Salter Bain Papers, Binder L62.
8   Robert P. Tristram Coffin was the author of *Kennebec, Cradle of the Americas* and *Ballads of Square-Toed Americans.*
9   *Collected Poems of Robert P Tristram Coffin,* Macmillan, 1948, p. 389.
10 CHB-MMB Reminiscences, Binder R1, Chapter 5, p. 8.
11 CHB, Notes made at Coral Gables, Florida, 1973.
12 CHB-MMB Reminiscences, Binder R1, Chapter 5, p. 9–10.
13 CHB, Notes made at Coral Gables, Florida, 1973.
14 CHB, Notes made at Coral Gables, Florida, 1973.
15 CHB-MMB Reminiscences, Binder R1, Chapter 5, p. 11.
16 HBMB interview with Eleanor Mahar Hurst, Pembroke, Maine, 9 July 1993.
17 CHB, Notes made at Coral Gables, Florida, 1973.
18 Much of the information about Pembroke and West Pembroke (one mile away) comes from Carl and Frances Hersey, *Pembroke Sesquicentennial, 1832–1982,* Machias, Maine, 1982. The Herseys were close friends of the Bests. Gail Menzel, the secretary of the Pembroke Historical Society, and editor of its journal, *The Pemmaquon Call,* has been both patient and expert in answering my many queries.
19 CHB-MMB Reminiscences, Binder R1, Chapter 5, p. 10.
20 HBMB interview with Eleanor Mahar Hurst, Pembroke, Maine, 9 July 1993.
21 CHB, Notes made at Coral Gables, Florida, 1973.
22 First published 26 March 1870, in the Boston Commercial Bulletin.
23 CHB, "1915–1925," Second draft, 4 December 1967, Reminiscences, Chapter 6, Binder R1.

24   CHB, "1915–1925," Second draft, 4 December 1967, Reminiscences, Chapter 6, Binder R1.

25   CHB, "1915–1925," Second draft, 4 December 1967, Reminiscences, Chapter 6, Binder R1.

26   CHB, "Who I Am and Why I Came to College," ca. 1916, Joan Salter Bain Papers, Binder L63, p. 1.

27   OFB to EPJ, 26 February and 7 June 1917, Joslin Clinic Archives, Boston, Anna Best file

28   HHB to Lillian Hallam, 30 March 1918. Joan Salter Bain Papers, Binder L61.

29   CHB Dictation, 7 April 1955.

30   CHB, "1915–1925," Second draft, 4 December 1967, Reminiscences, Binder R1.

31   June to August 1918, Joan Salter Bain Papers, Binder L63.

32   *Eastport Sentinel,* 28 August 1918, Joan Salter Bain Papers, Binder L62.

33   September 1918, Joan Salter Bain Papers, Binder L63.

34   W.T. Hallam to HHB and LFB, 6 October 1918, Joan Salter Bain Papers, Binder L61.

35   October 1918, Joan Salter Bain Papers, Binder L63. The HMS *Donegal* was a 9,800-ton armoured cruiser. "Jake" is a slang term for "all right" or "satisfactory."

36   CHB, "1915–1925," Second draft, 4 December 1967, Reminiscences, Binder R1.

37   David P Silcox, *Painting Place: The Life and Work of David B Milne,* University of Toronto Press, 1996.

38   November 1918, Joan Salter Bain Papers, Binder L63.

39   CHB, "1915–1925," Second draft, 4 December 1967, Reminiscences, Chapter 6, Binder R1.

40   FCA Jeanneret, introducing CHB at a Friends of Israel Luncheon, 15 February 1961. University of Toronto, Thomas Fisher Rare Book Library, Book Room, Manuscript Group 241, Box 1.

41   December 1918, Joan Salter Bain Papers, Binder L63.

42   George Gould and RJE Scott, *The Practitioner's Dictionary,* Philadelphia: P Blakiston's Son, 1916.

43   January 1919, Joan Salter Bain Papers, Binder L63.

44   CHB Dictation, 14 April 1955.

45   CHB, "1915–1925," Second draft, 4 December 1967, Reminiscences, Chapter 6, Binder R1.

46   CHB, "1915–1925," Second draft, 4 December 1967, Reminiscences, Chapter 6, Binder R1.

47   CHB, "1915–1925," Second draft, 4 December 1967, Reminiscences, Chapter 6, Binder R1.

48   The unattributed quotes in this chapter are from Margaret Mahon's diaries: 1914 (A and B), 1918–1919, and 1919 (A and B).

49   *The Atlas of Prince Edward Island* (Charlottetown, 1880) gives a wealth of information about the island and its people, including the sixty- seven lots

into which the island had been divided in 1767 and the owners of each property in 1880. The spelling of names is not as important as many people believe, and various members of the family have signed Macleod, MacLeod, or McLeod.

50   Irena Murray, Edward and W.S. Maxwell, *Canadian Architectural Collection,* McGill University, 1986, p. 100, no. 133, House for Rev. Mr. Mahon, Country House (basement, two floors, five bedrooms).

51   E.M. Sanders, ed., *The Life and Letters of the Right Hon. Sir Charles Tupper Bart, KCMG.* Cassell & Co., 1916, Vol. 1, p. 154. Unpublished copy of article in the A.W. Mahon Family Papers.

52   Cairine Wilson became the first woman senator in Canada in 1930 as a result of the *Persons* case.

53   MMB, "1912–1924," Reminiscences, Binder R1, Section 7.

54   The original copy of the commission is in the Best Family Papers.

55   MMB Scrapbook, Series 2, Vol. 1, pp. 4 –5.

56   MMB Scrapbook, Series 2, Vol. 1, p. 5.

57   MMB, "1912–1924," Reminiscences, Binder R1, Section 7.

58   MMB, "1912–1924," Reminiscences, Binder R1, Section 7.

59   MMB, "1912–1924," Reminiscences, Binder R1, Section 7.

60   St. Andrew's Church, Toronto, Year Book, 1930, pp. 6–7.

61   Captain Adelaide Macdonald Sinclair was director of the women's Royal Canadian Naval Service during the Second World War; Lorena Wellwood was a teacher who also worked for CHB; Elizabeth Maclennan became a prominent Toronto lawyer; Frieda Fraser became a scientist; and Catherine MacLeod Scroggie was one of Margaret's closest friends.

62   Stop 81 was at Peter's Crossing, south of Keswick. I am indebted for information about the Yonge Street Radial Line to Raymond Corley, PEng, Scarborough, Ontario.

63   The Princess Theatre on King Street West was one of Toronto's major legitimate theatre houses in the early part of the last century. It was demolished in 1934. Bingham's was a popular restaurant operating the Palm Gardens and Tea Room at 146 Yonge Street.

64   Stop 96 was at Sedore, on the shore of Lake Simcoe between Roaches Point and Jackson's Point.

65   Ethel M. Dell, *Greatheart,* condensed by Barbara Cartland, Duckworth, 1978, p. 114.

66   Dr. Archibald Gowanlock Huntsman, MD, LLD, was professor of marine biology at the University of Toronto from 1905 to 1954. He was director of the Atlantic Biological Station in St Andrews, New Brunswick, which bears his name, from 1911 to 1934.

67   Michael Bliss, *The Discovery of Insulin,* Toronto: McClelland & Stewart, 1982.

68   Barbara E. Hazlett, "Historical Perspective: The Discovery of Insulin," in John K Davidson, *Clinical Diabetes Mellitus: A Problem-Oriented Approach,* 3rd ed, New York: Thieme, 2000, pp. 3–11.

69   Gerald A. Wrenshall, Geza Hetenyi, William R. Feasby, *The Story of Insulin: Forty Years of Success Against Diabetes,* Toronto: Max Reinhardt, 1962.

70   Bernard Leibel and Gerald A. Wrenshall, *Insulin,* Toronto: Canadian Diabetes Association, 1971.

71   Aleita H. Scott, *Great Scott: Ernest Lyman Scott's Work with Insulin in 1911,* Bogota, NJ: 1972. Also Dickinson Richards, MD, of Columbia University, "The Effect of Pancreas Extract in Depancreatized Dogs: Ernest L. Scott's Thesis of 1911," in *Perspectives in Biology and Medicine,* 1966 (Autumn), pp. 84–95, courtesy of Clifford F. Gastineau, MD, of the Mayo Clinic, Rochester, Minnesota.

72   Moses Barron, "Relations of the Islets of Langerhans to Diabetes with Reference to Cases of Pancreatic Lithiasis," in *Surgery, Gynecology, and Obstetrics,* 31, 5 (November 1920), pp. 437–438. Barron later published "The Discovery of Insulin," in *Minnesota Medicine,* 1966, Vol. 49 (April and June).Banting's copy of this article was on display for years in the now demolished Old Medical Building of U of T but has since disappeared.

73   FGB Notebook, original at the Academy of Medicine of Toronto. FGB's spelling has been retained.

74   FGB to AG, *Report on the Discovery of Insulin,* September 1922, p. 1, Binder D1, Section 3.

75   FGB to AG, *Report on the Discovery of Insulin,* September 1922, p. 2, Binder D1-Section 3.

76   See Victor C. Myers and Cameron V. Bailey, *Journal of Biological Chemistry,* Vol. 24, pp. 147–61, 1916; and S.R. Benedict, *Journal of Biological Chemistry,* 34, 203, 1918; reference taken from JJRM, *Carbohydrate Metabolism and Insulin,* London: Longmans, Green, 1926, pp. 201 and 203.

77   The following quotes are all from CHB's handwritten notes in unnumbered loose-leaf binders. The first few pages of these notes are missing. In the same notebook is a series of notes headed, "Endocrinology — Ductless Glands — Dr. Taylor — missed first lecture." Norman B. Taylor, MB, later a colleague of CHB's, was listed in the University of Toronto Calendar, 1920–1, as a demonstrator in physiology.

78   CHB was probably referring to Wilhelm Ebstein (1836–1912). See entry for "Ebstein's lesion" in Gould and Scott, *The Practitioner's Medical Dictionary,* 3rd Edition, Philadelphia: Blakinston's Son, 1916. Also, "Some More Landmarks in the History of Diabetes, 1881, W. Ebstein," in N.S. Papaspyros, *The History of Diabetes Mellitus,* p 78. However, JJRM refers to Epstein and Rosenthal in his text *Carbohydrate Metabolism and Insulin,* 1926, see p. 76.

79   Jacques Raphael Lépine, *Le Diabète sucré,* Paris: Felix Alcan, 1909. See JJRM, *Carbohydrate Metabolism and Insulin,* 1926.

80   JJRM, *Physiology and Biochemistry in Modern Medicine,* St Louis: Mosby, 1918, p. 682.

81 Information courtesy of Harold Averill of the University of Toronto Archives, A1989-0011/Roll F.

82 The four preceding quotations are from a letter from CHB to HHB, 3 June 1921, Binder L61, Joan Salter Bain Papers.

83 Nelles Silverthorne, interviewed by HBMB, 17 February 1991.

84 FGB, *The Story of Insulin*, copy of unpublished manuscript, London, 1940, p. 26.

85 CHB wrote a note to his parents on the back of a picture of him riding: "This is 'Fox Glove' from the Hunt Club. I rode her to get her tamed down a bit before the officer went out for drill. She is a steeple chaser."

86 FGB, *The Story of Insulin*, copy of unpublished manuscript, London, 1940, p. 28.

87 Colonel Gooderham, son of Sir Edward Gooderham of Gooderham and Worts Distillers, was a prominent business leader. He was an active member of the Board of Governors of the University of Toronto and chairman of the Insulin Committee of the board.

88 FGB to Colonel Gooderham, *Report on the Discovery of Insulin*, September 1922, p. 3, Binder D1-Section 3.

89 CHB to MMB, 8 July 1921, Binder L1, p. 27.

90 CHB to MMB, 9 July 1921, Binder L1, p. 28.

91 CHB to MMB, 10 July 1921, Binder L1, p. 29.

92 CHB to MMB, 13 July 1921, Binder L1, p. 31.

93 CHB to MMB, 17 July 1921, Binder L1, p. 34.

94 CHB to MMB, "Sunday," postmark is 8 August 1921, Binder L2, p. 2.

95 FGB to JJRM, 9 August 1921, typed copy of handwritten letter, Binder D1-Section 5.

96 FGB and CHB to JJRM, 9 August 1921, typed copy of CHB's handwritten letter, Binder D1-Section 5.

97 FGB to JJRM, 9 August 1921, typed copy of handwritten letter, Binder D1-Section 5.

98 FGB and CHB to JJRM, 9 August 1921, typed copy of CHB's handwritten letter, Binder D1-Section 5.

99 FGB to JJRM, 9 August 1921, typed copy of FGB's handwritten letter, Binder D1-Section 5. On the list, the number 10 was skipped and the last number listed is 16.

100 CHB to MMB, 10 August 1921, Binder L2, p. 3.

101 CHB to MMB, 11 August 1921, Binder L2, p. 4

102 CHB to MMB, 15 August 1921, Binder L2, p. 5.

103 CHB to HHB, 12 February 1922, Binder L61, Joan Salter Bain Papers.

104 MMB to CHB, 16 August 1921, Binder L7, p. 8.

105 The four preceding quotations are from a letter from JJRM to FGB, 23 August 1921, Binder D1-Section 5.

106 CHB to MMB, 6 September 1921, Binder L2, p. 10.

107 FGB, *The Story of Insulin*, copy of unpublished manuscript, London, England, 1940, pp. 32-3.

108 FGB to AG, *Report on the Discovery of Insulin*, September, 1922, p. 4, Binder D1-Section 3.

109 JJRM to EPJ, 21 November 1921, copy in Best Papers

110 Binder D2 contains the original manuscript, handwritten by MMB, CHB, and FGB. See also Binder D3 for related documents.

111 *The Journal of Laboratory and Clinical Medicine*, Vol. 7, No. 5 (February 1922), pp. 251-66. Binder CHB Articles, p 16A-B-C-D.

112 FGB and CHB, "The Internal Secretion of the Pancreas," *The Journal of Laboratory and Clinical Medicine*, Vol. 7, No. 5 (February 1922). Binder CHB Articles, p. 16E.

113 CHB, Introduction to "The Internal Secretion of the Pancreas," in *Selected Papers of Charles H. Best*, p. 42.

114 CHB to MMB, n.d., Binder L2, p. 12.

115 FGB, *The Story of Insulin*, copy of unpublished manuscript, London, January 1940, pp. 35-6. William Lipsett Robinson was consulting pathologist to the chief coroner and to the Toronto General Hospital.

116 FGB to AG, *Report on the Discovery of Insulin*, September 1922, Binder D1-Section 3.

117 FGB and CHB, *Pancreatic Extracts*, Journal of Laboratory & Clinical Medicine (May 1922).

118 Letter H.M. Tory to JBC, 29 August 1921, 68-9-144, H.M. Tory Papers, University of Alberta Archives, p. 2. Binder Collip Documents.

119 FGB to AG, *Report on the Discovery of Insulin*, September 1922, Binder D1-Section 3.

120 University of Toronto, Collip Papers, Scrapbook 1, 1892–1922.

121 FGB, *The Story of Insulin*, copy of unpublished manuscript, London, January 1940, pp. 46-7.

122 ELM to Bruce Morpeth Macleod, 22 December 1921, Mahon letters, Binder L25.

123 Margaret Mahon to Bruce Morpeth Macleod, 29 December 1921, Mahon letters, Binder L25

124 JJRM to AG, *History of the researches leading to the discovery of Insulin*, September 1922, p. 5. Binder D1-Section 5.

125 FGB, CHB, and JJRM, *American Journal of Physiology*, 59: 479P. See "A Canadian Trail of Medical Research," in CHB's *Selected Papers*, p. 8; "Frederick Grant Banting, 1891–1941," in CHB's *Selected Papers*, p. 299; and "Insulin," in CHB's *Selected Papers*, p. 325.

126 FGB to AG, *Report on the Discovery of Insulin*, September 1922, p. 6. Binder D1-Section 3.

127 EPJ, interview by WRF, in Boston, 22 November 1957.

128 FGB to AG, *Report on the Discovery of Insulin*, September 1922. Binder D1-Section 3.

129 CHB to AG, *A Report of the Discovery and the Development of the Knowledge of the Properties of Insulin*, September, 1922, p. 3. Binder D1-Section 4.

130 FGB and CHB, "Pancreatic Extracts," *Journal of Laboratory and Clinical Medicine,* Vol. 7 No. 8 (May 1922).

131 JJRM to AG, *History of the researches leading to the discovery of Insulin,* September 1922. Binder D1-Section 2.

132 CHB to AG, *A Report of the Discovery and the Development of the Knowledge of the Properties of Insulin,* September 1922, p. 4. Binder D1- Section 4.

133 JBC to H.M. Tory, 25 January 1922, 68-9-144, H.M. Tory Papers, University of Alberta Archives.

134 FGB to AG, *Report on the Discovery of Insulin,* September 1922, p. 7. Binder D1-Section 3.

135 FGB, *The Story of Insulin,* copy of unpublished manuscript, London, January 1940, p. 54.

136 JBC to H.M. Tory, 25 January 1922, 68-9-144, H.M. Tory Papers, University of Alberta Archives.

137 Alison I-Syin Li, *J.B. Collip and the Making of Medical Research in Canada,* doctoral thesis, University of Toronto, 1992, p. 51.

138 JJRM to AG, *History of the researches leading to the discovery of Insulin,* September 1922, p. 7. Binder D1-Section 2.

139 CHB to HHB, 12 February 1922, Binder L61, Joan Salter Bain Papers.

140 CHB to HHB, 12 February 1922, Binder L61, Joan Salter Bain Papers.

141 JJRM to J.J. Mackenzie, 19 July 1922, Binder Letters: Science Related, Vol. 1. John Joseph Mackenzie, professor of pathology and bacteriology at the University of Toronto, died in 1922. The senate of the university established the J.J. Mackenzie Fellowship in his memory. CHB won this award in 1925 for obtaining the highest grade in pathology.

142 JJRM, JGF, FGB, and CHB to Sir Robert Falconer, 25 May 1922, Binder Letters: Science Related, Vol. 1.

143 JJRM to J.J. Mackenzie, 19 July 1922, Binder Letters: Science Related, Vol. 1.

144 When Linda Mahon wanted to find a copy in 1975, in reply to a query from London asking for the date of publication and title, it was discovered that both the departmental and the university libraries had the thesis entered in their files, but listed as "missing."

145 JJRM to AG, *History of the researches leading to the discovery of Insulin,* September 1922, p. 11. Binder D1-Section 2.

146 CHB to AG, *A Report of the Discovery and the Development of the Knowledge of the Properties of Insulin,* September 1922, p. 3. Binder D1- Section 4.

147 FGB to AG, *Report of the Discovery of Insulin,* September 1922, p. 7. Binder D1-Section 3.

148 JJRM to AG, *History of the researches leading to the discovery of Insulin,* September 1922. Binder D1-Section 2.

149 FGB to AG, *Report on the Discovery of Insulin,* September 1922, p. 8.

150 CHB to AG, *Report of the Discovery and the Development of the Knowledge of the Properties of Insulin,* September 1922, p. 4.

151 Item 1 is a handwritten statement by JBC, undated, Collip Papers, Thomas Fisher Rare Book Library, University of Toronto. Item 2 is "The

Contribution Made by JB Collip to the Development of Insulin while He Was in Toronto 1921-22," undated, Collip Papers, Thomas Fisher Rare Book Library, University of Toronto. Original document is in the Regional History Department of the University of Western Ontario's Library, Manuscript Collection 396. The third description is the second page of an identified document in the Collip Papers, Thomas Fisher Rare Book Library, University of Toronto. Binder Collip Documents.

152 Board of Governors Report, p. 168, P78-0002 (05), University of Toronto Archives. Binder Collip Documents.

153 CHB and DA Scott, *The Preparation of Insulin Paper,1923* in CHB, *Selected Papers,* p. 122.

154 Alison I-Syin Li, *JB Collip and the Making of Medical Research in Canada,* doctoral thesis, University of Toronto, 1992, p. 51.

155 CHB and DA Scott, *The Preparation of Insulin Paper, 1923* in CHB *Selected Papers* p. 122.

156 JJRM, *Carbohydrate Metabolism and Insulin,* London: Longmans, Green, 1926, p. 73.

157 JJRM, *Carbohydrate Metabolism and Insulin,* p. 32.

158 Sir Robert Falconer to H.M. Tory, 26 January 1922, A67-0007/379, University of Toronto Archives. Binder Collip Documents.

159 H.M. Tory to Sir Robert Falconer, 30 January 1922, A67-0007/074 "Tory," University of Toronto Archives. Binder Collip Documents.

160 FGB, *The Story of Insulin,* copy of unpublished manuscript, London, January 1940, pp. 55-7.

161 CHB to HHB, 10 May 1922, Binder L61, Joan Salter Bain Papers.

162 Best first met Wall when they were working on the golf course in Georgetown in 1920. He later offered him a job and trained him for lab work. Wall named his son Charles Banting Wall.

163 FGB to A Gooderham, *Report on the Discovery of Insulin,* September 1922, p. 9. Binder D1-Section 3.

164 CHB to MMB, June 1, 1922, Binder L2, p. 13.

165 CHB to MMB, 31 December 1920, Binder L1, p. 24.

166 CHB, dictation, 10 May 1955.

167 CHB-MMB, Reminiscences, Chapter 7, p. 9.

168 ASW to CHB, 12 July 1922, p. 5, Binder Letters: Science Related, Vol. 1.

169 FGB to CHB, 12 July 1922, File Original FGB-CHB Documents. The "Pavilion" was the Private Patients' Pavilion of the Toronto General Hospital, now demolished.

170 ASW to CHB, 14 July 1922, Binder Letters: Science Related, Vol. 1.

171 ASW to CHB, 12 July 1922, p. 2, Binder Letters: Science Related, Vol. 1.

172 ASW to CHB, 17 July 1922, pp. 2-3, Binder Letters: Science Related, Vol. 1.

173 ASW to CHB, 12 July 1922, p. 3, Binder Letters: Science Related, Vol. 1.

174 ASW to CHB, 17 July 1922, pp. 3-4, Binder Letters: Science Related, Vol. 1.

175 The two preceding quotations are from G.H.A. Clowes to CHB, 26 July 1922, Binder Letters: Science Related, Vol. 1.

176   FGB to CHB, 21 July 1922, File Original FGB-CHB Documents.

177   Letter FGB to CHB, 27 July 1922, File Original FGB-CHB Documents.

178   Letter ASW to CHB, 30 July 1922, Binder Letters: Science Related Vol. 1.

179   Letter JJRM to J.J. Mackenzie, 19 July 1922, Binder Letters: Science Related, Vol. 1.

180   Quoted by Franklin B. Peck, Sr., "Greetings and Message," New York Diabetes Association, 40th Insulin Anniversary., 1961.

181   Letter CHB to MMB, 11 September 1922, Binder L2, p. 15.

182   Letter CHB to MMB, 19 September 1922, Binder L2,p 17.

183   Letter CHB to MMB, 21 September 1922, Binder L2, p. 18. The award was the Reeve Prize of the University of Toronto.

184   Sir William Osler, *The principles and practice of medicine, designed for the use of practitioners and students of medicine,* 8th ed. with the assistance of William Thomas McCrae, New York: Appleton, 1917. CHB may have used the 9th ed. of 1920.

185   Toronto Star 9 September 1922,

186   AG to FGB, 16 September 1922. Binder D1-Section 1.

187   FGB to AG, *Report on the Discovery of Insulin,* September 1922, p. 13. Binder D1-Section 3.

188   JJRM to AG, September 20 or 22, 1922, pp. 1-2. (Both letters appear identical.) Binder D1-Section 2.

189   JJRM to AG, *History of the Researches Leading to the Discovery of Insulin,* September 1922, p. 7. Binder D1-Section 2.

190   CHB to AG, *A Report of the Discovery and the Development of the Knowledge of the Properties of Insulin,* September 1922, p. 4. Binder D1-Section 4.

191   Barbara E. Hazlett, "Historical Perspective: The Discovery of Insulin," in John K. Davidson, *Clinical Diabetes Mellitus: A Problem-Oriented Approach,* 3rd ed, New York: Thieme, 2000, p. 9.

192   Barbara F. Hazlett to HBMB, 17 September 2001.

193   JJRM to JBC, 18 September 1922, Collip Papers, Item 1, Thomas Fisher Rare Book Library, University of Toronto. See also Collip Binder.

194   AG to FGB, 16 September 1922. Binder D1-Section 1.

195   HHD, "Harold Ward Dudley," *Obituary Notices of Fellows of the Royal Society,* 1932–1935, Vol. 1, pp. 595-606, see p. 598.

196   Letter CHB to MMB, 3 October 1922, Binder L2, p. 19.

197   Copy of notice in August Krogh file.

198   *Toronto Daily Star,* Wednesday, 1 November 1922, MMB Scrapbook, Series 1, Vol. 1, p. 5.

199   MMB Scrapbook, Series 1, Vol. 1, p. 10.

200   MMB Scrapbook, Series 1, Vol. 1, p. 9.

201   MMB Scrapbook, Series 1, Vol. 1, p. 10.

202   Dr. Donald Fraser, Jr., to HBMB, 26 February 2002.

203   Dr. Edward H. Mason (McGill, 1914).

204   CHB to MMB, 24 December 1922, Binder L2, p. 20. Dr. Israel M.

Rabinowitch, who signed his letters "Rab," had a very large and successful diabetic clinic.

205 *Mail & Empire,* Friday, 29 December 1922, Scrapbook Series 1, Vol. 1, p. 9.

206 Robert Bárány to JJRM, 3 January 1923. File Bárány.

207 CHB to MMB, postmark is 2 January 1923, Binder L2, p. 21.

208 JJRM and FGB, *The Beaumont Foundation Lectures,* 29-30 January 1923, St Louis: Mosby, 1923.

209 Toronto *Daily Star,* Wednesday, 14 February 1923, MMB Scrapbook, Series 1, Vol. 1, pp. 24 and 31.

210 House of Commons Debates, 27 February 1923, pp. 703-4. File T.L. Church.

211 Letter LBH to FGB, 6 March 1923, Binder Letters: Science Related, Vol. 1.

212 Letter FGB to LBH, 13 March 1923, Binder Letters: Science Related, Vol. 1.

213 Letter JJRM to JBC, 10 March 1923, Binder Letters: Science Related, Vol. 1.

214 Academy of Medicine, Toronto, Resolution by Council, passed 23 March, 1923. Moved by Dr. Harry Bertram Anderson, a well-known pathologist and consulting physician who was president of the Academy in 1915, and seconded by Dr. J. Harris McPhedran, of a well-known Toronto medical family who were parishioners of Rev A.W. Mahon. He would become president of the Academy for 1931–2.

215 Letter Sir William Mulock to Mackenzie King, 27 March 1923. Mulock/King correspondence in the National Archives of Canada, William Lyon Mackenzie King, MC26, J1, Vol. 91, pp. 77025-77047 (courtesy Michael Eamon).

216 Letter Sir William Mulock to Mackenzie King, 27 March 1923, Mulock/King correspondence, National Archives of Canada, William Lyon Mackenzie King, MC26, J1, Vol. 91, pp. 77025-77047.

217 HHB, handwritten statement, 22 February 1924. Binder L61, Joan Salter Bain Papers.

218 It was a copy of the account of the discovery of insulin prepared by Banting for Gooderham in September 1922. Mulock/King correspondence, the National Archives of Canada, William Lyon Mackenzie King, MC26, J1, Vol. 91, pp. 77025-77047.

219 Mulock/King correspondence in the National Archives of Canada, William Lyon Mackenzie King, MC26, J1,Vol. 91, pp. 77025-77047.

220 File FGB Annuity.

221 House of Commons Debates, 27 June 1923, p. 4439. TL Church file

222 JGF to Prime Minister W.L. Mackenzie King, 27 June 1923. File FGB Annuity.

223 Prime Minister W.L. Mackenzie King to JGF, 5 July 1923. File FGB Annuity

224 FGB to CHB, 29 June 1923. File Original FGB-CHB Documents.

225 CHB to FGB, 28 June 1923. File FGB Annuity.

226 FGB to CHB, 15 July 1923. File FGB Annuity; also File Original FGB-CHB Documents.

227 FGB to EC Drury, 4 April 1923. See EC Drury file.

228   Bill No. 200, 4th Session, 15th Legislature. See FGB Annuity.

229   CHB to FGB, 28 June 1923. File FGB Annuity.

230   CHB to MMB, 8 August 1923, Binder L2, p. 25.

231   CHB to MMB,10 August 1923, Binder L2, p. 27.

232   CHB to MMB, 29 August 1923, Binder L3, p. 3.

233   MMB to CHB, 26 October 1923, Binder L8, p. 1.

234   Actual wording of telegram: "At any meeting or dinner please read following stop I ascribe to Best equal share in discovery stop hurt that he is not so acknowledged by Nobel trustees stop will share with him Banting." Original in Box 62, Banting papers, Thomas Fisher Rare book Library, University of Toronto.

235   CHB to MMB, 28 October 1923, Binder L3, p. 13

236   MMB to CHB, 26 October 1923, Binder L8, p. 1.

237   Margaret Mahon to Bruce Morpeth Macleod, 25 November 1923, Mahon letters, Binder L25.

238   Letter JJRM to August Krogh, 27 October 1922. File Krogh.

239   JJRM to Dr. Leonard Hill, 22 November 1922, and JJRM to C D Christie, 24 November 1922 (copies in Best papers).

240   FGB, typed copy of memo, 24 November 1922, Binder Letters: Science Related, Vol. 1. A handwritten attendance list in Eli Lilly and Company archives is headed "Round Table Conference, Saturday, November 25, 1922, Library, Medical Building, University of Toronto" and contains one more name: H. Rawle Geyelin, a diabetic specialist who raised money in New York City to equip the insulin plant in Toronto.

241   Section 5, "Special Regulations Concerning the Distribution, etc. of Prizes from the Nobel-Foundation by the Caroline Medico-Chirurgical Institute Given 29 June 1920." Courtesy of the Western Reserve Historical Society. Binder Letters: Science Related, Vol. 1. Also, Code of Statutes of the Nobel Foundation and Special Regulations concerning the prize for physiology and medicine, translated from Swedish. Caroline Medico-Chirurgical Institute in Stockholm, 1921.

242   August Krogh to The Medical Nobel Committee, Copenhagen, 27 January 1923, Karolinska Institutet, Sweden, courtesy Ann-Margreth Jörnvall. Translation from Danish to English courtesy Mrs. Lene Stewart, Toronto. Thank you also to Dr. Bruce Stewart for translation assistance. Binder Letters: Science Related, Vol. 1.

243   George Washington Crile to The Medical Nobel Committee, No. 10, 3 November 1922, the Karolinska Institutet, Stockholm, Sweden. Copy of letter supplied by the Western Reserve Historical Society, 10825 East Blvd., Cleveland, Ohio is dated 1 November 1922. Binder Letters: Science Related, Vol. 1.

244   J.N. (should be G.N. — George Neil) Stewart to The Medical Nobel Committee, No. 55, dated USA 6 January 1922 [sic, year is 1923], typed copy from the Karolinska Institutet, Stockholm, Sweden. Binder Letters: Science Related, Vol. 1.

245   Francis G. Benedict to The Medical Nobel Committee, No. 56, 8 January 1923, typed copy from the Karolinska Institutet, Stockholm, Sweden. Binder Letters: Science Related, Vol. 1.

246   Gøran Liljestrand, *The Nobel Prize for Insulin*, Londby and Lundgrens, 1957, p. 6. Also the chapter entitled "The Prize in Physiology or Medicine," in *Nobel: The Man and His Prizes*, 1962, p. 225.

247   In 1991, the author conducted an interview in Washington DC with Professor Rolf Luft, then secretary for the Nobel Committee. Luft then sent a long letter to HBMB, 21 August 1991.

248   MMB to CHB, 26 October 1923, Binder L8, p. 1; CHB to MMB, 28 October 1923, Binder L3, p. 13.

249   JJRM to Professor L Darmstaedter, Preussische Staatsbioliothek, Berlin, Germany, sent on 24 November 1924 (copy in Best Papers).

250   JJRM, Nobel Lecture, 26 May 1925, Nobel Museum, Stockholm.

251   FGB, *Diabetes and Insulin: Nobel Lecture delivered at Stockholm on September 15th, 1925,* Stockholm: Isaac Marcus' Boktr-A-B, 1925, p. 4. Erratum note is pasted in the margin of reprints, published in Stockholm by Imprimerie Royale, P.A. Norstedt & Fils, 1925, file of FGB-CHB Original Documents.

252   JGF to CHB, 10 September 1925, MMB Scrapbook, Series 1, Vol. 8, p. 97.

253   Photo courtesy of the City of Toronto Archives, Reference SC 266, Item 1707. Thank you to Edna Hajnal and to the staff of the Thomas Fisher Rare Book Library of University of Toronto for their help identifying the people in the photograph; Banting Scrapbook 1:1:59.

254   *The University of Toronto Monthly*, Vol. 24, No. 3 (December 1923), p. 115.

255   Gerald A. Wrenshall, Geza Hetenyi, W.R. Feasby, *The Story of Insulin: Forty Years of Success against Diabetes*, Toronto: Max Reinhardt, 1962.

256   Geza Hetenyi, Jr., "{Why Can't We Get It Right? Notes on the Discovery of Insulin," *Annals of the Royal College of Physicians and Surgeons of Canada*, Vol. 31, No. 5 (August) 1998, pp. 237-239. Dr. Hetenyi also published an important article, "The Day After: How Insulin Was Received by the Medical Profession," in *Perspectives in Biology and Medicine*, Vol. 38, No. 3 (Spring) 1995, pp. 396-405. The two subsequent papers by M. Bliss that Hetenyi refers to are: "J.B. Collip, A Forgotten Member of the Insulin Team," in Mitchinson and Dickin McGinnis, eds, *Essays in Canadian History of Medicine,* Toronto: McClelland and Stewart, 1988; and, "Rewriting Medical History: Charles Best and the Banting and Best Myth," *Journal of the History of Medicine and Allied Sciences*, Vol. 28, 1993, pp. 253-74.

257   *Torontonensis: The Year Book of the Graduates of the University of Toronto*, Vol. 25 (1923).

258   Order of Service at the Marriage of Margaret Hooper Mahon to Charles Herbert Best in St Andrew's Church, Toronto, 3 September 1924. See File MMB-CHB Marriage.

259   MMB Scrapbook, Series 2, Vol. 1, p. 11.

260   MMB-CHB Reminiscences, Binder R1, Chapter 7, p. 10.

261 Gordon (Campbell) Cameron, MD, was an associate professor in the BBDMR from 1927 to 1931.

262 MMB-CHB Reminiscences, Chapter 7, p. 10.

263 MMB Scrapbook, Series 2, Vol. 1, pp. 10-16.

264 MMB-CHB Reminiscences, Chapter 7, p. 10.

265 Henry Mahon and his wife, Lydia Arnoldson, had recently returned from Dawson City, Yukon, where he had been director of education for two years. Photographs show them with their sled dogs.

266 Eventually the MB was changed to an MD. The caption under CHB's photograph in *Torontonensis* is a quotation from Wordsworth: "A Man he seems of cheerful yesterdays, And confident to-morrows." *Torontonensis*, Vol. 27 (1925).

267 Others who won the Ellen Mickle Fellowship included Jakob Markowitz in 1923, David W. Pratt in 1926, Henry Borsook in 1927, and O.M. Solandt in 1936. University of Toronto, Faculty of Medicine, Supplement to the Calendar, 1942-3, p. 31.

268 J.G. FitzGerald to President Falconer, 22 December 1924, Binder L29, letters CHB-FitzGerald 1923–1928.

269 FitzGerald was a member of IHB 1923–26 and of IHD 1931–34 and 1936–39.

270 Florence M. Read, IHB of the Rockefeller Foundation to J.G. FitzGerald, 19 January, 1925, Binder L29, letters CHB-FitzGerald, 1923–1928.

271 Floyd Lyle, IHB of the Rockefeller Foundation to CHB, 22 January 1925, Binder L29, letters CHB-FitzGerald, 1923–1928.

272 CHB to HHB, 8 July 1925, Joan Salter Bain papers.

273 CHB to HHB, 8 July 1925, Joan Salter Bain Papers.

274 The unattributed quotes in this chapter are from Margaret Best's diaries 1 to 4.

275 CHB to LFB, 10 July 1925, Joan Salter Bain Papers.

276 CHB to LFB, 19 July 1925, Joan Salter Bain Papers.

277 CHB to HHB, 3 August 1925, Joan Salter Bain Papers.

278 CHB to HHB, 22 July 1925, Joan Salter Bain Papers.

279 Dr. J.E. Barnard, FRS.

280 CHB to HHB, 27 July 1925, Joan Salter Bain Papers.

281 CHB to HHB, 31 July 1925, Joan Salter Bain Papers.

282 CHB Dictation, 27 December 1957.

283 CHB to HHB, 3 August 1925, Joan Salter Bain Papers.

284 CHB to HHB 14 August 1925, Joan Salter Bain Papers.

285 CHB to HHB, 22 July 1925, Joan Salter Bain Papers.

286 CHB to HHB, 3 August 1925, Joan Salter Bain Papers.

287 CHB to HHB, 23 August 1925, Joan Salter Bain Papers.

288 CHB Dictation, 30 June 1960, p. 2.

289 CHB to HHB, 29 August 1925, Joan Salter Bain Papers.

290 CHB to HHB, 4 September 1925, Joan Salter Bain Papers.

291 CHB to HHB, 29 August 1925, Joan Salter Bain Papers.

292 CHB to HHB, 5 August 1925, Joan Salter Bain Papers.
293 Nelson's *Loose Leaf Living Medicine*, prepared under the direction of an international advisory board, New York and London: WW Merrick, 1923–27.
294 CHB to HHB, 5 August 1925, Joan Salter Bain Papers.
295 CHB to LFB, 14 August 1925, Joan Salter Bain Papers.
296 CHB to HHB, 1 September 1925, Joan Salter Bain Papers.
297 CHB to HHB, 4 September 1925, Joan Salter Bain Papers.
298 DA Scott and CHB, "The Preparation of Insulin," *Industrial and Engineering Chemistry*, Vol. 17, No. 3 (1925) pp. 238-40.
299 CHB to HHB, 14 September 1925, Joan Salter Bain Papers.
300 CHB to HHB, 4 September 1925, Joan Salter Bain Papers.
301 MMB Theatre programmes, Binder T1, p. 16.
302 MMB Theatre programmes, Binder T1, p. 17.
303 CHB to LFB, 14 August 1925, Joan Salter Bain Papers.
304 MMB Theatre programmes, Binder T1, p. 22.
305 MMB Theatre programmes, Binder T1, p. 25.
306 FGB to CHB, 13 May 1926.
307 A.W. Mahon to CHB, 18 June 1926, Mahon Letters, Binder L25.
308 CHB Dictation, 22 June 1960.
309 Probably Emmerich
310 MMB Theatre programmes, Binder T1, p. 30.
311 MMB Theatre programmes, Binder T1, p. 28.
312 MMB Theatre programmes, Binder T1, p. 29.
313 HHD to JJRM, 25 June 1926, MMB Scrapbook Series 1, Vol. 13, p. 91. See also HHD file.
314 CHB to Clifford Wells, 26 January 1927, see Rockefeller 1925–27 file
315 CHB Dictation, 27 December 1957.
316 Dr. Nils Ringertz, Karolinska Insitutet, to HBMB, 21 August 1998.
317 Philemon E. Truesdale to CHB, 5 October 1927, Harvard University file.
318 EPJ to CHB, 7 January 1927, Harvard University file.
319 Copy of page 47 from FGB-CHB Notebook 1, Harvard University file. See also Binder D1.
320 Frances Mary Bowes-Lyon was a sister of the Duchess of York.
321 FJM Stratton, *Richard Arman Gregory, Obituary Notices of the Royal Society*, London.
322 In 1929 Percy Williams and Myrtle Cook were involved in doing tests for Best in Toronto.
323 CHB and Ruth C. Partridge, "Observations on Olympic Athletes," in *Selected Papers of Charles H. Best*, Toronto: University of Toronto Press, 1963, pp. 548-556.
324 Emma Linda Mahon to Bruce Morpeth MacLeod, 7 August 1928.
325 Sources of information on Canada's role in the Olympics include Henry Roxborough, *Canada at the Olympics*, Ryerson Press, 1963.
326 JGF to CHB, June-July 1928, Binder L29, pp. 38-40.

327 HHD to Andrew Hunter, 21 April 1928, see HHD-Correspondence file.

328 HHD to JJRM, 2 May 1928, see HHD-Correspondence file.

329 O. Klotz to Sir Robert Falconer, 5 May 1928, Binder N1.

330 G.S. Young was a consulting physician and chairman of the council of the Canadian Medical Association.

331 JGF to CHB, 6 June 1928, Binder L29, p. 38

332 JGF to CHB, 6 June 1928, Binder L29, p. 38.

333 CHB to JGF, 17 June 1928, Binder L29, p. 39A.

334 JJRM to Sir Robert Falconer, 19 June 1928, Binder N1.

335 CHB to JGF, 29 June 1928, Binder L29, p. 39B.

336 CHB to JGF, 29 June 1928, Binder L29.

337 CHB to JGF, 10 July 1928, Binder L29, p. 40.

338 Sir Frank Young, Charles Herbert Best 1899–1978 *Biographical Memoirs of Fellows of the Royal Society* Vol. 28, November 1982.

339 Omond Solandt interview 19 February 1991.

340 The unattributed quotes in this chapter are from Margaret Best's diaries 4 to 16, and from her children's series, books 1, 2, and 3.

341 A.L. Chute to W R Feasby, 19 July 1960; AL Chute interview with HBMB, 19 February 1991.

342 HBMB, conversation with Mrs. Scroggie, 1993.

343 Katherine Hale Garvin was a journalist and writer. Her best-known books include *This Is Ontario* and *Historic Houses of Canada.*

344 *A Record of the Proceedings at the Opening of the Banting Institute, University of Toronto,* 1930, University of Toronto Press, 1931, pp. 35 and 49.

345 JJRM to A.V. Hill, 3 November 1931 (A.V. Hill file).

346 HHD to CHB 18 January 1932, Sir Henry Dale Correspondence.

347 CHB to HHD, 15 December 1931.

348 Charles H. Best, "A Brief History of the Discover of the Lipotropic Factors" in Selected Papers, University of Toronto Press, 1963 pp. 367-374.

349 Sir Frank Young Charles Herbert Best 1899–1978, *Biographical Memoirs of Fellows of the Royal Society* Vol. 28 November 1982.

350 W. Stanley Hartroft, *Charles Herbert Best and Choline,* MSS. 1953.

351 Minutes of the meeting of 20 February 1933, University Court of the University of Edinburgh, p. 70. University of Edinburgh file 1933 offer.

352 CHB to Sir Norman Walker, 25 March 1933. University of Edinburgh file 1933 offer.

353 CHB to Sir Norman Walker, 5 May 1933. University of Edinburgh file1933 offer.

354 F.A. Mouré, Bursar and Secretary to the Board of Governors of the University of Toronto, to CHB, 17 May 1933. University of Edinburgh file 1933 offer.

355 MMB Theatre programmes, Binder T2, p. 25.

356 MMB Theatre programmes, Binder T2, p. 26.

357 MMB Scrapbook Series 2, Vol. 8, p. 24.

358 This reference and other information for this congress are taken from *History of the International Congresses of Physiological Sciences, 1889–1968,* Wallace O.

Fenn, editor, Sponsored by the International Union of Physiological Sciences and published by The American Physiological Society, p. 315.

359 In his book, Cannon coined the term "homeostasis" in 1926 to describe an organism's tendency to maintain physiological stability, Cambridge Dictionary of American Biography, 1995, p. 114.

360 K.J. Franklin, "A Short History of the International Congresses of Physiologists, 1889–1938," in *History of the International Congresses of Physiological Sciences, 1889–1968,* Wallace O. Fenn, editor, The American Physiological Society, 1968, p. 316.

361 HBMB interview with O.M. Solandt, 20 February 1991.

362 File Frederic Newton Gisborne Starr. Courtesy of Paula Wilson, Canadian Medical Association.

363 A five-gaited horse can walk, trot, pace, canter, and gallop on command.

364 Dr. Donald M. Barnett of the Joslin Clinic searched in the Countway Library of Medicine at Harvard in the Benedict papers but found nothing. I am indebted to Norma Reynolds of Machias, Maine, for information on Dr. and Mrs. Benedict, also about CHB's Woodworth relatives from Nova Scotia who moved to Maine.

365 CHB Dictation, 4 January 1957, pp. 4-5.

366 Anne Edwards, "Frederick March" in *Architectural Digest* April 1990, pp. 222-224.

367 Brendan Gill, "Western Star Tom Mix" in *Architectural Digest* April 1994, pp. 164-165.

368 Charles Foster to HBMB, email, 7 April 2002 ; see also Charles Foster, *Stardust and Shadows: Canadians in Early Hollywood,* Durndurn Press, 2000.

369 William Osler, *Science and Immortality*, Boston: Houghton, Mifflin and Company, 1905, p. 42.

370 CHB to MMB, 9-14 September 1937, Letters Vol. 3.

371 Information courtesy of Dr. Donald Barnett of the Joslin Clinic.

372 EPJ to CHB, 1 October 1937.

373 CHB to EPJ, 15 October 1937.

374 A member of Canada's Group of Seven landscape artists

375 A lot has been written about Banting as an artist. Edited by John Flood of Penumbra Press in Moonbeam, near Kapuskasing, Ontario, a 1979 issue of *Northward Journal* contains A.J. Casson's article, "The Doctor As an Artist" and five short articles by Banting: "Diary and Drawings of Eastern Arctic Expedition, 1927, with A.Y. Jackson"; "Diary and Drawings of Western Arctic Expedition, 1928, with A.Y. Jackson"; "Fifteen Drawings of Cobalt and Quebec"; "Excerpt from a Russian Diary, July 13, 1935"; and "Ten Drawings of Russia." Also reprinted is a CBC radio broadcast by A.Y. Jackson, "On Banting, February, 1943."

376 A.Y. Jackson, "On Banting: February, 1943," originally broadcast on CBC, Canadian Roundup, Monday, 22 February 1943, published in *Northward Journal*, John Flood, editor, Nos 14/15 (1979), p. 98.

377 The St. Botolph Club is a private dining club at Harvard University, founded

120 years ago. Members are drawn from the arts and literature but speakers may come from any field. Information courtesy of Dr. Donald Barnett of the Joslin Clinic.

378 Originally in *Lancet*, II, 1938, pp. 554-6; also in *Selected Papers of Charles H Best*, 1963, p. 661-9.

379 C.H. Best, *Selected Papers*, Toronto: University of Toronto Press, 1963, pp. 613-618.

380 D.W.G. Murray, L.B. Jaques, T.S. Perrett, C.H. Best, "Heparin and the Thrombosis of veins following injury," *Surgery*, Vol. 2 (1937) pp. 163-187.

381 W.G. Bigelow, *Mysterious Heparin: The Key to Open Heart Surgery*, Toronto: McGraw-Hill Ryerson, 1990, p. 185.

382 W.G. Bigelow, *Mysterious Heparin: The Key to Open Heart Surgery*, Toronto: McGraw-Hill Ryerson, 1990, pp. 7-22.

383 Bigelow, p. 26.

384 Bigelow, p. 50.

385 Bigelow, pp. 71-75.

386 Shelley McKellar, *The Career of Gordon Murray: Patterns of Change in Mid-Twentieth Century Medicine in Canada*, Toronto: University of Toronto Press, 1999, pp. 48-50.(Thesis later published as *Surgical Limits: The Life of Gordon Murray*, Toronto: U of T Press, 2002.)

387 Helen Chute to CHB, 6 August 1941, MMB Scrapbook Series 1, Vol. 6.

388 Al Chute and Helen Chute, interview by HBMB, 19 February 1991.

389 H.H. Dale, "Edward Mellanby," 1884–1955, FRS, Biographical Memoirs.

390 Alison Dale Todd to CHB, 25 April, 1938.

391 *Marching On — To What?* (Toronto, 1939), a booklet of five radio addresses by George McCullagh, p. 29, McCullagh Papers (Footnote 46 in Brian J. Young, "C. George McCullagh and the Leadership League" in *The Canadian Historical Review*, Vol. 17, No. 3, September, 1966, p. 214. In 1966, the McCullagh Papers were held by Mrs. George McCullagh.

392 HHD to CHB, 11 May 1939, Royal Society Archives.

393 Albert and Mariner Leighton were always referred to as "Mr. Albert" and "Mr. Mariner." Their wives, Keziah and Delia, were known as "Mrs. Albert" and "Mrs. Mariner."

394 C.H. Best, D.Y. Solandt and Jessie Ridout, "The Canadian Project for the Preparation of Dried Human Serum for Military Use," *Selected Paper of Charles H. Best*, University of Toronto Press, 1963, pp. 670-676.

395 Richard W. Kapp, "Charles H. Best, the Canadian Red Cross Society, and Canada's First National Blood Donation Program," CBMH, Vol. 12, 1995, pp. 33 & 35. Also, "Front Line Service in Canada: Blood Donation, Social Activism and national Identity on the Home Front, 1939–1945," 1996.

396 Lieutenant Colonel R.J.S. Langford, *Corporal to Field Officer*, 2nd edition amended up to date, Toronto: Copp Clark, 1939.

397 Ronald Christie, a Scot, was professor of medicine at St. Bartholomew's Hospital, also attached to the base hospital at St Albans. He later became head of the department of medicine at McGill University in Montréal.

398 Memo from CHB to AVH, 27 October 1939, "Problems of military significance in progress in the Departments of Physiology and Physiological Hygiene in the Section of Physiology and Biochemistry in the Connaught Laboratories, University of Toronto, Toronto, Canada." Binder RS Dale-Florey, Royal Society.

399 CHB to HHD, 16 November 1939, Binder RS Dale-Florey, Royal Society 93HD33.1.92.

400 HHD to CHB, 18 November 1939. (Original copy contains a P.S. about CHB receiving the Baly Medal for Physiology from the Royal College of Physicians, an award Dale received in 1921.) See also Binder RS Dale-Florey, Royal Society.

401 CHB to HHD, 23 December 1939, Binder RS Dale-Florey, Royal Society.

402 CHB to HHD, 14 February 1940, Binder RS Dale-Florey, Royal Society.

403 CHB to HHD, 19 February 1940, Binder RS Dale-Florey, Royal Society.

404 HHD to CHB, 8 March 1940, Binder RS Dale-Florey, Royal Society.

405 Jackson was a well-known English neurologist.

406 MMB's Theatre programmes, Binder T3, p. 15. *The Little Foxes*, by Lillian Hellman, was first performed in New York in 1939.

407 Surgeon Commodore Archie McCallum, *"Memo and Report" to all members of the Royal Canadian Navy*, 26 December 1951, p. 8, courtesy of Dr. Barbara McCallum Blake.

408 FGB War Diary, 19 May 1940, pp. 4-5. Banting Papers U of T Library.

409 FGB War Diary 19 May 1940 p. 77.

410 FGB War Diary 19 May 1940 p. 93.

411 FGB War Diary 19 May 1940, pp. 101-4.

412 MMB Theatre programmes, Binder T3, p. 16.

413 Lord Adrian, "Herbert Spencer Gasser 1888–1963," *Biographical Memories of Fellows of the Royal Society.*

414 Rockefeller Foundation, RF SD-IHD Minutes, 14 March 1941, p. 41024.

415 Wilbur A. Sawyer to Alan Gregg 10 July 1940, RF Health Commission, Personnel, Series 700 (D.P. O'Brien).

416 Wilbur A. Sawyer to Hugh H. Smith, 5 October 1940, RF Health Commission, Personnel ,Series 700 (HH Smith).

417 CHB to HHD, 6 January 1941, Binder RS Dale-Florey, Royal Society.

418 CHB to HHD, 17 January 1941, Binder RS Dale-Florey, Royal Society.

419 HHD to CHB, 14 February 1941, Binder RS Dale-Florey, Royal Society.

420 Rockefeller Foundation, RF SD-IHD Minutes, 14 March 1941, p. 41024.

421 Footnote 2 in Michael Bliss, "Rewriting Medical History: Charles Best and the Banting and Best Myth," *The Journal of the History of Medicine and Allied Sciences, Inc.*, 1993, pp. 253-74, p. 255: Interview with Dr. L.W. Billingsley, 30 November 1983, Notes in Bliss Insulin Papers, Thomas Fisher Rare Book Library, University of Toronto. Bliss typed transcript of Notes in Best Family Papers.

422 C.J. Mackenzie to A.G.L. McNaughton, 11 February 1941, in Mel Thistle,

ed., *The Mackenzie-McNaughton Wartime Letters*, Toronto: University of Toronto Press, 1975, p. 62.

423   CHB to HHD 17 January 1941, Letters H.H. Dale & Florey, Royal Society.

424   C.J. Mackenzie to A.G.L. McNaughton, 11 February 1941, in Mel Thistle, ed, *The Mackenzie-McNaughton Wartime Letters*, Toronto: University of Toronto Press, 1975, pp. 66-7.

425   John Bryden, *Deadly Allies: Canada's Secret War, 1937–1947*, Toronto: McClelland & Stewart, 1989, p. 36.

426   C.J. Mackenzie, 25 February 1941, Meeting of the War Technical and Scientific Development Committee, National Research Council, quoted in John Bryden, *Deadly Allies: Canada's Secret War, 1937–1947,* Toronto: McClelland & Stewart, 1989, p. 81.

427   Bryden, *Deadly Allies,* p. 44.

428   "Account of Research Activities of the RCN Medical Research Division and the Associate Committee on Naval Medical Research." NRC, in *The Journal of Canadian Medical Services,* Vol. 3, No. 4, May 1945, p. 311.

429   CHB, "A Canadian Trail of Medical Research," speech given at Washington University, St Louis, Missouri, 21 November 1957.

430   CHB, "The Division of Naval Medical Research, Royal Canadian Navy," *Selected Papers of Charles H Best,* 1963.

431   The unattributed quotes in this chapter are from Margaret Best's diaries Vols. 16–24.

432   MMB Scrapbook, Series 1, Vol. 3, p. 29.

433   Rockefeller Foundation, RF SD-IHD Diary of WAS, 15 March 1941.

434   Rockefeller Foundation, RF SD-IHD Minutes, 14 March 1941, p. 41024.

435   Rockefeller Foundation, RF SD-IHD Minutes, 12 September 1941, p. 41146.

436   MMB to CHB Letters 7 March 1941, Binder L09.

437   MMB to CHB Letters 9 May 1941, Binder L09.

438   University of Toronto Staff Report, Annuities/Salary file

439   Memoirs of CC Lucas, pp. 9-1 to 9-3, courtesy of Dean C Robert Lucas, Memorial University, St. John's, Newfoundland.

440   *Festschrift: Charles Herbert Best,* 1968, p. iv.

441   Memoirs of C.C. Lucas, courtesy of Dean C. Robert Lucas, Memorial University, St. John's, Newfoundland. CHB and Irving B. Fritz, *History of the Banting and Best Department of Medical Research,* manuscript copy. Published article: C.H. Best and C.C. Lucas, "Choline — Chemistry and significance as a dietary factor." *Vitamins and Hormones,* Vol. 1, 1943, pp. 1–58.

442   MMB to CHB, 10 June 1940, vol. L09.

443   CHB to MMB, 8 May 1941, Binder L4

444   On 26 August 1940, Best had received a commission as a lieutenant in the Royal Canadian Army Medical Corps, but he did not wear an army uniform. He was transferred to the navy active list on 15 October 1941. He was promoted to surgeon commander in 1942 and surgeon captain in 1943.

445   Gaëtan Gervais, *Les Jumelles Dionne et l'Ontario français (1934–1944)*, 2000, pp. 49, 60, 169.

446   Rockefeller Foundation, RF SD-IHD Minutes, 20 June 1941, p. 41069.

447   Rockefeller Foundation, RF SD-IHD Minutes, 12 September 1941, p. 41097.

448   MMB Theatre Programmes, Binder T3, p. 20.

449   GP Thomson, "Charles Galton Darwin," *Biographical Memoirs of Fellows of the Royal Society*, 1963.

450   James Campbell to CHB, 28 June 1962.

451   EL Scott published "On the Influence of Intravenous Injections of an Extract of the Pancreas on Experimental Pancreatic Diabetes," in 1912 in the *American Journal of Physiology* (29:306). His story is told in Aleita H. Scott's *Great Scott: Ernest Lyman Scott's Work with Insulin in 1911*, published in 1972.

452   Rockefeller Foundation, RF SD-IHD, Diary of WAS, 3 October 1941.

453   CHB and MMB, Letters and telegrams, Binder L4.

454   CHB to MMB, received 19 November 1941, Binder L4.

455   CHB to MMB, 2 November 1941, Binder L4.

456   MMB to CHB, 23 October 1941, L10.

457   Andrew Duffy, "Franks' Incredible Flying Suit," *The Ottawa Citizen Weekly*, 4 November 2001, pp. 1–5.

458   CHB, "First Trip to England During WWII," see "1941A," p. 1, Binder L26.

459   CHB, handwritten notes, see "1941B," p. 1, Binder L26.

460   CHB and DYS, "Report to the Sub-Committee on Naval Medical Research of the Associate Committee on Medical Research of the National Research Council of Canada," p. 1, ca. 1942, Binder L26.

461   Surgeon Lieutenant Commander Eddy Amos carried out examinations of sailors re night lighting.

462   CHB, "First Trip to England During WWII," see "1941A," pp. 2–3, Binder L26.

463   Surgeon Lieutenant Commander Best read *The Northern Garrisons, Iceland, and the North Atlantic Islands*, by Eric Linklater, an official publication of the British War Office, 1941. Linklater was a major, commanding the Orkney Fortress between 1939 and 1941, and with the Directorate of Public Relations, War Office, between 1941 and 1945.

464   CHB, "First Trip to England During WWII," "1941A," p. 5, Binder L26.

465   CHB, "First Trip to England During WWII," "1941A," p. 7–8, Binder L26. David J. Bercuson and Holger H. Herwig, *The Destruction of the Bismarck*, Toronto: Stoddart, 2001.

466   CHB, "First Trip to England During WWII," "1941A," p. 8, Binder L26.

467   Duff Hart-Harris, *Peter Fleming* (1907–1971) *A Biography*, Jonathan Cape, 1974, p. 224.

468   CHB, "Scattered Notes, 1941," p. 1–3, Binder L26.

469   HG Wells, 1866–1946, one of the best-known writers in the English language was not a severe diabetic. His scientific fantasies such as *The Time*

Machine and serious socio-political works such as *The Outline of History* were among the most widely read of his books. See Norman and Jeanne MacKenzie, *HG Wells: A Biography*, New York: Simon and Schuster, 1973.

470   CHB, "Scattered Notes, 1941," p. 4–5, Binder L26.

471   CHB, handwritten notes, "1941B," p. 3, Binder L26.

472   Wilbur A. Sawyer to CHB, 6 October 1941.

473   CHB, "Part 2 — Scattered Notes," 1941, Binder L26.

474   Rockefeller Foundation, Annual Report 1943.

475   MMB Scrapbook, Series 1, Vol. 3, p. 39

476   CHB and DYS, "Report to the Sub-Committee on Naval Medical Research of the Associate Committee on Medical Research of the National Research Council of Canada," p. 5, 1942, Binder L26.

477   CHB, "Part 2 — Scattered Notes, 1941," Binder L26.

478   CHB, "Part 2 — Notes, 1941," pp. 1–7, Binder L26.

479   CHB, handwritten notes, "1941B," p. 4, Binder L26.

480   MMB Scrapbook, Series 1, Vol. 3, p. 36.

481   Rockefeller Foundation, RF Annual Report 1941, p. 69.

482   Rockefeller Foundation, RF SD-IHD, Diary of WAS, 26 February 1942. Note: CHB was Surgeon Lieutenant-Commander of the Royal Canadian Naval Volunteer Reserve.

483   Rockefeller Foundation, RF SD-IHD, Minutes, 13 March 1942, p. 42042.

484   Rockefeller Foundation, IHD Newsletter, 1 April 1942, p. 18.

485   MMB's Theatre Programmes, Binder T3, p. 22.

486   MMB's Theatre Programmes, Binder T3, p. 23.

487   ELM, Binder ELM Poetry.

488   Dr. Barbara Blake to HBMB, 23 May 1996.

489   CHB to MMB, 8 September1942, Binder L4

490   MMB's Theatre Programmes, Binder T3, p 24.

491   Edgar McInnis, *Canada: A Political and Social History*, Holt, Rinehart and Winston, 1947.

492   Pemmican: "North American Indian food of lean meat dried, pounded, mixed into paste with melted fat and pressed into cakes; beef similarly treated and frequently flavoured with currants etc. for Arctic and other travellers." Oxford Illustrated Dictionary, London: Oxford University Press, 1963, p. 605.

493   Brigadier General Delmar H. Denton, file Henry Macleod Mahon.

494   CHB to MMB, 5 March 1943, Binder L4.

495   CHB to MMB, 16 March 1943, Binder L4.

496   George W Spinney, CMG, president, Bank of Montreal and chairman, National War Finance Committee.

497   "William Wilfred Campbell," *Encyclopedia Canadiana*, Vol. 2, pp. 176–177. Some of his published works include *Collected Poems*, 1905; as editor, *Oxford Book of Canada Verse*, 1911; with Rev. George Bryce, *Scotsmen in Canada*, 1911.

498   ELM, Cape Breton Diaries, 1943.

499   James Donald Gillis (1870–1965), *The Cape Breton Giant: A Truthful Memoir*, Halifax: TC Allen, 1919. Angus McAskill (1825–1863).

500   Robert Browning, Epilogue from *Asolando*: "One who never turned his back but marched breast-forward/Never doubted clouds would break/Never dreamed, though right was worsted/Wrong would triumph."

501   FDR to CHB, 16 September 1943.

502   CHB, "Description of Second Trip to England During World War II," 1943 p. 3, Binder L26

503   CHB, "Second Trip to England During World War II, Continued," 1943, pp. 1–3.

504   Rockefeller Foundation, SD-IHD, Minutes, 12 November 1943, p. 43102.

505   Rockefeller Foundation, SD-IHD, Minutes, 12 November 1943, pp. 43147 to 43152.

506   RG24, Vol. 8165, File NSS, 1700-100/25, HZ Sable, A/Surgeon Lt Commander, RCNVR, A/Director, CMID, 1 November 1945. File JL Little.

507   Howard Florey, with Ernst Chain, made penicillin, discovered by Alexander Fleming, available for human use. The three scientists received the Nobel Prize in 1945.

508   CHB, "Second Trip to England During World War II, Continued," 1943, pp. 4–5, Binder L26

509   J.L. "Lew" Little to CHB, 28 November 1943.

510   Aside from the sources already mentioned, information on CHB's wartime activities can be gleaned from G.H. Ettinger's report for the National Research Council, entitled "History of the Associate Committee on Medical Research," written in 1946, and *Scientists at War*, by Wilfrid Eggleston, a press censor during the war who became head of the journalism programme at Carleton College in Ottawa. The *Official History of the Canadian Medical Services, 1939–1945, Volume Two, Clinical Subjects*, edited by Lieutenant Colonel W.R. Feasby, provides a lot of information, but often neglects, probably on purpose, to mention who was involved in what. Surgeon Captain C.H. Best is mentioned as one of eight advisers, along with six brigadiers and Surgeon Commodore Archie McCallum. The May 1946 issue of the *Journal of the Canadian Medical Services*, entitled "Account of Research Activities of the RCN Medical Research Division and the Associate Committee on Naval Medical Research — NRC," gives a great deal of information on the many problems facing naval personnel.

511   C.J. Mackenzie, Navy Medical Research Diary, Reference: 4-1943-10-7, CJ1, 1-15, 10 December. Courtesy of Bill Rawling, Directorate of History, Dept. of National Defence, Ottawa.

512   W.R. Feasby, *Official History of the Canadian Medical Services, Volume 2: Clinical Subjects*, Ottawa: Queen's Printer, 1953, pp. 347–9.

513   W.R. Feasby, *Official History of the Canadian Medical Services, Volume 2: Clinical Subjects*, Ottawa: Queen's Printer, 1953, p. 333. CHB, draft

report, "Medical Research in the Royal Canadian Navy," probably for Commodore McCallum.

514 W.R. Feasby, *Official History of the Canadian Medical Services, Volume 2: Clinical Subjects*, Ottawa: Queen's Printer, 1953, p. 343.

515 DRB, Briefings (Secret) 9th meeting of the DMRAC, 20 February 1959

516 MMB Scrapbook, Series 1, Vol. 4, pp. 33–36: numerous newspaper articles, photographs, and copy of speech by HJ Cody, launch took place 20 December 1943.

517 Rockefeller Foundation, IIID Newsletter, 1 January 1944, p. 14.

518 J.W. Pickerskill, editor, *The Mackenzie King Record, Volume 1, 1939–1944*, University of Toronto Press, 1959.

519 MMB to CHB, 3 February 1944, Binder L11.

520 Emily Carr to CHB, 13 July 1944.

521 In June 2002 the painting was nowhere to be found and its whereabouts are unknown.

522 A.N. Drury to CHB, 20 September 1944, MMB Scrapbook, Series 1, Vol. 4, p. 69.

523 C.H. Best, D.Y. Solandt and Jessie Ridout, "The Canadian Project for the Preparation of Dried Human Serum for Military Use," *Selected Papers of Charles H. Best*, University of Toronto Press, 1963, pp. 670–676.

524 Newspaper clippings: "Nobel Prizes Given in U.S. First New World Ceremony," *Toronto Telegram*, 11 December 1944, MMB Scrapbook, Series 1, Vol. 4, p. 67.

525 HBMB, Interview with Dr. Virgilio Foglia of Argentina, who was a graduate student at McGill University in the 1930s, IDF Congress, Washington, 1991.

526 CHB, Banting Memorial Lecture "Insulin and Diabetes — in Retrospect and in Prospect," *The Canadian Medical Association Journal*, Vol. 53, pp. 204–12 (1945).

527 Martin G. Goldner, "The First Vial of Insulin in the Hands of Prof. Oscar Minkowski," 1959.

528 CHB, Banting Memorial Lecture, "Insulin and Diabetes — in Retrospect and in Prospect," The Canadian Medical Association Journal, Vol. 53, pp. 204–12 (1945).

529 Raymond B Fosdick to CHB, 15 January 1946.

530 Rockefeller Foundation, RF SD-IHD, Inter-Office Correspondence, "Functions of the Board of Scientific Directors of the IHD," 4 January 1946.

531 MMB Scrapbook, Series 1, Vol. 4, p. 91: Premier George A Drew to Col WE Phillips, 10 April 1946, notation "copy for Dr. Best."

532 See Markowitz Papers, Thomas Fisher Rare Book Library, University of Toronto.

533 CHB to MMB, 19 June 1946, Binder L6.

534 Her late husband King George V was a diabetic.

535 CHB to MMB, 21 June 1946, Binder L6.

536 CHB's first two honorary degrees were from University of Chicago (1941) and the Sorbonne (1945).

537 CHB to MMB, 23 June 1946, Binder L6.

538 CHB to MMB, 27 June 1946, Binder L6.

539 Archives of Churchill College, Cambridge, The Royal Society Empire Scientific Conference Report, 1946, Vol. J, pp. 19–23.

540 The Bests' trip to South Africa in 1949 was funded by this foundation.

541 CHB to MMB, 3 July 1946, Binder L6.

542 CHB to MMB, 4 July 1946, Binder L6.

543 CHB to JM Manson, National Research Council, 11 April 1946, Royal Society Empire Scientific Conference, University of Toronto Library.

544 Archives of Churchill College, Cambridge, The Royal Society Empire Scientific Conference Report, 1946, Vol. J, p. 49.

545 CHB to MMB, 6 July 1946, Binder L6.

546 CHB to MMB, 5 July 1946, Binder L6.

547 CHB to MMB, 6 July 1946, Binder Letters L6, p. 40. See also e-mail from Dr. Philippe Hoet to HBMB, 1 February 2000, regarding the situation of diabetics, including himself, in Belgium during the Second World War.

548 CHB to MMB, 8 July 1946, Binder L6.

549 CHB to MMB, 8 July 1946, Binder L6.

550 SES, "Addresses of Welcome," Proceedings of the American Diabetes Association, Vol. 6 (1946), p. 47.

551 All unidentified quotes in this chapter are from MMB diaries 26–41.

552 Seale Harries, *Banting's Miracle*, Toronto: JM Dent, 1946.

553 Dr. Eugene Opie at the beginning of the twentieth century had predicted the crucial importance of the islands of Langerhans in diabetes.

554 Proceedings of the American Diabetes Association, Vol. 6 (1946) p. 87.

555 CHB to Charles Burns, 25 April 1947.

556 CHB, "Diabetes and Insulin," and "The Lipotropic Factors," Beaumont Lecture, Wayne County Medical Society, Springfield, Illinois: Charles C. Thomas, 1948.

557 Captain D.J. Goodspeed, *A History of the Defence Research Board of Canada*, Ottawa: Queen's Printer, 1958, p. 41.

558 CHB to Lt-Gen Charles Foulkes, 6 December 1945, p. 1, OMS file.

559 OMS to CHB, 21 December 1945. OMS file Best papers.

560 Also, Dr. Paul E. Gagnon, head of chemistry at Laval; Col. Robert Dickson Harkness, vice-president of Northern Electric in Montréal; Dr. John Hamilton Lane Johnstone, head of physics at Dalhousie; Dr. Otto Maass, chairman of chemistry at McGill; Dean C.J. Mackenzie; Wilfrid Gordon Mills, deputy minister of national defence; Dr. Donald Charles Rose, scientific adviser to the chief of the general staff at National Defence; and Dr. Gordon Merritt Shrum, head of physics at the University of British Colombia.

561 Goodspeed, p. 100.

562 Goodspeed, p. 227.

563 Goodspeed, p. 228.

564 HBMB, Speech to the Academy of Medicine of Toronto, 24 April 1996.

565 Omond Solandt to CHB, 4 April 1949. MMB Scrapbook Series 1, Vol. 5, p. 114.

566 Rockefeller Foundation, RF SD-IHD, George K. Strode Diary, 18 April 1947, p. 73.

567 "Citation for the Legion of Merit, Degree of Officer: Surgeon Captain Charles H. Best," June 1947. PAC Records (DRB).

568 John A. Logan to CHB, February 12, 1948.

569 "Progress in Malaria Research," Annual Report, 1949, International Health Division, Rockefeller Foundation, New York, p. 1. Courtesy of the Rockefeller Archive Center.

570 Amir Attaran, Director of the Malaria Project in Washington, "Malaria experts oppose 2007 DDT ban," *Globe and Mail,* 2 September 1999, p. A21.

571 CHB to MMB, 5 July 1946, Binder L6.

572 Professor Vaughan was medical officer in charge, North West London Blood Supply Depot for the Medical Research Council during the war.

573 Lord Stamp was a pathologist who during the war was attached to the Ministry of Supply.

574 Rockefeller Foundation, RF SD-IHD, George K. Strode Diary, 22 September 1947, p. 157.

575 Transcript of recording of speeches at IBM luncheon, 1948.

576 CHB and Irving Fritz, "History of the Banting and Best Department of Medical Research," ca 1968, pp. 32-4.

577 Transcript of taped letter to HBMB by Dr. Ronald R. Tasker, undated.

578 Rockefeller Foundation, RF SD-IHD, Minutes, 25 October 1948, p. 48150.

579 MMB's Theatre Programmes, Binder T3, p. 39.

580 Rebecca Sisler, *The Girls: A Biography of Frances Loring and Florence Wyle,* Toronto: Clarke, Irwin.

581 Dr. Nils Ringertz, Karolinska Institutet, to HBMB, 21 August 1998.

582 CHB to HHD, 23 March 1949, p. 2, Binder Nobel Re-Visited.

583 Gøran Liljestrand to HHD, 9 December 1948, Binder Nobel Re-Visited.

584 HHD to CHB, 16 April 1949, Binder Nobel Re-Visited.

585 BAH to CHB, 29 December 1949, Binder Nobel Re-Visited.

586 Reference to No. 41, To the Nobel Committee for Physiology and Medicine, Royal Caroline Institute Stockholm, 5 January 1950, signed BAH, 28 December 1949.

587 Reference No. 41, To the Nobel Committee for Physiology and Medicine, Royal Caroline Institute, Stockholm, 5 January 1950, signed BAH, 28 December 1949.

588 HHD to CHB, 9 January 1950, Binder Nobel Re-Visited.

589 Reference No. 48, to the Members of the Nobel Prize Committee of the Caroline Institute, Stockholm, 14 January 1950, signed Henry H. Dale, 9 January 1950.

590 Reference No. 48, to the Members of the Nobel Prize Committee of the Caroline Institute, Stockholm, 14 January 1950, signed Henry H. Dale, 9 January 1950.

591   Reference No. 48, To the Members of the Nobel Prize Committee of the Caroline Institute, Stockholm, 14 January 1950, signed Henry H. Dale, 9 January 1950.

592   Reference No. 94, To the Nobel Committee for Physiology and Medicine, Karolinska Institutet, Stockholm, 26 January 1950, signed Mario L De Finis, Asunción, 13 January 1950. Courtesy of Ann-Margreth Jörnvall, Administrator of the Nobel Committee to HBMB, 9 April 2001, with attachments.

593   MacKinley Helm, *John Marin*, Boston: The Institute of Contemporary Art, 1948.

594   BOAC — British Overseas Airways Corporation, later British Airways.

595   Hugh M. Urquhart, *Arthur Currie, a Biography of a Great Canadian*, J.M. Dent, 1950, Foreword by Jan Christiaan Smuts.

596   CHB, 6 February 1950, South Africa file.

597   The Nuffield Foundation, extract of Minutes: Thirty-First Meeting, Paper F. 31 (II.236 ii), 31 March 1950.

598   Letter from the Clerk of the Nuffield Foundation to HBMB, 22 April 1999.

599   Goodspeed, *A History of the Defence Research Board of Canada*, pp. 156–7.

600   John Bryden, *Deadly Allies: Canada's Secret War 1937–1947*, Toronto: McClelland and Stewart, 1989, p. 253.

601   Defence Medical Research Co-Ordinating Committee, 2nd Meeting, 3 November 1951, p. 2.

602   Jock de Marbois, *Surf of the Past: Adventures of Little Joe Buggins*, by Jock McGurkin, pseud. Unpublished manuscript at the Thomas Fisher Rare Book Library, University of Toronto.

603   *Toronto Telegram*, 13 March 1950. MMB Scrapbook Series 2, Vol. 4, pp. 4-5.

604   Frederick F. Tisdall, OBE, MD, was director of Research Laboratories, Department of Pediatrics, University of Toronto and the Hospital for Sick Children. He was best known as the person who developed Pablum.

605   Conversation between HHD and HBMB, London, July, 1950.

606   CAB to HBMB, 14 June 1950, MMB Scrapbook Series 1, No. 6.

607   CHB and Irving Fritz, "History of the BBDMR," ca 1968, p. 39.

608   E-mail from Philippe Hoet to HBMB, February 2000.

609   Axel Wenner-Gren, founder of the Electrolux Corporation in 1919, was a wealthy industrialist who donated large amounts of money for scientific research.

610   HHD to CHB, 31 December 1950, MMB Scrapbook, Series 1, Vol. 6, p. 91.

611   Section 33 of CHB's *Selected Papers* was taken from the draft of the monograph.

612   CHB to HHD, 4 January 1951, Binder Nobel Re-Visited.

613   HHD to CHB, 12 January 1951, Binder Nobel Re-Visited

614   CHB to HHD, 19 January 1951, Binder Nobel Re-Visited.

615   *El Comercio*, Lima, 26 February 1951, MMB Scrapbook, Series 1, Vol. 6, p. 49.

616   *La Prensa*, Lima, 28 February 1951, MMB Scrapbook, Series 1, Vol. 6, p. 50.

617 *The Standard*, Buenos Aires, 9 March 1951, MMB Scrapbook Series 1, Vol. 6, p. 54.

618 CHB meeting with the Hon. Paul Martin, 19 October 1951.

619 CHB, "An Account of My Meeting with the Rt Hon Louis St-Laurent, Prime Minister of Canada," November 1951.

620 A.L. Chute to CHB, 11 November 1951, MMB Scrapbook Series 1, Vol. 6.

621 J.G.L. Jackson, *RDL — A Splendid Life* (unpublished manuscript, biography of Robert "Robin" Daniel Lawrence), ca 1996, p. 49, Binder RDL.

622 Dr. C.N.H. Long was professor of physiological chemistry at Yale, a McGill MD who had worked in London at the same time as Best.

623 Arnold Joseph Toynbee and K.P. Kirkwood, *Turkey*, New York: Scribner, 1927.

624 W.A.E. Karunaratne C.M.G., introduction of CHB, Colombo, Ceylon ,23 July 1952. MMB Scrapbook Series 1, Vol. 7, p. 31.

625 Claude Bissell, "A Common Ancestry: Literature in Australia and Canada," *University of Toronto Quarterly,* 1956 (January), pp. 131–42.

626 Ewen Downie to CHB, 8 July 1952, MMB Scrapbook Series 1, Vol. 7, p. 39.

627 G.W. Cooper to CHB, 4 August 1952, MMB Scrapbook Series 1, Vol. 7, p. 38.

628 Ronald McKie, "He helped to take death out of diabetes" in Sydney *Daily Telegraph,*, 16 August 1952, MMB Scrapbook, Series 1, Vol. 7, p. 43.

629 CHB talk "What is most needed in medicine?" 3 August 1952, Australian Broadcasting Commission, MMB Scrapbook Series 1, Vol. 7, p. 41.

630 Ruby W. Board to CHB 16 August 1952, MMB Scrapbook Series 1, Vol. 7, p. 42.

631 Sir Cedric Stanton Hicks to CHB, 10 July 1952.

632 C.A. Gardner, *West Australia Wild Flowers*, Perth, 1951.

633 Bruce Hunt to CHB & MMB, 23 September 1952, MMB Scrapbook Series 1, Vol. 7,p. 59.

634 CHB to HHD 16 January 1953, letters H.H. Dale and Florey, Royal Society Binder.

635 All unidentified quotes from MMB diaries 42–63, or from ELM "Dear Jessie" letters, 1960.

636 CHB, Opening Plenary Remarks, see File XIXth International Physiological Congress, Montréal, 31 August 1953.

637 Wallace O. Fenn, *History of the International Congresses of Physiological Sciences 1889–1968*, American Physiological Society, 1968, Nineteenth Congress, p. 38.

638 The proceedings of the gathering were published and also appeared in a sixty-page reprint from the ADA's journal, *Diabetes,* Vol. 3, No. 1 (1954).

639 DRB "Organization of Defence Medical Research," revised 18 June 1951: report of first meeting of the Defence Medical Research Co- Ordinating Committee, 30 May 1951; and, DRB, "Medical Research Advisory Committee," Minutes, 6 March 1951: "Applications Recommended for Approval by MRAC and Approved as Consolidated Grants to finance the Research for the Next Two Years," (#223, Best Institute, #86, Sellers).

640   Letter from Otto Loewi to CHB, 1 January 1953, Binder Nobel Re-Visited.

641   File Nobel Prize 1953.

642   HHD to CHB, 20 February 1953.

643   Letter from Professor Hubert A Lechevalier, a retired colleague of Waksman, to HBMB, 19 August 2001. Also, "The Search for Antibiotics at Rutgers University," in John Parascandola, editor, *The History of Antibiotics, A Symposium*, Madison, Wisconsin: American Institute of the History of Pharmacy, 1980, pp. 113–123; headline, "Did McCandless woman get fair shake for role in discovery of streptomycin?" *Pittsburgh Post Gazette*, 15 April 2001, pp. A1-A5; Milton Wainwright, "Streptomycin: Discovery and Resultant Controversy," *Hist Phil Life Sci*, 13 (1991) pp. 97-124.

644   CHB to HHD, 5 January 1954, Royal Society; also Binder Nobel Re-Visited.

645   HHD to CHB, 11 January 1954, Royal Society; also Binder Nobel Re-Visited.

646   Goran Liljestrand, "The Prize in Physiology or Medicine" in *Nobel: The Man & His Prizes*, Stockholm: Nobel Foundation, 1950.

647   HHD to CHB 5 November 1953, letters H.H. Dale and Florey, Royal Society.

648   HHD to CHB, 16 February 1954, letters H.H. Dale and Florey, Royal Society.

649   CHB to HHD, 22 February 1954, letters H.H. Dale and Florey, Royal Society.

650   HHD to CHB, 1 March 1954, letters H.H. Dale and Florey, Royal Society.

651   Dicumarol is a constituent of rat poison.

652   Margaret Best was not the only person to find James Ensor's work "weird." He caused much furor in the art world during his career. His most famous work was *The Entry of Christ into Brussels*, painted in 1888, but not shown in public until 1929. See *A Dictionary of Twentieth-Century Art*, Oxford, 1999, p. 194.

653   CHB, "Donald Young Solandt, 1907–1955" *Proceedings of the Royal Society of Canada*, 1955. Note: My thanks to the late Barbara Garrard Solandt Griffin for much of the information about her first husband and to Barrie Solandt Maxwell for her memories of her father.

654   CHB, The Croonian Lecture, "The Lipotropic Agents in the Protection of the Liver, Kidney, Heart and Other Organs of Experimental Animals," *Proceedings of the Royal Society*, B, No. 145 (1956), pp. 151–169.

655   William Stirling, *Some Apostles of Physiology: Being an account of their lives and labours: Labours that have contributed to the advancement of the healing art as well as to the prevention of disease*, 1902.

656   Corneille Heymans, professor of pharmacology at the University of Ghent, won the Nobel Prize in 1938; Bernardo Houssay of Buenos Aires, Argentina, Nobel Prize 1947; Alex von Muralt, physiologist, Rector University of Berne, Switzerland, 1955–56; Maurice de Visscher, Head of Dept of Physiology, University of Minnesota.

657   Omond Solandt interview, 19 February 1991.

658 JKW Ferguson to HBMB, 20 July 1988.

659 CHB, 15 September 1956, Poetry file.

660 CHB Dictation,16 November 1956.

661 Dr. Feasby worked for several years on a biography of C.H. Best before ill health obliged him to stop. The result was several chapters that are of considerable interest, sometimes for his conclusions, but also for his interviews with people who are no longer available. It is obvious that he took great pains not to offend CHB, and particularly, MMB.

662 Recorded conversation CHB with Dr. W.R. Feasby, 1957.

663 Letter from CHB to W.R. Feasby , 6 May 1957, Binder Nobel Re-Visited.

664 Michael J Williams, "JJR Macleod: The Co-Discoverer of Insulin," *Proceedings of the Royal College of Physicians of Edinburgh*, July 1993, Vol. 23, No. 3, Supplement No. 1. Articles by Williams include: "In Memory of Macleod," *Balance*, British Diabetic Association, No. 113, October/November 1989, pp. 70–1; and "The Nobel Prize and Diabetes," *Balance*, British Diabetic Assocation, No. 117, June/July, 1990, pp. 12–4. Dr. and Mrs. Williams were very hospitable when the author visited Aberdeen in 1993.

665 CHB to W.R. Feasby, 15 July 1957.

666 Oslerian Oration: "The Discovery of Insulin," given 12 July 1957, Binder Oslerian Oration.

667 Dr. Ian Macdonald to CHB, 11 May 1959, CAB file.

668 CHB to Leslie McFarlane, 31 October 1955, see NFB files for additional documentation.

669 EJB interview, 2 August 2000.

670 Proceedings of the British Society for Endocrinology, 23 June 1959, *Journal of Endocrinology*, 19, pp. i–xvii.

671 Fortnum and Mason's elegant emporium on Piccadily owned by Canadian Garfield Weston owner of Weston Bakeries and Loblaw Supermarket chain.

672 CHB, "Unfinished Researches," *Quarterly Bulletin*, Northwestern University Medical School, Vol. 33, No. 4, p. 300, (Winter Quarter) Chicago, 1959, Copy in CHB Articles Binder, No. 8.

673 Yousuf Karsh, *Portraits of Greatness*, Toronto: U of T Press, 1959.

674 Karsh file.

675 Otto and Anka Sirek, interview 20 February 1991.

676 EJB interview, 2 August 2000.

677 All quotations for this trip are taken from the "Dear Jessie" letters, ELM to JHR, 2 November to 15 December 1960.

678 Royal Society of London, Obituary Notice of *Sir Thomas Lewis*, 1945, p. 200.

679 Multimillionaire industrialist, inventor of Electrolux.

680 The lectures were published in Swedish, but not in English. Best modified his text for the Dickson Memorial Lecture of the Royal Society of Medicine in London in May 1962.

681 Rolf Luft, Professor Emeritus at the Karolinska Institutet, to HBMB, 28 May 2002, confirmed that he had arranged for Professor Tor Hiertonn to look after MMB.

682   ELM to JHR 2 November–15 December 1960.

683   All further unattributed quotes are from MMB's diaries 56–63.

684   CHB to Claude Bissell, 27 April 1961. File BBDMR — 1961 Letter unsent.

685   CHB Dictation, 23 November 1961.

686   In June 2002 the painting was nowhere to be found.

687   Recently Dr. Donald M. Barnett, a staff physician at the Joslin Clinic for thirty-five years, published a well-written informative book about Joslin. Donald M. Barnett, *Elliott P Joslin, MD: A Centennial Portrait*, Joslin Diabetes Center, 1998.

688   Valerie Knowles, *First Person: A Biography of Cairine Wilson, Canada's First Woman Senator*, Toronto: Dundurn Press, 1988, p. 159.

689   EJB interview , 2 August 2000.

690   EJB interview 2 August 2000.

691   JBC, "Reminiscences on the Discovery of Insulin," *The Canadian Medical Association Journal*, Vol. 87, 17 November 1962. See Item 43 in CHB Articles Binder.

692   Ayala and Sam Zacks were well-known collectors and patrons of the arts in Toronto.

693   Dr. Thomas Doxiadis, personal physician to the Queen of Greece, director of the "Evangelismos" Medical Centre, Athens.

694   EJB interview, 2 August 2000.

695   MMB to HBMB, 19 September 1964.

696   EJB Interview, 2 August 2000.

697   Omond Solandt interview, 19 February 1991.

698   Aldwyn Stokes to John Hamilton, 3 November 1964. Copy sent to Dr. Ray Farquharson, courtesy of Dr. H.A.M. "Nell" Farquharson, Ray Farquharson's daughter. File CHB illness.

699   Michael Bliss, Interview with Allan Walters, 9 March 1981. Courtesy of Bernard Leibel; Leibel and Allan Walters file.

700   J.K.W. Ferguson to HBMB, 20 July 1988.

701   All unattributed quotes in this chapter from MMB diaries 63–73.

702   CHB to John D. Hamilton, 15 February 1965. File CHB illness.

703   Morley Whillans to CHB, 18 May 1965.

704   Omond Solandt interview, 19 February 1991.

705   BA Houssay in Leibel and Wrenshall, "On the Nature and Treatment of Diabetes," *Excerpta Medica, 1965. Proceedings of the Fifth Congress of the IDF,* International Diabetes Federation, 1964.

706   Gerald Wrenshall, Memo, 30 October 1965, p. 1, BBDMR

707   Gerald Wrenshall, Memo, 30 October 1965, pp. 2–3.

708   Unknown author, Memo, 5 April 1966. BBDMR — Reorganization/Hopes and Plans.

709   G.R. Williams interview, 9 June 1994.

710   David Naylor to HBMB, 4 March 2002, BBDMR.

711   ADA *Forecast* November-December 1966.

712 ADA, *The Journey and the Dream: A History of the American Diabetes Association,* 1990, p. 41.

713 OMS, *Festschrift: Charles Herbert Best,* Canadian Journal of Physiology and Pharmacology, c. 1968, p. iii.

714 ALC, *Festschrift: Charles Herbert Best,* Canadian Journal of Physiology and Pharmacology, c. 1968, p. iv.

715 Letter BAH to CHB, 10 February 1969.

716 Gilles Vigueault, *Ce que je dis c'est en passant,* 1970.

717 Jean Victor Allard, chief of the general staff; Charles Best; James Alexander Corry, principal of Queen's University; Donald Gordon of the CNR; Duncan Graham of the Toronto General Hospital; diplomat Arnold Heeney; scientist Gerhard Herzberg; artist Paul Lemieux; Hector McKinnon, ex-federal official; former prime minister Lester B. Pearson; Louis Rasminsky, governor of the Bank of Canada; and Robert Stanfield.

718 *John Ramsay of Kildalton: Being an Account of his Life in Islay and including the Diary of his trip to Canada in 1870.* Toronto: Peter Martin Associates Limited, 1969. John Ramsay of Kildalton was Janna's great-grandfather.

719 George Morland was an eighteenth-century English painter of country scenes.

720 Sailen Mookerjea to HBMB, 1 May 2001. Special thanks to Dr. Mookerjea for his informative letter.

721 CHB, "Perspectives: Past and Future," in Irving B. Fritz, ed., *Insulin Action: The Proceedings of a Symposium on Insulin, 25–27 October 1971,* p. 609.

722 CHB account of CH investiture by HM Queen Elizabeth II, 17 December 1971.

723 ELM to Jessie Ridout, 25 December 1971.

724 ELM to Jessie Ridout, 26 December 1971.

725 "The History, Discovery and Present Position of Insulin," *Commentarii,* Vol 2, No 57, Pontifical Academy of Sciences, 1972.

726 Stefan S. Fajans to HBMB, 13 December 1999.

727 In 1959, Murray Westgate played FGB and Ted Follows played CHB. In 1972, Michael J. Reynolds played FGB and Richard McKenna played CHB.

728 CHB and Irving B. Fritz, *History of the Banting and Best Department of Medical Research,* nd, p. 37.

729 *Globe and Mail Weekend Magazine,* 27 October 1973, pp. 14–16.

730 CHB, c.v. of MMB, August 1976.

731 Susan's half-sister Margaret Cairine Best.

732 CHB, "Schooner Cove Farm," 2 December 1963, unpublished, p. 1.

733 CHB, "Schooner Cove Farm," 2 December 1963, unpublished, p. 15.

734 Barry Penhale, pp. 2–3 of final section of interview with CHB, OMA Oral History Project, 1977.

735 In 2001 Dr. Cahill sent to HBMB the shingle from Dr. Herbert Best's office which he had found leaning against a back wall of the house in 1977.

736   CHB, *The Fascination of Medical Research: Recollections of the Past Fifty Years*, February 1978, BFP.

737   All unattributed quotes from MMB diaries volumes 73 to 75.

738   Dr. Douglas Stewart, "Remarks at the Memorial Service for Charles Alexander (Sandy) Best," 31 March 1978.

739   Fred W Whitehouse, Grosse Point, Michigan, to HBMB, 13 February 2000.

740   ADA, *The Journey and the Dream: A History of the American Diabetes Association*, 1990, pp. 208–9.

741   Eventually, Henry inherited most of these items and decided to include them in the material to be given to the Thomas Fisher Rare Book Library of the University of Toronto. He also arranged for some items, such as medals and some of the forty-six sets of CHB's university notes, to go on semi-permanent loan for display to the dean of medicine, the head of physiology, and the head of the Banting and Best Department of Medical Research.

742   International Biochemical Association Journal, Vol. 57, No. 6.

743   Draft of letter from MMB to Randall Sprague, ca 1980. See Michael Bliss file, BFP.

744   MMB, Notes about meetings with Michael Bliss, BFP.

745   Article submitted by ELM to the *Biographical Encyclopaedia of the World*, 8 May 1980. It was never published.

Index